T0329784

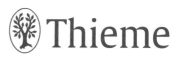

Learning Pharmacology through Clinical Cases

Mario Babbini, MD, PhD
Professor
Department of Pharmacology
Ross University School of Medicine
Portsmouth, Dominica, West Indies

Sandeep Bansal, MBBS, MD
Research Associate Professor
Course Director of Pharmacology
University of Illinois College of Medicine
Urbana-Champaign, Illinois, USA

Thieme
New York • Stuttgart • Delhi • Rio de Janeiro

Acquisition Editor: Delia K. DeTurris
Managing Editor: Kenneth Schubach
Director, Editorial Services: Mary Jo Casey
Production Editor: Kenny Chumbley
In-House Production Editor: Naamah Schwartz
International Rights Director: Heike Schwabenthan
International Production Director: Andreas Schabert
Editorial Director: Sue Hodgson
International Marketing Director: Fiona Henderson
International Sales Director: Louisa Turrell
Director of Sales, North America: Mike Roseman
Senior Vice President and Chief Operating Officer: Sarah
   Vanderbilt
President: Brian D. Scanlan

Cover image: AdobeStock, ©pikselstock

Library of Congress Cataloging-in-Publication Data

Names: Babbini, Mario, author. | Bansal, Sandeep, author.
Title: Thieme test prep for the USMLE[a] : learning pharmacology
   through clinical cases / Mario Babbini, Sandeep Bansal.
Other titles: Learning pharmacology through clinical cases
Description: New York : Thieme, [2018]
Identifiers: LCCN 2017047835| ISBN 9781626234239 (softcover)
   | ISBN 9781626234246 (eISBN)
Subjects: | MESH: Pharmacological Phenomena | Examination
   Questions | Case Reports
Classification: LCC RM301.13 | NLM QV 18.2 | DDC 615.1076--
   dc23
LC record available at https://lccn.loc.gov/2017047835

Important note: Medicine is an ever-changing science undergoing continual development. Research and clinical experience are continually expanding our knowledge, in particular our knowledge of proper treatment and drug therapy. Insofar as this book mentions any dosage or application, readers may rest assured that the authors, editors, and publishers have made every effort to ensure that such references are in accordance with **the state of knowledge at the time of production of the book.**

Nevertheless, this does not involve, imply, or express any guarantee or responsibility on the part of the publishers in respect to any dosage instructions and forms of applications stated in the book. **Every user is requested to examine carefully** the manufacturers' leaflets accompanying each drug and to check, if necessary in consultation with a physician or specialist, whether the dosage schedules mentioned therein or the contraindications stated by the manufacturers differ from the statements made in the present book. Such examination is particularly important with drugs that are either rarely used or have been newly released on the market. Every dosage schedule or every form of application used is entirely at the user's own risk and responsibility. The authors and publishers request every user to report to the publishers any discrepancies or inaccuracies noticed. If errors in this work are found after publication, errata will be posted at www.thieme.com on the product description page.

Some of the product names, patents, and registered designs referred to in this book are in fact registered trademarks or proprietary names even though specific reference to this fact is not always made in the text. Therefore, the appearance of a name without designation as proprietary is not to be construed as a representation by the publisher that it is in the public domain.

© 2018 Thieme Medical Publishers, Inc.
Thieme Publishers New York
333 Seventh Avenue, New York, NY 10001 USA
+1 800 782 3488, customerservice@thieme.com

Thieme Publishers Stuttgart
Rüdigerstrasse 14, 70469 Stuttgart, Germany
+49 [0]711 8931 421, customerservice@thieme.de

Thieme Publishers Delhi
A-12, Second Floor, Sector-2, Noida-201301
Uttar Pradesh, India
+91 120 45 566 00, customerservice@thieme.in

Thieme Publishers Rio de Janeiro, Thieme Publicações Ltda.
Edifício Rodolpho de Paoli, 25º andar
Av. Nilo Peçanha, 50 – Sala 2508
Rio de Janeiro 20020-906, Brasil
+55 21 3172 2297

Cover design: Thieme Publishing Group
Typesetting by Prairie Papers

Printed in India by Replika Press Pvt Ltd.
ISBN 978-1-62623-423-9

Also available as an e-book:
eISBN 978-1-62623-424-6

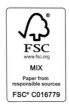

Table of Contents

Preface vii

1   Acromegaly 1

2   Acute Lymphoblastic Leukemia 9

3   Asthma... 17

4   Atrial Fibrillation... 25

5   Bipolar Disorder 37

6   Breast Cancer 43

7   Cardiogenic Shock 51

8   Crohn's Disease 59

9   Chronic Kidney Disease 69

10 Chronic Obstructive Pulmonary Disease 79

11 Drug Abuse 87

12 Epilepsy.. 95

13 Essential Hypertension... 105

14 General Anesthesia 115

15 Glaucoma 125

16 Gout... 133

17 Graves' Disease 143

18 Growth Retardation and Hypogonadism................................... 153

19 Heart Failure 163

20 Hematopoietic Cell Transplantation 175

21 Hodgkin's Lymphoma 183

22 Hormonal Contraception 191

23 Human Immunodeficiency Virus Infection 201

24 Infective Endocarditis 211

25 Iron Deficiency Anemia 219

26 Liver Cirrhosis 227

27 Lung Cancer 237

28 Megaloblastic Anemia...245

29 Migraine..251

30 Myasthenia Gravis..259

31 Myocardial Infarction..269

32 Parkinson's Disease...281

33 Peptic Ulcer Disease...291

34 Perimenopause and Osteoporosis..299

35 Pheochromocytoma...309

36 Pneumonia...319

37 Polycystic Ovarian Syndrome..327

38 Primary Adrenal Deficiency (Addison's Disease)..337

39 Prostate Cancer...347

40 Psoriasis..355

41 Pulmonary Embolism..363

42 Rheumatoid Arthritis..371

43 Schizophrenia..383

44 Solid Organ Transplantation..393

45 Stroke..401

46 Systemic Lupus Erythematosus...411

47 Torsade de Pointes..419

48 Type 1 Diabetes Mellitus..425

49 Type 2 Diabetes Mellitus..435

50 Urinary Tract Infection...445

Index..451

Preface

This book is a collection of clinical cases designed to promote the learning of pharmacology by using case studies. Working with cases is the best way to involve students in the learning process because:

▶ Every case shows a real situation, very close to those seen in every day practice.
▶ Every case can elicit several problems that must be solved. In other words, it is a problem-based learning process.
▶ Every case not only requires the knowledge of several disciplines but also the application of this knowledge to specific clinical situations.

The format of each case is the following:

▶ Each case provides relevant data (presenting complaint and its history, past medical history, family history, drug history, physical examination, lab findings, diagnosis, pharmacotherapy) to identify the main features of the case, along with a set of statements that describe the case follow-up.
▶ Each case has a series of multiple-choice questions.
  – Some questions address the knowledge of basic disciplines (mainly, physiology, pathology, and microbiology) the student needs to assess the case.
  – Other questions are related to the pharmacotherapy of the disease. These questions encompass the pharmacokinetics, mechanism of action, adverse effects, contraindications, and the interactions of all drugs used for the pharmacotherapy of the case.

The questions are designed to prepare students for the United States Medical Licensing Examinion (USMLE) Step 1 and Step 2. Four to six choices are provided for each question, but for all questions there is only one best answer.

Each question has a learning objective, the correct answer, and an explanation. The learning objective is a brief behavioral statement written using an action verb. If a student can perform the action, then he or she should be able to answer the question correctly. The explanation includes both the reasons why a given answer is correct and why the distractors are wrong.

Many questions are related to the highest levels of Bloom's taxonomy (e.g., interpretation of data and the solution of problems) rather than being simple recall questions.

The rationale for this book is related to the current trend in medical education. Today, it is more and more evident that the mere memorization of information provided by books is insufficient for meaningful learning. In other words "knowledge that cannot be used is useless." It is the application of knowledge that counts. A vast array of medical problems is available in the literature today, but there are few books related to the pharmacology of clinical cases. The driving idea of this book is to link the clinical case to the application of basic knowledge, primarily in physiology, pathology, and microbiology, as well as to explain the reasons for using specific drugs in real clinical problems, with the goal of promoting critical thinking skills.

The main audience of the book is medical school students. However, the book could also be useful for students in other medical fields, including pharmacists, physician assistants, and nurses.

Pharmacology and clinical medicine are fast-evolving disciplines. The authors have referred to reliable sources in order to provide information in accordance with currently accepted standards. However, the authors are aware that in several instances, the pharmacotherapy of disease is still controversial. We have tried, as much as possible, to avoid questions addressing controversial issues.

This book is not intended to be a substitute for pharmacology textbooks. Students are strongly advised to consult their textbooks of pharmacology for more in-depth coverage of the subject matter.

Mario Babbini, MD, PhD
Sandeep Bansal, MBBS, MD

Case 1   Acromegaly

G.A., a 40-year-old man, complained to his physician of difficulty seeing objects in the periphery, excessive sweating, and gradual enlargement of his hands and feet. His shoe size had increased by two sizes in the last 2 years, and his wedding ring also had to be resized. He had recently started snoring, and he would waken in the morning with a headache. His facial skin had also become oilier.

Physical examination showed a man with a slightly protruding lower jaw. His vital signs were as follows: blood pressure 130/88 mm Hg, pulse 80 bpm, respirations 22/min.

The patient's skin was thickened, and excessive perspiration was noted on his hands and feet. Visual field examination revealed temporal hemianopia. Dental examination showed increased dental spacing.

Pertinent laboratory results on admission were as follows:

Blood hematology

► Blood glucose, fasting: 130 mg/dL (normal, 70–110)
► Growth hormone (GH) suppression test: GH 20 ng/mL (normal, < 2)
► Insulin-like growth factor 1 (IGF-1) 890 ng/mL (normal, 138–410)
► Prolactin: 50 ng/mL (normal, < 20)
► Free testosterone: 2.5 pg/mL (normal for age 40, 6.8–21.5)
► Luteinizing hormone (LH): 2.2 U/L (normal 6–23)
► Follicle-stimulating hormone (FSH): 1.3 U/L (normal 4–25)

MRI scan of the head

Pituitary macroadenoma encroaching on the optic chiasma.

Colonoscopy

Normal, with no evidence of tumor growth.

The diagnosis was acromegaly due to GH-secreting adenoma. G.A. was scheduled for transsphenoidal resection of the adenoma.

Six weeks postsurgery, G.A. felt much better, and his peripheral vision had also improved. However, a lab exam showed that his GH and IGF-1 levels were still high due to the extrasellar invasion of the adenoma. He was thus started on therapy with a somatostatin analogue and a dopamine agonist.

Questions

1. G.A. was diagnosed with a growth hormone–secreting adenoma. Which of the following types of cells constitute a major part of this adenoma?

A. Basophilic cells

B. Acidophilic cells

C. Chromophobe cells

D. Null cells

2. G.A. was found to have increased fasting glucose levels. Which of the following was most likely the cause of this finding?

A. Suppression of glucagon secretion

B. Increased glycogenesis

C. Antagonism of insulin action

D. Decreased excretion of glucose in urine

E. Increased cortisol levels

3. G.A. was found to have decreased blood levels of testosterone. Which of the following was most likely the cause of this decrease?

A. GH-induced inhibition of Leydig cell function

B. Prolactin-induced increase of gonadotropin release

C. Increased somatostatin release

D. GH-induced impairment of Sertoli cell function

4. G.A. felt well after surgical resection of his adenoma. However, because of the residual tumor, his GH and IGF-1 levels were still high. He started a therapy with a somatostatin analogue. Which of the following drugs was most likely prescribed?

A. Octreotide

B. Lansoprazole

C. Somatropin

D. Sunitinib

E. Leuprolide

5. Which of the following signal transduction pathways best describes the molecular mechanism of octreotide action to suppress somatotroph function?

A. Stimulation of adenylyl cyclase

B. Closure of potassium channels

C. Activation of mitogen-activated protein kinase

D. Inhibition of adenylyl cyclase

E. Opening of calcium channels

6. G.A. was prescribed a dopamine agonist. Which of the following drugs was most likely administered?

A. Bromocriptine

B. Cabergoline

C. Olanzapine

D. Sumatriptan

E. Buspirone

7. Nausea is a common adverse effect of dopamine agonists. Which of the following brain structures is most likely the primary site of the action that mediates this adverse effect?

A. Frontal cortex

B. Amygdala

C. Area postrema

D. Paraventricular nucleus

E. Vestibular nuclei

8. Which of the following could most likely develop as an adverse effect of octreotide early in the course of treatment of acromegaly?

A. Kyphosis

B. Cholelithiasis

C. Hyperprolactinemia

D. Esophageal varices

E. Abdominal pain

9. G.A. did not respond adequately to the octreotide and cabergoline therapy. He was subsequently prescribed pegvisomant. Which of the following phrases best describes the mechanism of action of pegvisomant?

A. Inhibition of growth hormone release

B. Blockade of somatostatin receptors

C. Activation of insulin-like growth factor 1 receptors

D. Activation of growth hormone receptor

E. Blockade of growth hormone receptors

10. Which of the following signs and symptoms of acromegaly are unlikely to resolve with drugs that reduce growth hormone release or its action?

A. Soft tissue changes

B. Prognathism

C. Hyperglycemia

D. Oiliness of skin

E. Hyperhidrosis

Answers and Explanations

▶ *Learning objective:* Describe the histology of the anterior pituitary gland.

1. Answer: B

The cells of the anterior pituitary gland are classified as acidophils or basophils, depending on their affinity for acidic or basic histology dyes, respectively. Acidophilic cells look red and basophilic cells look blue under the microscope. The five types of anterior pituitary cells can be subdivided as follows:

- ▶ Somatotrophs (GH-secreting cells): acidophilic
- ▶ Lactotrophs (prolactin-secreting cells): acidophilic
- ▶ Corticotrophs (adrenocorticotropic hormone [ACTH]-secreting cells): basophilic
- ▶ Gonadotrophs (FSH- and LH-secreting cells): basophilic

- ▶ Thyrotrophs (thyroid-stimulating hormone [TSH]-secreting cells): basophilic

A See correct answer explanation.

C Chromophobe cells are cells that stain poorly with histology dyes and look pale under the microscope.

D Null cells are lymphocytes that lack characteristic surface markers that are found on B and T lymphocytes. They are not the hormone-secreting cells of the anterior pituitary.

▶ *Learning objective:* Describe the effects of growth hormone on glucose metabolism.

2. Answer: C

Growth hormone antagonizes the function of insulin, resulting in decreased peripheral utilization of glucose and increased gluconeogenesis. Normally, GH release peaks during sleep, and, in concert with other hormones, such as cortisol, helps to maintain glucose levels within the normal range to provide a continuous supply of glucose to the vital organs. However, in cases of GH-secreting adenoma, GH levels are constantly high, which results in increased blood glucose levels that could lead to diabetes mellitus. G.A.'s fasting glucose levels were above the normal range of 70 to 110 mg/dL, indicating the antagonizing effects of GH on insulin activity.

A Glucagon secretion is not suppressed by growth hormone. Moreover, suppression of glucagon secretion would not cause increased blood glucose levels.

B Glycogenesis is decreased, not increased, due to antagonism of insulin actions.

D Glucose is normally filtered by the glomerulus and is completely reabsorbed by the renal tubules. When blood glucose is > 200 mg/dL, it exceeds the renal reabsorption capacity, and glucose starts appearing in the urine. Decreased renal excretion of glucose cannot occur in the presence of high blood glucose.

E Increased cortisol levels could cause hyperglycemia, but cortisol levels are not increased by GH-secreting adenoma. Actually, the anterior pituitary adenoma could compress the surrounding corticotroph cells and impair corticotropin release to decrease cortisol synthesis in the adrenal cortex.

▶ *Learning objective:* Describe the likely causes of decreased gonadal function in a patient with a pituitary mass.

3. Answer: A

A pituitary tumor mass, especially a macroadenoma (functional or nonfunctional) can press against other cell types in the anterior pituitary to impact their function. In case of a nonfunctional pituitary adenoma, usually the first cells impacted are GH-secreting cells, and then in sequential order, gonadotrophs, thyrotrophs, and corticotrophs are impacted. G.A. had a GH-secreting macroadenoma that possibly had caused pressure effects to impair gonadotroph function, resulting in decreased gonadotropin (LH and FSH) secretion. Decreased gonadotropin levels result in decreased stimulation of Leydig cells to synthesize and release testosterone.

B G.A. had hyperprolactinemia. However, high prolactin levels would inhibit gonadotropin-releasing hormone (GnRH) from the hypothalamus, which in turn would impair, not increase, gonadotropin release.

C Somatostatin release is not increased in acromegaly due to GH-secreting adenoma. Moreover, somatostatin does not impact Leydig cell function.

D GH does not impact Sertoli cell function. Moreover, Sertoli cells have to do with spermatogenesis, and not with testosterone synthesis and release.

▶ *Learning objective:* Describe the pharmacology of somatostatin analogues.

4. Answer: A

Growth hormone release from the somatotrophs of the anterior pituitary is regulated by hypothalamic hormones: GH-releasing hormone (GHRH) and somatostatin (SST). GHRH stimulates and SST inhibits the release of GH.

Somatostatin has a half-life of 1 to 3 minutes, making it unsuitable for long-term treatment of acromegaly. Therefore, somatostatin analogues are used for the treatment of acromegaly. Octreotide, and the long-acting agent lanreotide, are commonly used somatostatin analogues. These are small peptide drugs that are administered by subcutaneous or intramuscular injection. Octreotide elimination half-life is approximately 80 minutes, compared to 1 to 3 minutes for somatostatin, thus making it a more suitable agent for therapeutic indications. It is usually administered subcutaneously three times a day, but its long-acting, slow-release form can be administered intramuscularly every 4 weeks. Lanreotide is a longer-acting somatostatin analogue. The sustained-release formulation of lanreotide is administered intramuscularly every 10 to 14 days, and the extended-release formulation is administered every 4 weeks. The goal of the therapy is to reduce the symptoms, reduce GH levels to < 2.5 ng/mL with GH suppression test (normal, < 2 ng/mL), and bring the insulin-like growth factor 1 (IGF-1) levels within the age- and gender-specific normal limits.

Although surgery (transsphenoidal resection of adenoma) is the first-line treatment for most patients with acromegaly, its effectiveness depends on factors such as (1) size of the tumor, (2) the tumor's invasiveness, and (3) the skill of the surgeon. Initial remission with surgery can be achieved in about 80% of patients who have microadenoma and about 40 to 60% with macroadenoma. Drug therapy is attempted for patients who do not respond well to surgery and for initial responders with recurrence of signs and symptoms. In patients with acromegaly with an invasive tumor invading the cavernous sinus or the nearby optic chiasma, surgery helps in debulking the tumor and rapidly relieving the signs and symptoms, such as temporal hemianopia, caused by compression of the tumor mass on the surrounding structures. However, it is difficult to remove the entire invasive adenoma; thus increased GH levels and signs and symptoms of acromegaly can appear soon after initial debulking of tumor. Drug therapy is used for further management of these patients, as was initiated for G.A.

B Lansoprazole is a H^+/K^+ adenosine triphosphatase (ATPase) (gastric proton pump) inhibitor that is used for the treatment of acid-peptic disease.

C Somatropin is a recombinant human growth hormone used as a replacement therapy to treat short stature caused by GH deficiency.

D Sunitinib is an inhibitor of receptor tyrosine kinase, which is used in the treatment of renal cell carcinoma and gastrointestinal stromal tumor.

E Leuprolide is a gonadotropin-releasing hormone (GnRH) analogue that stimulates gonadotropin secretion when administered in a pulsatile manner, and inhibits gonadotropin secretion when administered using a depot formulation for continuous release into the circulation.

▶ *Learning objective:* Describe the molecular mechanism of action of octreotide.

5. Answer: D

Somatostatin and its analogues bind to SST receptors (SSTRs), which are membrane-bound G-protein coupled receptors. There are five subtypes of SSTRs. SSTR-2 and 5 are the most abundant subtypes on somatotrophs. Somatostatin analogues have high selectivity for SSTR-2 and SSTR-5.

SSTRs are linked to multiple signaling pathways. One pathway involves the inhibitory G proteins ($G_{i/o}$). Binding of SST or its analogues to SSTRs leads to activation of the inhibitory G proteins to cause inhibition of adenylyl cyclase, resulting in decreased cyclic adenosine monophosphate (cAMP) levels. Another pathway involves potassium channels directly coupled to the receptor. Activation of SSTRs by SST or SST analogues opens potassium channels. Exit of potassium ions from the cell leads to hyperpolarization, which in turn causes closure of voltage-gated calcium channels. This results in decreased calcium entry into the cells, causing inhibition of exocytosis of GH. These two mechanisms—lowering of intracellular cAMP and calcium ions—are the most important mechanisms known that are involved in suppressing GH hormone secretion.

Inhibition of GH secretion by somatostatin analogues primarily works through SSTR-2. SSTR-2 and SSTR-5 are also physiologically important subtypes in the pancreatic islets. Somatostatin, mainly the locally produced somatostatin in the pancreas, inhibits insulin and glucagon secretions by interacting with SSTR-5 and SSTR-2, respectively. Because of their greater affinity for SSTR-2, octreotide and lanreotide are effective in controlling GH hypersecretion without much disturbance of insulin secretion and carbohydrate metabolism.

A Octreotide inhibits, rather than stimulates, adenylyl cyclase.

B, E Octreotide has no direct effects on potassium channels.

C SSTRs also modulate mitogen-activated protein kinase (MAPK), but this mechanism appears to mediate antiproliferative effects of somatostatin on tumor cells, not GH secretion.

E Octreotide has no direct effects on calcium channels.

▶ *Learning objective:* Describe the pharmacology of dopamine agonists used in the treatment of acromegaly and prolactinoma.

6. Answer: B

Both bromocriptine and cabergoline are dopamine agonists. Therapy with dopamine agonists is the first-line treatment for a prolactinoma, in contrast to transsphenoidal surgery being the first-line treatment for a GH-secreting adenoma, as was initially done in G.A.'s case. Dopamine agonists bind to dopamine receptors present on the surface of lactotrophs to reduce prolactin release and shrink the size of the prolactinoma. Bromocriptine is short acting, so it needs to be administered orally 2 to 4 times a day in divided doses. Cabergoline, a longer-acting dopamine agonist, is administered orally 1 to 3 times a week. The drug appears to be more effective than bromocriptine and has fewer adverse effects compared to bromocriptine. Because of these advantages, cabergoline is largely preferred today over bromocriptine for the long-term treatment of prolactinoma and acromegaly.

In about 20–30% of patients with acromegaly, lactotrophs are also present in the GH-secreting adenomas. Such patients benefit from the concomitant dopamine agonist therapy along with a somatostatin analogue. G.A.'s blood tests revealed hyperprolactinemia, indicating the presence of lactotrophs in his GH-secreting macroadenoma. Also, it has been shown that activation of dopamine receptors on the pituitary of acromegalic patients can suppress (for unknown reason) GH release. The octreotide/cabergoline combination therapy has been found to be more effective than either drug alone to shrink the size of the GH-secreting adenoma, reduce GH and IGF-1 levels, and resolve the signs and symptoms of acromegalic patients. These are the reasons for adding cabergoline to G.A.'s therapy.

A Both bromocriptine and cabergoline are dopamine agonists, but cabergoline is longer acting and appears to have fewer adverse effects, so it is preferred for therapeutic purposes.

C Olanzapine is an atypical antipsychotic drug.

D Sumatriptan is a serotoninergic agonist that is used in the treatment of acute attack of migraine.

E Buspirone is an anxiolytic drug that is used for the treatment of generalized anxiety disorder.

▸ *Learning objective:* Describe the mechanism of development of nausea and vomiting as adverse effects of dopamine agonists.

7. Answer: C

Up to 29% of patients on therapy with dopamine agonists develop nausea. Dopamine agonists can activate D2 receptors present in the chemoreceptor trigger zone (CTZ), a brain center located within the area postrema at the bottom of the fourth ventricle. The area postrema is outside the blood–brain barrier and is thus accessible to emetogenic stimuli caused by drugs carried in the blood.

Activation of D2 receptors by dopamine agonists cause CTZ to transmit signals to the vomiting center, resulting in the development of nausea.

A, B, C, E These structures can transmit signals to the vomiting center, but they are not activated by dopamine agonists.

D The paraventricular nucleus is present in the hypothalamus. Many neurons

from the nucleus project to the posterior pituitary, where they release oxytocin or vasopressin. The nucleus does not transmit signals to the vomiting center.

▸ *Learning objective:* Describe the common adverse effects of octreotide.

8. Answer: E

Approximately 50% of patients taking octreotide experience gastrointestinal adverse effects, such as nausea, abdominal pain, and diarrhea, soon after initiation of therapy. In most of the patients these symptoms subside over time and cessation of therapy is not needed.

A Kyphosis can occur as an adverse effect of growth hormone replacement therapy in children with growth retardation.

B Cholelithiasis (gallstones) develops in about 25% of patients on octreotide therapy, usually after 6 months of continued treatment with the drug. It is not an early adverse effect of octreotide.

C Hyperprolactinemia can occur as an adverse effect of dopamine antagonists. Dopamine agonists are actually used as the first-line treatment of a prolactinoma.

D Octreotide has a therapeutic role in the management of portal hypertension and bleeding esophageal varices; it does not cause esophageal varices.

▸ *Learning objective:* Describe the mechanism of action of pegvisomant.

9. Answer: E

Pegvisomant is a GH receptor antagonist. It binds to GH receptor and inhibits binding of GH to it, thus inhibits GH receptor dimerization and its activation. Unlike the action of somatostatin analogues, pegvisomant does not inhibit GH release from the somatotrophs. By inhibiting the action of GH, pegvisomant blocks generation of IGF-1. Therefore, in the presence of pegvisomant, levels of IGF-1 would decrease, but the levels of GH would remain high. In contrast, the levels of both GH and IGF-1 would decrease in response to octreotide.

Therapy with somatostatin analogues has been shown to provide clinical improvement in about 75% of patients with acromegaly. Clinical improvement increases by adding cabergoline to the treatment in responsive patients. Pegvisomant, administered daily as subcutaneous injections, is mainly used in patients who have failed therapy with somatostatin analogues. It has been shown to reduce IGF-1 levels to normal in more than 90% of patients.

A This would be the mechanism of action of somatostatin analogues.

B Somatostatin receptor inhibitors are not yet available for any therapeutic indication.

C IGF-1 activates insulin-like growth factor-1 receptors.

D This would be the action of somatostatin and its analogues.

▶ *Learning objective:* Identify the sign that cannot be reversed in acromegalic patients undergoing appropriate therapy.

10. Answer: B

With successful reduction in growth hormone hypersecretion or its actions on the GH receptors, patients would undergo cessation of bone overgrowth. However, the bony changes that have already occurred would not reverse. Therefore, changes such as protruding jaw (prognathism) and increased spacing of teeth do not resolve.

A, C, D, E With successful therapy, patients experience reduction in soft tissue bulk of the extremities and cessation of hyperhidrosis and oily skin. Reversal of hyperglycemia and headache is also seen.

Case 2

Acute Lymphoblastic Leukemia

S.W., a 7-year-old boy, was admitted to the hospital with a 2-week history of intermittent fever, sore throat, tiredness, easy bruising, headache, and bone pain. The patient's past medical history was unremarkable. His family history revealed that 10 years ago his father suffered from a non-Hodgkin's lymphoma that was completely cured after anticancer chemotherapy.

Physical examination showed an alert, interactive, but ill-appearing boy. His skin was pale with random macular bruises just inferior to the hairline and over the proximal upper extremity. A petechial-appearing rash was present over the buttock and lower left flank. Hepatomegaly was evident 2 cm below the costal margin with no splenomegaly. The rest of the physical examination was normal.

Pertinent laboratory results on admission were as follows:

Blood hematology

- ► Erythrocyte sedimentation rate (ESR): 65 mm/h (normal < 20)
- ► Red blood cell count (RBC): $3.8 \times 10^6/\mu L$ (normal, children 4.0–6.0)
- ► Hemoglobin (Hgb): 8.5 g/dL (normal 12–16)
- ► Hematocrit (Hct): 33% (normal 36–48)
- ► White blood cell count (WBC): $45 \times 10^3/\mu L$ (normal 4–10)
- ► Differential WBC count: 72% lymphocytes (normal, 30–40%), 7% neutrophils (normal, 50–60%), and 11% blasts
- ► Platelet: $85 \times 10^3/\mu L$ (normal 130–400)

Blood chemistry

- ► Creatinine: 0.8 mg/dL (normal 0.6–1.2)
- ► Blood urea nitrogen: 22 mg/dL (normal 8–25)
- ► Uric acid, 6.8 mg/dL (normal, 2.5–8);
- ► Alkaline phosphatase: 160 U/L (normal 25–100)

Bone marrow exam

- ► Histology: 35% blasts (identified as lymphoblasts by immunophenotyping)
- ► Cytogenetic analysis: reciprocal translocation t(8;14)
- ► Lumbar puncture: normal

A diagnosis of acute lymphoblastic leukemia was made, and a multidrug treatment was started with vincristine, prednisolone, and asparaginase. In addition S.W. received intrathecal chemotherapy for central nervous system (CNS) prophylaxis.

On the day after starting the anticancer treatment the following pertinent laboratory values were obtained:

- ▶ WBC: $15 \times 10^3/\mu L$ (normal 4–10)
- ▶ Potassium (K^+): 6.6 mEq/L (normal, 3.5–5.5)
- ▶ Phosphorus (P): 6.8 mg/dL (normal, 2.5–5.5)
- ▶ Uric acid: 12.8 mg/dL (normal, 2.5–8)
- ▶ Calcium (Ca): 6.0 mg/dL (normal, 9.0–11.5)
- ▶ Creatinine: 1.8 mg/dL (normal, 0.6–1.2)

An appropriate therapy was started to control this oncological emergency. Treatment included the administration of rasburicase and sevelamer.

Questions

1. S.W. was diagnosed with acute lymphoblastic leukemia, the most common cancer in children. Which of the following exam results for this patient is most indicative of his disease?

A. Peripheral lymphocytes: 72%

B. Reciprocal translocation: t(8;14)

C. Peripheral neutrophils: 4%

D. Peripheral blasts: 11%

E. Bone marrow lymphoblasts: 35%

2. Which of the following pairs of symptoms in S.W.'s recent medical history are most common in the clinical presentation of a child with acute lymphoblastic leukemia?

A. Fever–Tiredness

B. Headache–Easy bruising

C. Easy bruising–Tiredness

D. Fever–Easy bruising

E. Fever–Headache

F. Tiredness–Headache

3. Acute lymphoblastic leukemia is today a curable disease. Which of the following is most likely the cure rate of this disease in children?

A. 20%

B. 30%

C. 40%

D. 50%

E. 70%

F. > 90%

4. After diagnosis S.W. started an anticancer treatment. Which of the following phrases best defines the phase of his therapy?

A. CNS prophylaxis

B. Remission induction

C. Postremission consolidation

D. Maintenance

5. S.W.'s chemotherapy included vincristine. Which of the following molecular actions most likely mediated the therapeutic effect of the drug in the patient's disease?

A. Intercalation between DNA trands

B. Inhibition of microtubule disassembly

C. Inhibition of microtubule assembly

D. Alkylation of nucleophilic groups on DNA bases

E. Inhibition of tyrosine kinases

6. Which of the following adverse effects could most likely occur because of vincristine treatment?

A. Epileptic seizures

B. Acute glomerulonephritis

C. Acute hepatitis

D. Heart failure

E. Peripheral neuropathy

7. S.W.'s chemotherapy included asparaginase. Which of the following molecular actions most likely mediated the therapeutic effect of the drug in the patient's disease?

A. Inhibition of asparagine synthesis in tumor cells

B. Increased asparagine synthesis in normal cells

C. Hydrolysis of circulating asparagine

D. Increased asparagine breakdown in tumor cells

E. Inhibition of asparagine breakdown in normal cells

8. Which of the following is an adverse reaction that can occur in > 10% of cases during asparaginase therapy, and can be (rarely) life-threatening?

A. Pulmonary embolism

B. Stroke

C. Bone marrow depression

D. Hypersensitivity reaction

E. Disseminate intravascular coagulation

F. Acute renal failure

9. S.W. also received intrathecal chemo-therapy for CNS prophylaxis. Which of the following anticancer drugs was most likely given?

A. Etoposide

B. Methotrexate

C. Vinblastine

D. Bleomycin

E. Imatinib

F. Dacarbazine

10. On the day after starting the anticancer treatment S.W.'s lab values indicated hyperkalemia, hypocalcemia, hyperphosphatemia, and hyperuricemia. Which of the following was the most likely cause of these abnormal values?

A. Worsening of leukemia

B. Asparaginase overdose

C. Tumor lysis syndrome

D. Vincristine-induced kidney failure

E. Fanconi's syndrome

11. Rasburicase was given to S.W. Which of the following actions most likely mediated the therapeutic effect of the drug in the patient's disease?

A. Inhibition of uric acid synthesis

B. Stimulation of renal excretion of K^+

C. Inhibition of renal reabsorption of uric acid

D. Inhibition of intestinal absorption of phosphate

E. Conversion of uric acid to allantoin

F. Inhibition of renal reabsorption of phosphate

12. Sevelamer was given to S.W. Inhibition of which of the following actions most likely mediated the therapeutic effect of the drug in the patient's disease?

A. Intestinal phosphate absorption

B. Renal K^+ excretion

C. Renal phosphate reabsorption

D. Renal Ca^{2+} excretion

E. Triphosphate synthesis

Answers and Explanations

▶ *Learning objective:* Identify the exam result that is most indicative of acute lymphoblastic leukemia.

1. Answer: E

A diagnosis of acute lymphoblastic leukemia generally requires that at least 20 to 30% of the cells in the bone marrow are lymphoblasts, as in the present case. Under normal circumstances, blasts are never more than 5% of bone marrow cells.

A, C, D All these results may suggest leukemia, but the disease usually is not diagnosed without looking at a sample of bone marrow cells.

B A reciprocal translocation involving the long arms of chromosomes 8 and 14, designated t(8;14), is present in about 16% of patients with lymphoblastic leukemia but is also present in a high proportion of Burkitt's cell tumors of both African and non-African origin.

▶ *Learning objective:* Identify the pairs of symptoms that are most common in the clinical presentation of a child with acute lymphoblastic leukemia.

2. Answer: C

Easy bruising and tiredness are common symptoms of acute lymphoblastic leukemia in children because thrombocytopenia (causing easy bruising) occurs in > 70% of cases, and anemia (causing tiredness) occurs in > 50% of cases.

A, B, D, E, F The incidence of fever and headache in children with acute lymphoblastic leukemia is < 10%.

▶ *Learning objective:* Identify the correct cure rate of acute lymphoblastic leukemia in children

3. Answer: F

Recent studies have shown that children with acute lymphoblastic leukemia have a survival rate of more than 90%. The survival rates increased for girls and boys of all racial and ethnic groups and for all age groups except infants under 1 year old. Researchers attribute the improved survival rates to the best drugs and dosages to treat children with acute lymphoblastic leukemia. Survival rates for infants did not increase as much with improvements in drug use because more infants died from side effects of their treatment.

A, **B**, **C**, **D**, **E** See correct answer explanation.

▶ *Learning objective:* Describe the phases of acute lymphoblastic leukemia treatment.

4. Answer: B

The treatment of acute lymphoblastic leukemia includes the following four phases:

▶ **Induction:** The induction is the first phase of chemotherapy. It is done to achieve remission, which means that no leukemic cells can be found in the blood, and bone marrow must have < 5% lymphoblasts.
▶ **CNS prophylaxis**: All treatment protocols for childhood acute lymphoblastic leukemia use some form of CNS preventive therapy to avoid the invasion of CNS by leukemic cells.
▶ **Consolidation:** this is a period of dose-intensive postremission chemotherapy aimed to intensify the achieved remission.
▶ **Maintenance**: This refers to the continuation of treatment to sustain the complete remission achieved from induction and consolidation chemotherapy. Early trials have shown that, without maintenance treatment, the majority of patients will relapse. In people treated for acute lymphoblastic leukemia, maintenance usually lasts many years, and then they are considered cured.

Since S.W.'s anticancer chemotherapy was the first after diagnosis it was an induction chemotherapy.

A, C, D See correct answer explanation.

▶ *Learning objective:* Identify the most likely mechanisms of anticancer action of vincristine.

5. Answer: C

Vincristine and vinblastine are vinca alkaloids. These drugs bind specifically to beta-tubulin, the structural protein that forms microtubules, and block its polymerization with alpha-tubulin to form microtubules, thus preventing microtubule assembly. In this way they cause an arrest of the mitotic cycle in metaphase.

A This would be the mechanism of action of anthracyclines.
C This would be the mechanism of action of taxanes.
D This would be the mechanism of action of alkylating drugs.
E This would be the mechanism of action of imatinib.

▶ *Learning objective:* Identify a common adverse effect of vincristine.

6. Answer: E

Vinca alkaloids have certain toxicities in common (i.e., nausea and vomiting, diarrhea, alopecia), but other adverse effects differ. Vincristine causes a dose-limiting neurotoxicity but is a mild myelosuppressive, whereas vinblastine causes negligible neurotoxicity but gives rise to a severe, dose-limiting myelosuppression. Virtually all patients receiving vincristine have some degree of neuropathy, and approximately 25 to 30% of children treated with the drug will develop clinically significant peripheral neuropathy requiring dose reduction or treatment discontinuation. The neuropathy involves both sensory and motor fibers and can manifest as paresthesias, loss of reflexes, weakness, and autonomic neuropathies. Vincristine neuropathy is usually reversible, but improvement is gradual and may take up to several months.

The exact mechanism of vincristine-induced peripheral neuropathy is still uncertain but is most likely related to the impaired microtubule function involved in axonal transport. Intact microtubules are required for axonal transports, and neuronal survival and function depend on these transport processes.

A Vincristine can cause neurotoxicity, but seizures are rare because the drug poorly crosses the blood–brain barrier.

B, **C**, **D** Vincristine cannot cause these adverse effects.

▶ *Learning objective:* Explain the mechanism of action of asparaginase.

7. Answer: C

Asparaginase is a cornerstone of treatment protocols for acute lymphoblastic leukemia and is used (as a drug of the multidrug treatment) for remission induction and intensification treatment in all pediatric regimens. The drug is an enzyme that hydrolyzes circulating asparagine. Because tumor cells in acute lymphoblastic leukemia have very low levels of asparagine synthetase, they require an exogenous source of asparagine for growth. Asparaginase depletes the existing supply of asparagine, thereby inhibiting protein synthesis in the tumor cells. In contrast, normal cells can synthesize asparagine and are therefore less susceptible to the cytotoxic action of asparaginase. An increased asparagine synthetase activity of tumor cells is the cause of resistance to asparaginase.

A Tumor cells cannot synthesize asparagine.

B, **E** Asparagine synthesis or breakdown in normal cells is not affected by asparaginase.

D Asparaginase can increase the breakdown of circulating asparagine, not of asparagine already taken by in tumor cells.

▶ *Learning objective:* Identify a frequent, and sometimes serious, adverse effect of asparaginase.

8. Answer: D

Asparaginase is a large protein molecule. Therefore it can cause hypersensitivity reactions in about 14% of patients (up to 35% when given intravenously), including life-threatening anaphylaxis.

A, **B**, **C**, **E**, **F** Asparaginase can cause all these adverse reactions, but their occurrence is < 1%.

▶ *Learning objective:* Identify the drug administered intrathecally to children with acute lymphoblastic leukemia for prevention of leukemic relapse.

9. Answer: B

Before CNS preventive therapy was routine, the CNS was the most common site of leukemic relapse in children with acute lymphoblastic leukemia. Today, preventive therapy is performed with intracranial irradiation and intrathecal administration of anticancer drugs. Methotrexate (with or without cytarabine and corticosteroids) is the most common drug administered intrathecally to prevent relapse.

A Etoposide is an inhibitor of topoisomerase II, used mainly in lung cancers and lymphomas.

C Vinblastine is an inhibitor of microtubule assembly, used mainly in breast cancer and lymphomas.

D Bleomycin is an anticancer antibiotic that acts by breaking DNA and is used mainly in lymphomas and solid tumors.

E Imatinib is a tyrosine kinase inhibitor, used mainly in chronic myelogenous leukemia.

F Dacarbazine is an alkylating agent, used mainly in sarcomas and lymphomas.

▶ *Learning objective:* Identify the most likely cause of metabolic abnormalities that occurred soon after starting induction chemotherapy for acute lymphoblastic leukemia.

10. Answer: C

Tumor lysis syndrome is an oncological emergency that is caused by anticancer-induced massive tumor cell lysis with the release of large amounts of potassium, phosphate, and nucleic acids into the systemic circulation. These molecules are mainly concentrated intracellularly. Moreover, the phosphate concentration in malignant cells is up to four times higher than in normal cells. Thus rapid tumor breakdown often leads to hyperphosphatemia, which can cause secondary hypocalcemia. Catabolism of the nucleic acids to uric acid leads to hyperuricemia, and the marked increase in uric acid excretion can result in the precipitation of uric acid in the renal tubules and can also induce renal vasoconstriction, impaired autoregulation, decreased renal blood flow, and inflammation, resulting in acute kidney injury. This injury in turn can amplify the metabolic abnormalities caused by tumor cell lysis. The tumors most frequently associated with tumor lysis syndrome are clinically aggressive non-Hodgkin's lymphoma and acute lymphoblastic leukemia.

A, B, D All these events have a negligible risk of acute kidney failure.

E Fanconi's syndrome is due to inadequate reabsorption in the proximal renal tubules of the kidney. Signs include hypokalemia, not hyperkalemia, and hypophosphatemia, not hyperphosphatemia.

▶ *Learning objective:* Describe the mechanism of action of rasburicase.

11. Answer: E
Rasburicase and pegloticase are recombinant urate oxidase (also named uricase). This enzyme, absent in humans, converts uric acid to allantoin, a product very soluble and easily eliminated by the kidney. Rasburicase has been approved by the U.S. Food and Drug Administration for the treatment of hyperuricemia in patients with tumor lysis syndrome. The drug is preferred to allopurinol because it causes a rapid reduction in serum uric acid. In contrast allopurinol decreases uric acid formation and therefore has no effect on the uric acid already formed and cannot acutely reduce the serum uric acid concentration. Uricosuric drugs (e.g., probenecid)

are contraindicated because of the tumor lysis–induced acute kidney injury.

A Inhibition of uric acid synthesis would be the mechanism of action of allopurinol.

B Stimulation of renal excretion of K^+ would be an action of several diuretics.

C Inhibition of renal reabsorption of uric acid would be the mechanism of action of uricosuric drugs like probenecid.

D Inhibition of intestinal absorption of phosphate would be the mechanism of action of phosphate-binding drugs.

▶ *Learning objective:* Describe the mechanism of action of sevelamer.

12. Answer: A
Hyperphosphatemia remains a major problem in tumor lysis syndrome and can cause acute kidney injury. Strategies aimed at lowering serum phosphate levels (aggressive hydration and phosphate binder therapy) should be used. Sevelamer is a phosphate binder that ties dietary phosphate within the gastrointestinal tract. Amine groups in the sevelamer molecule cross-link with phosphate in the gut, thereby preventing phosphate absorption. This action decreases serum phosphate concentrations.

B Inhibition of renal K^+ excretion would be the mechanism of action of K^+-sparing diuretics.

C Inhibition of renal phosphate reabsorption would be a mechanism of action of parathyroid hormone.

D Inhibition of renal excretion of Ca^{2+} would be a mechanism of action of parathyroid hormone.

E Triphosphate synthesis is not inhibited by sevelamer.

Case 3

Asthma

S.T., a 10-year-old boy, was accompanied by his mother to his pneumologist for a follow-up evaluation of his asthma. The boy reported he had to use his albuterol meter-dose inhaler 1 to 2 times per week during the past month, but now he had to use it once daily. He also stated that his shortness of breath was increased and often occurred even at rest. Last week he was awakened twice during the night by cough. The patient's asthma was diagnosed at the age of 9 and defined as "intermittent." Until recently the disease was well controlled with albuterol as needed.

S.T.'s past medical history was significant for allergic rhinitis in the spring and summer for 4 years. He had been living at home with his parents, a brother of 6, a dog, and a cat. The patient's father also had asthma during childhood, but his asthma has since resolved completely.

S.T.'s vital signs were as follows: blood pressure 110/66 mm Hg, heart rate 65 bpm, respirations 26/min. Physical examination showed a boy in moderate respiratory distress with audible expiratory wheezes, occasional coughing, and a prolonged expiratory phase.

Pertinent laboratory results on admission were as follows:

Spirometry

▸ Forced expiratory volume in the first second of expiration (FEV_1): 65% of predicted
▸ Repeated FEV_1 after albuterol: 85% of predicted

From the patient's history, physical examination, and lab results a diagnosis of "moderate persistent asthma" was made. The current therapy was changed by adding inhaled fluticasone twice daily to albuterol as needed. S.T.'s mother was concerned about the adverse effects of glucocorticoids, but the pneumologist told her that systemic adverse effects of inhaled fluticasone were extremely rare.

Two weeks later S.T. returned to the pneumologist's office for follow-up evaluation. His mother said that recently she noticed several white spots on her son's mouth. S.T. stated that his shortness of breath was decreased, but he still had to use his albuterol inhaler almost every day. Physical examination showed several white plaques on the oral mucosa, palate, and tongue. Spirometry yielded an FEV_1 of 72% predicted. The pneumologist explained to the mother that the oral thrush was due to candidiasis, most likely related to fluticasone therapy. He also said that the asthma was not completely controlled, but he did not want to increase the fluticasone dose. The therapy was updated by adding oral montelukast, one tablet daily, and clotrimazole lozenges for 2 weeks.

Questions

1. S.T. had been suffering from asthma. Which of the following is most likely the primary pathological condition underlying this disease?

A. Hyperreactivity of airways to stimuli

B. Chronic progressive bronchial infection

C. Widespread pulmonary fibrosis

D. Multiple pulmonary microemboli

E. Increased alveolar wall destruction

2. Both asthma and chronic obstructive pulmonary disease (COPD) are obstructive lung disorders and therefore have several features in common. Which of the following disease features can best distinguish asthma from COPD?

A. Airway inflammation

B. Episodic exacerbation of airflow obstruction

C. Full recovery of respiratory function over time

D. Reduction in maximum expiratory flow

E. Reduction in ratio of FEV_1 to forced vital capacity (FVC)

3. S.T.'s spirometry yielded an FEV_1 of 70% predicted, and repeat spirometry after albuterol resulted in an FEV_1 of 85% predicted. The result of this test indicates most likely which of the following pathological features of lung disease?

A. Bronchial infection

B. Pulmonary thromboembolism

C. Bronchial hyperreactivity

D. Pulmonary fibrosis

E. Pulmonary hypertension

4. Spirometry is commonly used to help diagnose asthma. Which of the following lung volumes and capacities can be measured by spirometry?

A. Total lung capacity (TLC)

B. Functional residual capacity (FRC)

C. Residual volume (RV)

D. Forced vital capacity (FVC)

5. The production of which of the following antibodies most likely played a primary role in the evolution of S.T.'s disease?

A. IgA

B. IgE

C. IgG

D. IgM

E. IgD

6. Which of the following sets of cells most likely played a primary role in the pathogenesis of S.T.'s asthma?

A. T_h2 helper cells–red blood cell–eosinophils

B. Red blood cells–T_h2 helper cells–mast cells

C. Red blood cells–natural killer cells–eosinophils

D. T_h2 helper cells–mast cells–eosinophils

E. T_h2 helper cells–red blood cells–natural killer cells

F. Mast cells–natural killer cells–eosinophils

7. Which of the following inflammatory mediators was most likely the most important for triggering S.T.'s bronchoconstriction?

A. Histamine

B. Prostaglandin D2

C. Interleukin 13

D. Leukotriene D4

E. Platelet-activating factor

8. S.T. was using inhaled albuterol as needed. Which of the following molecular actions most likely mediated the effectiveness of the drug in the patient's disease?

A. Increased phosphorylation of myosin light chain

B. Activation of myosin light chain kinase

C. Increased formation of the $Ca^{2+}/$ calmodulin complex

D. Inhibition of cyclic adenosine monophosphate (cAMP)-dependent protein kinase

E. Increased synthesis of cAMP

9. Fluticasone was prescribed to S.T. The inhibition of which of the following enzymes most likely contributed to the anti-inflammatory effect of the drug in the patient's disease?

A. Phospholipase A_2

B. Cyclooxygenase I

C. Dihydrofolate reductase

D. Epoxygenase

E. Peptidyl transferase

10. The physician told S.T.'s mother that systemic adverse effects of inhaled fluticasone are extremely rare. Which of the following statements best explains the reason for this low toxicity?

A. The dose reaching the systemic circulation is very small.

B. Most of the drug is quickly excreted by the kidney.

C. The drug is completely metabolized by the lung.

D. The drug is completely eliminated with the exhaled air.

E. The drug cannot get through the duodenal wall.

11. Glucocorticoids can exert useful molecular actions on receptors involved in asthma pathogenesis. Which of the following is most likely one of these actions in the bronchial tree?

A. Decrease activation of nicotinic neuronal acetylcholine receptors

B. Decrease activation of muscarinic M_3 receptors

C. Decreased activation of adenosine A_1 receptors

D. Prevent desensitization of histamine H_1 receptors

E. Prevent desensitization of β_2-adrenoceptors

12. Montelukast was prescribed to S.T. Which of the following molecular actions most likely mediates the effectiveness of the drug in the patient's disease?

A. Activation of β_2 adrenoceptors

B. Inhibition of 5-lipoxygenase

C. Competitive blockade of leukotriene receptors

D. Inhibition of phospholipase A_2

E. Competitive blockade of M_3 receptors

F. Inhibition of phosphodiesterase

13. S.T. was diagnosed with oral candidiasis. Which of the following is the correct definition of this disease?

A. Endemic fungal infection

B. Endemic protozoan infection

C. Endemic bacterial infection

D. Opportunistic fungal infection

E. Opportunistic protozoan infection

F. Opportunistic bacterial infection

14. S.T's physician believed that candidiasis was a consequence of fluticasone therapy. Which of the following actions of the drug most likely contributes to the patient's disorder?

A. Increased plasma levels of free fatty acids

B. Increased gluconeogenesis

C. Reduced macrophage-mediated production of tumor necrosis factor (TNF)

D. Increased protein synthesis in the liver

E. Decreased Ca^{2+} absorption from the intestine

15. Clotrimazole lozenges for 2 weeks were prescribed for S.T. Which of the following molecular actions most likely mediated the therapeutic effect of the drug in the patient's candidiasis?

A. Inhibition of conversion of squalene to lanosterol
B. Formation of artificial pores in the fungal membrane
C. Inhibition of fungal mitosis
D. Inhibition of squalene synthesis
E. Inhibition of conversion of lanosterol to ergosterol

Answers and Explanations

▸ *Learning objective:* Identify the primary pathological condition underlying asthma.

1. Answer: A

The fundamental abnormality in asthma is an airway hyperreactivity to a variety of stimuli. Because of this the disease is characterized by bronchoconstriction, airway edema, inflammation, and remodeling.

▸ *Learning objective:* identify the disease feature that can best distinguish asthma from COPD.

2. Answer: C

Asthma resolves in many children, although for as many as 1 in 4 the disease persists in adulthood. COPD, on the other hand, can be controlled but not cured, and it causes an inexorable loss of respiratory function over time.

A, B, D, E All these features can occur in both asthma and COPD.

▸ *Learning objective:* Identify the pathological condition of a patient showing a 20% increase in FEV1 in response to albuterol.

3. Answer: C

Bronchial hyperreactivity is present in virtually all persons with asthma, including those with mild disease. Bronchial hyperreactivity is defined as either a 20% decrease in FEV_1 in response to a provoking factor (including inhalation of a broncho-constricting agent, such as methacholine), or a 20% increase in FEV_1 in response to a bronchodilating agent, such as albuterol, as in the present case.

A, B, D, E These pathological features of lung disease do not have a 20% increase in FEV_1 in response to a bronchodilating agent.

▸ *Learning objective:* Identify the lung volumes and capacities that can be measured by spirometry.

4. Answer: D

Residual volume (RV) cannot be measured by spirometry. Therefore any lung volume or capacity that includes RV cannot be measured by spirometry. Forced vital capacity (FVC) is the volume of air that can be forcibly expired after a maximal inspiration. It is the sum of inspiratory reserve volume (IRV), tidal volume (TV), and expiratory reserve volume (ERV). Because FVC does not include RV, it can be measured by spirometry.

A TLC = IRV + TV + ERV + RV. It includes RV, so it cannot be measured by spirometry.

B FRC = ERV + RV. It includes RV, so it cannot be measured by spirometry.

C RV cannot be measured by spirometry.

▸ *Learning objective:* Identify the immunoglobulin (Ig) that plays a primary role in the evolution of allergic asthma.

5. Answer: B

The patient's history of an allergic rhinitis indicates that his asthma was most likely atopic, that is, allergic in nature. Indeed more than 80% of asthmatic patients have a concomitant diagnosis of allergic rhinitis. Atopy is a genetic predisposition for the production of IgE antibodies in response to allergens. Atopy is the strongest predisposing factor in the development of asthma. The IgE is present in relatively low serum concentration. Most is adsorbed on the surface of mast cells and eosinophils. Linking of IgE on mast cell surfaces by antigen triggers the release of leukotrienes, prostaglandins, and histamine, leading to the immediate allergic responses.

A IgA is an antibody that plays a crucial role in the immune function of mucous membranes. IgA is involved in the pathogenesis of some diseases, including IgA nephropathy, celiac disease, and Henoch–Schönlein's purpura.

C IgG is the main type of antibody found in blood and extracellular fluid, enabling it to control infection of body tissues by binding many kinds of pathogens.

D IgM is the first antibody to appear in response to initial exposure to an antigen. It is particularly effective at complement activation.

E IgD is an antibody that is usually coexpressed with another cell surface antibody called IgM. IgD is thought to have important immunological functions, including activation of several immunocompetent cells.

► *Learning objective:* Describe the three types of blood cells most likely involved in the pathogenesis of allergic asthma.

6. Answer: D

In atopic asthma most cells of the airways are involved and become activated. These include the following:

► **T$_h$2 helper cells** that are activated by the initial encounter with allergens. They are referred to as helper cells because they are instrumental in helping other leucocytes to respond.

► **Mast cells** are cells of connective tissue that reside throughout the wall of the respiratory tract. An increased number of these cells (up to fivefold) have been described in the airways of atopic asthmatics. Mast cells remain inactive until an allergen binds to IgE already coating these cells. This causes the degranulation of mast cells, leading to the release of several mediators. This release elicits the **acute-phase reaction** (also called the immediate asthmatic response) that occurs within minutes after the exposure to an allergen. Mast cells also release cytokines that promote the influx of other leukocytes, particularly eosinophils.

► **Eosinophils** circulate in blood and migrate to inflammatory sites in tissues, where they are activated by cytokines released from T$_h$2 helper cells. Following activation, eosinophils can release several mediators locally. Eosinophils and other cells, including macrophages and epithelial cells, mediate the **late-phase reaction** (also called the late asthmatic response) that usually starts 3 to 6 hours after the immediate phase.

A, B, C, E, F Natural killer cells are cells that can kill virus-infected and tumor cells. These cells are minimally involved in the pathogenesis of asthma.

► *Learning objective:* Identify the most important mediator that triggers bronchoconstriction in asthmatic patients.

7. Answer: D

Today leukotrienes are thought to be the most effective bronchoconstricting agents. They are a thousand times more potent than histamine, both in vitro and in vivo. They are released following mast cell degranulation and cause prolonged bronchoconstriction as well as increased microvascular permeability and increased mucus secretion.

A, B Both histamine and prostaglandin D2 are bronchoconstricting agents, but their role in allergic asthma appears to be relatively minor because their potency is much lower than that of leukotrienes.

C, E These mediators are involved in the pathogenesis of asthma, but they are not bronchoconstricting agents.

► *Learning objective:* Identify the molecular action mediating the therapeutic effect of albuterol in asthmatic patients.

8. Answer: E

Albuterol is a β_2 receptor agonist. Activation of β_2-adrenoceptors in all smooth muscle cells of the body increases the synthesis of cAMP, which in turn activates the cAMP-dependent protein kinase. This enzyme accelerates the inactivation of myosin light chain kinase. The decreased availability of this enzyme decreases the phosphorylation of myosin light chain, which is a needed step for smooth muscle contraction. In summary, the activation of β_2-adrenoceptors will cause relaxation of all smooth muscle cells.

C Increased formation of Ca^{2+} calmodulin complex would increase, not decrease, the smooth muscle contractility.

A, **B**, **D** β_2-Adrenoceptor activation leads to effects opposite to those listed.

▶ *Learning objective:* Identify the enzyme whose inhibition mediates the anti-inflammatory effect of fluticasone.

9.   Answer: A

Fluticasone is a synthetic glucocorticoid. These drugs are effective inhibitors of phospholipase A_2, the enzyme that releases arachidonic acid from membrane-bound phospholipids. Arachidonic acid is the precursor of prostaglandins, leukotrienes, and platelet-activating factor. This action of glucocorticoids most likely involves the gene expression mediated induction of the synthesis of lipocortin, an enzyme that acts as an inhibitor of phospholipase A_2. The inhibition of phospholipase A_2 causes decreased synthesis of all prostaglandins and leukotrienes, which are powerful inflammatory mediators. The inhibition of leukotriene synthesis is especially important because they are the most powerful bronchoconstricting agents in asthma.

B By inhibiting the synthesis of phospholipase A_2, glucocorticoids also inhibit the synthesis of cyclooxygenase I, but this enzyme is not involved in the inflammatory process.

C, **D**, **E** These enzymes are not inhibited by glucocorticoids, and they are not involved in the inflammatory process.

▶ *Learning objective:* Explain why adverse effects of inhaled glucocorticoids are extremely rare.

10.   Answer: A

The reason for the low toxicity of inhaled glucocorticoids such as fluticasone is related to their specific pharmacokinetics. Approximately 80 to 90% of an inhaled dose is deposited in the oropharynx, swallowed, and subsequently absorbed by the gastro-

intestinal tract. This fraction undergoes first-pass metabolism in the liver, which is quite high (the oral bioavailability of fluticasone is < 1%). Approximately 10 to 20% of an inhaled dose enters the lung. This fraction exerts the local therapeutic effect and is then absorbed into the systemic circulation. Therefore, when given by the inhalatory route, the drug can achieve in the lung a concentration that is adequate for the local therapeutic effect but too small for systemic adverse effects.

B Glucocorticoids are > 95% eliminated by liver biotransformation, not by kidney excretion.

C The drug is completely metabolized by the liver, not by the lung.

D Exhaled air cannot eliminate fluticasone because the drug has already permeated the bronchial mucosa.

E The drug can get through the duodenal wall quite easily (all glucocorticoids can permeate the cell membranes) but cannot reach the systemic circulation because of a very large first-pass loss.

▶ *Learning objective:* Identify a useful action of glucocorticoids on receptors involved in asthma pathogenesis.

11.   Answer: E

Glucocorticoids are the most effective agents to treat asthma. Daily medication of low-dose inhaled glucocorticoids is considered the first step for chronic therapy of persistent asthma. The principal advantages of this route of administration are their pronounced local effects and their low systemic toxicity. Glucocorticoid actions useful to treat asthma include the following:

▶ The anti-inflammatory activity that reduces mucus hypersecretion and airway edema
▶ Prevention of desensitization of β_2-adrenoceptors
▶ Reduction of bronchial hyperreactivity

Owing to the mechanism that modifies gene expression, the time required to see a particular effect depends on the time required for new protein synthesis. General biochemical effects start immediately, but varying amounts of time are required to produce a clinical response. In asthmatic patients response to β_2-adrenoceptor stimulation is usually decreased, likely due to tolerance related to continuous activation. Restoration of normal responsiveness to endogenous catecholamines as well as to exogenous β_2-agonists occurs within 2 to 4 hours of glucocorticoid administration.

A, B, C All these actions would cause bronchodilation, but glucocorticoids do not exhibit these actions.

D Prevention of desensitization of histamine H_1 receptors would be an adverse effect in an asthmatic patient.

▶ *Learning objective:* Explain the molecular mechanism of action of montelukast.

12. Answer: C

Montelukast and zafirlukast are competitive leukotriene receptor antagonists used in the treatment of asthma. Although these drugs are not as effective as glucocorticoids, they are used especially when a glucocorticoid dose cannot be increased because of adverse effects, as in the present case.

A Activation of β_2-adrenoceptors would be the mechanism of action of albuterol.

B Inhibition of 5-lipoxygenase would be the mechanism of action of zileuton.

D Inhibition of phospholipase A_2 would be a mechanism of action of glucocorticoids.

E Competitive blockade of M_3 receptors would be the mechanism of action of ipratropium and tiotropium.

F Inhibition of phosphodiesterase would be a mechanism of action of theophylline.

▶ *Learning objective:* Explain the meaning of opportunistic infection.

13. Answer: D

Candidiasis is an opportunistic fungal infection. An opportunistic infection is an infection caused by bacterial, viral, fungal, or protozoan pathogens that take advantage of a host with a weakened immune system or an altered microbiota (such as a disrupted gut flora). Many of these pathogens do not cause disease in a healthy host who has a normal immune system. A compro-

mised immune system, however, presents an opportunity for the pathogen to infect. In the present case the glucocorticoid therapy most likely caused a local immunosuppressive effect that triggered the oral candidiasis, a common fungal infection in immunocompromised patients.

A, B, C Endemic refers to an infection that is maintained in the population due to sustained transmission without the need for external inputs. Candidiasis is not an endemic infection.

E, F Candidiasis is a fungal, not a bacterial or protozoal infection.

▶ *Learning objective:* Identify a glucocorticoid action that can contribute to the development of drug-induced oral candidiasis.

14. Answer: C

Glucocorticoids can trigger several infection diseases because of their anti-inflammatory and immunosuppressive effects. These drugs inhibit the synthesis of almost all known proinflammatory cytokines, including the macrophage-mediated production of TNF. This cytokine has proinflammatory, oncostatic, and chemotactic properties, which play interacting roles in immune system function.

A, B, D, E Glucocorticoids can exert all these actions, but they do not contribute significantly to the anti-inflammatory and immunosuppressive effects of these drugs.

▶ *Learning objective:* Explain the molecular mechanism of action of clotrimazole.

15. Answer: E

Clotrimazole is an antifungal drug of the azole subclass. Azoles inhibit cytochrome P450 enzymes. This inhibition impairs the activity of a P450-dependent lanosterol demethylase that converts lanosterol to ergosterol. The ultimate effect is an inhibition of ergosterol synthesis in fungal cells, which leads to disruption of fungal cell membranes. The specificity of azole drugs results from their greater affinity for fungal than for mammalian cytochrome P450 enzymes. Oral candidiasis usually responds to topical treatment with lozenges slowly. The lozenges are completely dissolved in the mouth 4 to 5 times daily for 14 days.

A This would be the mechanism of action of terbinafine.

B This would be the mechanism of action of amphotericin B.

C This would be the mechanism of action of griseofulvin.

D No antifungal drugs can inhibit the synthesis of squalene. In mammalian cells this synthesis can be inhibited by 3-hydroxy-3-methylgutaryl coenzyme A (HMG-CoA) reductase inhibitors (named statins) through an inhibition of the synthesis of mevalonate.

Case 4

Atrial Fibrillation

B.B., a 52-year-old Caucasian man, was admitted to the hospital because of a persistent increase of his cardiac rate. The patient reported that 2 weeks prior he had noticed intermittent episodes of lightheadedness and a fluttering sensation in his chest. These episodes had occurred four times since then. Each time the symptoms occurred suddenly, lasted no more than 1 minute, and were accompanied by a sinking feeling in the chest but not by shortness of breath or chest pain. The patient noticed that, during the attacks, his pulse was fast and irregular and he felt anxious, but once they were over he felt just fine. He also noticed that, after the attacks, he had an urgent need to urinate and would pass a large amount of urine. One week ago he noticed that his cardiac frequency was persistently increased.

B.B.'s past medical history was negative for ischemic heart disease, diabetes, myocardial infarction, and hypertension. He quit smoking 1 year ago, after smoking heavily for 32 years. The patient denied the use of illicit drugs but admitted drinking one or two glasses of wine daily for the past 20 years.

Physical examination showed a well-developed and nourished Caucasian male who looked his age and was in no acute distress. He was 180 cm tall and weighed 75 kg. The patient's vital signs on admission were as follows: blood pressure: lying 135/84 mm Hg, sudden standing 130/82 mm Hg; pulse 122 bpm and grossly irregular; respirations 18/min and regular. Chest auscultation revealed some expiratory wheezes and prolonged forced expiration. Heart examination showed apical heart beats 144/min, irregularly irregular rhythm, no murmurs or gallop. The remainder of the physical examination was unremarkable.

Results of laboratory exams on admission were as follows:

Blood hematology

All standard parameters were within normal limits.

Electrocardiogram

Irregular R–R intervals, undulating baselines without definitive P waves, normal width of the QRS complexes, and ventricular rate of 140 beats/min.

Chest X-ray

Localized radiolucency with attenuation of vascular marking in lower lung fields.

From the patient's examination and electrocardiogram (ECG) data a diagnosis of atrial fibrillation (AF) was made. An echocardiogram revealed no valvular disease, but the left atrium was slightly enlarged.

Further lab tests gave the following results:

Thyroid function tests

► Free thyroxine (fT_4) 1.9 pmol/L (normal 0.7–1.8)
► Free triiodothyronine (fT_3) 0.6 pmol/L (normal 0.2–0.5)

▶ Thyrotropin (TSH) 0.1 mIU/mL (normal 0.5–5.0)

Arterial blood gas analysis

▶ pH 7.35 (normal 7.35–7.45)
▶ PCO_2 45 mm Hg (normal 35–45)
▶ PO_2 72 mm Hg (normal 75–100)

Spirometry

▶ Forced expiratory volume in the first second of expiration/forced vital capacity (FEV_1/FVC): 65 (% predicted)
▶ FEV_1: 60 (% predicted)
▶ Total lung capacity (TLC): 58 (% predicted)

B.B. was placed on anticoagulant therapy with warfarin and was given diltiazem. The next day his heart rate was 90 bpm, and the patient was dismissed from the hospital with a post-discharge therapy that included both warfarin and diltiazem.

One month later B.B. returned to the hospital for a control visit. He reported no symptoms, and his physical examination was unremarkable. The ECG showed AF with a ventricular rate of 85 bpm. All lab exams were within normal limits. The therapy was maintained for another month, and then the patient returned to the hospital for conversion of his AF to normal sinus rhythm. The cardiologist explained the electrical cardioversion to B.B. but the patient was afraid of the procedure and refused the therapy. After further exams the pharmacological cardioversion was chosen for this patient.

B.B. received an ibutilide infusion for 10 minutes. A few minutes later a normal sinus rhythm was seen on the monitor. The patient was later discharged from the hospital with an appropriate therapy to maintain the normal sinus rhythm.

Questions

1. B.B. was diagnosed with AF. Which of the following phrases best describes the atrial rhythm that is typical of this disorder?

A. The atria contract rapidly and regularly at rates of 240 to 400 beats/min.

B. The atria contract rapidly and irregularly at rates of 400 to 600 beats/min.

C. All atrial impulses are transmitted to the ventricles, causing tachycardia.

D. Abnormal atrial impulses can reenter the atria through accessory pathways.

E. The atria contract rapidly and regularly at rates of 200 to 600 beats/min.

2. B.B. was diagnosed with AF. Which of the following phrases best describes the cardiac electrical impulses that primarily occur in this disorder?

A. Continuous and chaotic reentry of electrical impulses within the atrial myocardium

B. Continuous reentry of electrical impulses through the Kent bundle

C. Continuous and fast reentry of electrical impulses within the atrial myocardium

D. Increased electrical impulse frequency from the sinoventricular node

E. Complete block of electrical impulse transmission through the AV node

3. It is known that left atrial contraction contributes to left ventricular filling, which in turn contributes to cardiac output. In AF the atrial contraction is profoundly impaired. Which of the following could be, at rest, the maximum decrease of cardiac output in B.B.?

A. 2%

B. 4%

C. 10%

D. 20%

E. 50%

4. B.B. complained of lightheadedness during the episodes of palpitation. Which of the following is most likely cause of this symptom?

A. Transient increase in brain blood flow

B. Adrenergic discharge due to anxiety

C. Transient decrease in cardiac output

D. Decreased firing of vagus nerve

E. Transient impairment of the baroreceptor reflex

5. B.B. noticed that after the attack he had an urgent need to urinate, and he passed a large amount of urine. Which of the following actions most likely cause this symptom?

A. Increased blood flow to the bladder

B. Sympathetic firing to the detrusor muscle

C. Renin secretion from the macula densa

D. Secretion of atrial natriuretic peptide

E. Secretion of antidiuretic hormone (ADH) from the pituitary

6. From B.B.'s history and exam results, which of the following pairs of disorders most likely contributed to the appearance of AF in this patient?

A. Chronic heart failure and hypothyroidism

B. Chronic obstructive pulmonary disorder and hyperthyroidism

C. Essential hypertension and chronic heavy alcohol intake

D. Pulmonary embolism and hypertrophic cardiomyopathy

E. Transient ischemic attack and exertional angina

7. B.B. was prescribed warfarin. The main reason for this therapy was most likely to prevent which of the following disorders?

A. Ischemic colitis

B. Wolff–Parkinson–White's syndrome

C. Heart failure

D. Ischemic stroke

E. Ventricular tachycardia

8. Which of the following steps of B.B.'s coagulation cascade was specifically inhibited by warfarin?

A. Factor IV activation

B. Breakdown of fibrin

C. Factor XII activation

D. Factor II synthesis

E. Factor IV synthesis

F. Factor II activation

9. The inhibition of which of the following enzymes most likely mediated the efficacy of warfarin in the patient's disease?

A. Cyclooxygenase

B. Epoxide reductase

C. Serine protease

D. Transaminase

E. Neuraminidase

10. Which of the following lab exams should be performed frequently during warfarin therapy?

A. Bleeding time

B. International normalized ratio

C. Platelet count

D. Plasmin blood level

E. Fibrinolysis time

11. Which of the following drugs should be used as an antidote if B.B.'s lab exams indicate an overdosage of warfarin?

A. Vitamin B_{12}

B. Bivalirudin

C. Alteplase

D. Protamine

E. Vitamin K

F. Desmopressin

12. B.B. was prescribed diltiazem. Which of the following was most likely the main reason for this drug being prescribed for the patient?

A. Restore the normal sinus rhythm

B. Increase the coronary blood flow

C. Control the ventricular rate

D. Prevent pulmonary embolism

E. Prevent heart failure

13. Which of the following molecular actions most likely mediated the antiarrhythmic effect of diltiazem in the patient's disease?

A. Activation of cardiac M_2 muscarinic receptors

B. Decreased formation of Ca^{2+}/calmodulin complex

C. Blockade of cardiac β-receptors

D. Increased Ca^{2+} release from sarcoplasmic reticulum

E. Blockade of cardiac Ca^{2+} channels

14. It is known that the affinity of an antiarrhythmic drug for its target channels depends upon the state of the channel. Which of the following sets of actions best describes the affinity of diltiazem for its target channels?

Diltiazem affinity for cardiac Ca^{2+} channels

	Resting	Activated	Inactivated
A.	Low	High	High
B.	Low	Low	High
C.	High	High	Low
D.	Low	High	Low
E.	High	Low	High

15. Which of the following cardiac regions was most likely the primary site of action of diltiazem in this patient?

A. SA node

B. Atrial myocytes

C. AV node

D. Purkinje fibers

E. Ventricular myocytes

16. After the successful control of his ventricular rate, B.B. was discharged from the hospital with an appropriate post-discharge therapy. Which of the following drugs was most likely included in the patient's prescription?

A. Losartan

B. Heparin

C. Levothyroxine

D. Ipratropium

E. Propranolol

17. B.B. received a pharmacological cardioversion with ibutilide. The blockade of which of the following cardiac ion channels most likely mediated the therapeutic effect of the drug in the patient's disease?

A. Activated Na^+ channels

B. Resting Na^+ channels

C. Activated K^+ channels

D. Resting K^+ channels

E. Activated Ca^{2+} channels

F. Resting Ca^{2+} channels

18. An appropriate postdischarge therapy was prescribed to B.B. in order to maintain the normal sinus rhythm after cardioversion. Which of the following drugs should be appropriate for this purpose?

A. Mexiletine

B. Lidocaine

C. Sotalol

D. Flecainide

E. Amiodarone

Answers and Explanations

► *Learning objective:* Identify the statement that best describes AF.

1. Answer: B

AF is an atrial arrhythmia characterized by two main features:

► The atrial rate is very fast (400–600 beats/min).

► The heart rate is irregularly irregular. In other words there is no pattern, and when the pulse is felt, it seems very fast and quite chaotic, with beats happening haphazardly.

A This would be the primary feature of atrial flutter, where the atria contract rapidly but regularly at rates of 240 to 400 beats/min.

C Except for the connection through the atrioventricular (AV) bundle, the atrial muscle mass is separated from the ventricular muscle mass by fibrous tissue. Therefore impulses from the atria can enter the ventricles only through the AV bundle. When the atria are fibrillating, impulses arrive from the atrial muscle to the AV node rapidly and irregularly. Because the AV node will not pass a second impulse for about 0.35 seconds after a previous one, at least 0.35 seconds must elapse between one ventricular contraction and the next. An additional but variable interval of 0 to 0.6 seconds occurs before one of the fibrillatory impulses can enter the AV node. Thus the interval between successive ventricular contractions varies from a minimum of about 0.35 seconds to a maximum of about 0.95 seconds. The conclusion is that only some of the atrial impulses can pass through to the ventricles in a haphazard way. Therefore the ventricles contract anywhere between 50 and 180 times a minute, but usually between 140 and 180 times a minute.

D This would be the mechanism of reentrant supraventricular tachycardia.

E See correct answer explanation.

► *Learning objective:* Recognize the statement that best describes the cardiac electrical impulses occurring in AF.

2. Answer: A

AF results from cardiac impulses that go mad within the atrial muscle mass, stimulating first one portion of the atrial muscle, then another portion, then another, and eventually feeding back onto itself to reexcite the same atrial muscle over and over. When this occurs many small portions of the atrial muscle will be contracting at the same time while other portions will be relaxing.

The background conditions that can trigger AF can be subdivided into two groups:

- ▶ All conditions that increase the excitability of some portion of the atrial myocardium (i.e., all conditions that make the resting membrane potentially less negative)
- ▶ All conditions that favor the reentry of cardiac impulses

In fibrillation many separate waves spread at the same time in different directions over the cardiac muscle. Therefore the reentrant impulses in fibrillation are not simply a single impulse moving in a circle—they have degenerated into a series of multiple wave fronts that have the appearance of a chain reaction.

B This would be the pathogenesis of Wolff–Parkinson–White's syndrome.

C This would be the pathogenesis of atrial flutter.

D This would be the pathogenesis of sinus tachycardia.

E An AV block is always present in AF but is not complete, because some atrial impulses pass into the ventricle.

▶ *Learning objective:* Define the maximum decrease in cardiac output that can be caused by AF.

3. Answer: D

Atrial contraction normally accounts for a percent of left ventricular filling when a person is at rest because most of ventricular filling occurs prior to atrial contraction as blood passively flows from the pulmonary veins, into the left atrium, then into the left ventricle through the open mitral valve. The contribution of left atrial systole to left ventricular filling is highly dependent on age and varies between ~ 20% (age < 35) and ~ 50% (age > 60) in persons at rest. These data do have clinical implications. When atrial contraction is impaired because of AF, cardiac output can be decreased by as much as 20%.

A, B, C, D See correct answer explanation.

▶ *Learning objective:* Explain the most likely reason of lightheadedness in a patient with AF.

4. Answer: C

The lightheadedness can be a symptom during an acute attack of tachycardia; if the heart is going too fast the diastolic time is decreased and ventricular filling is reduced. Therefore, even if cardiac output is usually directly proportional to the heart rate, it can decrease in spite of an increased heart rate when preload is reduced. The transient decrease in cardiac output causes mild cerebral ischemia, which in turn would decrease brain oxygen supply, the ultimate cause of lightheadedness.

A, B, D All these factors would cause an increase, not a decrease, of brain oxygen supply.

E The baroreceptor reflex is not involved in AF-induced tachycardia.

▶ *Learning objective:* Explain the most likely reason of urinary urgency after a tachycardia episode.

5. Answer: D

The need to urinate after a tachycaedia episode is the consequence of an increase in the urine formation by the kidney, due to the secretion of the atrial natriuretic peptide (ANP). The atria and other tissues contain a family of peptides with diuretic, natriuretic, and vasodilator properties. The ultimate stimulus for the release of ANP from the atria is the atrial stretch. ANP acts by activating specific receptors whose second messenger is cyclic guanosine monophosphate (cGMP). In general, ANP actions, as they relate to renal Na^+ and water excretion, antagonize those of the renin–angiotensin–aldosterone system. The ultimate effect is an increase in the excretion of Na^+ and water by the kidney. The ANP-induced increase in cGMP also causes vasodilation (mainly on capacitance vessels), which in turn leads to a hypotensive effect.

A, B As mentioned earlier, the need to urinate is due to an increase in urine formation by the kidney (i.e., increased diuresis). Increased blood flow to the bladder and increased sympathetic firing to the bladder have nothing to do with diuresis.

C Renin secretion is decreased, not increased, by ANP.

E ADH secretion from the pituitary is decreased, not increased, by ANP.

▶ *Learning objective:* Identify the pairs of the patient's disorders that contributed to the appearance of AF.

6. Answer: B

The patient's spirometry showed a reduction in FEV_1 and TLC. Blood gas analysis indicated a slight decrease in PO_2 and a borderline normal PCO_2. All these data and the smoking history are consistent with a chronic obstructive pulmonary disorder (COPD) of moderate degree. Thyroid exam results indicated that B.B. was suffering from unrecognized hyperthyroidism. Both disorders can increase the risk of AF and should be considered in every patient with recent onset of AF.

A vast array of diseases can increase the risk of AF, including ischemic heart disease, hypertension, chronic heart failure, cardiac surgery, Wolff–Parkinson–White's syndrome, COPD, pulmonary embolism, cerebrovascular accident, thyrotoxicosis, sudden emotional stress, and chronic heavy intake of alcohol.

From this list it can be seen that AF can present in three distinct clinical circumstances:

▶ As a secondary arrhythmia associated with structural heart disease
▶ As a secondary arrhythmia owing to systemic abnormality
▶ As a primary arrhythmia in the absence of a definable disease (the so-called lone AF, which is more frequent in healthy young adults and usually has a more benign course)

Therefore the clinical presentation ranges from a minimally symptomatic or asymptomatic incidental finding (the lone AF) to acute pulmonary edema in patients with heart failure. Between these extremes, AF may

▶ herald the presence of a noncardiac disorder (e.g., thyrotoxicosis),
▶ alert to the significance of another cardiac disorder (e.g., Wolff–Parkinson–White's syndrome),
▶ constitute a complicating factor of another cardiovascular disorder (e.g., myocardial infarction, hypertension).

AF can be paroxysmal (isolated attacks of rapid and irregular atrial rhythm that come and go abruptly) or persistent (sustained episodes of rapid and irregular atrial rhythm lasting more than 1 week). A paroxysmal AF can become persistent over time, as in the present case.

A Chronic heart failure is a risk factor for AF, but hypothyroidism is not.

C Both disorders are risk factors for AF, but B.B. did not suffer from them (two glasses of wine daily cannot be considered heavy drinking).

D, E These disorders are risk factors for AF, but B.B. did not have them.

▶ *Learning objective:* Recognize the disease that can be prevented by warfarin therapy in a patient with AF.

7. Answer: D

The two primary goals of treatment of AF are to control the ventricular response rate and to reduce the risk of stroke. In fact, AF is the leading cause of systemic emboli (45% of cardiogenic emboli in the United States occur in patients with AF), and patients with AF have a greater than fivefold increase in risk of stroke compared to control populations. Emboli likely arise from atrial mural thrombi that may form because of the circulatory stasis. Warfarin is an oral anticoagulant that blocks the synthesis of several vitamin K–dependent clotting factors. The benefit of anticoagulation with warfarin in the reduction of ischemic stroke in AF patients has been convincingly demonstrated in multiple well-controlled, randomized clinical trials. However, since the margin between adequate therapy and hemorrhage is relatively narrow, the efficacy of preventing embolic events must be considered against the risk of bleeding. The mean reduction in stroke was about 70% (from 4–5% per year to 1–2% per year) with an incremental risk of serious bleeding of less than 1% per year. Aspirin has also proved effective in preventing stroke, though less so than warfarin. Therefore an appropriate policy would be to use aspirin in settings where the risk of stroke is low or the risk of bleeding from warfarin is high.

A Ischemic colitis is due to a reduced blood flow to the colon but is not an embolic disease.

B, C, E All these diseases may be associated with AF but are not due to embolus formation.

▶ *Learning objective: Describe a step of the coagulation cascade that is specifically inhibited by warfarin.*

8. Answer: D

Warfarin is a coumarin anticoagulant. These drugs inhibit the liver synthesis of several coagulation factors (II, VII, IX, and X) by decreasing the reduced form of vitamin K, which is required for the synthesis of these factors.

A, E Coagulation factor IV is calcium. Complex molecules, not simple ions, can be synthesized and activated.

B Breakdown of fibrin is accomplished by fibrinolytic drugs, not by anticoagulants.

C Factor XII is Hageman's factor. It is part of the coagulation cascade and is activated in vivo by contact with poly anions, not by warfarin. It is considered to have little effect on coagulation in vivo.

F Factor II is prothrombin. Warfarin can inhibit the synthesis of several coagulation factors but has no effect on the activation of already formed factors.

▶ *Learning objective: Describe the enzyme of vitamin K synthesis that is specifically inhibited by warfarin.*

9. Answer: B

The hepatic synthesis of clotting factors including ll (prothrombin), Vll, IX, and X, as well as the anticoagulant factors proteins C and S, is dependent on levels of reduced vitamin K. This synthesis involves the carboxylation of the amino terminal glutamate residues of the clotting factors. This carboxylation requires reduced vitamin K, which is maintained in the reduced form by the enzyme vitamin K epoxide reductase. Warfarin inhibits vitamin K epoxide reductase, thus blocking the carboxylation (i.e., the synthesis) of clotting factors.

A Cyclooxygenases are enzymes involved in the biosynthesis of prostaglandins and thromboxanes.

C Serine proteases are enzymes that cleave peptide bonds in proteins. They are involved in various physiological functions, including digestion, immune response, and blood coagulation.

D Transaminases (also called aminotransferases) are enzymes that catalyze a type of reaction between an amino acid and an α-keto acid. Measuring their concentrations in the blood is important for the diagnosis of diseases.

E Neuraminidases are glycoside hydrolase enzymes that cleave the glycosidic linkages of neuraminic acids. The best-known neuraminidase is the viral neuraminidase, a drug target for the prevention of the spread of influenza infection.

▶ *Learning objective: Describe the lab exam that should be performed frequently during warfarin therapy.*

10. Answer: B

Laboratory tests used to assess hemostasis include the following:

▶ Activated partial thromboplastin time (aPTT), which is prolonged when there is a defect in either the intrinsic or the common pathway. This test is more sensitive to heparin, likely because heparin accelerates the neutralization of many coagulation factors of the intrinsic pathway.

▶ International normalized ratio (INR), which is prolonged when there is a defect in either the extrinsic or the common pathway. This test is more sensitive to warfarin, likely because warfarin inhibits the synthesis of factor VII, a key factor in the extrinsic pathway.

Because the warfarin anticoagulant effect can be strongly influenced by several factors, the INR test must be performed frequently, and the dose must be adjusted to maintain the test within a recommended range of 2 to 3 in most patients with medical conditions increasing thrombotic risk, as in the present case.

A Bleeding time is a lab test to assess platelet function. It is prolonged when the level of platelets is decreased or when platelets are abnormal. It is rarely used today, but it is still the most reliable way of assessing clinical bleeding in patients with uremia.

C Platelet count is used for assessing bleeding disorders due to thrombocytopenia, liver disease, or bone marrow failure. It cannot assess the activity of anticoagulant drugs.

D Plasmin is the enzyme that causes proteolytic digestion of fibrin. Its plasma level cannot measure the activity of anticoagulant drugs.

E Fibrinolysis time is tested to evaluate fibrinolytic activity. It cannot assess the activity of anticoagulant drugs.

▶ *Learning objective:* Identify the drug to be used as an antidote in case of a warfarin overdose.

11. Answer: E

When an excessive anticoagulant effect of warfarin is suggested by a high INR, the standard treatment is the administration of vitamin K. The drug accelerates the formation of factor II, VII, IX, and X, thereby "reversing" the effects of warfarin.

A Vitamin B$_{12}$ is used to treat megaloblastic anemia due to vitamin B$_{12}$ deficiency.

B Bivalirudin is a parenteral anticoagulant that acts as a direct thrombin inhibitor.

C Alteplase is a fibrinolytic drug used in myocardial infarction, stroke, and pulmonary embolism.

D Protamine is the antidote for heparin overdose.

F Desmopressin is a vasopressin analogue that increases factor VIII activity and is used in patients with hemophilia A or von Willebrand's disease.

▶ *Learning objective:* explain the reason for the use of diltiazem in AF.

12. Answer: C

A main goal of AF therapy is to reduce the high ventricular rate in order to avoid the risks related to tachycardia. This can be achieved in two ways:

▶ By giving drugs that depress conduction and increase refractoriness in the AV node, so that fewer impulses can reach the ventricle (the so-called rate control)
▶ By restoring the normal sinus rhythm (the so-called rhythm control)

The rate control is usually instituted first because this control may cause a dramatic decrease in the patient's symptoms. Appropriate drugs include beta-blockers, calcium channel blockers, and digoxin. The choice among these agents depends on the concomitant disease (e.g., digoxin is indicated if the heart contractility is impaired, calcium channel blockers must be avoided if an accessory pathway is present, etc.). In the present case beta-blockers should be the agents of choice because the patient has hyperthyroidism. However, beta-blockers are contraindicated in patients with COPD, and the choice of a calcium channel blocker, such as diltiazem, was more appropriate for this patient.

It is important to note that the rate control with antiarrhythmic drugs does not avoid the need for chronic anticoagulation because the patient remains in AF.

When the rate control is successfully achieved, a rhythm control can be attempted with either electrical or pharmacological cardioversion.

Electrical cardioversion (EC) is largely preferred today because of the adverse effects and the risk of proarrhythmia of most antiarrhythmic drugs. EC is accomplished with a single strong electric shock, which throws the entire heart into refractoriness for a few seconds. A normal sinus rhythm usually follows a few seconds later.

Pharmacological cardioversion can be accomplished with many antiarrhythmic drugs, including ibutilide, flecainide, and amiodarone, but today ibutilide is largely preferred.

Both electrical and pharmacological cardioversion can be complicated by systemic embolism. Therefore therapeutic anticoagulation should be given for at least 3 weeks prior to cardioversion and continued for 4 week after cardioversion.

It is important to note that restoration to normal sinus rhythm can be achieved easily (in over 90% of patients after cardioversion) but is difficult to maintain (sinus rhythm remains for 12 months in only 30–50%).

A Some antiarrhythmic drugs can be used to restore the normal sinus rhythm (pharmacological cardioversion), but Ca^{2+} channel blockers are not effective converters.

B Diltiazem causes coronary vasodilation, but this was not the reason for the administration of the drug to B.B.

D When the rate control is achieved, the atrium is still fibrillating; therefore, the risk of thromboembolism is not prevented.

E Diltiazem can decrease cardiac contractility and therefore can facilitate, not prevent, heart failure.

▶ *Learning objective:* Explain the mechanism of action of diltiazem.

13. Answer: E

Diltiazem is a Ca^{2+} channel blocker. Dihydropyridine Ca^{2+} channel blockers, such as nifedipine, block the voltage-gated L-type calcium channels almost exclusively in smooth muscles (mainly arteriolar smooth muscle), leading to vasodilation. Nondihydropyridine Ca^{2+} channel blockers, such as diltiazem and verapamil, can block voltage-gated L-type Ca^{2+} channels, both in smooth muscle and in the heart, leading to arteriolar vasodilation and to antiarrhythmic effect.

A, C Ca^{2+} channel blockers do not have these actions.

B By decreasing the cytosolic availability of Ca^{2+}, diltiazem decreases the formation of Ca^{2+}/calmodulin complex, but this occurs in smooth muscle, not in the heart, where Ca^{2+} binds to troponin, not to calmodulin.

D Because less Ca^{2+} is available in the cytoplasm, the release of Ca^{2+} from sarcoplasmic reticulum would be decreased, not increased.

▶ *Learning objective:* Describe the affinity of diltiazem for its target channels.

14. Answer: A

The affinity of a channel blocker for its ion channel depends on the state of the channel. In general affinity is low when the channel is on the resting state, but it is high when the channel is activated or inactivated. This rule can explain why channel blockers act as antiarrhythmic drugs, because channel activation mediates the upstroke of the action potential.

B, C, D, E See correct answer explanation.

▶ *Learning objective:* Identify the site of action of diltiazem in AF.

15. Answer: C

The main goal in AF and flutter is to achieve the "rate control, " so as to prevent the tachycardia induced by too many impulses reaching the ventricle. This can be done with any drug that can decrease AV conduction (e.g., beta-blockers, Ca^{2+} channel blockers acting on the heart, and digoxin). Diltiazem can decrease AV conduction; therefore, the main site of action of the drug in patients with AF or flutter is the AV node.

A Diltiazem can decrease heart frequency by acting on the sinoatrial (SA) node, but this is not the mechanism of the action of this drug in AF because, in the fibrillating atrium, the SA node is no longer the main pacemaker. In fact, in AF multiple microreentrant circuits can lead to chaotic activation of the atrium.

B, D, E These parts of the heart (i.e., right bundle branch, left bundle branch, and interventricular septum) are formed by the so-called fast fibers, whose conduction is Na^+ dependent. Ca^{2+} channel blockers have minimal activity on fast fibers.

▶ *Learning objective:* Recognize a drug used to treat COPD

16. Answer: D

B.B. was found to have COPD of moderate degree. Some quaternary anticholinergic drugs, such as ipratropium, tiotropium, and aclidinium, are commonly used in COPD because they relax bronchial smooth muscle through competitive inhibition of muscarinic receptors with negligible effects on bronchial secretions. Ipratropium is the anticholinergic drug most frequently used.

A Losartan is an angiotensin II antagonist used mainly as an antihypertensive, but B.B. did not have hypertension.

B B.B. was already receiving warfarin; there is no need to add another anticoagulant.

C This drug is contraindicated in a patient with hyperthyroidism.

E This drug is contraindicated in a patient with COPD.

▸ *Learning objective:* Describe the ion channels primarily blocked by ibutilide.

17. Answer: C

Ibutilide is a class III antiarrhythmic drug. The hallmark of this drug class is the blockade of cardiac K^+ channels. In addition ibutilide seems also to activate an inward Na^+ current. Both mechanisms could likely contribute to the prolongation of action potential duration.

A Blockade of activated Na^+ channels is the mechanism of a class Ia antiarrhythmic drug.

E Blockade of activated Ca^{2+} channels is the mechanism of a class IV antiarrhythmic drug.

B, **D**, **F** Antiarrhythmic drugs do not block resting ion channels.

▸ *Learning objective:* Identify the drug to be used for maintenance of normal sinus rhythm after cardioversion.

18. Answer: D

In order to prevent recurrences of AF after cardioversion many drugs can be used, including procainamide, flecainide, sotalol, and amiodarone. None seems clearly superior, and the choice is dependent on a number of clinical variables. Flecainide is contraindicated in patients with structural heart disease, but B.B. did not present symptoms of ischemic heart disease or heart failure; therefore the drug should be an appropriate choice in this case.

C Sotalol is a nonselective β-adrenoceptor antagonist. These drugs are contraindicated in patients with a bronchospastic disorder like COPD, as in the present case.

E Amiodarone is contraindicated in this patient because of hyperthyroidism.

A, **B** Antiarrhythmic drugs of class Ib, such as mexiletine and lidocaine, cannot maintain normal sinus rhythm after cardioversion.

Case 5

Bipolar Disorder

C.Z., a 26-year-old woman, was accompanied by her mother on a visit to the local psychiatric hospital, following the advice of their family physician. The mother reported that her daughter had been acting increasingly strange over the last month. She had been staying up later and later at night and her radio was played loudly all that time. During the day she often started singing in a loud voice. She also began repeatedly buying new suits and jewelry, and she admitted to her mother that she had started drinking a lot of alcohol and using cocaine because doing so made her very happy. C.Z. was employed as a waiter in a restaurant, but 2 weeks prior she had quit her job because her boss did not believe she was the best waiter and that she was about to receive a national prize for her work. She told her mother that she had a new job and it was going to make her a millionaire.

C.Z. was not married and was living at home with her parents. She had had a boyfriend, but he died 1 year ago in a car accident. The medical history of C.Z. and her family was unremarkable.

Examination showed a woman dressed flamboyantly in a brightly colored robe. She looked her age and was evidently in an elevated ad expansive mood. During the interview C.Z. was pacing up and down, waving her hands in the air and speaking in an elated, loud, sing-song voice. When asked about her new job she became angry and replied, "Why don't you trust me? I had documents to prove it, but vampires live in this city and destroyed my documents." During the conversation C.Z. had a rapid, unstoppable flow of speech. She constantly shifted from one theme to another and kept repeating, "My thoughts are racing, they are going too fast." C.Z. was suspicious and stated that people around her were plotting against her, since she kept hearing the voice of her dead boyfriend saying, "They want to kill you."

A diagnosis of bipolar I disorder was made. C.Z. was admitted to the hospital, underwent several lab tests, and started a treatment with lithium, valproate, and olanzapine. During the following 3 weeks the manic episode gradually subsided. Some adverse effects of the therapy were controlled by titrating the drug doses. One week later C.Z. was dismissed from the hospital with the same postdischarge therapy. She was informed that dehydration, fever, and vomiting could lead to an increase in her lithium levels. She was also instructed to ask her physician before taking any drug because some drugs could also increase her lithium levels.

Questions

1. C.Z. was diagnosed with a bipolar disorder. Which of the following sets of lifetime prevalence and mean age of onset is most likely correct for this disorder?

Set	LTP	MAO
A.	1–3%	40–50
B.	4–5%	40–50
C.	1–3%	20–30
D.	4–5%	40–50
E.	4–5%	20–30

LTP: lifetime prevalence
MAO: mean age onset (years)

2. According to the Diagnostic and Statistical Manual of Mental Disorders (DSM-5), a manic episode of bipolar I disorder can include psychotic features. Which of the following of C.Z.'s symptoms most likely indicate that psychotic features were present in her manic episode?

A. Decreased need for sleep

B. Inflated self-esteem

C. Auditory hallucinations

D. Racing thoughts

E. Greater talkativeness than usual

3. C.Z. started drinking a lot of alcoholic beverages. Alcohol and substance abuse can occur in patients with bipolar disorder. Which of the following is the reported percentage of bipolar patients who are abusing alcohol and illicit drugs?

A. 5%

B. 10%

C. 20%

D. 30%

E. > 40%

4. C.Z. started a treatment program that included lithium, a drug usually classified as a mood stabilizer. Which of the following is most likely the percent of overall success for both achieving remission of the manic phase and preventing a relapse of bipolar episodes?

A. < 50%

B. 55–58%

C. 60–80%

D. 85–90%

E. > 95%

5. The precise mechanism of antimanic action of lithium is still unknown. However, a major current working hypothesis relates the therapeutic effect of the drug to which of the following actions on signal transduction pathways?

A. Inhibition of inositol signaling

B. Activation of glycogen-kinase 3 signaling

C. Activation of cyclic adenosine monophosphate (cAMP) signaling

D. Inhibition of cyclic guanosine monophosphate (cGMP) signaling

E. Inhibition of tyrosine kinase signaling

6. It is well known that lithium can cause a vast array of adverse effects, most likely related to its narrow margin of safety. Which of the following pairs of adverse effects could most likely occur during the first days of C.Z.'s therapy?

A. Hand tremor–constipation

B. Insomnia–hand tremor

C. Insomnia–polyuria

D. Constipation–insomnia

E. Hand tremor–polyuria

F. Constipation–polyuria

7. After 2 weeks of therapy a lab test showed a normal renal function and a plasma lithium level of 1.8 mEq/L. The psychiatrist believed that this level was most likely the reason for some adverse effects reported by C.Z. and decided to withhold lithium for a while. Lithium has a half-life of about 20 hours. Which of the following would be the hours to withhold lithium in order to reach a safer, yet likely therapeutic, level of 0.75 mEq/L?

A. 20
B. 100
C. 80
D. 10
E. 30
F. 40

8. C.Z.'s treatment included valproate, an anticonvulsant drug that was found to have effective mood-stabilizing properties. Which of the following anticonvulsant drugs could be used as a second-line agent in treatment-resistant patients experiencing a manic episode?

A. Ethosuximide
B. Carbamazepine
C. Phenobarbital
D. Gabapentin
E. Levetiracetam

9. C.Z.'s treatment included olanzapine. The blockade of which of the following pairs of brain receptors most likely mediates the therapeutic effect of the drug in the patient's disorder?

A. 5-HT_{2A}–β_2
B. N-methyl-D-aspartate (NMDA)–D_2
C. β_2–D_2
D. 5-HT_{2A}–NMDA
E. D_2–5-HT_{2A}
F. β_2–NMDA

10. C.Z. was told that some drugs could increase her lithium level. Drugs from which of the following pairs of drug classes can most likely have this effect?

A. Macrolide antibiotics–nonsteroidal anti-inflammatory drugs (NSAIDs)
B. NSAIDs–thiazide diuretics
C. Antiviral drugs–macrolide antibiotics
D. Thiazide diuretics–macrolide antibiotics
E. Antiviral drugs–thiazide diuretics
F. NSAIDs–antiviral drugs

Answers and Explanations

▸ *Learning objective:* Identify the lifetime prevalence and the mean age of onset of bipolar disorder.

1. Answer: C

Bipolar disorder occurs in about 1–3% of the global population. It may begin in childhood, but most cases occur in the third decade of life.

A, B, D, E See correct answer explanation.

▸ *Learning objective:* Identify the primary symptom that can differentiate between manic and hypomanic episode.

2. Answer: C

C.Z. had auditory hallucinations (hearing the voice of her dead boyfriend) and delusions (vampires live in this city). A bipolar I disorder can include psychotic features (i.e., hallucinations, delusions).

A, B, D, E All these symptoms are typical of a manic episode but are not psychotic symptoms.

▶ *Learning objective:* Identify the percentage of bipolar patients taking alcohol and illicit drugs.

3. Answer: E

Alcohol and substance abuse is common among patients with bipolar disorder, and this can have a significant impact on the course of the illness and response to treatment. Bipolar patients often self-medicate with alcohol or cocaine during episodes, resulting in further impairment of judgment, poor impulse control, and worsening of the clinical course.

A, B, C, D See correct answer explanation.

▶ *Learning objective:* Identify the percentage of bipolar patients who can be treated effectively with lithium.

4. Answer: C

Lithium is a drug currently used in bipolar disorders, both to abort an acute manic or hypomanic episode and to prevent relapses. The overall success rate for achieving remission of the manic phase can be as high as 80%, and the drug can prevent recurrence of the manic phase or the bipolar depression in about two-thirds of patients.

A, B, D, E, F See correct answer explanation.

▶ *Learning objective:* Identify the action on signal transduction pathway that most likely mediates the antimanic effect of lithium.

5. Answer: A

The precise mechanism of lithium therapeutic effect is unknown but is most likely related to the direct inhibition of inositol signaling. Lithium inhibits inositol monophosphatase, the rate-limiting enzyme involved in inositol recycling. This leads to depletion of phosphatidylinositol 4,5-bisphosphate (PIP_2), which is the precursor of inositol 1,4,5-triphosphate (IP_3) and diacylglycerol (DAG). Over time the effects of these transmitters on the cell diminish in proportion to the depletion of PIP_2.

B Lithium causes inhibition, not activation, of glycogen synthase kinase-3, a protein kinase that regulates signal pathways involved in apoptosis.

C Lithium causes inhibition, not activation, of cAMP signaling.

D, E The action of lithium on these signaling pathways is negligible or none.

▶ *Learning objective:* Describe the adverse effects of lithium.

6. Answer: E

Hand tremor is an adverse effect of lithium that is dose dependent and can occur in up to 60% of patients receiving high doses. When tremor is not disturbing, treatment is not necessary. Otherwise a concomitant treatment with a beta-blocker can help.

Polyuria and polydipsia are common adverse effects of lithium, occurring in up to 40% of patients receiving the drug, and are due to lithium-induced diabetes insipidus. The mechanism of this disorder is thought to be related to the renal handing of lithium. In the collecting tubule lithium is reabsorbed through the Na^+ channels and is therefore concentrated inside the principal cells. In those cells vasopressin activates V_2 receptors, which in turn stimulate adenylyl cyclase. The resulting increase in cAMP triggers an increased rate of insertion of aquaporins into the apical membrane, thereby increasing water permeability. The high concentration of lithium in the principal cells blocks the action of vasopressin, likely by inhibiting adenylyl cyclase, thereby causing nephrogenic diabetes insipidus.

A, D, F Lithium tends to cause diarrhea, not constipation.

B, C, D Lithium tends to cause drowsiness, not insomnia.

▶ *Learning objective:* Calculate the time to withhold lithium therapy in case of presumed overdose toxicity.

7. Answer: F

Lithium has a narrow therapeutic window. The minimum effective concentration of the drug is about 0.6 mEq/L, and toxicity can occur with more than 1.5 mEq/L. Definite lithium intoxication usually occurs when concentration is higher than 2 mEq/L.

By definition the plasma concentration of a drug halves every half-life. Therefore the plasma level will be 0.9 mEq/L after one half-life and 0.45 mEq/L after 2 half-lives, or after 40 hours.

A, **B**, **C**, **D**, **E** See correct answer explanation.

▶ *Learning objective:* Identify the anticonvulsant drug that can be used as a second-line agent in the treatment of a manic episode.

8. Answer: B

Carbamazepine is approved for both acute and maintenance therapy of bipolar disorder. The mechanism of action of the drug in this disorder is not known. Carbamazepine is generally reserved for lithium-refractory patients, rapid cyclers, or mixed states. Other anticonvulsant drugs used in bipolar disorder are lamotrigine, which is approved for maintenance treatment, and valproate, which is used in Europe for maintenance treatment.

A Ethosuximide is used as a first-line agent in absence seizures.

C Phenobarbital is used as a second-line agent in partial and generalized tonic-coclonic seizures.

D Gabapentin is used as an adjunct in partial and generalized tonic-coclonic seizures.

E Levetiracetam is used as an adjunct in partial and generalized tonic-coclonic seizures.

▶ *Learning objective:* Identify the brain receptors most likely blocked by olanzapine.

9. Answer: E

Olanzapine is an atypical antipsychotic drug. Several agents of this subclass are approved for the treatment of a manic episode. They are especially effective when the episode includes psychotic features like delusions and hallucinations, as in the present case. Most atypical antipsychotic drugs can block both D_2 and $5-HT_{2A}$, and this could be the reason for the better therapeutic profile of these drugs.

A, **B**, **C**, **D**, **F** Olanzapine has negligible blocking activity on NMDA glutamate receptors and β_2-adrenoceptors.

▶ *Learning objective:* Identify the drugs that can increase lithium plasma levels.

10. Answer: B

Thiazide diuretics can reduce up to 25% the clearance of lithium. This is because lithium is 80% reabsorbed in the proximal tubule (but not in the other part of the nephron) by the same mechanism as Na^+. Thiazides or loop diuretics can cause a depletion of salt and water, which in turn triggers an enhanced reabsorption of Na^+ in the proximal tubule. This is accompanied by enhanced lithium reabsorption that can lead to increased lithium plasma levels, causing toxicity.

NSAIDs interfere with renal prostaglandin production and can reduce the renal clearance of lithium. This effect can develop over 5 to 10 days and can result in up to 150% increase in lithium plasma levels.

A, **C**, **D** Macrolide antibiotics do not affect lithium levels.

C, **E**, **F** Antiviral drugs do not affect lithium levels.

Case 6

Breast Cancer

V.A., a 61-year-old woman, complained to her physician of a painful lump in the upper, outer quadrant of her right breast, noted 3 days earlier.

Past medical history of the patient indicated that 5 years earlier she was diagnosed with hyperthyroidism and underwent thyroid ablation with radioactive iodine, followed by treatment with levothyroxine since then. Last year V.A. was diagnosed with deep venous thrombosis, which disappeared after an appropriate treatment.

V.A.'s menarche occurred when she was 13, and she entered menopause at the age of 45. She was married with one son, born when she was 23. Her last mammogram, taken 1 year ago, was negative. Family history of the patient was significant in that her mother died of breast cancer at the age of 55. The patient denied the use of illicit drugs but admitted drinking one glass of wine daily during meals.

Physical examination showed a thin woman, with a body mass index (BMI) of 20, who appeared her age with the following vital signs: blood pressure 135/82, heart rate 72 bpm, respirations 16/min, body temperature 98.2°F (36.8°C). Right breast examination showed skin retraction with arm elevated, without nipple retraction. Edema was noted on the skin in the right upper outer quadrant with no associated erythema. A hard, tender, 3 × 3 cm mass was palpated in the right upper outer quadrant; it was not fixed to the skin and was without ulceration. A 2 cm firm, tender mass was palpated in the right armpit. The left breast was without mass or lymphadenopathy. The rest of the physical examination was unremarkable.

Pertinent laboratory results on admission were as follows:

Blood hematology

- Erythrocyte sedimentation rate (ESR): 43 mm/h (normal < 20)
- Red blood cell count (RBC): $4.2 \times 10^6/\mu L$ (normal, women 4.0–6.0)
- Hemoglobin (Hgb): 13.5 g/dL (normal 12–16)
- Hematocrit (Hct): 30% (normal 36–48)
- White blood cell count (WBC): $9 \times 10^3/\mu L$ (normal 4–10)
- Platelet: $280 \times 10^3/\mu L$ (normal 130–400)
- Creatinine: 0.9 mg/dL (normal 0.6–1.2)
- Blood urea nitrogen: 22 mg/dL (normal 8–25)
- Alkaline phosphatase: 132 U/L (normal 25–100)

Bilateral mammography

The right breast showed a spiculated mass with some infiltration of the surrounding fatty tissue. The mass measured approximately 2 × 4 × 3 cm and was associated with interductal calcifications. The left breast showed no abnormality.

Ultrasound of right breast and right axilla

An ill-defined mass was hypoechoic and had abnormal vascularity. There was skin thickening and some suggestion of soft tissue edema associated with it.

Within the right axilla there were two lymph nodes that were abnormal in appearance.

Needle aspiration biopsy

- ▶ Right breast: Infiltrating ductal carcinoma, poorly differentiated, estrogen and progesterone receptors positive.
- ▶ Right axillary lymph nodes: Cytomorphology was similar to that seen in the breast aspiration material.

Positron emission tomography scan

There was no suggestion of metastases in liver, bones, or other organs.

Cytogenetic analysis

Human epidermal growth factor receptor 2 (ERBB2) positive

A diagnosis of breast cancer was made, and V.A. underwent partial mastectomy. Seven days after the operation she was discharged from the hospital with a postdischarge therapy that included raloxifene and trastuzumab.

Three years later V.A. was still cancer free, and the oncologist decided to stop the ongoing therapy and to start anastrozole.

Questions

1. V.A. was diagnosed with breast cancer. Which of the following events of the patient's history and physical exam was most likely a strong risk factor for the development of her breast cancer?

A. Alcohol consumption

B. Body mass index

C. Mother's death of breast cancer

D. Age of patient's pregnancy

E. Age of patient's menarche

F. Thyroid hormone therapy

2. From V.A.'s symptoms and signs, which of the following was most likely the stage of her breast cancer?

A. Stage 0

B. Stage I

C. Stage II

D. Stage III

E. Stage IV

3. Which of the following is most likely the single most important prognostic factor in breast cancer?

A. Age

B. Extent of lymph node involvement

C. Tumor grade

D. Presence of estrogen receptors

E. Presence of ERBB2 protein

4. V.A.'s ultrasound of the right axilla and the needle aspiration biopsy indicated that the cancer was present in two axillary lymph nodes. The increase of which of the following tumor cell receptors was most likely primarily responsible for the lymph node metastases?

A. Estrogen receptors

B. Epidermal growth factor receptors

C. Tumor necrosis factor receptors

D. Laminin receptors

E. Interleukin-1 receptors

5. The cytogenetic analysis of V.A.'s biopsy turned out to be ERBB neu positive. Which of the following phrases best explains this result?

A. Overexpression of antiapoptotic oncogene Bcl-2

B. Mutation of tumor suppressor gene p53

C. Overexpression of epidermal growth factor receptor gene

D. Mutation of tumor suppressor gene Rb

6. V.A.'s postdischarge therapy included raloxifene. Which of the following lab results of this patient best explains the reason for raloxifene treatment?

A. Increased alkaline phosphatase

B. Involvement of axillary lymph nodes

C. Tumor mass of 2 × 4 × 3 cm

D. Presence of tumor estrogen receptors

E. Presence of ERBB2 protein

7. Which of the following phrases correctly defines the receptor activity of raloxifene?

A. Selective estrogen receptor agonist

B. Selective progestin receptor agonist

C. Selective estrogen receptor antagonist

D. Selective estrogen receptor modulator

E. Selective progestin receptor antagonist

8. Taking into account V.A.'s medical history and raloxifene therapy, the risk of which of the following disorders was most likely increased in this patient?

A. Liver failure

B. Venous thromboembolism

C. Atrial fibrillation

D. Acute glomerulonephritis

E. Ulcerative colitis

F. Gouty arthritis

9. A drug currently used in breast cancer is tamoxifen. Which of the following statements best explain why the oncologist prescribed raloxifene instead of tamoxifen for this patient?

A. Tamoxifen can cause disturbing hot flashes.

B. Raloxifene can decrease the risk of endometrial cancer.

C. Tamoxifen can worsen the patient's osteoporosis.

D. Raloxifene is far more effective than tamoxifen.

E. Tamoxifen can increase the risk of deep venous thrombosis.

10. V.A. was treated with trastuzumab. The binding to which of the following proteins most likely mediated the therapeutic effect of the dug in the patient's disease?

A. Antioncogene p53

B. ERBB2 receptors

C. Vascular endothelial growth factor

D. CD 20 phosphoprotein

E. Cancer tyrosine kinase

11. Which of the following is the most serious and potentially fatal adverse effect of trastuzumab?

A. Ischemic stroke

B. Pseudomembranous colitis

C. Liver failure

D. Heart failure

E. Hypertensive crisis

F. Chronic obstructive pulmonary disease

12. V.A. was treated with anastrozole. The inhibition of which of the following enzymes most likely mediated the therapeutic effect of the drug in the patient's disease?

A. Transpeptidase

B. DNA polymerase

C. Aromatase

D. Ribonucleotide reductase

E. Topoisomerase II

F. 5α-reductase

13. Which of the following adverse effects could be most likely expected during anastrozole treatment?

A. Anemia

B. Skin ulcer

C. Bone fractures

D. Vaginal dryness

E. Deep venous thrombosis

F. Increased sweating

Answers and Explanations

▶ *Learning objective:* Identify a strong risk factor for the development of the patient's breast cancer.

1. Answer: C

A strong family history of breast cancer represents a compelling risk factor of breast cancer. Having a first-degree relative (mother, sister, or daughter) with breast cancer almost doubles a woman's risk.

A Drinking alcohol is clearly linked to an increased risk of developing breast cancer. The risk increases with the amount of alcohol consumed but is quite small in women who have 1 to 2 alcoholic drinks a day, as in the present case.

B Obesity (defined as a BMI > 30) is associated with a small increased risk of breast cancer. However, the present patient had a normal BMI.

D, E Women who have had more menstrual cycles because they started menstruating early (before age 12) and/or because they went through menopause later (after age 55) have a slightly higher risk of breast cancer. The increased risk may be due to a longer lifetime exposure to the hormones estrogen and progesterone. However, neither early menarche nor late menopause occurred in the present patient.

F Thyroid hormone has estrogen like effects at high levels, but a replacement therapy with the right dose of thyroid hormone is not a risk factor for the development of breast cancer.

▶ *Learning objective:* Identify the stage of breast cancer from the patient's symptoms and signs.

2. Answer: C

Breast cancer is usually subdivided into the following stages:

▶ **Stage 0:** there is no evidence of cancer cells or noncancerous abnormal cells breaking out of the part of the breast in which they started, or getting through to or invading neighboring normal tissue.

▶ **Stage I (divided into IA and IB):** in stage IB there is invasive breast cancer (cancer cells are breaking through to or invading normal surrounding breast tissue). The tumor is no larger than 2 centimeters, and there are small groups of cancer cells in the lymph nodes.

▶ **Stage II (divided into IIA and IIB):** in stage IIB the tumor is larger than 2 centimeters but no larger than 5 centimeters and has spread to 1 to 3 axillary lymph nodes.

▶ **Stage III (divided into IIIA, IIIB and IIIC):** in stage IIIC the cancer has spread to 10 or more axillary lymph nodes or to the chest wall.

▶ **Stage IV:** in this stage the cancer has spread beyond the breast and nearby lymph nodes to other organs of the body, such as the lungs, bones, liver, or brain.

Because V.A. has a tumor larger than 2 cm that has spread to two axillary lymph nodes her cancer should be classified as stage II.

A, B, D See correct answer explanation.

▶ *Learning objective:* Identify the most important prognostic factor in breast cancer.

3. Answer: B

Many factors can affect the course of breast cancer, but the involvement of lymph nodes correlates with disease-free and overall survival better than other prognostic factors. For node-negative patients the overall survival rate is > 80%. For patients with 1 to 3 positive nodes the survival rate is 40%, and for those with > 10 positive nodes the rate is 15%.

A, C, D, E All these factors can affect the prognosis of breast cancer but are less important than the extent of lymph node involvement.

▶ *Learning objective:* Identify the tumor cell receptor whose increase is most likely responsible for tumor metastases.

4. Answer: D

In order to metastasize, the tumor cells must first become less adhesive and detach from the primary site, and then attach elsewhere. Laminins are high-molecular-weight proteins of the extracellular matrix. They are an important and biologically active part of the cell basal lamina, influencing cell differentiation, migration, and adhesion. Tumor cells tend to have many more laminin receptors than do normal cells, allowing them to attach more readily to basement membranes at distant sites.

A, B, C, E All these receptors can be present in breast cancer cells, but they do not play a significant role in tumor metastasis.

▶ *Learning objective:* Explain the reason for a ERBB2 positive result.

5. Answer: C

Human epidermal growth factor receptor 2 (HEBB2) is a member of the human epidermal growth factor receptor (EGFR) family. Activation of these receptors initiates a variety of signaling pathways that promote cell proliferation and oppose apoptosis. Therefore they must be tightly regulated to prevent the occurrence of uncontrolled cell growth. Amplification or overexpression of the gene that makes these receptors has been shown to play an important role in the development and progression of certain types of cancer, including breast cancer. About 30% of breast cancers overexpress the ERBB2 receptor protein due to amplification on chromosome 17, and this is strongly associated with increased disease recurrence and a poor prognosis. However, the presence of ERBB2 in the breast cancer identifies women who might benefit from treatments directed against the ERBB2 receptor protein.

A The overexpression of this oncogene can lead to the development of B-cell follicular lymphoma.

B Mutation of this antioncogene has been found in many human tumor cells.

D Mutation of this antioncogene can lead to the development of retinoblastoma.

▶ *Learning objective:* Identify the primary reason for the use of raloxifene in breast cancer.

---

6. Answer: D

Raloxifene is a drug acting on estrogen receptors. More than half of breast cancers require the estrogens to grow, whereas other breast cancers are able to grow without estrogens. Estrogen-dependent breast cancer cells produce proteins called hormone receptors, which can be estrogen receptors, progesterone receptors, or both. If hormone receptors are present within a woman's breast cancer, she is likely to benefit from treatments that lower estrogen levels or block the actions of estrogen. These treatments are referred to as hormone therapies, and such tumors are referred to as hormone-responsive or hormone receptor positive. In contrast, women whose tumors do not contain estrogen or progesterone receptors do not benefit from endocrine therapy, which is therefore not recommended.

A, B, C, E All these exam results indicate the presence of a tumor but do not explain the reason for hormonal therapy.

▶ *Learning objective:* Identify the correct definition of the receptor activity of raloxifene.

---

7. Answer: D

Raloxifene is a selective estrogen receptor modulator (SERM). Drugs of this class act as either agonists or antagonists, depending on the estrogen receptor involved and the expression of estrogen-dependent genes. In this way they can produce beneficial estrogenic action in certain tissues (e.g., bone, brain, liver), but antagonistic activity in other tissues (e.g., breast) where estrogenic action may be deleterious.

A Selective estrogen receptor agonists are drugs that are able to activate estrogen receptors only (ethinyl estradiol, mestranol).

B Selective progestin receptor agonists are drugs that are able to activate progestin receptors only (norethindrone, norgestrel).

C Selective estrogen receptor antagonists are drugs that are able to block estrogen receptors only (fulvestrant).

E Selective progestin receptor antagonists are drugs that are able to block progestin receptors only (mifepristone).

▶ *Learning objective:* Identify the disorder whose risk was increased because of raloxifene treatment.

---

8. Answer: B

Raloxifene acts as an estrogen receptor agonist on most organs, tissues, and metabolic pathways, including the clotting cascade. Estrogens increase plasma levels of factor II, VII, VIII, IX, X, and XII and decrease plasma levels of antithrombin III, thereby increasing blood coagulation. Since the patient had already been treated for deep venous thrombosis she was most likely at increased risk for raloxifene-induced venous thromboembolism.

A, C, D, E, F The risk for these disorders is not increased by raloxifene therapy.

▶ *Learning objective:* Describe the main advantage of raloxifene over tamoxifen in hormonal therapy for breast cancer.

---

9. Answer: B

Tamoxifen and raloxifene are the only selective estrogen receptor modulators approved by the U.S. Food and Drug Administration for the treatment of hormone receptor–positive breast cancer. However, in vitro tamoxifen acts as an estrogen receptor antagonist on the breast but as a receptor agonist on the endometrium, whereas raloxifene acts as a receptor antagonist on both breast and endometrium. Clinically the risk of endometrial cancer of raloxifene users is less than that of nonusers, whereas tamoxifen users have a risk of developing endometrial cancer three times higher than that of raloxifene users, particularly in women over age 50 years. This can explain the oncologist's choice.

A Both tamoxifen and raloxifene can cause disturbing hot flashes.

C Both tamoxifen and raloxifene can improve, not worsen, osteoporosis because both act as estrogen receptor agonists on bone.

D Raloxifene is as effective as tamoxifen in reducing the risk of invasive breast cancer.

E Both tamoxifen and raloxifene can increase the risk of deep venous thrombosis.

▶ *Learning objective:* Explain the mechanism of action of trastuzumab.

10. Answer: B

Trastuzumab is a monoclonal antibody to a cell surface protein called human epidermal growth factor receptor 2 (ERBB2), which may be overexpressed in breast carcinoma. The normal biological response to HER2 signaling is stimulation of cell division. Trastuzumab binds with high affinity to ERBB2 receptor, thus preventing the binding of human epidermal growth factor to the same receptor. In this way tumor growth is inhibited. Trastuzumab is the only HER2-directed agent that results in a survival benefit when administered to a patient with HER2-positive breast cancer, as in the present case.

A The antioncogene p53 is a protein, encoded by the p53 tumor suppressor gene, which is a powerful apoptosis promoter. Inhibition of this protein would cause an increase, not a decrease, of tumor growth.

C Inhibition of vascular endothelial growth factor would be the mechanism of anticancer action of bevacizumab.

D Inhibition of CD 20 phosphoprotein would be the mechanism of anticancer action of rituximab.

E Inhibition of tyrosine kinase would be the mechanism of anticancer action of tyrosine kinase inhibitors (imatinib, erlotinib, sunitinib).

▶ *Learning objective:* Identify the most serious and potentially fatal adverse effect of trastuzumab.

11. Answer: D

Trastuzumab, as monotherapy or as combination therapy, is associated with a four- to sixfold increase in symptomatic myocardial dysfunction compared to patients not receiving trastuzumab. Clinical signs of heart failure can occur in about 1% of patients treated with trastuzumab alone, but can occur in up to 20% of patients who receive the drug plus anticancer chemotherapy. The reason for this cardiotoxicity is still unknown, but HER2 antigen is highly expressed in the development of the heart during embryogenesis.

A, B, C, E, F There are no reports of these adverse effects in patients treated with trastuzumab.

▶ *Learning objective:* Identify the enzyme specifically inhibited by anastrozole.

12. Answer: C

Anastrozole is a selective aromatase inhibitor. The enzyme aromatase is found in a number of human tissues and cells, including ovarian granulosa cells, the placental-trophoblast, adipose and skin fibroblasts, bone, and the brain. Fibroblasts at the tumor site in breast cancer tend to synthesize higher levels of the enzyme. Aromatase converts androgens to estrogens. The estrogen found at low levels in postmenopausal women are produced by aromatization of adrenal and ovarian androgens. Aromatase inhibitors cause almost total suppression of estrogen levels in postmenopausal women. Therefore they are preferentially used in postmenopausal women with a hormone receptor–positive breast cancer, either as a first-line therapy or in patients who completed 3 to 5 years of SERM, as in the present case.

A DD-transpeptidase (also called D-alanyl-D-alanine carboxypeptidase) is a bacterial enzyme that cross-links the peptidoglycan chains to form rigid cell walls.

The enzyme is inhibited by beta-lactam antibiotics.

B DNA polymerases are enzymes that synthesize DNA molecules from deoxyribonucleotides. The bacterial DNA polymerase is inhibited by rifamycin antibiotics.

D Ribonucleotide reductase is an enzyme that catalyzes the formation of deoxyribonucleotides from ribonucleotides. The enzyme is inhibited by some anticancer drugs, such as fludarabine.

E Topoisomerase II is an enzyme that relieves the torsional strain caused by the unwinding of the DNA during the replication. The enzyme is inhibited by some anticancer drugs, such as topotecan.

F 5α-reductases are enzymes involved in the metabolism of steroid hormones. An isoenzyme of this class is inhibited by finasteride, a drug used in prostate cancer.

▶ *Learning objective:* Identify a frequent adverse effect of anastrozole.

13.   Answer: C

Compared to SERM, aromatase inhibitors like anastrozole have been associated with a significantly lower incidence of vaginal bleeding, hot flashes, ischemic cerebrovascular events, and thromboembolic events. However, these drugs are associated with a higher incidence of bone fractures, which occurs in about 10% of patients receiving the drug. Numerous reports have demonstrated that aromatase suppression leads to clinically significant bone demineralization, resulting in increased rates of osteopenia, osteoporosis, and fractures. The mechanism of this adverse effect is most likely related to estrogen deficiency because there is a well-known association between postmenopausal estrogen deficiency and the development of osteoporosis.

A, B, D, E, F All these listed adverse effects can occur during anastrozole therapy, but their incidence is < 3%.

Case 7 — Cardiogenic Shock

D.E., a 58-year-old Caucasian man, was admitted to the intensive cardiac unit (ICU) after four-vessel coronary artery bypass surgery. He had a 10-year history of hypertension and of two myocardial infarctions 5 years and 6 months before surgery. Home medications included aspirin, captopril, metoprolol, and lovastatin. The patient was sedated, intubated, and had a pulmonary artery catheter in place. His vital signs in the ICU were stable, with a blood pressure of 120/80 mm Hg and a heart rate of 75 bpm.

One hour after admission to the ICU, the patient's blood pressure fell, and now he had the following hemodynamic profile and clinical parameters:

Parameter		Patient's values	Normal values
Blood pressure (BP) (mm Hg)	Systolic	85	120–140
	Diastolic	50	70–90
Heart rate (bpm)		110	60–80
Cardiac output (CO) (L/min)		2.5	4–6
Cardiac index		1.9 L/min/m²	2.8–4.2
Pulmonary capillary wedge pressure (PCWP) (mm Hg)		22	< 12
Total peripheral resistance (TPR) (dyne·sec·cm⁻⁵)		1,540	800–1,400
Respiratory rate (min)		26	12–20
Urine output (mL/h)		3	30–80
Temperature (°F)		96.8	95.3–98.4

The cardiologist made the diagnosis of cardiogenic shock, and an intermediate dose of dopamine (4 µg/kg/min) was initiated by intravenous (IV) infusion and maintained for the next 2 hours. The following changes in the hemodynamic profile were recorded.

Parameter		Previous values	Present values
Blood pressure (BP) (mm Hg)	Systolic	85	105
	Diastolic	50	65
Heart rate (bpm)		110	134
Cardiac output (CO) L/min		2.5	3.5
Cardiac index		1.9 L/min/m^2	2.3 L/min/m^2
Pulmonary capillary wedge pressure (PCWP) (mm Hg)		22	20
Total peripheral resistance (TPR) (dyne sec·cm^{-5})		1,540	1,515
Respiratory rate (min)		26	20
Urine output (mL/h)		3	20
Temperature °F		96.8	97.5

The cardiologist realized that the patient's stroke volume increased very little after dopamine administration. Thus the major increase in CO was caused by the chronotropic, rather than the inotropic, effect of dopamine. This suggested the addition of dobutamine to the ongoing treatment.

An IV infusion of dobutamine was started at low dosage and titrated up to 7 µg/mL/min. At the same time dopamine was tapered down to 2 µg/mL/min.

Three hours later the therapy yielded the following hemodynamic profile.

Parameter		Previous values	Present values
Blood pressure (BP) (mm Hg)	Systolic	105	122
	Diastolic	65	60
Heart rate (bpm)		134	105
Cardiac output (CO) L/min		3.5	4.8
Cardiac index		1.9 L/min/m^2	2.4 L/min/m^2
Pulmonary capillary wedge pressure (PCWP) (mm Hg)		20	13
Total peripheral resistance (TPR) (dyne·sec·cm^{-5})		1,515	1,230
Respiratory rate (min)		20	18
Urine output (mL/h)		20	50
Temperature °F		97.5	97.5

The patient remained stable with the infusion of dobutamine and dopamine for the past 4 hours. The drugs were tapered slowly, and 2 days later the patient was dismissed from the ICU.

Questions

1. D.E. was diagnosed with cardiogenic shock. Which of the following sets of cardiovascular parameters shown in the following table most likely suggested this diagnosis?

Set	CO	PCWP	TPR
A.	↓	↓	↑
B.	↑	↔	↓
C.	↓	↑	↑
D.	↑	↓	↔
E.	↓	↔	↓

↓ = increased ↓ = decreased ↔ = negligible change

2. Taking into account the patient's initial hemodynamic profile and the diagnosis of cardiogenic shock, which of the following therapeutic interventions would be appropriate for the patient at this stage?

A. Volume replacement (IV saline infusion)

B. Inotropic drugs

C. Vasodilating drugs

D. Thiazide diuretics

3. Which of the following actions could be expected from the dosage of dopamine administered to D.E.?

A. Activation of the chemoreceptor trigger zone

B. Decreased preload

C. Increased renal Na⁺ reabsorption

D. Decreased renin secretion

E. Increased afterload

4. Dopamine was given to D.E. by IV infusion. Which of the following statements best explains the reason for this administration route?

A. The drug can cause nausea and vomiting if given as IV bolus.

B. The drug has a half-life of about 2 minutes.

C. The drug can damage tissues if given intramuscularly (IM).

D. The drug has a large volume of distribution.

E. The drug has a very large first-pass loss.

5. The minimum effective dose (MED) of dopamine is about 0.5 µg/kg/min, and the minimum toxic dose (MTD) is about 15 mg/kg/min. Which of the following statements correctly defines the dosage range between MED and MTD?

A. Therapeutic index

B. Drug potency

C. Drug efficacy

D. Median therapeutic dose

E. Therapeutic window

6. Which of the following was most likely the time (in minutes) needed to achieve practically the steady-state plasma concentration of dopamine in this patient?

A. 24

B. 16

C. 8

D. 6

E. 2

F. 12

7. The cardiologist realized that the patient's stroke volume increased very little after dopamine administration. Which of the following was most likely this increase (in mL/beat)?

A. 20

B. 2

C. 6

D. 10

E. 12

F. 3

8. Which of the following statements best explains the effect of dopamine infusion on the oxygen consumption of the patient's heart?

A. Increased < 10%

B. Decreased < 10%

C. Decreased > 30%

D. Increased > 30%

E. Not changed substantially

9. Dobutamine was given to D.E. Which of the following molecular actions most likely mediated the dobutamine-induced increase in heart contractility?

A. Opening of voltage-gated Ca^{2+} channels

B. Opening of ligand-gated K^+ channels

C. Increased synthesis of diacylglycerol

D. Increased synthesis of cyclic guanosine monophosphate (cGMP)

E. Inhibition of cyclic adenosine monophosphate (cAMP)-dependent protein kinase A

10. Dobutamine infusion significantly enhanced D.E.'s urine output. The increase of which of the following hemodynamic parameters most likely mediated this enhancement?

A. Blood pressure

B. Cardiac preload

C. Cardiac afterload

D. Heart rate

Answers and Explanations

▶ *Learning objective:* Identify the changes in cardiovascular parameters that can define a cardiogenic shock.

1. Answer: C

Cardiogenic shock is caused by a reduction in cardiac output due to a primary cardiac disorder. Because the pumping activity of the heart is substantially depressed, the decrease in cardiac output is pronounced, and the cardiac index is concomitantly lowered. A cardiac index < 2 is indicative of cardiogenic shock.

PCWP, which provides an indirect measure of the left atrial pressure (which in turn is an index of preload) is increased because of the decreased pumping activity of the heart. A PCWP > 18 is indicative of cardiogenic shock.

TPR is increased because of the activation of the sympathetic system.

A, B, D, E See correct answer explanation.

▶ *Learning objective:* Describe the most appropriate emergency therapy for a patient with cardiogenic shock.

2. Answer: B

The very low cardiac index of the patient indicates that the shock is severe. The low cardiac output, in spite of an increased heart rate, indicates that the stroke volume is low (CO = SV × HR); that is, the contractility of the heart is substantially decreased. This could be due to several reasons, but the most common after a bypass surgery is a "stunned" myocardium. If blood flow is returned to an area of heart muscle after a period of ischemia, the heart muscle may not pump normally for a period of days following the event. This is referred to as stunned myocardium.

In case of severe pumping failure the most appropriate intervention to improve cardiac output is inotropic support.

A The patient has a high PCWP, which indicates that preload is already high. An attempt to increase the intravascular volume would further increase preload, which in turn would increase the workload of a heart that is already unable to pump. Moreover, an increase in intravascular volume might increase the pulmonary vascular pressure, adding the risk of pulmonary edema.

C Vasodilating drugs would decrease the afterload, thereby improving the cardiac output. However, the major risk of vasodilator therapy is further reduction of an already low systolic arterial pressure. Therefore vasodilator therapy should be attempted only when the systolic blood pressure is > 90 mm Hg.

D Diuretics decrease the intravascular volume, thereby decreasing preload. However, this is the case only if a sufficient glomerular filtration rate (GFR) is operative. In this case the very low urine output indicates that the perfusion of the kidney is badly compromised, and therefore the diuretic action would be very limited.

▶ *Learning objective:* Describe the action caused by a low dose of dopamine.

3. Answer: B

The dose given to the patient is an intermediate dose that is able to activate D_1-adrenoceptors in the splanchnic vascular bed and kidney, as well as β_1-adrenoceptors. In addition, this dose can cause a release of norepinephrine from the adrenergic terminals.

By activating β_1-adrenoceptors in the heart, dopamine increases the stroke volume and heart rate, which in turn increases cardiac output. Activation of D_1-adrenoceptors in the kidney vascular bed increases renal blood flow and decreases reabsorption of Na^+ from the proximal tubule. These effects increase the diuresis, which in turn decreases the intravascular volume. The improved heart pumping performance and the decreased intravascular volume lead to a decreased preload.

A Activation of D_2-adrenoceptors in the chemoreceptor trigger zone is usually caused by high doses, not intermediate doses, of dopamine.

C By activating D_1-adrenoceptors in the proximal tubule, dopamine decreases rather than increases Na^+ reabsorption.

D By activating β_1-adrenoceptors in the macula densa, dopamine increases rather than decreases renin secretion.

E The systemic vascular resistance is not much affected by an intermediate dose of dopamine because the D_1-mediated vasodilation of the splanchnic and renal beds is counteracted by the vasoconstriction caused by the release of norepinephrine. Therefore afterload should not change significantly. Actually, in the present patient the TPR was slightly decreased and therefore cardiac afterload would be decreased, not increased.

▶ *Learning objective:* Explain the main pharmacokinetic reason for the administration of dopamine by IV infusion.

4. Answer: B

When a drug has a very short half-life and a sustained action is required, the drug must be given in a form that allows a slow, continuous absorption (IV infusion, transdermal patch, depot preparation, etc.). In an emergency situation the IV infusion is the best drug administration route for drugs with a very short half-life.

A Dopamine can cause nausea and vomiting, but this is related to the dose, not to the administration procedure.

C Dopamine can cause ischemic necrosis if given in large doses, but this is not the reason why it is not given IM (other sympathomimetics, e.g., epinephrine, which can also cause ischemic necrosis, are nevertheless administered IM).

D The volume of distribution has nothing to do with the administration route.

E First-pass loss refers to oral drug administration. Dopamine is not effective when given orally because it is completely metabolized by the liver (i.e., it has a complete first-pass loss), but this is not the reason for its administration by IV infusion.

▶ *Learning objective:* Define the therapeutic window of a drug.

5. Answer: E

The range between the MED and the MTD of a drug is called the therapeutic window. It defines the ranges of doses with a high chance of efficacy and a low chance of adverse effects, that is, the range of doses which have a high probability of therapeutic success.

A The therapeutic index is the ratio between a harmful dose and an effective dose of a drug.

B Drug potency refers to the dose of a drug needed to produce a given effect. The lower the dose, the higher the potency.

C Drug efficacy is the maximal effect a drug can produce, irrespective of the dose given.

D The median therapeutic dose is the dose of a drug that can produce a given effect in 50% of the population under study.

▶ *Learning objective:* Calculate the time needed to reach the steady-state plasma concentration of dopamine given by IV infusion.

6. Answer: C

The half-life of dopamine is about 2 minutes. For every drug that follows a first-order elimination kinetics and is administered at fixed intervals, the time needed to achieve the steady-state plasma concentration (exactly 94% plasma concentration) is equal to 4 half-lives. This time is independent of the dose and the dosing intervals (provided that this interval is less than 4 half-lives).

A, B, D, E See correct answer explanation.

▶ *Learning objective:* Calculate the patient's increase in stroke volume after dopamine administration.

7. Answer: F

Knowing that CO = SV × HR, the patient's initial stroke volume was

▶ 2,500 mL/min / 110 beat/min = 23 mL/beat.

The patient's stroke volume after 2 hours of dopamine administration was

▶ 3,500 mL/min / 134 beat/min = 26 mL/beat.

Therefore the increase was only 3 mL/beat.

A, B, C, D, E See correct answer explanation.

▶ *Learning objective:* Calculate the change of cardiac oxygen consumption, knowing the patient's systolic blood pressure and the heart rate.

8. Answer: D

A widely used index of cardiac oxygen consumption is the so-called double product (also called the pressure-rate product), which is the product of systolic blood pressure and heart rate. This product correlates closely with the oxygen consumption of the heart. In D.E. the product was

▶ 85 × 110 = 9,350 before dopamine infusion
▶ 105 × 134 = 14,070 after dopamine infusion

Therefore a > 30% increase in oxygen consumption has occurred after dopamine infusion. This suggests that dopamine has likely affected adversely the myocardial oxygen supply/demand ratio.

A, B, C, E See correct answer explanation.

▶ *Learning objective:* Describe the molecular mechanism of action of dobutamine.

9. Answer: A

Dobutamine is a β_1-adrenoceptor agonist. Activation of these receptors leads to an increased synthesis of cAMP, which in turn activates the cAMP-dependent protein kinase A. This enzyme mediates the following two actions, which can affect cardiac contractility:

Increased opening of voltage-gated Ca^{2+} channels (which increases contraction)

Increased Ca^{2+} reuptake by the sarcoplasmic reticulum (which increases relaxation)

Thus the activation of cAMP-dependent protein kinase A serves to increase both the speed of contraction and the speed of relaxation.

B Opening of ligand-gated K^+ channels would cause hyperpolarization of the cardiac muscle membrane, adversely affecting heart contractility.

C Increased synthesis of diacylglycerol can follow the activation of α_1-adrenoceptors, not of β_1-adrenoceptors.

D Increased synthesis of cGMP can follow the activation of some peptide receptors, not of β_1-adrenoceptors.

E cAMP-dependent protein kinase A is activated, not inhibited, by the activation of β_1-adrenoceptors.

▶ *Learning objective:* Identify the hemodynamic parameter that mediates the increase in urine output after dopamine infusion in a patient with cardiogenic shock.

10. Answer: A

Dobutamine is a selective β_1-adrenoceptor agonist and therefore is expected to increase the stroke volume. This action is usually greater than that of dopamine. Selectivity is not absolute, and at higher doses the drug may also activate β_2- and α_1-adrenoceptors. For reasons that are still uncertain, dobutamine appears to cause only a small increase in heart rate; therefore the increase in CO is mainly due to the increase in stroke volume. The pronounced oliguria of the patient was mainly due to the fall in blood pressure, which in turn decreased sharply the hydrostatic pressure in the glomerular capillaries and the GFR. By increasing CO and arterial pressure dobutamine is expected to increase the GFR, which in turn increases diuresis.

B. By improving cardiac contractility dobutamine decreases, not increases, preload.

C, **D** In cardiogenic shock the low cardiac output causes a reflex activation of the sympathetic system, which in turn increases TPR and heart rate. By improving cardiac contractility dobutamine offsets this activation and therefore decreases, not increases, these hemodynamic parameters.

Case 8

Crohn's Disease

G.H., a 32-year-old man, was admitted to the hospital because of a 3-week history of inter-mittent cramping pain in the right lower abdominal quadrant associated with an increased frequency of bowel movements (up to eight each day). Stools were semiformed with no blood. He tried to control diarrhea with an over-the-counter preparation of loperamide, with little success. The patient also reported that he had lost 16 pounds and that 3 days ago he became feverish (100°F, 37.8°C). The patient denied alcohol or illicit drug use, but he had been smoking one pack of cigarettes daily for the past 15 years.

The patient's vital signs on admission were as follows: blood pressure 130/75 mm Hg, pulse 88 bpm, respirations 22/min. His physical examination was essentially normal except for an abdominal tenderness on palpation on the right lower quadrant. Pertinent lab results on admission were as follows:

Blood hematology

- ► Hematocrit 28% (normal 36–48%)
- ► Hemoglobin (Hgb) 8.5 g/dL (normal 12–16)
- ► White blood cell count (WBC) 16×10^3 mL (normal 4.5–10.5)
- ► Erythrocyte sedimentation rate (ESR) 65 mm/h (normal < 15).

Stool test

Stools were loose, watery, and positive for occult blood.

Endoscopy

A cobblestoned-appearing terminal ileum and ascending colon, with areas of normal tissue separated by areas of ulcerated mucosa.

Intestinal biopsy

A patchy acute and chronic inflammatory infiltrate, crypt abscesses, and several noncaseating granulomas.

A diagnosis of moderate Crohn's disease (CD) was made, and G.H. started therapy with mesalamine and prednisone (25 mg/d). One week later he was dismissed from the hospital with the same postdischarge therapy. After 1 month of prednisone G.H. experienced no evi-dent improvement of his disease. He had fewer bowel movements (3–4 each day), but his appetite and weight were not increased, and he still had intermittent abdominal pain and a low-grade fever. The gastroenterologist decided to add methotrexate and metronidazole to the therapy. Five weeks into the new therapy all the symptoms disappeared, and the predni-sone dosage was tapered to 10 mg/daily.

After 9 months of remission G.H. was hospitalized for an acute exacerbation of his dis-ease. He was treated with high-dose prednisone, and an infliximab infusion was started. The therapy was effective, and G.H. was dismissed from the hospital with the infliximab treatment to be given every 8 weeks.

The therapy kept him symptom free for 6 months, but later Crohn's symptoms reemerged, and the gastroenterologist decided to substitute infliximab with another monoclonal antibody. The new drug was quite effective, but, after 10 months of remission, G.H. was hospitalized because of severe abdominal pain associated with abdominal distension and vomiting. A computed tomographic (CT) scan indicated partial small bowel obstruction at the terminal ileum. G.H. was scheduled for surgery and had 50 cm of the terminal ileum removed, along with the ascending colon to the hepatic flexure.

After the operation G.H. was treated with azathioprine, and 1 week later he was discharged from the hospital with the same postdischarge therapy. Azathioprine worked well for several months. G.H.'s only complaints were mild abdominal pain and occasional diarrhea. The patient also noticed that his feces had an oily appearance and were especially foul smelling.

One year later G.H. was readmitted to the hospital for another acute exacerbation of his disease. Because G.H. had an inadequate response to conventional CD therapies, the gastroenterologist decided to prescribe natalizumab.

Questions

1. G.H. was diagnosed with CD. Which of the following features of bowel inflammation is unique to this disease?

A. Ulcerative

B. Granulomatous

C. Spread transmurally

D. Uniform and diffuse

2. G.H. was diagnosed with CD. Which of the following phrases best explains the anatomical site of this disease?

A. Distal ileum and colon

B. Colon and rectum

C. Any part of the gastrointestinal tract

D. Duodenum only

E. Rectum only

3. Which of the following of G.H.'s symptoms and signs was diagnostic for his disease?

A. Abdominal pain

B. Diarrhea

C. Weight loss

D. Noncaseating granulomas

E. Crypt abscesses

F. Areas of ulcerated mucosa

4. G.H. tried to control his diarrhea with loperamide. Direct activation of which of the following receptors most likely mediated the therapeutic effect of the drug in this patient?

A. β_2-adrenergic

B. Nicotinic neuronal (Nn) cholinergic

C. 5-HT$_3$ serotoninergic

D. α_2-adrenergic

E. μ-opioid

F. M$_3$ muscarinic

5. G.H.'s hematocrit was 28%. Which of the following disorders most likely accounts for this result?

A. Adrenal insufficiency

B. Iron deficiency anemia

C. Impaired erythropoiesis

D. Hemolytic anemia

E. Increased WBC count

6. G.H. lost 16 pounds in 3 weeks. Which of the following was most likely the primary cause of this weight loss?

A. Dehydration

B. Increased body metabolism

C. Malabsorption

D. Intestinal bacterial overgrowth

E. Intestinal ischemia

7. Mesalamine was prescribed to G.H. Which of the following molecular actions most likely mediates the therapeutic effect of the drug in the patient's disease?

A. Inhibition of activation of T cells

B. Inhibition of prostaglandin synthesis

C. Inhibition of tumor necrosis factor α (TNF-α)

D. Increased synthesis of interleukin-10 (IL-10)

E. Increased synthesis of lipocortin

8. Which of the following molecular actions most likely contributes to the therapeutic effect of prednisone in G.H.'s disease?

A. Increased catabolism of prostaglandins

B. Increased activation of phospholipase A2

C. Decreased lipocortin biosynthesis

D. Increased activation of the complement system

E. Decreased cytokine production

9. Methotrexate was added to G.H.'s therapy. Which of the following actions best explains the effectiveness of methotrexate in the patient's disease?

A. Antineoplastic

B. Anti-inflammatory

C. Immunosuppressive

D. Immunostimulant

E. Analgesic

10. Methotrexate can kill most rapidly proliferating cells. The killing of which of the following cells primarily mediates the therapeutic effect of methotrexate in G.H.'s disease?

A. Granulocytes

B. Plasma cells

C. T-helper cells

D. Mast cells

E. Myeloid cells

11. The inhibition of which of the following enzymes most likely mediates the therapeutic effect of methotrexate in G.H.'s disease?

A. Topoisomerase

B. RNA polymerase

C. Calcineurin

D. Dihydropteroate synthetase

E. Dihydrofolate reductase

12. Metronidazole was added to G.H.'s therapy in order to reduce the role of the intestinal flora in the inflammatory process. Which of the following classes of microorganisms are sensitive to metronidazole?

A. Mycoplasmas

B. Plasmodia

C. Bacteroides

D. Neisseriae

E. Rickettsiae

13. Which of the following molecular actions on bacterial cells most likely mediated the therapeutic effect of metronidazole in G.H.'s disease?

A. Damage of bacterial DNA

B. Inhibition of cell wall synthesis

C. Inhibition of relaxation of supercoiled DNA

D. Synthesis of abnormal proteins

E. Inhibition of purine synthesis

14. Infliximab was given to G.H. The inhibition of which of the following cytokines most likely mediated the therapeutic effect of the drug in the patient's disease?

A. Interferon-α (IFN-α)

B. IL-10

C. Granulocyte colony stimulating factor

D. IL-1

E. TNF-α

15. Which of the following is a potentially lethal adverse effect that can occur soon after infliximab administration?

A. Acute heart failure

B. Toxic epidermal necrolysis

C. Erythema multiforme

D. Pulmonary edema

E. Acute infusion reaction

F. Stevens–Johnson's syndrome

16. Because infliximab was no longer effective, the gastroenterologist decided to substitute it with another monoclonal antibody. Which of the following drugs was most likely prescribed?

A. Abciximab

B. Trastuzumab

C. Adalimumab

D. Basiliximab

E. Ustekinumab

F. Canakinumab

17. Azathioprine was prescribed to G.H. after the operation to maintain postoperative remission. Which of the following molecular actions most likely mediated the prophylactic effect of the drug in this patient?

A. Blockade of TNF-α receptors
B. Inhibition of clonal expansion of T and B lymphocytes
C. Inhibition of antigen presentation by dendritic cells
D. Stimulation of genetic expression of IL-2
E. Stimulation of macrophage phagocytic activity

18. After the operation G.H. noticed that his feces had an oily appearance and were especially foul smelling. Which of the following was most likely the cause of the patient's steatorrhea?

A. Increased liver bile acid pool
B. Decreased secretion of gastrin
C. Increased pancreatic secretion of lipase
D. Increased chylomicron formation in the intestinal lumen
E. Lack of micelle formation in the intestinal lumen

19. Natalizumab was prescribed to G.H. The blockade of which of the following endogenous compounds most likely mediated the therapeutic effect of the drug in this patient?

A. TNF-α
B. Integrins
C. IL-2 receptors
D. Epidermal growth factor receptors
E. Vascular endothelial growth factor

Answers and Explanations

▶ *Learning objective:* Identify the feature of bowel inflammation that is unique to CD.

1. Answer: C

CD is a chronic inflammatory bowel disease that begins with crypt inflammation and abscesses and progresses to focal ulcers. The distinguishing feature of the disease is that the inflammation is transmural (i.e., the inflammation spans the entire depth of the intestinal wall). In other inflammatory bowel diseases (e.g., ulcerative colitis, pseudomembranous colitis, etc.) the inflammation is seen only in the surface mucosa.

A The CD inflammation is ulcerative, but this feature is shared by other inflammatory bowel diseases, such as ulcerative colitis.

B The CD inflammation is granulomatous, but this feature is shared by several other inflammatory diseases.

D The CD inflammation is patchy, not diffuse, with discrete ulceration separated by normal-appearing mucosa.

▶ *Learning objective:* Identify the anatomical site of CD.

2. Answer: C

CD can affect any part of the gastrointestinal tract.

A CD usually affects the distal ileum and colon, but, as already explained, a unique feature of this disease is that it may occur in any part of gastrointestinal tract.

B These parts of the intestine are classically affected by ulcerative colitis. The disease does not involve other parts of the gastrointestinal tract.

D Disease involving the duodenum is usually related to duodenal diverticula.

E Disease involving the rectum only (proctitis) usually results from infection or radiation.

▶ *Learning objective:* Describe the result of intestinal biopsy that is diagnostic for CD.

3. Answer: D

In up to 50% of cases noncaseating granulomas are detected in the bowel wall by an intestinal biopsy. When detected, they are diagnostic for CD, as in the present case. However, they are not detected in about half of patients with CD.

A, B, C Most patients with CD present with the classic symptom triad of abdominal pain, diarrhea, and weight loss. These symptoms, however, are not specific, and many patients are first seen with an acute abdomen that simulates acute appendicitis.

E, F These signs are often present in CD, but they are also seen in ulcerative colitis.

▶ *Learning objective:* Explain the molecular mechanism of action of loperamide.

4. Answer: E

Loperamide is the most common over-the-counter preparation to treat diarrhea. The drug is an opioid agonist that directly activates μ-receptors in the enteric nervous system. This activation of both enteric neurons and smooth muscles ultimately causes a decrease in contraction of intestinal longitudinal muscles but a marked increase in contraction of circular muscles. Therefore propulsive peristaltic waves are diminished and tone is increased, thus relieving diarrhea. The drug cannot cross the blood–brain barrier and is therefore free of central properties and potential for addiction.

A Activation of β_2-adrenoceptors can cause relaxation of smooth muscle, but β_2-adrenoceptor agonists are not used to treat diarrhea.

B Nn receptors are located in the autonomic ganglia. Activation of these receptors would increase both sympathetic and parasympathetic firing. Because the parasympathetic is predominant in the gastrointestinal system, its activation would increase intestinal peristalsis, an adverse effect in patients with diarrhea.

C Serotonin causes contraction of nonvascular smooth muscle. Activation of serotoninergic receptors in the gastrointestinal system would increase intestinal peristalsis, an adverse effect in patients with diarrhea.

D Activation of α_2-adrenoceptors can cause relaxation of intestinal smooth muscle, but α_2-adrenoceptor agonists are not used to treat diarrhea.

F Muscarinic receptors are parasympathetic. Activation of these receptors in the gastrointestinal system would increase intestinal peristalsis, an adverse effect in patients with diarrhea.

▶ *Learning objective:* Identify the disease that can cause low hematocrit.

5. Answer: B

The low hematocrit is usually an indication of anemia. G.H.'s anemia is most likely due to chronic blood loss (see the Hgb value and the positive occult blood in the feces). An anemia due to chronic blood loss is an iron deficiency anemia.

A, C, D These disorders can cause low hematocrit, but G.H.'s clinical picture does not suggest any of these disorders.

E An increased WBC count cannot cause low hematocrit.

▶ *Learning objective:* Explain the reasons of weight loss in patients with CD.

6. Answer: C

There are two main causes of weight loss in CD. The first is malabsorption (i.e., the inadequate assimilation of dietary substances due to defects in digestion, absorption, or transport). A vast array of disorders can cause malabsorption, but in CD the cause is related to the chronic inflammation of the small intestine, which prevents adequate absorption of nutrients. The second cause is decreased oral intake since patients with bowel strictures feel better when they do not eat.

A, B, D, E All these disorders can cause weight loss, but G.H.'s clinical picture does not suggest any of these disorders.

▸ *Learning objective:* Explain the molecular mechanism of action of mesalamine.

7. Answer: B

Mesalamine (5-ASA) is the 5-amino derivative of salicylic acid. Even if the efficacy of mesalamine in CD is limited or marginal, given its favorable effect profile, the drug is often tried as an initial therapy for mild to moderate CD.

Aminosalicylates are believed to work topically in areas of injured gastrointestinal mucosa. These drugs likely act by inhibiting cyclooxygenases, thus decreasing prostaglandin synthesis. In support of prostaglandins as the mediators for inflammatory bowel disease are reports of disease exacerbation after oral administration of misoprostol, a prostaglandin derivative. However, specific inhibitors of prostaglandins are less effective than mesalamine and related compounds. Thus the exact mechanism of action of mesalamine is still uncertain.

Other potential mechanisms of aminosalicylates are related to their inhibition of the production of proinflammatory cytokines. 5-ASA inhibits the activation of nuclear transcription factor κB (NFκB), which regulates the transcription of proinflammatory cytokines.

Mesalamine is well absorbed through the small intestine and does not reach the distal small bowel or colon in appreciable quantities. To overcome this problem a number of pharmaceutical formulations (sulfasalazine, olsalazine, etc.) have been designed to deliver the drug to various distal segments of the small bowel or the colon. Mesalamine itself is formulated in various ways (time-release granules, tablets with a pH-dependent coating, etc.) to deliver the drug to different segments of the GI tract.

A Inhibition of activation of T cells would be the mechanism of action of cyclosporine, an immunomodulatory drug sometimes used in CD.

C Inhibition of TNF-α would be the mechanism of action of several drugs, including etanercept and infliximab. These drugs are sometimes used in CD.

D IL-10 is an anti-inflammatory cytokine. The gene expression–mediated induction of synthesis of anti-inflammatory cytokines contributes to the anti-inflammatory effect of glucocorticoids.

E Lipocortin is an enzyme that acts as an inhibitor of phospholipase A2, the enzyme that catalyzes the synthesis of eicosanoids. Glucocorticoids increase the synthesis of lipocortin, thereby inhibiting the synthesis of eicosanoids. The outcome is an anti-inflammatory effect.

▸ *Learning objective:* Identify the molecular action that can mediate the therapeutic effect of glucocorticoids in CD.

8. Answer: E

Glucocorticoids inhibit the synthesis of almost all known proinflammatory cytokines and can stimulate the synthesis of some anti-inflammatory cytokines (e.g., IL-10). Especially important seems the inhibition of the anti-inflammatory IL-1, IL-6, IL-12, and TNF-α.

A Glucocorticoids inhibit prostaglandin biosynthesis but have no effect on the metabolism of prostaglandins.

B, C Glucocorticoids increase, not decrease, the biosynthesis of lipocortin, which in turn inhibits, not enhances, the activity of phospholipase A2.

D The complement system is an important mediator of host defense and has proinflammatory activity. Glucocorticoids inhibit, rather than activate, this system.

▸ *Learning objective:* Identify the action that mediates the effectiveness of methotrexate in CD.

9. Answer: C

Methotrexate is an antineoplastic drug often used as an immunosuppressive. Many agents that kill proliferative cells appear to work at a similar level in immune response. Methotrexate can cause and maintain remission in patients with CD, as in the present case.

A See correct answer explanation.

B Even if methotrexate is used to treat an inflammatory disease (CD), the action of the drugs is primarily immunosuppressive rather than anti-inflammatory.

D See correct answer explanation.

E By definition an analgesic is a drug whose main effect is to diminish or abolish pain independently from the cause that elicits it. Methotrexate can reduce only the pain related to neoplastic or immunological disorders.

▶ *Learning objective:* Identify the cell type the killing of which by methotrexate most likely mediates the therapeutic effect of the drug in CD.

10. Answer: C

T-helper cells are the major effector cells in several autoimmune diseases. Killing these cells represents an important goal of any immunosuppressive treatment.

A, B, D These cells are not dividing and therefore are not the target for methotrexate.

E Myeloid cells do not play a significant role in autoimmune disease. These cells are killed because they are rapidly proliferating, and this explains myelosuppression, which is a major toxic effect of methotrexate.

▶ *Learning objective:* Describe the enzyme inhibition by methotrexate, which most likely mediates the therapeutic effect of the drug in CD.

11. Answer: E

Methotrexate inhibits dihydrofolate reductase, the enzyme that catalyzes the reduction of folate to dihydrofolate and the reduction of dihydrofolate to tetrahydrofolate. The decreased synthesis of tetrahydrofolate, which is a one-carbon-unit carrier, inhibits the synthesis of purines and pyrimidines, which are essential for the synthesis of ribonucleotides.

A Inhibitors of topoisomerase of cancer cells include etoposide and topotecan. Inhibitors of topoisomerase of bacterial cells are the fluoroquinolone antibiotics.

B Rifamycin antibiotics are inhibitors of bacterial RNA polymerase.

C Immunosuppressive drugs such as cyclosporine and tacrolimus are inhibitors of calcineurin enzyme.

D Sulfonamides are inhibitors of bacterial dihydropteroate synthetase.

▶ *Learning objective:* Describe the bacteria that are sensitive to metronidazole.

12. Answer: C

Metronidazole has a potent bactericidal activity against obligate anaerobes, including *Bacteroides*, the most common anaerobes of normal intestinal flora. The fact that in the normal adult colon 96 to 99% of bacterial flora consists of anaerobes explains why metronidazole is especially useful in reducing this flora. Some patients with CD improve symptomatically while taking metronidazole, but the improvement seems only transient in most cases.

A Mycoplasmas are facultative anaerobes and therefore not sensitive to metronidazole.

B Plasmodia are protozoa and therefore not sensitive to metronidazole.

D Neisseriae are aerobes and therefore not sensitive to metronidazole.

E Mycobacteria are aerobes and therefore not sensitive to metronidazole.

▶ *Learning objective:* Describe the molecular mechanism of action of metronidazole.

13. Answer: A

Metronidazole is an antibiotic active against most microaerophilic and anaerobic bacteria and anaerobic protozoa. These microorganisms, unlike their aerobic counterparts, contain electron transport components, called ferredoxins, that can donate electrons to metronidazole. This donation forms a highly reactive nitro radical anion that damages bacterial DNA. The ultimate effect is bactericidal.

B Inhibition of cell wall synthesis would be the mechanism of action of beta-lactam antibiotics.

C Inhibition of relaxation of supercoiled DNA would be the mechanism of action of fluoroquinolones.

D Synthesis of abnormal proteins would be part of the mechanism of action of aminoglycoside antibiotics.

E Inhibition of purine synthesis would be the mechanism of action of trimethoprim-sulfamethoxazole.

▶ *Learning objective:* Identify the endogenous compound that is specifically destroyed by infliximab.

14. Answer: E

TNF-α is a proinflammatory cytokine that is an important mediator of several inflammatory diseases. Infliximab is a monoclonal antibody targeted against TNF-α and is the first monoclonal antibody to be approved by the U.S. Food and Drug Administration for the treatment of CD. A single infusion of the drug has been shown to induce a clinical response or remission in 65% of patients with moderate to severe treatment-resistant CD. Short-term benefits after a single infusion may persist for up to 12 weeks, but a number of serious adverse effects can occur.

A Interferons are cytokines used as antiviral and anticancer agents.

B IL-10 is a cytokine with pronounced anti-inflammatory activity. Inhibition of this cytokine in CD would be irrational.

C Granulocyte colony stimulating factor is a cytokine used primarily in stem cell transplantation.

D IL-1 is a proinflammatory cytokine but is not inhibited by infliximab.

▶ *Learning objective:* Describe a potentially lethal adverse effect that can occur soon after infliximab administration.

15. Answer: E

All infusion reactions involve the immune system; however, some (anaphylactic, caused by subsequent exposure) are allergic in nature and usually mediated by immunoglobulin E (IgE). Symptoms and signs include rash, coughing, sneezing, wheezing, difficulty breathing, urticaria, angioedema, abdominal cramping, hypotension, and palpitations. Other reactions (anaphylactoid, caused by first exposure) are not true allergic reactions and are mediated by cytokine release (the so-called cytokine-release syndrome). Symptoms and signs include high fever, chills, myalgia, joint pain, tremor, confusion, hallucinations, and seizures. The clinical manifestations of both syndromes are almost the same, and in nontypical cases differentiation between the two syndromes can be

difficult. Both reactions can be lethal and can be minimized by pretreatment with a high dose of glucocorticoids.

Acute infusion reactions occur in about 20% of patients treated with monoclonal antibodies and represent the most serious adverse effect of these drugs.

A, B, C, D, F All these adverse effects have been associated with infliximab administration in postmarketing reports, but their frequency is very low, and often a causal relationship to infliximab cannot be established.

▶ *Learning objective:* Identify the monoclonal antibody that can be substituted for infliximab in the treatment of CD.

16. Answer: C

Infliximab is usually the first TNF-α inhibitor to be used in CD. When the drug is poorly tolerated or not effective, it can be replaced by another TNF-α inhibitor because it has been shown that patients unresponsive to infliximab may have a good response to the second inhibitor. The TNF-α inhibitors approved for the treatment of CD in patients with inadequate responses to infliximab are adalimumab and certolizumab (not listed).

A, B, D, E, F These monoclonal antibodies are not TNF-α inhibitors and are not used in CD.

▶ *Learning objective:* Describe the molecular mechanism of action of azathioprine.

17. Answer: B

Azathioprine is an immunosuppressive agent used for induction and maintenance of remission in CD. It is a prodrug that is converted in the body to mercaptopurine, an antimetabolite anticancer drug that blocks purine biosynthesis, forming a false nucleotide that is incorporated into DNA. This leads to cytotoxicity, mainly toward cells with a high turnover rate, which includes T and B lymphocytes. The proliferation of these lymphocytes is inhibited, and therefore both cell-mediated and antibody-mediated immune responses are inhibited. Azathioprine, however, appears to be a more effective immunosuppressive than mercaptopurine itself. The basis for this superiority is unknown.

The drug can consistently prevent postoperative CD recurrence for up to 2 years. However, the long-term benefit of treatment beyond 2 years has not been established.

A Azathioprine has no blocking activity on receptors of TNF-α.

C Antigen presentation by different antigen-presenting cells is an early step in the adaptive immune response. This step is not inhibited by azathioprine.

D, E These two actions would actually increase, not decrease, the immunological response of the body.

▶ *Learning objective:* Describe the physiological cause of steatorrhea.

18. Answer: E

Steatorrhea is a common symptom of patients who have undergone the removal of the terminal ileum, which is the principal site of bile salt absorption in men. Normally the reabsorbed bile salts recirculate to the liver to maintain the bile-acid pool. Because of this, new synthesis of bile acid is needed only to replace the small portion of bile salts lost in the feces. With ileal resection most of the bile acids secreted are not reabsorbed, and the liver pool is significantly diminished. Bile acids are needed for micelle formation in the intestinal lumen to solubilize products of lipid digestion so that they can be absorbed. The excessive loss of bile salts causes a lack of micelle formation, which in turn prevents the absorption of the product of lipid digestion, causing steatorrhea.

A Increased liver bile acid pool would decrease, not increase, steatorrhea.

B Gastrin is a peptide hormone that stimulates secretion of gastric acid by the parietal cells of the stomach. It does not affect lipid absorption.

C Pancreatic lipase is an enzyme secreted from the pancreas that hydrolyzes (breaks down) dietary fat molecules. Increased availability of this enzyme would favor, not hinder, lipid absorption.

D Increased chylomicron formation in the intestinal lumen would favor, not hinder, lipid absorption.

▶ *Learning objective:* Describe the molecular mechanism of action of natalizumab.

19. Answer: B

Natalizumab is a monoclonal antibody that blocks leukocyte migration from the blood vessels to sites of inflammation by inhibiting the action of cell adhesion molecules called integrins. Cell adhesion molecules represent a heterogeneous group of transmembrane molecules expressed on numerous cell types, including endothelial cells and leukocytes. Cell adhesion molecules promote the transmigration of leukocytes across the endothelial cell. The particular adhesion molecule targeted by natalizumab is α4 integrin, which is expressed on all circulating leukocytes except neutrophils. Natalizumab is effective in increasing rates of remission and maintaining symptom-free status in patients with CD. Natalizumab may be appropriate in patients who failed other forms of therapy, as in the present case. Unfortunately the drug can cause, in about 0.4% of patients, a progressive multifocal leukoencephalopathy, a demyelinating disease of the central nervous system that occurs almost exclusively in immunosuppressed individuals and is fatal in most cases. Because of this, the drug is approved only through a carefully restricted program. Approximately 50% of patients respond to initial therapy with natalizumab.

A TNF-α is blocked by several antibodies used as immunosuppressive agents.

C IL-2 receptors are blocked by daclizumab, a monoclonal antibody used to prevent rejection in renal transplant patients.

D Epidermal growth factor receptors are blocked by trastuzumab, a monoclonal antibody used to treat breast cancer.

E Vascular endothelial growth factor is blocked by bevacizumab, a monoclonal antibody used to treat lung and colon cancers.

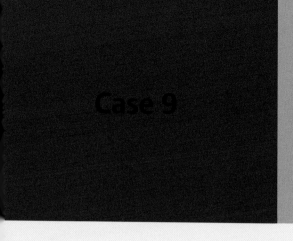

Case 9

Chronic Kidney Disease

M.N., a 45-year-old man, presented to his physician because he noticed that his urine was cloudy and red. He stated that urination was otherwise normal, without burning sensation or pain. He also denied any abrupt sensation that urination was imminent, but he recently noticed he started voiding several times during the night. M.N. stated he had been experiencing diminished appetite and easy fatigability for the past 2 months, and he had also been complaining of some flank and abdominal pain for the last 3 weeks.

Medical history of the patient indicated that 3 years ago he suffered from renal colic due to a small calculus obstructing the ureter. At that time a radiograph disclosed two small cysts in the right kidney. The patient had been suffering from tension headaches from time to time and was taking, episodically, different nonsteroidal anti-inflammatory drugs (NSAIDs) to relieve the pain. M.N.'s father died at age 62 from kidney failure. A sister, aged 47, is living and well. A brother died at age 52 from kidney failure. M.N. reported occasional alcohol consumption on weekends. He did not smoke and denied illicit drug use.

M.N. was admitted to the hospital for further investigation and treatment. Physical examination on admission showed a well-developed and nourished white male (weight 72 kg) who looked his age and was in no acute distress. Vital signs were as follows: blood pressure 158/92 mm Hg, heart rate 76 bpm, respirations 12/min and regular. Pain was elicited by a brisk percussion on the costovertebral angles of both sides, just below the 12th rib. The prostate appeared normal on rectal examination.

Pertinent laboratory results on admission were as follows:

Blood hematology

- ▶ Red blood cell count (RBC): $3.1 \times 10^6/\mu L$ (normal 4.0–6.0)
- ▶ Hemoglobin (Hgb): 9 g/dL (normal 12–16)
- ▶ Hematocrit (Hct): 25% (normal 36–48)
- ▶ White blood cell count (WBC): $8 \times 10^3/\mu L$ (normal 4–10)
- ▶ Platelet: $220 \times 10^3/\mu L$ (normal 130–400)

Blood chemistry

- ▶ pH: 7.30
- ▶ PCO_2 26 mm Hg (normal 33–45)
- ▶ Bicarbonate 15 mEq/L (normal 22–28)
- ▶ Serum creatinine (SCr): 4 mg/dL (normal 0.6–1.2)
- ▶ Blood urea nitrogen (BUN): 40 mg/dL (normal 8–25)
- ▶ Uric acid: 11 mg/dL (normal 4–8.5)
- ▶ Sodium: 138 mEq/L (normal 135–146)
- ▶ Potassium: 6.8 mEq/L (normal 3.6–5.3)
- ▶ Calcium: 5.5 mg/dL (normal 8.5–10.5)
- ▶ Phosphate: 5.9 mg/dL (normal 2.8–4.5)

- Magnesium: 3.1 mEq/L (normal 1.5–2.4)
- Total cholesterol: 170 mg/dL (normal < 200)
- Low-density lipoprotein (LDL) 90 mg/dL (normal < 100)
- High-density lipoprotein (HDL) 45 mg/dL (normal > 40)
- Triglycerides: 120 mg/dL (normal < 150)

Urinalysis (24-hour urine collection)

- Total urine volume: 2.8 L. Appearance: cloudy, red.
- Osmolality: 300 mOsm/kg
- pH: 7.1
- Proteinuria: +++
- Hematuria: ++++
- Glucose: negative
- Ketones: negative
- Bilirubin: negative
- Nitrite: negative
- WBC: 15/HPF (high power field) (normal < 5)
- Eosinophils: absent
- RBC: 100/HPF (high power field) (normal < 3)
- Sediment: several double refractile lipid bodies, no bacteria.

A diagnosis of chronic kidney disease/failure (CKD) was made, and M.N. underwent further exams to clarify the cause of his disease. These exams provided the following additional information:

Electrocardiography

Prolonged PR interval, widened QRS complex, peaked T wave

Renal ultrasonography

The left kidney was enlarged, with two cysts of about 2.5 cm. The right kidney was enlarged with multiple small cysts scattered throughout the cortex and the medulla.

Computed tomographic scan

The renal computed tomogram was in agreement with the renal ultrasonogram. The liver tomogram disclosed some small cysts disseminated throughout the parenchyma.

From the patient's history and examination, a final diagnosis was made and an appropriate therapy was implemented. M.N. received intravenous (IV) calcium gluconate and then was treated with a combination of insulin-dextrose and albuterol to rapidly reduce serum potassium levels. The insulin-dextrose therapy was repeated, and 3 days later, the serum K^+ level was 5.1. One week later, M.N. was discharged from the hospital with a postdischarge therapy directed to

- control the high blood pressure
- treat the anemia
- correct the hyperphosphatemia
- manage the secondary hyperparathyroidism
- avoid nephrotoxic drugs such as NSAIDs

Questions

1. M.N. was diagnosed with CKD. Which of the following pairs of serum values are the best indicators of his disease?

A. BUN and potassium

B. Potassium and calcium

C. Creatinine and BUN

D. Calcium and creatinine

E. Potassium and creatinine

F. BUN and calcium

2. Which of the following would be the most likely range of M.N.'s estimated GFR (in mL/min)?

A. 10–15

B. 20–30

C. 40–50

D. 60–70

E. 80–90

F. 100–120

3. Chronic kidney disease (CKD) is usually classified in stages, according to the value of GFR. M.N.'s kidney disease most likely belongs to which of the following stages?

A. Stage 1

B. Stage 2

C. Stage 3

D. Stage 4

E. Stage 5

4. M.N. noticed that he started voiding several times during the night. The patient's measured daily urine output was 2.8 L. Which of the following phrases best explains a primary reason for the patient's polyuria?

A. Decreased GFR

B. Increased Na^+ reabsorption by the proximal tubule

C. Increased K^+ reabsorption by the collecting tubule

D. Increased Mg^{2+} reabsorption by the thick ascending limb of Henle

E. Loss of kidney concentrating ability

5. M.N. was found to have serum pH of 7.30. Which of the following would be most likely the acid–base disorder of this patient?

A. Respiratory acidosis

B. Respiratory alkalosis

C. Metabolic acidosis

D. Metabolic alkalosis

E. Mixed acidosis

6. M.N. was found to have serum pH of 7.30. The impairment of which of the following kidney functions is the primary reason for the patient's acid–base disorder?

A. Increased phosphoric acid excretion

B. Decreased ammonia secretion

C. Increased tubular K^+ excretion

D. Decreased renal synthesis of calcitriol

7. M.N. was found to have serum K^+ of 6.7 mEq/L and serum magnesium of 3.1 mEq/L. Which of the following phrases best explains the main reason for the patient's hyperkalemia and hypermagnesemia?

A. Decreased aldosterone secretion

B. Increased flow rate in the collecting tubule

C. More negative electrical potential in the collecting tubule

D. Critical reduction in GFR

E. Increased dietary K^+ intake

8. M.N. received calcium gluconate IV. Which of the following statements best explains the primary reason for this therapy?

A. To speed up K^+ elimination by the kidney

B. To increase K^+ entry into cells

C. To counteract K^+-induced cardiac toxicity

D. To offset the secondary hyperaldosteronism

E. To counteract K^+-induced skeletal muscle toxicity

9. M.N. received insulin and albuterol to rapidly reduce the serum K^+ level. Which of the following is the most likely molecular mechanism of both drugs leading to this reduction?

A. Increased K^+ excretion by the kidney

B. Decreased K^+ entry into cells

C. Decreased intestinal K^+ absorption

D. Decreased secondary hyperaldosteronism

E. Increased Na^+/K^+ adenosine triphosphatase (ATPase) activity

10. M.N. was found to have serum phosphate of 5.9 mg/dL. Which of the following phrases best explains the main reason for the patient's hyperphosphatemia?

A. Low parathyroid hormone (PTH) serum level

B. Hypocalcemia

C. Decreased GFR

D. Hyperkalemia

E. High dietary phosphate intake

11. M.N. was found to have serum calcium of 5.5 mg/dL. Which of the following represents a main cause of the patient's hypocalcemia?

A. Hyperkalemia

B. Hyperphosphatemia

C. Increased calcitriol synthesis

D. Hypermagnesemia

E. Low PTH serum level

12. Which of the following was the most likely cause of the M.N.'s hematuria?

A. Nephritic syndrome

B. Kidney cancer

C. Benign prostatic hyperplasia

D. Bladder cancer

E. Nephrolithiasis

F. Urinary tract infection

G. Polycystic kidney disease (PKD)

13. The treatment of M.N.'s disease included a tight control of his high blood pressure. Which of the following pairs of antihypertensive drugs would be appropriate for the control of blood pressure in this patient?

A. Propranolol and fenoldopam

B. Propranolol and losartan

C. Propranolol and hydrochlorothiazide

D. Losartan and fenoldopam

E. Losartan and hydrochlorothiazide

F. Fenoldopam and hydrochlorothiazide

14. The treatment of M.N.'s disease included treatment of his anemia. Which of the following pairs of drugs would be appropriate for this patient?

A. Erythropoietin and folic acid

B. Iron and cyanocobalamin

C. Folic acid and cyanocobalamin

D. Iron and erythropoietin

E. Iron and folic acid

F. Erythropoietin and cyanocobalamin

15. The treatment of M.N.'s disease included the correction of his hyperphosphatemia. Which of the following drugs would be appropriate for this purpose?

A. Prednisone

B. Cholestyramine

C. Sevelamer

D. Cholecalciferol (vitamin D_3)

E. Teriparatide

16. M.N. was instructed to avoid nephrotoxic drugs, such as NSAIDs. This toxicity is primarily due to the impairment of renal synthesis of which of the following pairs of endogenous compounds?

A. Prostaglandin E_2–leukotriene B_4

B. Prostaglandin E_2–bradykinin

C. Prostaglandin E_2–prostacyclin

D. Leukotriene B_4–bradykinin

E. Leukotriene B_4–prostacyclin

F. Prostacyclin–bradykinin

Answers and Explanations

▶ *Learning objective:* Identify the two lab tests that best indicate CKD.

1. Answer: C

Patients with CKD are often asymptomatic, and renal dysfunction can be detected only by laboratory testing. M.N.'s abnormal values for SCr and BUN, as well as hyperkalemia and hypocalcemia, hyperphosphatemia, and hypermagnesemia are all consistent with CKD. However, SCr is the primary marker for renal function. Creatinine is derived from creatine and phosphocreatine, major constituents of muscle. Once creatinine is released from muscle into plasma, it is excreted almost exclusively by glomerular filtration and a decrease in glomerular filtration rate (GFR) results in an increase of SCr.

BUN measures the nitrogen portion of urea. Urea forms in the liver and constitutes the final product of protein metabolism. Urea is excreted by the kidney, and a markedly increased BUN can indicate an impaired renal function.

SCr and BUN levels, when considered together, are reliable indicators of renal failure.

A, F BUN alone is not an indicator of CKD because BUN may be normal with as much as 50% reduction in the GFR. Moreover, BUN may be elevated not only by renal disease but also by extrarenal disorders.

A, B, E Potassium is not a good test for detecting early renal dysfunction. Hyperkalemia is usually present in later stages of CKD but can be found in many other extrarenal disorders.

B, D, F Hyperparathyroidism is one of the pathological manifestations of CKD but can be found in other extrarenal disorders.

▶ *Learning objective:* Calculate the GFR of a patient, given sufficient data.

2. Answer: B

Because creatinine is cleared almost exclusively by glomerular filtration, creatinine clearance (CrCL) can be used as a clinically useful measure of a patient's GFR. Several formulas have been proposed to estimate CrCL from SCr. A commonly used formula is that of Cockcroft and Gault. For adult males the formula is as follows:

$$CrCL = (140 - age)\ by\ body\ weight\ (in\ kg) / SCr\ (72)$$

In the present case

$$CrCL = (140 - 45) \times 72\ /\ (4 \times 72)$$
$$= 23.75\ mL/min$$

A, C, D, E, F See correct answer explanation.

▶ *Learning objective:* Estimate the stage of CKD from the value of GFR.

3. Answer: D

The stages of CKD are mainly based on estimated GFR. There are five stages classified as follows:

▶ Stage 1: GFR ≥ 90 mL/min: kidney function is normal, but urine findings or structural abnormalities or genetic traits point to kidney disease.

▶ Stage 2: GFR 60 to 89 mL/min: mildly reduced kidney function and other findings (as for stage 1) point to kidney disease.

▶ Stage 3: GFR 30 to 59 mL/min: moderately reduced kidney function.

▶ Stage 4: GFR 15 to 29 mL/min: severely reduced kidney function.

▶ Stage 5: GFR < 15 mL/min: end-stage kidney failure.

Because the estimated GFR of M.N. is 23.75, he can be classified as having stage 4 kidney disease.

A, B, C, E See correct answer explanation.

▶ *Learning objective:* Explain the reason of initial polyuria in a patient with CKD.

4. Answer: E

In general, with the progression of CKD, the urine output will decline gradually. However, in several cases, the patients may experience polyuria for a period. This polyuria seems primarily related to loss of kidney concentrating ability.

CKD results from irreversible loss of a large number of functioning nephrons. Decreased renal function interferes with the kidneys' ability to maintain fluid and electrolyte homeostasis. The ability to concentrate the urine declines early and causes obligatory polyuria, which is mainly related to the decrease of tubule function. The kidney tubule reabsorbs normally about 99% of the filtered fluid. In the present patient the GFR is about 23 mL/min, which means 33.1 L/d. If the tubular function were normal the kidney would excrete only 1/100 of that filtrate, namely 331 mL of urine daily. However, if the concentrating ability of the kidney is decreased because of loss of nephrons, less water will be reabsorbed in the thin descending limb of Henle's loop, and this explains why polyuria can occur when there is a significant decrease in kidney concentrating ability.

A, B, C, D In all these cases oliguria, not polyuria, would be present.

▶ *Learning objective:* Identify the reason for the acid–base disorder in CKD.

5. Answer: C

The patient has low pH, low PCO_2, and low bicarbonate. This pattern indicates that the acid–base disorder is metabolic acidosis.

A Respiratory acidosis would have low pH, high PCO_2, and high bicarbonate.

B Respiratory alkalosis would have high pH, low PCO_2, and low bicarbonate.

D Metabolic alkalosis would have high pH, high PCO_2, and high bicarbonate.

E Mixed acidosis would have low pH, high PCO_2, and low bicarbonate.

▶ *Learning objective:* Explain the primary reason for low serum pH in patients with CKD.

6. Answer: B

Metabolic acidosis is commonly associated with CKD. As the number of functioning nephrons declines in CKD, acid excretion is initially maintained by an increase in the ammonia secreted per nephron. However, total ammonium excretion begins to fall when the GFR is below 40 to 50 mL/min. At this level of renal function, ammonia secre-

tion per total GFR is three to four times above normal, suggesting that the impairment in ammonia secretion is caused by too few functioning nephrons rather than impaired function in the remaining nephrons.

As a result, CKD leads to retention of hydrogen ions.

A In addition to the fall in ammonium excretion, there is a diminished, not increased, excretion of titratable acids (primarily as phosphoric acid). This decrease may also play a role in the pathogenesis of metabolic acidosis in patients with advanced kidney disease.

C In CKD, tubular excretion of K^+ is decreased, not increased, due to loss of nephrons. Moreover, hypokalemia would cause metabolic alkalosis, not acidosis.

D In CKD there is decreased renal synthesis of calcitriol, which in turn can cause hypocalcemia. However, hypocalcemia is usually associated with alkalosis, not acidosis.

▶ *Learning objective:* Explain the causes of hyperkalemia and hypermagnesemia in CKD.

7. Answer: D

In the kidney potassium excretion is determined by the sum of three processes:

▶ The rate of potassium filtration
▶ The rate of potassium reabsorption by the proximal tubule (about 65%) and by the loop of Henle (about 25%)
▶ The rate of potassium secretion by the distal and collecting tubules. Changes in potassium secretion in these sites account for most of the daily variation in potassium excretion.

In renal failure patients generally maintain potassium balance within normal limits until GFR decreases to less than 25% of normal value. This is called potassium adaptation. Mechanisms involved in this process include

▶ Increased aldosterone levels
▶ Polyuria, which promotes higher distal tubule flow rates
▶ A more negative luminal electrical potential caused by the increased

concentration of phosphate and sulfate, two highly impermeable anions

Impairment of these adaptive mechanisms and a critical reduction in GFR can lead to progressive hyperkalemia.

The kidney closely regulates magnesium excretion by changing tubular reabsorption. When the GFR is substantially reduced, the amount of filtered magnesium is low, and all magnesium is reabsorbed, leading to hypermagnesemia. Moreover, decreased extracellular fluid calcium concentration leads to a decrease in magnesium excretion.

A In CKD there is almost always a secondary hyperaldosteronism.

B, **C** These two actions would cause an increase, not a decrease, of K+ excretion.

E An increased dietary K^+ intake can contribute to a high serum potassium level in a patient with CKD, but it is not the main cause of hyperkalemia. Moreover, there is no evidence of an increased intake in the patient's history.

▶ *Learning objective:* Explain the reason for calcium administration in a patient with hyperkalemia and significant electrocardiographic (ECG) abnormalities.

8. Answer: C

Hyperkalemia with ECG changes, as in the present case, requires urgent treatment. Three therapeutic modalities are available (in descending order):

▶ Drugs that antagonize the cardiac effects of hyperkalemia (calcium salts)
▶ Drugs that shift potassium from the extracellular to the intracellular space (insulin and $β_2$-agonists)
▶ Drugs or procedures that enhance potassium elimination (sodium polystyrene, loop or thiazide diuretics, hemodialysis)

Calcium antagonizes the cardiotoxicity of hyperkalemia by stabilizing the cardiac cell membrane against undesirable depolarization. Onset of effect is rapid ($≤ 15$ minutes) but relatively short-lived. This agent is the first-line treatment for severe hyperkalemia, when the ECG shows significant abnormalities, as in the present case.

A, **B** Calcium has no effect on the serum level of potassium. It does not speed up K^+ elimination by the kidney and does not increase K^+ entry into cells. For that reason, administration of calcium is usually accompanied by other therapies that actually help lower serum potassium levels.

D, **E** Calcium administration can have these effects, but they are not the primary reason for administering calcium IV to M.N.

▶ *Learning objective:* Explain the mechanism of insulin and albuterol in the treatment of hyperkalemia.

9. Answer: E

Insulin-dextrose IV and albuterol (often by nebulization) are sometimes used together to treat hyperkalemia because they have an additive effect. Both drugs act to increase K^+ entry into cells by increasing Na^+/K^+ ATPase activity. In addition, $β_2$-adrenoceptor activation in skeletal muscle also activates the inwardly directed $Na^+/K^+/2 Cl^-$ cotransporter, which may account for as much as one-third of the uptake response. The albuterol dose for treating hyperkalemia (10 mg) is substantially higher than the usual dose for the treatment of bronchospasm, and the use of β-adrenergic agonists remains somewhat controversial, in spite of their effectiveness.

A Increased K^+ excretion by the kidney is an action of many diuretics, including thiazides and loop diuretics.

B Both insulin and albuterol increase, not decrease, K^+ entry into cells.

C Intestinal K^+ absorption is not affected by insulin or albuterol.

D Secondary hyperaldosteronism occurs in chronic renal failure, but insulin and albuterol do not affect this disorder.

▶ *Learning objective:* Explain the primary cause of hyperphosphatemia in chronic kidney disease.

10. Answer: C

The renal tubules have a normal "transport maximum" for reabsorbing phosphate, and when more than this maximum is present in the glomerular filtrate, the excess is excreted.

In CKD, the smaller population of surviving nephrons leads to a reduction of GFR, which in turn decreases the amount of filtered phosphate. Initially, the consequent small increase in serum phosphate leads to a reciprocal small decrease in serum ionized calcium concentration, which in turn stimulates PTH secretion (secondary hyperparathyroidism). PTH diminishes fractional phosphate reabsorption by the kidney, lowering the elevated serum phosphate to its initial level. When GFR is < 30 mL/min, PTH fails to achieve its effect because of the critically low number of surviving nephrons, and hyperphosphatemia develops.

A In CKD, the PTH serum level is high, not low.

B Hypocalcemia is a consequence, not a cause, of hyperphosphatemia.

D Potassium turnover does not affect serum phosphate level.

E High dietary phosphate intake decreases, not increases, phosphate reabsorption.

▶ *Learning objective:* Explain the causes of hypocalcemia in CKD.

11.   Answer: B

In CKD hypocalcemia occurs mainly because of the following:

▶ Hyperphosphatemia decreases ionized calcium concentration because calcium phosphate salts are deposited in several body tissues. PTH, the secretion of which is stimulated by hypocalcemia, can initially restore normal calcium concentration. However, when the number of surviving nephrons is very low, hyperphosphatemia ensues and calcium phosphate salts are deposited in tissues, furthering the development of secondary hyperparathyroidism.

▶ Reduced nephron mass decreases the renal biosynthetic capacity, leading to a decreased synthesis of calcitriol ($1,25(OH)^2$). Because calcitriol augments intestinal calcium

absorption, low serum calcitriol level can cause hypocalcemia.

A, D Potassium and magnesium turnover does not affect serum calcium level.

C In CKD calcitriol synthesis is decreased, not increased.

E In CKD the PTH serum level is high, not low.

▶ *Learning objective:* Identify the disorder that most likely caused hematuria in a patient with CKD.

12.   Answer: G

Several pieces of evidence point out that the patient's hematuria was most likely due to a ruptured cyst of the patient's polycystic kidney.

PKD is a systemic hereditary disorder transmitted most frequently by an autosomal dominant gene (ADPKD). It is characterized by renal cysts that reduce functional renal tissue, commonly by hepatic cysts, and less frequently by malformation of selected vasculature. The incidence of the disease is 1:200 to 1:1000, which makes it the most common hereditary disorder in the United States. Clinical onset of ADPKD is in early or middle adult life, and the disease progresses to end-stage renal failure over a period of many decades in approximately 50% of the affected persons.

The evidence indicating that the patient's disease was most likely ADPKD includes the following factors:

▶ The family history, which is invaluable in the diagnosis of ADPKD. In the present case direct information is lacking, but the father and a brother died of kidney failure. In both cases the failure could be due to an undiagnosed or unreported ADPKD.

▶ The cysts, which were detected on imaging studies.

▶ The kidney failure, which develops in about 40% of patients as the disease progresses.

▶ The hematuria, which occurs in 30 to 50% of patients with ADPKD.

▶ The flank and back pain, which is the most common complaint (~ 50%) in patients with symptomatic ADPKD.

The mechanism of pain has not been defined but is likely related to the stretching of the pain-sensitive renal capsule.

▶ The double refractory lipid bodies, which may originate in cysts and are found in the urine of 60% of patients with ADPKD. While hematuria and proteinuria are nonspecific signs, double refractory lipid bodies are highly indicative of a cystic disease of the kidney.

A, B, C, D All these diseases can cause hematuria, but the patient has no symptoms suggesting any of these disorders.

E Nephrolithiasis can cause hematuria, but the patient history of a single episode of renal colic due to a kidney stone makes this diagnosis quite unlikely.

F Urinary infection can cause hematuria, but the patient has no bacteria in the urine.

▶ *Learning objective:* Identify the appropriate pair of drugs for the treatment of hypertension in a patient with CKD.

13. Answer: E

Mild to moderate hypertension is the most common abnormality identified in the physical examination of ADPKD patients. It has been consistently shown that lowering systolic blood pressure to levels below 130 mm Hg among CKD patients with high proteinuria can significantly slow the progression of the disease. Angiotensin-converting enzyme (ACE) inhibitors or angiotensin blockers, such as losartan, have demonstrated favorable effects in slowing the progression of renal disease in both diabetic and nondiabetic patients. The combination with a thiazide diuretic increases the antihypertensive effect of these agents and counteracts the potential hyperkalemia that can occur when agents interfering with the angiotensin system are given alone. Therefore, these agents are given usually with a thiazide diuretic, as in the present case.

A, D, F Fenoldopam is a dopamine D_1-antagonist used only in hypertensive emergencies.

B, C Nonselective β-blockers (e.g., propranolol) are no longer first-line agents for the treatment of hypertension because it has been shown that they are inferior to renin-angiotensin inhibitors and are less well tolerated. Moreover they can worsen hyperkalemia by blocking β_2-induced K^+ entry into cells.

▶ *Learning objective:* Identify the appropriate pairs of drug for the treatment of anemia in a patient with CKD.

14. Answer: D

Anemia is a common feature in many patients with CKD. The anemia is hypoproliferative, normocytic, and normochromic and is due primarily to reduced production of erythropoietin by the kidney (a presumed reflection of the reduction in functioning renal mass). Anemia due to renal dysfunction generally develops when the GFR declines to < 30 mL/min, as in the present case. The anemia slowly responds to erythropoietin, which remains the treatment of choice. Patients with CKD are commonly iron deficient, and adequate iron stores are essential for achieving maximum benefit from erythropoietin administration. Therefore, iron supplementation is usually given prior to initiation of erythropoietin treatment.

A, B, C, E, F Drugs such as folic acid and cyanocobalamin are given in case of megaloblastic anemias that are rare in chronic kidney disease.

▶ *Learning objective:* Identify the appropriate drug for the control of hyperphosphatemia in CKD.

15. Answer: C

Hyperphosphatemia in CKD must be treated; it has been shown that a normal serum phosphate level significantly decreases mortality among CKD patients. Sevelamer is a phosphate binder. It binds dietary phosphate within the gastrointestinal tract. Amine groups in the sevelamer molecule cross-link with phosphate in the gut, thereby preventing phosphate absorption. When taken with meals, sevelamer lowers both serum phosphate and PTH. The drug is used for the management of hyperphosphatemia in patients with stage 4 to 5 CKD. Because the drug is not absorbed, adverse effects are limited to the gut (nausea, dyspepsia, diarrhea, abdominal pain).

A Glucocorticoids tend to decrease the calcium serum level. Therefore, they are contraindicated in this patient because he already has hypocalcemia.

B Cholestyramine is a bile acid binder, not a phosphate binder.

D Cholecalciferol (vitamin D_3) is commonly given to patients with CKD to correct hypocalcemia. However, the drug would increase intestinal phosphate absorption and therefore is not the best drug to manage hyperphosphatemia.

E Teriparatide is a recombinant PTH. In the normal person PTH can decrease serum phosphate, but in severe CKD hyperphosphatemia is related to the critically low number of surviving nephrons and PTH does not work.

▶ *Learning objective:* Identify the pairs of endogenous compounds whose renal synthesis was inhibited by NSAIDs, thereby causing renal toxicity.

16.   Answer: C

The major renal eicosanoid products are prostaglandin E_2 and prostacyclin. Prostaglandins play important roles in maintaining normal renal function through their local vasodilating effects, particularly in marginally functioning kidneys. This prostaglandin-mediated renal blood flow in turn maintains GFR, inhibits tubular Na^+ reabsorption, and favors Na^+ excretion in the collecting ducts. All these functions can be decreased by drugs that inhibit prostaglandin biosynthesis, such as NSAIDs. The renal toxicity of these drugs is negligible in a normal person (unless huge doses are given) but can be quite important for patients with CKD.

A, **D**, **E** Leukotriene synthesis is not affected by NSAIDs.

B, **D**, **F** Bradykinin synthesis is not affected by NSAIDs.

Chronic Obstructive Pulmonary Disease

Q.R., a 52-year-old woman, was admitted to the hospital with a chief complaint of worsening of her chronic productive cough and increasing shortness of breath, especially with exertion. She stated she typically awakened each morning with a cough that lasted about 1 hour and that she was not able to walk up a flight of stairs without dyspnea. She described her symptoms as very disturbing and interfering with her ability to work around the house.

Q.R. had a smoking history of one pack of cigarettes per day since age 18. She quit smoking 1 year ago when she was diagnosed with chronic obstructive pulmonary disease (COPD). She had been taking inhaled albuterol as needed since that time, and the therapy was well tolerated, although she sometimes had an annoying hand tremor. Her other medical problem was a 9-year history of hypertension, presently treated with hydrochlorothiazide and losartan.

The patient's vital signs on admission were as follows: blood pressure 138/85, pulse 85 bpm, respirations 26/min. Physical examination showed a patient in no apparent distress. The lungs were hyperexpanded on percussion, and auscultation revealed scattered rhonchi throughout both lung fields and diffuse wheezing.

Pertinent laboratory results on admission were as follows:

Chest radiography

Slightly enlarged cardiac shadow, thickened bronchial wall, and multiple avascular zones surrounded by thin wall.

Spirometry

Forced expiratory volume in the first second of expiration (FEV_1) was 65% predicted.

Sputum Gram's stain

Numerous polymorphonuclear leukocytes and mixed bacterial flora

From the results of the physical examination and laboratory tests it was concluded that Q.R.'s COPD was significantly worsened and that a change in therapy was needed. The patient was instructed to maintain inhaled albuterol as needed and to add inhaled ipratropium daily.

Q.R. followed the therapy carefully and her chronic cough and dyspnea lessened significantly. She seemed to do reasonably well for 2 years. However, during the last 2 months she noticed increasing dyspnea and productive cough and was readmitted to the hospital for evaluation.

Q.R.'s vital signs on admission were as follows: blood pressure 175/95, pulse 85 bpm, respiration 28 breaths/min. Physical examination showed a patient in obvious respiratory distress with a barrel chest and the use of accessory muscles and retraction. Spirometry yielded an FEV_1 of 48% predicted. Lab exams on admission also included serum pH, PaO_2, $PaCO_2$, and SaO_2.

The patient was hospitalized for 7 days. During that time she received oxygen therapy, nebulized bronchodilator therapy, and systemic glucocorticoids. She was discharged from the hospital with the following postdischarge therapy: albuterol inhalations as needed, salmeterol two inhalations daily, ipratropium three inhalations daily, and oral sustained-release theophylline two tablets daily. Her antihypertensive therapy was changed by adding nifedipine to her previous regimen.

Questions

1. Q.R. had been suffering from COPD. Which of the following pairs of respiratory disorders were most likely present in the patient's disease?

A. Chronic bronchitis–bronchiectasis

B. Chronic bronchitis–lung abscess

C. Lung abscess–emphysema

D. Bronchiectasis–lung abscess

E. Chronic bronchitis–emphysema

F. Bronchiectasis–emphysema

2. Q.R.'s lung auscultation found diffuse wheezes. Which of the following is most likely the primary cause of these high-pitched whistling noises?

A. Decreased bronchial secretion

B. Decreased bronchial blood flow

C. Turbulent airflow through small airways

D. Turbulent airflow through larynx

E. Increased mucociliary clearance

F. Decreased mucociliary clearance

3. COPD is an obstructive lung disorder. Which of the following variations in lung volumes and capacities can be most likely expected in patients suffering from COPD?

A. Decreased total lung capacity (TLC)

B. Increased peak expiratory flow (PEF)

C. Increased forced vital capacity (FVC)

D. Decreased residual volume (RV)

E. Decreased FEV_1

4. Spirometry is the gold standard diagnostic test for COPD. The decrease of which of the following pairs of spirometry values is most indicative of the severity of this disease?

A. FEV_1–FEV_1:FVC ratio

B. FEV_1–TLC

C. TLC–FEV_1:FVC ratio

D. RV–TLC

E. RV–FEV_1:FVC ratio

F. RV–FEV_1

5. In COPD, inhalational exposures can trigger an inflammatory response in airways and alveoli that can lead to disease in genetically susceptible people. The increased activity of which of the following lung enzymes most likely contributed to Q.R.'s disease?

A. α_1-antitrypsin

B. Peptidase inhibitor 3

C. Monooxygenases

D. Dihydrofolate reductase

E. Neutrophil elastase

6. Q.R. had occasional hand tremor during albuterol treatment. Which of the following molecular actions most likely mediated this adverse effect?

A. Increased K^+ exit from cells

B. Increased sequestration of cytosolic Ca^{2+}

C. Decreased activity of Ca^{2+}/Na^+ exchanger

D. Decreased availability of cyclic adenosine monophosphate (cAMP)

E. Inhibition of adenylyl cyclase

7. Q.R.'s antihypertensive therapy included oral losartan. Which of the following molecular actions most likely mediated the therapeutic effect of the drug in the patient's disease?

A. Blockade of angiotensin-converting enzyme (ACE)

B. Release of nitric oxide from endothelial vascular cells

C. Activation of D_1-receptors in the mesenteric vascular bed

D. Blockade of vasopressin V_1-receptors all over the body

E. Blockade of angiotensin II receptors all over the body

F. Blockade of Ca^{2+} channels in vascular smooth muscle

8. Inhaled ipratropium was prescribed to Q.R. The beneficial effect of the drug is likely mediated by the blockade of which pairs of receptors in the bronchial tree?

A. Histaminergic H_1–nicotinic neuronal (Nn)

B. Histaminergic H_1–muscarinic M_3

C. Histaminergic H_1–adrenergic α_1

D. Nicotinic neuronal (Nn)–muscarinic M_3

E. Nicotinic neuronal (Nn)–adrenergic α_1

F. Muscarinic M_3–adrenergic α_1

9. Which of the following adverse effects was Q.R. most likely to suffer from ipratropium treatment?

A. Constipation

B. Tremor

C. Xerostomia

D. Urinary retention

E. Insomnia

F. Palpitations

10. When readmitted to the hospital, Q.R. underwent several lab tests. Which of the following sets of blood test results shown in the attached table was most likely found at that time?

Set	pH	PaO_2	$PaCO_2$	SaO_2
A.	↓	↑	↑	↑
B.	↓	↓	↑	↓
C.	↑	↑	↓	↓
D.	↑	↑	↑	↑
E.	↓	↓	↑	↑

PaO_2: Arterial oxygen tension

$PaCO_2$: Arterial carbon dioxide tension

SaO_2: Arterial oxygen saturation

↑ increased, ↓ decreased

11. The postdischarge therapy for Q.R. included the concurrent administration of salmeterol and ipratropium. Which of the following statements best explains the primary reason for this combined treatment?

A. Ipratropium increases salmeterol bioavailability.

B. Ipratropium increases salmeterol half-life.

C. Ipratropium counteracts salmeterol-induced headache.

D. Salmeterol and ipratropium can have synergistic effects.

E. Salmeterol counteracts ipratropium-induced xerostomia.

F. Salmeterol decreases ipratropium metabolism.

12. Theophylline was prescribed to Q.R. Which of the following is a proposed mechanism for the bronchodilating action of theophylline?

A. Inhibition of phosphodiesterase enzyme

B. Activation of cell surface receptors for adenosine

C. Inhibition of catecholamine release from adrenergic terminals

D. Stimulation of nitric oxide release from vascular endothelium

E. Activation of α_2-receptors in bronchial smooth muscle

13. Which of the following actions most likely occurred during the first days of the-ophylline therapy?

A. Decreased cardiac contractility

B. Dilatation of cerebral blood vessels

C. Decreased diuresis

D. Increased gastric secretion

E. Depression of the respiratory center

14. Q.R.'s postdischarge therapy included diltiazem. Which of the following actions most likely mediated the antihypertensive effect of the drug in the patient's disease?

A. Arterial vasodilation

B. Venous vasodilation

C. Decreased cardiac output

D. Decreased central adrenergic tone

E. Inhibition of angiotensin II biosynthesis

Answers and Explanations

▶ *Learning objective:* Identify the two respiratory disorders that are most frequently associated with COPD.

1.   Answer: E

COPD is an intentionally imprecise term used to denote a partially reversible air flow limitation caused by a bronchial inflammatory response to inhaled toxins, most often cigarette smoke.

The disease most often combines

▶ **chronic bronchitis:** clinically defined as a chronic cough for at least 3 months for 2 consecutive years.

▶ **emphysema:** pathologically defined as alveolar wall destruction leading to loss of elastic recoil and airspace enlargement.

Q.R. has features of both disorders (see the patient's symptoms and the X-ray result).

A, B, C, D, F Bronchiectasis and lung abscess can occur in COPD but are far less common than chronic bronchitis and emphysema. Bronchiectasis may indicate the presence of more advanced airway dysfunction. Lung abscess results from bacterial colonization.

▶ *Learning objective:* Explain the mechanism of the wheezing sounds that can be heard in patients suffering from COPD.

2.   Answer: C

Airflow through a narrowed segment of a small airway becomes turbulent, causing vibration of the airway walls. This vibration produces the sound of wheezing. Wheezes are more common during expiration, because the increased intrathoracic pressure during this phase narrows the small airways.

A Increased, not decreased, bronchial secretion can cause narrowing of small airways.

B Increased, not decreased, bronchial blood flow can cause narrowing of small airways.

D Turbulent flow of air through a narrowed segment of the large extrathoracic airways (epiglottis, larynx, etc.) produces a loud sound of constant pitch called stridor. This sound is predominantly inspiratory.

E, F Mucociliary clearance describes the self-clearing mechanism of the bronchi. This clearance can be severely inhibited, not increased, in COPD as a consequence of chronic inflammation, but this inhibition is not the primary cause of wheezing sounds.

▶ *Learning objective:* Identify the variations in lung volumes and capacities that can be expected in patients suffering from COPD.

3.   Answer: E

The FEV_1 is the most useful parameter in diagnosing and monitoring patients with obstructive lung disease. The amount of FEV_1 decrease is commonly used to assess the severity of obstructive lung disease.

A TLC is the amount of air in the lungs after maximum inflation. TLC is normal or most often increased, not decreased, in obstructive lung disorders.

B PEF is the highest forced respiratory flow. PEF is decreased, not increased, in obstructive lung disorders.

C FVC is the maximum amount of air forcibly expired after maximum inspiration. FVC is normal or decreased, not increased, in obstructive lung disorders.

D RV can be expressed as RV = TLC − FVC. Residual volume is increased, not decreased, in obstructive lung disorders.

▸ *Learning objective:* Identify the two spirometry values that are decreased in COPD.

4. Answer: A

Spirometry is the best laboratory test for making the diagnosis of COPD. In this disease FEV_1 is decreased, FVC is normal or decreased, and the FEV_1:FVC ratio is decreased. FEV_1 and FVC are easily measured with office spirometry. FEV_1 and the FEV_1:FVC ratio values best define the severity of the disease, because they correlate with symptoms and mortality.

B, C, D TLC is normal or increased in obstructive lung disease.

D, E, F RV is increased, not decreased, in obstructive lung disorders.

▸ *Learning objective:* Identify the lung enzyme whose activity is increased in COPD.

5. Answer: E

The inflammation of COPD is thought to be mediated by an increase in protease activity and a decrease in antiprotease activity. Lung proteases, such as neutrophil elastase, break down elastin and connective tissue in the normal process of tissue repair. Their activity is normally balanced by antiproteases (primarily α_1-antitrypsin). In patients with COPD, activated neutrophils release proteases as part of the inflammatory process. Protease activity exceeds antiprotease activity and tissue destruction results, causing emphysema.

A, B α_1-Antitrypsin and peptidase inhibitor 3 (also called elafin) are antiproteases, not proteases. Their activity is decreased, not increased, in COPD. Cigarette smoke can also inactivate endogenous antiproteases, including α_1-antitrypsin, increasing the risk of tissue damage.

C, D These enzymes are not proteases.

▸ *Learning objective:* Explain the likely mechanism of albuterol-induced tremor.

6. Answer: B

Tremor is the most frequent adverse effect of β_2-agonists (up to 40% of patients). It likely occurs because β_2-adrenoceptor activation accelerates the sequestration of cytosolic Ca^{2+} (by opening Ca^{2+} channels in the sarcoplasmic reticulum of skeletal muscle). The decreased availability of cytoplasmic Ca^{2+} cannot sustain the contraction of skeletal muscle, and tremor occurs.

A β_2-Agonists stimulate Na^+/K^+ adenosine triphosphatase (ATPase). This action facilitates K^+ entry, not exit, into cells.

C Decreased activity of the Ca^{2+}/Na^+ exchanger would increase, not decrease, the availability of cytoplasmic Ca^{2+}.

D By activating β_2-adrenoceptors, availability of cAMP is increased, not decreased.

E Adenylyl cyclase is activated, not inhibited, by albuterol.

▸ *Learning objective:* Explain the mechanism of action of losartan.

7. Answer: E

Losartan is an angiotensin II receptor blocker. These drugs are selective blockers of angiotensin II receptor 1, and the antagonism is often insurmountable. Therefore these drugs inhibit both in vitro and in vivo, most of the biological effects of angiotensin II. Angiotensin blockers seem to reduce the activity of angiotensin II receptors more effectively than do ACE inhibitors. This is likely because ACE inhibitors do not inhibit alternative, non-ACE, angiotensin II–generating pathways. Because angiotensin blockers act on receptors, the action of angiotensin II is inhibited regardless of the biochemical pathway leading to angiotensin II formation.

A Blockade of ACE would be the mechanism of action of ACE inhibitors, such as captopril.

B Release of nitric oxide from endothelial vascular cells would be the mechanism of action of several vasodilating drugs, including nitrates, nitroprusside hydralazine, and histamine.

C Activation of D_1-receptors in the mesenteric vascular bed would be the mechanism of action of fenoldopam.

D Blockade of vasopressin V_1-receptors all over the body would be the mechanism of action of a subclass of diuretic drugs named vaptans.

F Blockade of Ca^{2+} channels in vascular smooth muscle would be the mechanism of action of Ca^{2+} channel blockers, such as nifedipine.

▶ *Learning objective:* Identify the two receptors that are blocked by ipratropium.

8.   Answer: D

Ipratropium is a quaternary ammonium compound that belongs to the class of antimuscarinic drugs. Unlike tertiary amines, quaternary ammonium antimuscarinic drugs block mainly muscarinic receptors but also have significant blocking activity on nicotinic neuronal (Nn) receptors. Therefore inhaled ipratropium can block both M_3 receptors and Nn receptors located in small parasympathetic ganglia within the bronchial tree. Both actions can contribute to the final bronchodilating effect of the drug.

A, B, C Ipratropium has no effect on histaminergic H_1 receptors.

C, E, F Ipratropium has no effect on α_1-adrenoceptors.

▶ *Learning objective:* Identify the most common adverse effect of ipratropium.

9.   Answer: C

Ipratropium is given by inhalatory route as an aerosol. When a drug is given by aerosol, a significant amount of the drug is deposited on the oral mucosa, causing local effects. Dry mouth is the most common adverse effect of inhaled ipratropium. It can occur in up to 25% of patients and is most likely due to blockade of muscarinic receptors in salivary glands.

A, B, D, E, F All these are systemic adverse effects. They occur very rarely with inhaled ipratropium because the inhaled bioavailability of the drug is < 5%.

▶ *Learning objective:* Identify the blood gas test results of a patient suffering from severe COPD.

10.   Answer: B

The pronounced decrease of Q.R.'s FEV_1 found on readmission indicates an exacerbation of her disease. When COPD becomes severe, pH decreases because of respiratory acidosis, arterial oxygen tension

decreases, and arterial carbon dioxide tension increases. Oxygen saturation decreases because of emphysema, which impairs gas exchange from destruction of alveolar walls and the pulmonary capillary bed.

A, C, D, E See correct answer explanation.

▶ *Learning objective:* Explain the rationale for the use of a combination of salmeterol and ipratropium in COPD.

11.   Answer: D

Salmeterol is a long-acting β_2-agonist; ipratropium is an anticholinergic drug. It has been shown that the combination of two long-acting bronchodilators, such as salmeterol and ipratropium, provides better bronchodilation than the individual agents. It is a general rule in pharmacology that a synergism can occur when two drugs with different mechanisms of action are given concomitantly, and the current guidelines recommend combining long-acting bronchodilators with differing mechanisms of action for the control of COPD.

A, B Ipratropium does not have these effects. Moreover these effects refer to the systemic absorption of the drug that would be counterproductive during inhalational therapy, where local effects are needed.

C Headache is the most common adverse effect of salmeterol reported from clinical studies (up to 28%). However, ipratropium cannot counteract salmeterol-induced headache.

E, F Salmeterol does not have these effects.

▶ *Learning objective:* Describe a proposed mechanism of the bronchodilating action of theophylline.

12.   Answer: A

Theophylline is a methylxanthine. All drugs of this class have bronchodilating activity, albeit less pronounced than that of the $\beta2$-agonists or anticholinergic agents. The molecular basis for this action is still uncertain, but the two main proposed mechanisms are as follows:

1. Nonspecific inhibition of phosphodiesterase enzymes.

Inhibition of phosphodiesterase 4, which appears most directly involved in the airways actions of these drugs, causes a rise in the intracellular cAMP concentration, which in turn leads to smooth muscle relaxation. Therefore the bronchodilating effect of methylxanthines results from perturbation of the same pathway that is initiated by β_2-agonists, although methylxanthines act downstream of β_2-adrenoceptor stimulation.

2. Blockade of adenosine receptors. Adenosine acts as a local hormone and a transmitter with myriad biological actions, including bronchoconstriction in patients with bronchospastic disease.

B Methylxanthines block, not activate, cell-surface receptors for adenosine.

C Methylxanthines stimulate, not inhibit, catecholamine release from adrenergic terminals.

D, E Methylxanthines do not cause these effects.

▶ *Learning objective:* Describe the main adverse effects of theophylline.

13. Answer: D

Methylxanthines (e.g., theophylline) stimulate gastric secretion, which can explain the abdominal discomfort that frequently occurs after the intravenous administration of theophylline. The effect on gastric secretion is most likely due to theophylline-induced inhibition of phosphodiesterase, which in turn increases intracellular cAMP, thereby causing an activation of H^+/K^+ ATPase.

A, B, C, E Actually theophylline causes effects opposite to those listed.

▶ *Learning objective:* Describe the action mediating the antihypertensive effect of diltiazem.

14. Answer: A

Diltiazem is a Ca^{2+} channel blocker. All drugs of this class relax arterial smooth muscle, and this accounts for their antihypertensive action. In addition, some drugs of this class (including diltiazem and verapamil) can decrease cardiac contractility and rate, an action that contributes to their antihypertensive effect.

B Ca^{2+} channel blockers have little effect on the venous bed and hence do not affect cardiac preload significantly.

C Diltiazem does not affect cardiac output appreciably, because the direct depressive effect on cardiac contractility and rate is balanced by a reflex increase in the same parameters, due to vasodilation.

D Diltiazem does not affect significantly the central adrenergic tone.

E Diltiazem does not affect significantly angiotensin II biosynthesis.

Case 11

Drug Abuse

C.K., a 24-year-old woman, was admitted unconscious to the emergency department of the local hospital. The woman was well known by hospital personnel, because she had been admitted several times in recent years for symptoms related to drug abuse.

The patient's chart record indicated that she was a homeless person whose long history of polydrug abuse began when she was 14. She smoked marijuana regularly and sniffed or smoked cocaine almost daily. Other illicit drugs the patient used when they were available included "ecstasy" (methylenedioxymethamphetamine), "angel dust" (phencyclidine), "acid" (LSD), "benzos" (benzodiazepines), and "dope" (heroin).

Physical examination showed an unconscious patient with the following vital signs: blood pressure 100/50, heart rate 95 bpm, respirations 5/min, temperature 95.5°F (35.2°C). Examination also showed a diffuse cyanosis, pinpoint pupils, absent bowel sounds, one fresh needle puncture wound, and several healed scars from needle puncture wounds in the cubital fossa area.

A diagnosis of heroin overdose was made, and emergency therapy was started. The patient was ventilated and given oxygen through a bag-valve mask, and intravenous (IV) naloxone was given.

A few minutes later the patient regained consciousness, and her blood pressure and respiration gradually normalized. The patient was then transferred to a rehabilitation center for further therapy and detoxification.

Questions

1. C.K. was a polydrug abuser. Most licit and illicit recreational drugs act by increasing dopamine concentration primarily in which of the following brain structures?

A. Locus ceruleus

B. Amygdala

C. Nucleus accumbens

D. Substantia nigra

E. Hippocampus

2. C.K. smoked marijuana regularly. The activation of which of the following brain receptors most likely mediated the rewarding effects of the patient's smoking?

A. N-methyl-D-aspartate (NMDA) receptors

B. α_2-adrenoceptors

C. 5-HT receptors

D. Cannabinoid receptors

E. γ-aminobutyric acid (GABA) receptors

F. Opioid receptors

3. Which of the following sets of symptoms and signs did C.K. most likely experience shortly after smoking her marijuana cigarette?

A. Relaxed euphoria–pinpoint pupils–tachycardia

B. Pinpoint pupils–tachycardia–nausea

C. Nausea–red eyes–relaxed euphoria

D. Tachycardia–red eyes–relaxed euphoria

E. Red eyes–pinpoint pupils–nausea

4. The most active compound of marijuana is the Δ^9-tetrahydrocannabinol. From lab research and medical reports, which of the following is the approximate ratio of lethal dose/effective dose (i.e., the therapeutic index) of Δ^9-tetrahydrocannabinol?

A. 15

B. 50

C. 100

D. 1,000

E. 5,000

F. > 20,000

5. C.K. sniffed cocaine almost daily. Which of the following actions on the neuronal synapses most likely mediated the rewarding (i.e., pleasant) effects of this drug?

A. Inhibition of monoamine oxidase

B. Blockade of α_2-adrenoceptors

C. Blockade of 5-HT receptors

D. Activation of 5-HT reuptake

E. Blockade of β_2-adrenoceptors

F. Inhibition of monoamine reuptake

6. Cocaine can cause addiction. Which of the following daily exposures to smoked or intravenous cocaine may be sufficient to cause addiction?

A. 1–2

B. 4–5

C. 15–20

D. 25–30

E. > 30

7. C.K. sniffed or smoked cocaine almost daily. Which of the following sets of symptoms and signs would most likely occur if the patient smoked a large amount of cocaine?

A. Mydriasis–cold sweating–decreased body temperature

B. Ravenous appetite–cold sweating–mydriasis

C. Hallucinations–mydriasis–cold sweating

D. Hallucinations–ravenous appetite–decreased body temperature

E. Mydriasis–hallucinations–ravenous appetite

8. C.K. sometimes used methylenedioxymethamphetamine. Which of the following is most likely the primary neurotransmitter that mediates the action of this drug?

A. Acetylcholine

B. Serotonin

C. Norepinephrine

D. GABA

E. Histamine

9. C.K. sometimes used phencyclidine. Which of the following brain receptors most likely mediated the actions of this drug?

A. Cholinergic

B. Noradrenergic

C. Serotoninergic

D. GABAergic

E. Glutamatergic

10. Phencyclidine overdose can cause several adverse effects. Which of the following symptoms and signs is considered a hallmark of phencyclidine intoxication?

A. Profound hypotension

B. Bradycardia

C. Nystagmus

D. Pain hypersensitivity

E. Hypothermia

F. Decreased respiratory rate

11. C.K. sometimes used LSD. Which of the following brain receptors most likely mediates the central nervous system effects of this drug?

A. Cholinergic

B. Noradrenergic

C. GABAergic

D. Serotoninergic

E. Glutamatergic

12. C.K. was diagnosed with heroin overdose and exhibited the classic signs of this intoxication, including pinpoint pupils. The stimulation of which of the following brain nuclei most likely mediated this drug effect?

A. Locus ceruleus

B. Nucleus ambiguus

C. Edinger–Westphal's nucleus

D. Area postrema

E. Nucleus accumbens

F. Nucleus basalis of Meynert

13. A sign of heroin overdose showed by C.K. was a respiratory rate of 5 breaths/min. Which of the following was most likely the primary mechanism of opioid-induced respiratory depression?

A. Increased activation of the pneumotaxic center

B. Blockade of cholinergic receptors of the diaphragm

C. Increased activation of the apneustic center

D. Reduced sensitivity of the respiratory center to PCO_2

E. Increased tone of the bronchial smooth muscles

14. It is known that most effects of heroin undergo tolerance after chronic use. Which of the following two effects exhibit negligible opioid tolerance?

A. Miosis–constipation

B. Respiratory depression–vomiting

C. Miosis–respiratory depression

D. Constipation–vomiting

E. Miosis–vomiting

F. Constipation–respiratory depression

15. C.K. received a naloxone injection that rapidly reversed the signs of heroin overdose. Which of the following molecular mechanisms most likely mediated this drug effect?

A. Partial agonist at μ-opioid receptors

B. Partial agonist at dopamine adrenoceptors

C. Antagonist at μ-opioid receptors

D. Agonist at kappa opioid receptors

E. Antagonist at dopamine adrenoceptors

Answers and Explanations

▶ *Learning objective:* Identify the brain structure that most likely mediates the reinforcing (i.e., pleasant) property of drugs.

1. Answer: C

The median forebrain bundle is a bundle of axons running from the midbrain to the basal forebrain and connects many limbic, hypothalamic, and midbrain structures with one another. It contains ascending catecholaminergic and serotoninergic neurons. Dopaminergic neurons from the ventral tegmentum, which travel in the median forebrain bundle, synapse with cells of the nucleus accumbens, a basal ganglia nucleus located just in front of the hypothalamic preoptic area. This system has been called the reward system of the brain, because it has been shown that reinforcement produced by pleasurable stimuli (e.g., food, water, sexual behavior, and even social interactions) can be modulated by manipulation of this tegmental–accumbens dopaminergic circuit.

The reinforcing (i.e., pleasant) properties of drugs seem associated with their ability to increase the levels of dopamine in the nucleus accumbens region. Most recreational drugs reliably activate the brain reward system, and it is therefore likely that the euphoric effects of drugs (and therefore their addiction liability) are mediated by increased dopamine extracellular levels in the nucleus accumbens reward system.

A The locus ceruleus is a nucleus located in the pons and involved with physiological responses to stress and panic. It is the principal site for brain synthesis of norepinephrine.

B The amygdala is a region of the brain located deep within the temporal lobes, responsible for detecting fear and preparing for emergency events.

D The substantia nigra is a basal ganglia nucleus located in the midbrain that plays an important role in reward and movement.

E The hippocampus is a region of the brain located within the brain's medial temporal lobes, primarily responsible for regulating memory—in particular long-term memory.

▶ *Learning objective:* Identify the brain receptors most likely activated by marijuana smoking.

2. Answer: D

The rewarding effects of marijuana smoking are thought to be related to the activation of cannabinoid receptors by Δ^9-tetrahydrocannabinol, the main psychoactive substance of cannabis leaves. Two types of cannabinoid receptors have been found in the human brain and some peripheral tissues. They are named CB1 and CB2, and both are G-protein-coupled receptors. Endogenous ligands (anandamide, 2-arachidonoylglycerol) for these receptors have been identified, and they act as neurotransmitters. Cannabinoid receptors are widely distributed in the cerebral cortex, hippocampus, striatum, and cerebellum and are mainly located presynaptically, where they inhibit the release of either glutamate or GABA. The physiological role of these receptors and their endogenous ligands is still incompletely understood, but they are likely to have important functions because of their wide location. For example, in the hippocampus they may contribute to induction of synaptic plasticity during memory formation.

A NMDA receptors are thought to be blocked by some drugs of abuse (e.g., phencyclidine and ketamine).

B α_2-Adrenoceptors are activated by brain norepinephrine and epinephrine. This activation is related to some withdrawal effects of drug of abuse but does not seem primarily involved in the rewarding effect of these drugs.

C 5-HT receptors are involved in some central and peripheral effects of psychedelic drugs.

E GABA receptors are involved in the rewarding effects of drugs like ethanol, barbiturates, and benzodiazepines.

F Opioid receptors are involved in the rewarding effects of opioids.

▶ *Learning objective:* Identify the set of
symptoms and signs that most likely occur
shortly after smoking marijuana.

3. Answer: D

The two most common somatic signs that occur after smoking marijuana are tachycardia and dilation of conjunctival vessels (red eyes). The most prominent psychological effect is a relaxed euphoria that is associated with easy laughing, impaired memory and concentration, social withdrawal, sensation of slowed time, impaired motor coordination, and increased appetite.

A, B, E Marijuana tends to cause mydriasis, not pinpoint pupil.

B, C, E Marijuana has antiemetic activity; therefore nausea is quite unlikely.

▶ *Learning objective:* Identify the therapeutic
index of cannabinoids.

4. Answer: F

Cannabinoids are among the least toxic drugs known. No report of cannabinoid-induced death has been reported in the literature, even when huge doses of cannabinoids are consumed by drug users. Studies in several animal species conclude that the ratio of lethal dose to effective dose is 20,000:40,000. In lay terms this means that is impossible to die from a cannabinoid overdose.

A, B, C, D, E See correct answer explanation.

▶ *Learning objective:* Identify the molecular
action of cocaine that most likely mediates
its rewarding effects.

5. Answer: F

It has been shown that cocaine is able to block monoamine transporters—that is, the different transport proteins that carry catecholamines and serotonin through the membrane of neuron synaptic terminals. By blocking catecholamine transport proteins, the drug prevents the reuptake of dopamine into the presynaptic neurons, increasing the concentrations of the neurotransmitter in the synaptic cleft of dopamine neurons. The increased dopamine availability in the nucleus accumbens most likely mediates the rewarding (i.e., pleasant) effects of cocaine.

A Inhibition of monoamine oxidase is an effect of some antidepressant drugs (e.g., phenelzine).

B By inhibiting monoamine reuptake, cocaine can cause (indirectly) activation, not blockade, of α_2-adrenoceptors.

C By inhibiting monoamine reuptake, cocaine can cause (indirectly) activation, not blockade, of 5-HT receptors.

D Cocaine blocks, not activates, 5-HT reuptake.

E By inhibiting monoamine reuptake, cocaine can cause (indirectly) activation, not blockade, of β_2-adrenoceptors.

▶ *Learning objective:* Identify the number
of daily smoked or intravenous cocaine
exposures that may be sufficient to cause
cocaine addiction.

6. Answer: B

Cocaine is one of the most addictive drugs. It is thought that 4 to 5 daily exposures to intravenous or smoked cocaine may be sufficient to trigger addiction to the drug.

The greater abuse potential of intravenous or smoked cocaine is attributed to the faster rate of drug delivery to the brain (within 10 seconds), and the faster onset of a more intense pleasurable effect.

A, C, D, E See correct answer explanation.

▶ *Learning objective:* Identify the set of
symptoms and signs caused by cocaine
overdose.

7. Answer: C

Cocaine produces end-organ toxicity in virtually every organ system in the body. This is because the drug can increase the availability of both catecholamines (dopamine, norepinephrine) and indolamines (serotonin) in the synaptic space of several tissues. Symptoms and signs of cocaine overdose are mediated by this increased availability and depend on the prevalence of receptors for that specific neurotransmitter in a given organ/tissue. Peripheral symptoms include mydriasis (due to of α_1-adrenoceptor activation in the radial muscle of the iris), cold (because of α_1-mediated skin vasoconstriction), and sweating (mediated by central activation of the sympathetic nervous system). Central symptoms include hallucinations (mainly tactile "bugs crawling under the skin").

B, D, E Cocaine causes poor, not ravenous, appetite.

A, D Cocaine causes an increase, not a decrease, in body temperature.

▶ *Learning objective:* Identify the neurotransmitter that most likely mediates the actions of methylenedioxymethamphetamine.

8. Answer: B

Methylenedioxymethamphetamine is an amphetamine analogue with both psychostimulant and psychedelic properties. The drug is used globally along with rave culture. Methylenedioxymethamphetamine causes the release of monoamines by reversing the action of their respective transporters. It has a preferential affinity for serotonin transporters, and the release of this neurotransmitter is so great that there is a marked intracellular depletion for 24 hours after a single dose.

A Acetylcholine is the brain neurotransmitter that mediates the therapeutic action of some drugs (e.g., donepezil and rivastigmine) used in Alzheimer's disease.

C Norepinephrine is the brain neurotransmitter that mediates some actions (increased arousal, reduced sleep) of amphetamines and cocaine.

D GABA is the neurotransmitter that mediates the rewarding effect of drugs like ethanol, barbiturates, and benzodiazepines.

E Histamine is the neurotransmitter involved in the central effects of first-generation antihistamine antagonists.

▶ *Learning objective:* Identify the neurotransmitter that most likely mediates the actions of phencyclidine.

9. Answer: E

Phencyclidine is a drug with both psychostimulant and psychedelic properties that binds with high affinity and blocks the NMDA subtype of glutamate receptors in the brain. A closely related drug, ketamine, seems to act in a similar way and is used as a general anesthetic agent but is sometimes abused (street name "special K").

A Central cholinergic receptors are activated (indirectly) by some cholinesterase inhibitors (e.g., donepezil and rivastigmine) used in Alzheimer's disease.

B Central noradrenergic receptors mediate some actions (increased arousal, reduced sleep) of amphetamines and cocaine and the therapeutic action of some antidepressant drugs.

C Central serotoninergic receptors mediate the therapeutic action of some antidepressants, such as selective serotonin reuptake inhibitors (SSRIs).

D Central GABAergic receptors mediate the therapeutic action of sedative-hypnotic drugs, such as benzodiazepines and barbiturates.

▶ *Learning objective:* Identify the sign that is considered a hallmark of phencyclidine intoxication.

10. Answer: C

Phencyclidine overdose may cause agitation and hostile and assaultive behavior (unlike classical psychedelic drugs that very rarely cause such behavior). The action of the drug on the autonomic nervous system becomes more prominent and is characterized by a confusing combination of adrenergic, cholinergic, and dopaminergic effects. A hypertensive response is typically encountered. Tachycardia, tachypnea, hyperthermia, and miosis (or more rarely mydriasis) may also be noted, but vertical, horizontal, or rotatory nystagmus is considered a hallmark of phencyclidine intoxication, because it is present in up to 69% of cases.

A, B, D, E, F Phencyclidine intoxication usually causes signs opposite to those listed.

▶ *Learning objective:* Identify the brain receptors primarily activated by LSD.

11. Answer: D

LSD is a semisynthetic ergot alkaloid, classified as a psychedelic drug. The primary action of this drug class is to alter cognition and perception. Extensive studies have shown that the drug (like most ergot derivatives) interacts with several 5-HT receptor subtypes in the brain (mainly, 5-HT1A, 5H-T2A, and 5-HT2C) as a full or partial agonist. It appears to act as a full agonist at 5-HT1A presynaptic autoreceptors of raphe neurons, thereby decreasing the release of 5-HT, which normally exerts an inhibiting influence on cortical neurons by filtering the incoming sensory information.

A Central cholinergic receptors mediate the action of some cholinesterase inhibitors (e.g., donepezil and rivastigmine) used in Alzheimer's disease.

B Central noradrenergic receptors mediate some actions (increased arousal, reduced sleep) of amphetamines and cocaine and the therapeutic action of some antidepressant drugs.

C Central GABAergic receptors mediate the therapeutic action of sedative-hypnotic drugs, such as benzodiazepines and barbiturates.

E Central glutamatergic receptors are involved in the action of some psychedelic drugs, such as phencyclidine.

▶ *Learning objective:* Identify the brain nucleus that mediates heroin-induced miosis.

12. Answer: C

Heroin is an opioid agonist. Opioids can stimulate Edinger-Westphal's nucleus (also known as the accessory oculomotor nucleus), which is the accessory parasympathetic cranial nerve nucleus of the oculomotor nerve. Neurons of this nucleus innervate the sphincter muscle of the iris (causing miosis) and the ciliary muscle (causing increased lens curvature). Therefore prominent miosis can be caused by virtually all opioid agonists. Tolerance to this opioid effect is negligible.

A The locus ceruleus is a nucleus located in the pons and is involved with physiological responses to stress and panic. It is the principal site for brain synthesis of norepinephrine.

B The nucleus ambiguus is a group of large motor neurons, situated deep in the medullary reticular formation. It is one of the nuclei of the vagus nerve.

D The area postrema is a structure located on the floor of the fourth ventricle. It contains the chemoreceptor trigger zone, a nucleus that triggers vomiting in response to emetic drugs.

E Nucleus accumbens is a basal ganglia nucleus located just in front of the hypothalamic preoptic area.

F The nucleus basalis of Meynert is a group of neurons in the substantia innominata of the basal forebrain, which has wide projections to the neocortex. Its primary function is to modulate the ratio of reality and virtual reality components of visual perception.

▶ *Learning objective:* Describe the primary mechanism of opioid-induced respiratory depression.

13. Answer: D

Opioid can cause respiratory depression primarily by reducing the sensitivity of the brainstem respiratory center to PCO_2, one of the most potent physiological stimuli to ventilation.

A, C Opioids can depress, not activate, these centers, but this is not the primary mechanism of opioid-induced respiratory depression.

B Depression of the respiratory center causes, of course, a decrease in diaphragm activity, but opioids do not block diaphragm cholinergic receptors.

E Large doses of opioid can cause bronchoconstriction, but respiratory depression induced by this drug is central, not peripheral.

▶ *Learning objective:* Identify the two effects of opioids for which tolerance is negligible.

14. Answer: A

Most effects of opioids undergo tolerance, including the lethal effect. Notable exceptions are the effects on the eye (which lead to miosis and cyclospasm) and the effects on the enteric smooth muscle (which lead to constipation) for which tolerance is negligible.

B, C, D, E, F Respiratory depression and vomiting undergo tolerance after chronic use.

▸ *Learning objective:* Describe the mechanism of action of naloxone.

15.   Answer: C

Naloxone is an opioid antagonist that can bind and block all opioid receptors, even if it has a greater affinity for μ-opioid receptors. The major clinical application of naloxone is in the treatment of acute opioid overdose, as in the present case. The drug completely reverses the opioid effects within 2 to 3 minutes. The action of the drug is short, and a severely depressed patient may recover after a single dose and appear normal after 1 to 2 hours. Naloxone should not be given to a dependent subject who appears normal when taking opioids, because it almost instantaneously precipitates an abstinence syndrome.

A Partial agonists at μ-opioid receptors include some opioid drugs (e.g., buprenorphine).

B Partial agonists at dopamine adrenoceptors include drugs like aripiprazole, used as antipsychotic agents.

D Agonists at kappa opioid receptors include some opioid drugs (e.g., pentazocine).

E Antagonists at dopamine adrenoceptors include most antipsychotic drugs.

Case 12

Epilepsy

F.H., a 16-year-old girl, was accompanied by her mother to the neurologic clinic for routine follow-up of her epileptic seizures.

Medical history of the patient indicated that her birth was normal, but she was diagnosed with cerebral palsy and serious mental retardation when she was 1 year old. Seizures developed during infancy. She was diagnosed with epilepsy and was admitted several times to the neurologic clinic. F.H.'s past medical records indicated that her seizures began with an outcry followed by loss of consciousness and contraction of her arms and legs, followed by shaking. Consciousness returned slowly, and the patient was drowsy and agitated afterward.

Many anticonvulsants were tried over the years, including phenytoin, carbamazepine, valproic acid, topiramate, and levetiracetam. Other antiepileptic drugs were sometimes added to the main treatment as adjunctive therapy. All these drugs were eventually discontinued because either they were not effective or they caused intolerable adverse effects. The patient had never been seizure-free. For the past 6 months F.H. suffered, on average, five to eight seizures per month. The patient had been taking lamotrigine because the drug appeared somewhat effective, although the overall control of the patient's seizures was far from satisfactory.

F.H. never attended school and required close supervision by family or nurses. Both F.H.'s parents were alive and well. A brother of 12 was in good health. The family history was negative for seizures.

Physical examination showed a young girl sitting in a wheelchair. She was unable to walk, and her fine motor control was poor. Her talking was extremely slow, and a severe intellectual disability was evident.

During the examination the patient suddenly underwent a seizure that lasted about 8 minutes. An emergency therapy was started, which included intravenous (IV) administration of an appropriate drug.

Questions

1 F.H. was diagnosed with epilepsy. Which of the following best defines this disorder?

A. Chronic irreversible deterioration of cognition

B. Sudden abnormal discharge of cortical neurons

C. Chronic disorder characterized by recurrent seizures

D. Acute seizure due to a localized ischemic brain disorder

E. Chronic disorder characterized by abnormal movements or behavior

2 Which of the following pairs of neurotransmitters are thought to be primarily involved in the pathogenesis of epilepsy?

A. γ-aminobutyric acid (GABA)–serotonin

B. GABA–glutamate

C. GABA–norepinephrine

D. Serotonin–glutamate

E. Serotonin–norepinephrine

F. Norepinephrine–glutamate

3 F.H. was diagnosed with epilepsy. Which of the following seizure types was F.H. most likely having?

A. Absence seizures

B. Tonic-clonic seizures

C. Myoclonic seizures

D. Atonic seizures

E. Complex partial seizures

4 Which of the following autonomic symptoms and signs likely occurred during the tonic-clonic phase of F.H.'s seizures?

A. Hyperpnea

B. Hypotension

C. Bradycardia

D. Pale skin

E. Loss of bladder control

5 F.H.'s past treatment included phenytoin. Which of the following brain cation channels was most likely the primary target of this drug?

A. Resting Na^+ channels

B. Inactivated Na^+ channels

C. Resting Ca^{2+} channels

D. Inactivated Ca^{2+} channels

E. Resting K^+ channels

F. Inactivated K^+ channels

6 Phenytoin exhibits dose-dependent elimination kinetics. Which of the following pharmacokinetic parameters of the drug most likely decreases by increasing the dose?

A. Half-life ($t_{1/2}$)

B. Clearance (CL)

C. Time to reach the steady state

D. Volume of distribution (Vd)

E. Oral bioavailability

7 Several antiseizure drugs can cause a dose-dependent impairment of the cerebellar–vestibular function. Which of the following is a common and early adverse effect of phenytoin that is related to this impairment?

A. Tremor

B. Nystagmus

C. Dystonic reaction

D. Drowsiness

E. Peripheral neuropathy

8 F.H.'s past treatment included carbamazepine. The inhibition of which of the following neurophysiologic actions most likely contributed to the therapeutic effect of the drug in the patient's disease?

A. Postsynaptic inhibitory potentials (PSIPs)

B. Posttetanic potentiation

C. K^+ conductance on neuronal cell membranes

D. Long term depression

E. Cl^- conductance on neuronal cell membranes

9. Which of the following adverse effects most likely prompted the neurologist to discontinue carbamazepine treatment?

A. Sinus bradycardia

B. Sialorrhea

C. Diarrhea

D. Nausea and vomiting

E. Hallucinations

10. F.H.'s past treatment included valproic acid. Which of the following sets of ionic currents shown in the attached table most likely mediated the therapeutic effect of the drug?

Set	Na^+ current	K^+ current	Ca^{2+} current	Cl^- current
A.	↓	↓	↑	↓
B.	↓	↓	↔	↑
C.	↔	↓	↑	↓
D.	↓	↓	↔	↑
E.	↓	↑	↓	↑

↑ increased ↓ decreased ↔ unchanged

11. Valproic acid can cause a very rare but life-threatening adverse effect on which of the following organs?

A. Brain

B. Heart

C. Liver

D. Lung

E. Kidney

12. F.H.'s past treatment included topiramate. A blockade of which of the following brain receptors most likely contributed to the therapeutic effect of the drug?

A. Muscarinic receptors

B. α-Amino-3-hydroxy-5-methyl-4-isoxazolepropionic acid (AMPA) receptors

C. D_2-receptors

D. $α_2$-adrenoceptors

E. 5-HT receptors

F. Opioid receptors

13. Levetiracetam was administered to F.H. The exact mechanism of antiseizure action of this drug is still unknown but is most likely related to the high affinity of this drug for which of the following brain molecular targets?

A. Na^+ channels

B. Synaptic vesicle protein

C. AMPA receptors

D. GABA receptors

E. Ca^{2+} channels

14. F.H.'s present treatment included lamotrigine. Blockade of which of the following pairs of brain ion channels most likely accounts for the antiseizure effect of this drug.

A. Na^+–Cl^- channels

B. Na^+–K^+ channels

C. Na^+–Ca^{2+} channels

D. K^+–Ca^{2+} channels

E. K^+–Cl^- channels

F. Ca^{2+}–Cl^- channels

15. Which of the following is a potential life-threatening adverse effect that may occur during lamotrigine therapy?

A. Myocardial infarction

B. Stroke

C. Kidney failure

D. Stevens–Johnson's syndrome

E. Liver cirrhosis

16. Which of the following antiseizure drugs administered to F.H. is a potent enzyme inducer that can affect its own drug metabolism?

A. Valproic acid

B. Topiramate

C. Carbamazepine

D. Levetiracetam

E. Lamotrigine

17. Some antiseizure drugs were administered to F.H. as adjunctive therapy. The mechanism of action of one of these drugs is thought to be related to blockage of voltage-gated N-type Ca^{2+} channels on presynaptic terminals, thus inhibiting the release of glutamate. Which of the following drugs likely has this mechanism of action?

A. Zonisamide

B. Ethosuximide

C. Gabapentin

D. Clonazepam

E. Phenobarbital

18. During the physical examination F.H. suddenly underwent a seizure that lasted about 8 minutes. Which of the following types of seizures was the patient most likely having?

A. Complex partial seizure

B. Absence seizure

C. Status epilepticus

D. Myoclonic seizure

E. Atonic seizure

F. Simple partial seizure

19. Which of the following drugs was most likely given IV to stop F.H.'s ongoing seizure?

A. Carbamazepine

B. Ethosuximide

C. Gabapentin

D. Diazepam

E. Topiramate

F. Levetiracetam

Answers and Explanations

▶ *Learning objective:* Give the correct definition of epilepsy.

1. Answer: C

Epilepsy must not be confused with seizures. A seizure is a sudden physical or mental disorder resulting from abnormal, paroxysmal, hypersynchronous electrical neuronal activity in the cerebral cortex. Epilepsy is a chronic disorder, the hallmark of which is recurrent, unprovoked seizures. Epilepsy is the third most common neurologic disorder worldwide, after dementia and stroke. The disease can rarely be cured permanently, but it can be controlled in more than 80% of cases with appropriate antiepileptic drugs.

A Epilepsy may cause a deterioration of cognition, but this is not at all a feature of all epileptic patients.

B This is the definition of seizure, not of epilepsy.

D A single acute seizure is not epilepsy. Moreover, an ischemic brain disorder can cause seizures but is not a necessary factor for the appearance of seizures.

E Some types of epilepsy can show abnormal movements or behavior, but several abnormal movements (e.g., dystonias) or abnormal behaviors (e.g., schizoid disorders) are not due to seizures.

▶ *Learning objective:* Identify the pairs of neurotransmitters that are thought to be primarily involved in the pathogenesis of epilepsy.

2. Answer: B

Epilepsy is a chronic recurrent disorder of cerebral function characterized by repeated seizures.

Seizures require three conditions:

▶ A population of pathologically excitable neurons (referred to as the primary focus)

▶ A genetic or pathology-induced increase in excitatory activity of glutamatergic neurons through recurrent connections in order to spread the discharge

▶ A genetic or pathology-induced decrease in the activity of the normally inhibitory GABA neurons

Just why the neurons in or near a focal cortical lesion discharge spontaneously and synchronously is not fully understood, but it is known that a damaged cell is in a state of partial depolarization because its cytoplasmic membrane has an increased ionic permeability. This can explain why these cells are susceptible to activation by hyperthermia, hypoxia, hypoglycemia, hypocalcemia, and hyponatremia, as well as by repeated sensory (e.g., photic) stimulation.

A, **D**, **E** Serotonin can contribute to the amplification of synaptic transmission during seizures but is not the primary neurotransmitter involved in epileptic seizures.

C, **E**, **F** Norepinephrine can contribute to the amplification of synaptic transmission during seizures but is not the primary neurotransmitter involved in epileptic seizures.

▶ *Learning objective:* From the patient's medical record, identify the type of seizure she was most likely having.

3.   Answer: B

F.H.'s medical records indicate that the patient was having tonic-clonic seizures. When these seizures are recurrent, the epilepsy is also referred to as grand mal. A tonic-clonic seizure is typically subdivided into tonic, clonic, and postictal phases.
The tonic phase lasts for 10 to 20 seconds. It begins with flexion of the trunk and elevation and abduction of the elbows. Subsequent extension of the back and neck is followed by extension of the arms and legs. This can be accompanied by apnea, which is secondary to laryngeal spasm.

The clonic phase begins with generalized movements that occur at a rate of about 4 to 8 per second. This is because phases of atonia alternate with repeated violent flexor spasms. This phase lasts for 30 to 120 seconds. The patient continues to be apneic during this phase.

The postictal phase includes a variable period of unconsciousness (usually 2 to 3 minutes), during which the patient becomes quiet and breathing resumes. The patient gradually awakens, often after a period of stupor or sleep, without recall of the seizure itself.

A Absence seizures (also known as petit mal seizures) consist of loss of consciousness for 5 to 30 seconds, with a blank stare and occasional motor symptoms, such as eyelid fluttering and lip smacking;

there is no fall or convulsion. The impairment of external awareness is so brief that the patient is unaware of it.

C Myoclonic seizures are brief, lightning-like jerks of a limb, several limbs, or the whole trunk. Consciousness is not lost.

D Atonic seizures are a brief, complete loss of muscle tone and consciousness.

E Complex partial seizures exhibit sensory hallucinations and mental distortion. Consciousness is altered but not lost.

▶ *Learning objective:* Identify an autonomic sign that can most likely occur during the tonic-clonic phase of an epileptic seizure.

4.   Answer: E

Several autonomic signs can occur during a tonic-clonic seizure, due to hyperactivity of both sympathetic and parasympathetic systems. The loss of bladder control is present in more than 50% of cases, and loss of bowel control sometimes occurs.

A During the tonic-clonic phase of the seizure, the patient is apneic.

B Hypertension, not hypotension, usually occurs during the tonic-clonic phase of the seizure.

C Tachycardia, not bradycardia, usually occurs during the tonic-clonic phase of the seizure.

D The skin is usually flushed or sometimes cyanotic, not pale, during the tonic-clonic phase of the seizure.

5.   Answer: B

The anticonvulsant effect of phenytoin most likely results from blockage of inactivated Na^+ channels, an action that is both voltage- (greater effect when the membrane is depolarized) and frequency-dependent (greater effect when Na^+ channels open and close at high frequency). The same effect is also seen with therapeutically relevant concentration of carbamazepine, valproic acid, topiramate, and lamotrigine and probably represents the primary mechanism of action of these drugs in partial and generalized tonic-clonic seizures.

A, **C**, **E** Antiseizure drugs have negligible effects on resting ion channels.

D, **F** Phenytoin can interact with these channels at high doses, but the contribution of this action to the antiseizure effect of the drug is uncertain.

▶ *Learning objective:* Identify the brain ion channel that is the primary target of phenytoin.

6. Answer: B

Virtually all phenytoin is eliminated by liver metabolism. The elimination is dose-dependent (i.e., first-order at low doses, but zero-order at higher doses), even if these doses are still within the therapeutic range. This means that when the maximum capacity of the liver to metabolize the drug is approached, even a small further increase in dosage may cause a very large increase in blood levels of the drug. For drugs that follow a zero-order kinetics, clearance decreases as the dose increases.

A The half-life of the drug is 0.7 Vd/CL. Because the Vd is unchanged and the CL is decreased, the half-life is increased, not decreased.

C The time to reach the steady state of a drug is dependent on the half-life only. Since the half-life is increased, the time to reach the steady state is increased, not decreased.

D The volume of distribution refers to the distribution of a drug. Dose-dependent elimination kinetics refers to the elimination of a drug. Distribution and elimination are independent pharmacokinetic parameters.

E Bioavailability refers to the fraction of the drug that reaches the systemic circulation. Because the maximum capacity of the liver to metabolize the drug is reached, this fraction, if anything, should be increased, not decreased.

▶ *Learning objective:* Identify an adverse effect of phenytoin that is related to a drug-induced impairment of the cerebellar–vestibular function.

7. Answer: B

Nystagmus is an early, dose-dependent adverse effect of phenytoin that is due to an impairment of vestibular function. It is common and frequently associated with ataxia, due to an impairment of cerebellar function.

A Tremor is not reported as an adverse effect of phenytoin. Moreover, the brain cir-

cuits involved in the pathogenesis of tremor do not include cerebellar–vestibular circuits.

C Dystonic reaction is not reported as an adverse effect of phenytoin, and its pathogenesis does not include cerebellar–vestibular circuits.

D Both drowsiness and insomnia can occur during phenytoin therapy, but they are not related to an impairment of cerebellar–vestibular function.

E Peripheral neuropathy (sensory peripheral polyneuropathy) can occur in patients receiving phenytoin, but it is not due to cerebellar-vestibular impairment.

▶ *Learning objective:* Select the inhibition of a neurophysiological action that can contribute to the therapeutic effect of carbamazepine.

8. Answer: B

Carbamazepine antiseizure action most likely involves an inhibition of posttetanic potentiation of central nervous system neurons surrounding the epileptic focus. Posttetanic potentiation is the production of enhanced postsynaptic potentials that occurs after a rapid (tetanizing) train of impulses in the presynaptic neuron. The inhibition of posttetanic potentiation likely explains why carbamazepine (and drugs with similar mechanism of action, like phenytoin) can prevent the spread of seizure discharge from the epileptic focus. The excessive discharge of the focus itself is not prevented, and therefore electroencephalographic alterations are not eliminated by the drug.

A The inhibition of PSIPs would favor, not inhibit, the spread of the discharge from the epileptic focus.

C The inhibition of K^+ conductance on neuronal cell membranes would depolarize the cell membranes, which in turn would favor, not inhibit, the spread of the discharge from the epileptic focus.

D Long-term depression is characterized by a decrease in synaptic strength. It is produced by slower stimulation of presynaptic neurons. Its inhibition would favor, not inhibit, the spread of the discharge from the epileptic focus.

E The inhibition of Cl⁻ conductance on neuronal cell membranes would depolarize the cell membranes, which in turn would favor, not inhibit, the spread of the discharge from the epileptic focus.

▸ *Learning objective:* Describe a common adverse effect of carbamazepine that can cause the discontinuation of the treatment.

9. Answer: D

Two of the most frequently observed adverse reactions associated with carbamazepine, particularly during the initial phases of therapy, are nausea (~ 20%) and vomiting (~ 15%).

A Carbamazepine causes atrial tachycardia, not bradycardia, in < 2% of patients receiving the drug. The syndrome can be severe.

B Carbamazepine causes xerostomia, not sialorrhea, in about 8% of patients receiving the drug.

C Carbamazepine causes constipation, not diarrhea, in about 10% of patients receiving the drug.

E Carbamazepine can cause hallucinations, but they occur very rarely and only after high doses.

▸ *Learning objective:* Describe the change in ionic currents that most likely mediates the anticonvulsant action of valproic acid.

10. Answer: E

Valproic acid is the antiseizure drug with the widest activity spectrum. The drug can be considered a first- or second-line therapy in most forms of epilepsy at all age groups. In addition, it is currently used to treat bipolar disorder and to prevent migraine headaches.

The mechanisms of action of valproic acid have not been fully established, but they are most likely multiple, including the following:

▸ Voltage- and frequency-dependent blockade of voltage-gated Na⁺ channels
▸ Blockade of T-type Ca²⁺ channels in thalamic neurons
▸ Opening K⁺ channels (at high doses)

▸ Increased GABA content in the brain, which in turn causes increased opening of Cl⁻ channels
▸ Blockade of N-methyl-D-aspartate (NMDA) receptors, which in turn causes a decreased opening of Ca²⁺ channels

These mechanisms of action follow the general rule that an antiseizure drug either decreases the depolarization of neuronal membranes (decrease of Na⁺ or Ca²⁺ currents) or increases the polarization of neuronal membranes (increase of K⁺ or Cl⁻ current).

A, B, C, D See correct answer explanation.

▸ *Learning objective:* Identify the body organ that can be the site of a very rare but life-threatening adverse effect of valproic acid.

11. Answer: C

Valproic acid can cause severe hepatotoxicity. Indeed, more than 100 fatal cases of acute or chronic liver injury due to valproate have been reported in the literature. Liver toxicity is always serious, is often lethal, and can have a fulminant course. Very young children or persons with mental retardation are especially at risk, as in the present case. Likely the appearance of F.H.'s prodromal symptoms and signs of liver toxicity (as a threefold increase of liver transaminases) prompted the neurologist to discontinue the drug.

A Valproic acid can cause various central adverse effects (drowsiness, asthenia, amblyopia, anxiety ataxia, etc.), but these effects are not life-threatening.

B Valproic acid can cause various cardiovascular adverse effects (bradycardia and tachycardia, postural hypotension, etc.), but these effects are not life-threatening.

D Valproic acid can cause various respiratory adverse effects (flulike syndrome, fungal infection, etc.), but these effects are not life-threatening.

E Valproic acid can cause some renal adverse effects (hyponatremia, etc.), but these effects are not life-threatening.

▶ *Learning objective:* Identify the brain receptor that is most likely blocked by topiramate.

12. Answer: B

Topiramate is a second-generation antiseizure drug that likely works with multiple mechanisms of action, including the following:

▶ Blockade of AMPA receptors, which in turn causes decreased opening of cation channels
▶ State- and frequency-dependent blockade of voltage-gated Na^+ channels
▶ Blockade of L-type Ca^{2+} channels
▶ Potentiation of the inhibitory effects of GABA

The drug is considered a broad spectrum antiepileptic drug, effective in most types of seizures.

In addition, it is used to treat bipolar disorder and certain types of neuropathic pain, and to prevent migraine headaches.

A Brain muscarinic receptors can be blocked by anticholinergic amines (e.g., atropine).

C Brain D_2-receptors can be blocked by antipsychotic drugs (e.g., haloperidol).

D Brain α_2-adrenoceptors can be blocked by clonidine.

E Brain 5-HT receptors can be blocked by some antipsychotic drugs (e.g., clozapine) or by some antiemetic drugs (e.g., ondansetron).

F Brain opioid receptors can be blocked by opioid antagonists (e.g., naloxone and naltrexone).

▶ *Learning objective:* Identify the most likely molecular target of levetiracetam.

13. Answer: B

Levetiracetam binds with high affinity to a synaptic vesicle protein. It is thought that this binding can prevent the release of excitatory neurotransmitters like glutamate. The drug is approved by the U.S. Food and Drug Administration as adjunctive therapy in the treatment of the following:

▶ Partial seizures
▶ Primary generalized tonic-clonic seizures
▶ Myoclonic seizures in patients with juvenile myoclonic epilepsy

A Antiseizure drugs like phenytoin and carbamazepine have high affinity for Na^+ channels.

C Topiramate has high affinity for AMPA receptors.

D Benzodiazepines have high affinity for GABA receptors.

E Ethosuximide has high affinity for Ca^{2+} channels.

▶ *Learning objective:* Identify the pairs of channels most likely blocked by lamotrigine.

14. Answer: C

Lamotrigine causes a voltage- and frequency-dependent blockade of both voltage-gated Na^+ and Ca^{2+} channels. The Na^+ channels blockade probably explains the efficacy of the drug in partial seizures and in generalized tonic-clonic seizures, whereas the Ca^{2+} channels blockade would account for its efficacy in absence seizures and myoclonic seizures. The drug is also used to treat bipolar disorders.

A, B, D, E, F See correct answer explanation.

▶ *Learning objective:* Identify a potential life-threatening adverse effect of lamotrigine.

15. Answer: D

Lamotrigine can cause a generalized skin rash that is the most frequent cause of discontinuation of the therapy. The rash is a hypersensitivity reaction, usually mild, but severely affected patients may develop Steven-Johnson syndrome or toxic epidermal necrolysis, two potentially lethal dermatitides. The incidence of skin rash is higher in children, and some studies suggest that a potentially life-threatening dermatitis develops in 1 to 2% of pediatric patients.

A, B, C, E Lamotrigine does not cause these adverse effects.

▶ *Learning objective:* Identify the antiseizure drug that can increase its own metabolism.

16. Answer: C

Carbamazepine is a potent enzyme inducer and can induce its own metabolism; this appears to be mediated via its effects on the hepatic cytochrome P-450 3A4 (CYP3A4) isoenzyme. Onset of enzyme induction is at about 3 days, with maximum effect at about 30 days. This autoinduction can cause pharmacokinetic tolerance, and the treatment dosage should be adjusted accordingly.

A Valproic acid is an inhibitor, not an inducer, of liver enzymes like CYP2C9 and glucuronosyltransferase.

B Topiramate is a mild inducer of CYP3A4 isoenzyme and does not affect its own metabolism.

D, E Levetiracetam and lamotrigine do not affect liver monooxygenases.

▶ *Learning objective:* Identify the anticonvulsant drug that can block voltage-gated N-type Ca2+ channels on presynaptic terminals.

17. Answer: C

The exact mechanism by which gabapentin exerts its antiseizure activity is not known, but it does not appear to be related to its development as a GABA analogue. Gabapentin binds with high affinity to voltage-gated N-type Ca^{2+} channels on presynaptic terminals, which in turn decreases the synaptic release of glutamate. Gabapentin is approved as adjunctive therapy in the treatment of partial seizures. It is also approved for the treatment of neuropathic pain (postherpetic neuralgia) and restless leg syndrome.

A Zonisamide acts by blocking primarily Na^+ channels. It is used as an adjunct drug in tonic-clonic seizures and certain myoclonias.

B Ethosuximide acts by blocking T-type Ca^{2+} channels. It is a first-line agent for absence seizures.

D Clonazepam is a benzodiazepine used mainly in absence seizures.

E Phenobarbital is a barbiturate used mainly in tonic-clonic and partial seizures.

▶ *Learning objective:* Select the appropriate definition of a seizure that lasts more than 5 minutes.

18. Answer: C

Status epilepticus is defined as an epileptic seizure lasting more than 5 minutes, or more than one seizure between which a patient does not fully regain consciousness. The syndrome is life-threatening, and the mortality rate can be up to 20% for adults but is more than 50% for the elderly.

A, B, D, E, F See correct answer explanation.

▶ *Learning objective:* Identify the drug that is commonly given to stop an ongoing epileptic seizure.

19. Answer: D

Diazepam and lorazepam are the two first-line agents for the treatment of status epilepticus. Usually the seizure ends 3 to 5 minutes after starting the IV treatment. Other antiseizure drugs that can be employed in the initial treatment are fosphenytoin (a more soluble prodrug of phenytoin) and phenobarbital. However, the peak effect of fosphenytoin is usually delayed; therefore this drug is used only following the initial treatment with diazepam or lorazepam. Phenobarbital may be used as an alternative to fosphenytoin after the initial control of status epilepticus in patients who cannot tolerate fosphenytoin or when fosphenytoin is not effective.

A, B, C, E, F See correct answer explanation.

Case 13

Essential Hypertension

A.B., a 66-yr-old Caucasian man, presented with a pounding occipital headache that started late in the day and worsened as the evening approached. He also complained of a persistent, productive cough and of some shortness of breath upon exertion.

A.B. had a 1-year history of hypertension and was treated with weight reduction, a low-sodium diet, and hydrochlorothiazide. The patient took medication for 6 months but stopped it on his own. Medical history showed that the patient had been suffering from chronic obstructive pulmonary disease (COPD) for 10 years and from toxic amblyopia for 2 years, both likely due to heavy smoking. He had also been suffering from prostatic hyperplasia for 3 years but refused the surgical treatment. Two months ago A.B. suffered from an acute episode of angioedema, apparently due to a hypersensitivity reaction. Family history indicated that A.B.'s father died of colon cancer at the age of 64, and his mother died of kidney failure at the age of 78.

A.B. was admitted to the hospital for further evaluation of cardiac function and lab tests. Drugs taken by the patient on admission were as follows: inhaled albuterol as needed and tamsulosin daily.

Physical examination showed a well-developed male who looked his age and was in no acute distress. He was 166 cm tall and weighed 72 kg. Vital signs were as follows:

▸ Blood pressure while lying: 174/98 mm Hg (left arm), 172/96 mm Hg (right arm)
▸ Blood pressure while standing: 168/96 mm Hg (left arm), 170/94 mm Hg (right arm)
▸ Heart rate (HR): 72 bpm and regular
▸ Respirations: 22/min and regular

Funduscopic examination revealed mild arterial narrowing, sharp disc, and no exudate or hemorrhage. Chest auscultation showed some expiratory wheezes and coarse breath sounds, which cleared after coughing. The remainder of the physical examination was unremarkable.

Pertinent laboratory results on admission were as follows:

Blood chemistry

▸ Fasting glucose 100 mg/dL (normal 65–110)
▸ Creatinine: 1.1 mg/dL (normal 0.6–1.2)
▸ Blood urea nitrogen (BUN): 22 mg/dL (normal 5–25)
▸ Sodium: 138 mEq/L (normal 135–146)
▸ Potassium: 3.8 mEq/L (normal 3.5–5.5)
▸ Total cholesterol: 270 mg/dL (normal < 200)
▸ Triglycerides: 230 mg/dL (normal < 150)
▸ High-density lipoprotein (HDL) cholesterol: 35 mg/dL (normal > 40; negative risk factor > 60)
▸ Low-density lipoprotein (LDL) cholesterol: 180 mg/mL (normal < 100 mg/mL)

Electrocardiography

Signs of mild left ventricular hypertrophy

Echocardiography

Cardiac output (CO) at rest: 5.2 L/min (normal 4–6)

The past diagnosis was essential hypertension, and the patient was instructed to follow a dietary restriction for weight reduction and to increase his physical activity. He was discharged from the hospital with the following postdischarge therapy: hydrochlorothiazide (12.5 mg once daily), amlodipine, inhaled albuterol (180 µg) as needed, tamsulosin (0.4 mg daily).

Two months later the patient returned to the hospital for a control visit. In spite of a careful adherence to the physician's instructions and to the prescribed therapy, A.B.'s blood pressure was still 170/98. It was decided to add a third drug to the therapy, and clonidine was prescribed. The therapy was effective, and 2 weeks later A.B.'s blood pressure was 142/85 mm Hg.

Three months later A.B. presented to the emergency department with a 2-day history of progressively increasing shortness of breath. He admitted he discontinued all medications 2 weeks ago because of some annoying adverse effects. He also complained he had not urinated over the last 24 hours. Physical examination revealed an anxious-appearing man who was alert, oriented, and in respiratory distress. Vital signs were as follows: blood pressure 228/130, pulse 120 bpm, respirations 32/min. Chest examination revealed decreased breath sounds and bilateral rales. Cardiac auscultation showed S3 an S4 gallop. A diagnosis of hypertensive crisis was made and emergency therapy was instituted that included intravenous (IV) infusion of a drug. One hour later A.B.'s blood pressure was 165/92 mm Hg.

Questions

1. Essential hypertension is a common disorder. Which of the following is the estimated percentage of adults Americans with hypertension?

A. 10%

B. 20%

C. 30%

D. 40%

E. 50%

2. A.B. was diagnosed with essential hypertension. According to the Eighth Joint National Committee (JNC 8) Hypertension Management Algorithm, which of the following would be the appropriate goal for blood pressure lowering in A.B.?

A. Systolic < 130; diastolic < 90

B. Systolic < 150; diastolic < 90

C. Systolic < 130; diastolic < 80

D. Systolic < 140; diastolic < 80

E. Systolic < 140; diastolic < 90

3. The mean blood pressure measured on A.B. indicates most closely the pressure present in which of the following tissues/organs?

A. Pulmonary arteries

B. Aorta

C. Arterioles

D. Capillaries

E. Venules

4. When the blood pressure increases, the baroreceptor reflex attempts to decrease the blood pressure toward normal. Which of the following statements best explains why the reflex was not able to decrease A.B.'s blood pressure?

A. Baroreceptors reset in chronic hypertension.

B. Baroreceptors cannot operate when diastolic pressure is > 90 mm Hg.

C. The vasomotor center is impaired in chronic hypertension.

D. The firing rate of carotid sinus nerve is impaired in chronic hypertension.

E. Baroreceptors cannot operate when systolic pressure is > 160 mm Hg.

5. A.B.'s mean blood pressure was about 20% above normal. Which of the following would most likely be the mean blood flow of the patient at that time?

A. Normal

B. 20% above normal

C. 20% below normal

D. > 20% above normal

E. > 20% below normal

6. A.B. was diagnosed with essential hypertension. Which of the following factors is most likely to be important in the development of his hypertension?

A. Increased catecholamine secretion from the adrenal medulla

B. Renal retention of excess sodium

C. Genetic defect in aldosterone metabolism

D. Renal artery stenosis

E. Increased production of atrial natriuretic factor

7. Which of the following cardiovascular functions was most likely the main determinant of A.B.'s hypertension?

A. HR

B. CO

C. Stroke volume (SV)

D. Systemic vascular resistance (SVR)

E. Venous return

8. A common cause of essential hypertension is narrowing of arterioles. This is a powerful cause of the increase in blood pressure because, according to Poiseuille's equation, resistance is inversely proportional to which power of the vessel radius?

A. 1st power

B. 2nd power

C. 3rd power

D. 4th power

E. 5th power

9. A.B.'s postdischarge therapy included hydrochlorothiazide. Which of the following actions most likely mediated the long-term therapeutic effect of this drug in the patient's disease?

A. Decreased cardiac output

B. Arteriolar vasodilation

C. Reduction of blood volume

D. Inhibition of angiotensin activity

E. Decreased central sympathetic tone

10. Which of the following actions on Na^+, K^+, and H^+ transport was most likely increased in A.B.'s kidney by hydrochlorothiazide treatment?

A. K^+ reabsorption in the proximal convolute tubule

B. Na^+ reabsorption in the thin ascending limb of the loop of Henle

C. H^+ excretion in the collecting tubule

D. K^+ excretion in the proximal convolute tubule

E. H^+ reabsorption in the thick ascending limb of the loop of Henle

11. A.B. was given amlodipine. Which of the following actions most likely mediates the antihypertensive effect of this drug?

A. Decreased central parasympathetic outflow

B. Increased venous capacitance

C. Decreased afterload

D. Increased volume of extracellular fluids

E. Decreased cardiac output

12. Today angiotensin-converting enzyme (ACE) inhibitors are a first-line treatment for essential hypertension. Which of the following A.B.'s disorders most likely contraindicated the use of these drugs?

A. COPD

B. Angioedema episode

C. Toxic amblyopia

D. Prostatic hyperplasia

13. A.B. was prescribed clonidine. Which of the following actions most likely mediated the antihypertensive effect of clonidine in this patient?

A. Decreased central sympathetic outflow

B. Decreased renin secretion

C. Decreased blood volume

D. Decreased heart contractility

E. Peripheral venous pooling

14. A.B.'s lack of blood pressure control was related to medication noncompliance, as is often the case. Which of the following adverse effects most likely made the patient discontinue all medications?

A. Angioedema

B. Sialorrhea

C. Tachypalpitations

D. Daytime sedation and drowsiness

E. Peripheral edema

15. Which of the following drugs was most likely given to manage A.B.'s hypertensive crisis?

A. Esmolol

B. Nitroprusside

C. Fenoldopam

D. Losartan

E. Verapamil

F. Minoxidil

16. Which of the following is most likely the molecular mechanism of action of the drug given to manage A.B.'s hypertensive crisis?

A. Blockade of α_1-adrenoceptors

B. Opening of potassium channels in vascular smooth muscle

C. Increased availability of nitric oxide

D. Blockade of calcium channels in vascular smooth muscle

E. Activation of dopamine D_1-receptors

17. Which of the following was most likely the specific reason for the choice of the drug used to treat A.B.'s hypertensive crisis?

A. The patient's heart failure

B. The very short half-life of the drug

C. The patient's refractory hypertension

D. The patient's prostatic hyperplasia

E. The patient's anuria

Answers and Explanations

▶ *Learning objective:* Identify the estimated percentage of American adults with essential hypertension.

1. Answer: C

It is estimated that approximately 30% of American adults have hypertension, which therefore represents the most frequently encountered medical condition in the United States. It is also one of the most significant risk factors for cardiovascular morbidity and mortality. Hypertension cannot be cured, but antihypertensive drug therapy can substantially reduce the risk of cardiovascular event and death.

A, B, D, E See correct answer explanation.

▶ *Learning objective:* Describe the correct blood pressure for a patient older than 60 with no significant concomitant diseases.

2. Answer: B

The JNC 8 report states that the goals for blood pressure lowering are based on age, diabetes mellitus (DM), and chronic kidney disease (CKD) as follows:

▶ Age < 60, no DM, no CKD: 140/90 mm Hg

▶ Age > 60, no DM, no CKD: 150/90 mm Hg

▶ All ages with DM or CKD: 140/90 mm Hg

A.B. is older than 60 with no DM (see blood glucose level) and no CKD (see creatinine and BUN plasma levels). Therefore the goal should be a systolic blood pressure < 150 and a diastolic blood pressure < 90.

A, C, D See correct answer explanation.

▶ *Learning objective:* Identify the organ whose arterial pressure is quite close to the measured mean blood pressure.

3. Answer: B

The heart pumps blood continuously into the aorta. Therefore the mean blood pressure in the aorta is high, averaging about 95 mm Hg. This is quite close to the mean blood pressure in a normal adult. This similarity also holds in cases of hypertension. The measured blood pressure of a hypertensive patient indicates most closely the pressure present in the patient's aorta. As the blood flows into the systemic circulation, its pressure falls progressively to about 0 mm Hg by the time it reaches the termination of the venae cavae in the right atrium of the heart.

A The mean blood pressure in the pulmonary arteries is typically 9 to 18 mm Hg.

C The mean blood pressure in the arterioles is about 50 mm Hg.

D The mean blood pressure in the capillaries is about 30 mm Hg.

E The mean blood pressure in the venules is 12 to 20 mm Hg.

► *Learning objective:* Explain why the baroreceptor reflex is not able to control the blood pressure of a chronic hypertensive patient.

4. Answer: A

The baroreceptor reflex is fully operative even during chronic hypertension but, for still unknown reasons, their set point is changed. In people with chronic hypertension the baroreceptors and their reflexes change, and they function to maintain the elevated blood pressure as if it is normal. In other words, baroreceptors become less sensitive to sudden changes in carotid sinus blood pressure.

B, E The sensitivity range of the baroreceptor reflex is 60 to 180 mm Hg.

C The vasomotor center is fully operative in chronic hypertension.

D The firing rate of the carotid sinus nerve is not compromised in chronic hypertension.

► *Learning objective:* Explain why the mean blood flow does not change in a patient with essential hypertension.

5. Answer: A

When the arterial pressure is suddenly increased, the blood flow increases for 1 to 2 minutes but then decreases to about 15% of the original control value. However, over a period of hours or days a long-term local blood flow regulation develops in addition to the acute regulation, and the blood flow through the tissues gradually comes back almost exactly to the normal value.
Because A.B.'s hypertension likely started more than 1 year previously, it can be concluded that the blood flow was essentially normal.

B, C, D, E See correct answer explanation.

► *Learning objective:* Explain a factor that is thought most important in the pathogenesis of essential hypertension.

6. Answer: B

The patient was diagnosed with essential hypertension. The cause of essential hypertension is still unknown, and it is unlikely that the disease has a single cause. Nevertheless, renal retention of excess sodium is thought to be important in initiating this form of hypertension. In fact the extracellular fluid volume increases in hypertensive patients when exposed to high dietary sodium intake, in spite of the expected natriuretic response. Sodium retention leads to an increased intravascular fluid volume, increased CO, and peripheral vasoconstriction.

A This would occur in pheochromocytoma and causes secondary, not essential, hypertension.

C This would cause primary hyperaldosteronism, which leads to secondary, not essential, hypertension.

D This would cause renovascular hypertension, a form of secondary, not essential, hypertension.

E Increased production of atrial natriuretic factor would reduce sodium retention and therefore would reduce blood volume.

► *Learning objective:* Describe the main cardiovascular determinant of essential hypertension.

7. Answer: D

Blood pressure can be defined by the following: BP = CO × TPR. A.B.'s CO was normal; therefore his hypertension must be due primarily to an increase in TPR, which is the most common cause of essential hypertension.

A, B A.B.'s heart rate and CO were within normal limits.

C Because CO = SV × HR, it can be concluded that stroke volume was also within normal limits.

E Venous return is defined as the flow of blood into the right atrium. In an intact circulation, venous return equals CO in the steady state because the circulation is a closed system of tubes. Because A.B.'s CO was normal, it can be concluded that his venous return was also normal.

▶ *Learning objective:* Identify the power of the vessel radius that is inversely proportional to vessel resistance.

▶ *Learning objective:* Identify the kidney ion transport that was most likely increased by thiazides.

8. Answer: D

According to Poiseuille's equation, blood vessel resistance is inversely proportional to the 4th power of the vessel radius. Because pressure is flow by resistance, a small decrease in vessel radius can cause a significant increase in blood pressure, in order to maintain a normal blood flow. Poiseuille's equation applies only to theoretical rigid, cylindrical tubes with laminar flow. Arterioles are elastic tubes, often with turbulent flow, and autoregulation does occur when flow is changed. Nevertheless Poiseuille's equation points out why narrowing of the arterioles can be such a powerful cause of hypertension.

A, B, C, E See correct answer explanation.

▶ *Learning objective:* Explain the main action that most likely mediates the long-term antihypertensive effect of thiazides.

9. Answer: B

The initial hypotensive effect of thiazides is associated with a reduction in plasma volume and CO. Peripheral vascular resistance is usually unaffected (or sometimes increased).

However, after 4 to 8 weeks of continuous therapy intravascular volume and CO return toward normal, whereas peripheral vascular resistance decreases due to arteriolar vasodilation.

The mechanism of this vasodilation is still poorly understood and is probably multifactorial. Likely a primary factor is related to a thiazide-induced depletion of body Na^+ stores, which leads to a fall in smooth muscle Na^+ concentration. This in turn decreases intracellular Ca^{2+} concentration by activating the Ca^2/Na^+ exchanger. The decreased availability of Ca^{2+} leads to vascular smooth muscle relaxation.

A, C These factors can explain the initial, but not the long-term, antihypertensive effect of thiazides.

D, E Thiazides do not affect angiotensin activity and do not act on the central nervous system (CNS).

10. Answer C

By blocking the Na^+/Cl^- symporter in the early distal tubule, thiazides increase the delivery of Na^+ to the collecting tubule. The consequent increased reabsorption of Na^+ creates a luminal negative potential, which favors both H^+ and K^+ excretion.

A K^+ is 80% reabsorbed in the proximal convolute tubule. Thiazides do not affect this reabsorption.

B All diuretics decrease, not increase, tubular Na^+ reabsorption.

D K^+ excretion in the collecting tubule, not in the proximal convolute tubule, is increased by thiazides.

E H^+ is not reabsorbed, but only excreted, by kidney tubules.

▶ *Learning objective:* Describe the main cardiovascular action that mediates the antihypertensive effect of amlodipine.

11. Answer: C

Dihydropyridine drugs like amlodipine block calcium channels in the smooth muscle cell membrane. This leads to a decrease in the availability of free intracellular calcium and therefore to a vasodilating effect. Vasodilation is limited to the arterioles (the effect on capacitance vessels is negligible) and causes a reduction of SVR, which in turn decreases afterload.

A Decreased central parasympathetic outflow can explain the antihypertensive effect of clonidine.

B Increased venous capacitance can explain the antihypertensive effect of venous vasodilators like nitrates.

D Increased volume of extracellular fluids would cause hypertension, not hypotension.

E Decreased cardiac output can explain the antihypertensive effect of β-blockers.

▶ *Learning objective:* Describe a primary contraindication to the use of ACE inhibitors.

▶ *Learning objective:* Describe the action mediating the antihypertensive effect of clonidine.

12. Answer: B

A previous episode of angioedema is an absolute contraindication to the use of ACE inhibitors. These drugs are known to cause angioneurotic edema in 0.1 to 0.3% of patients. This effect is not dose-related and nearly always develops within the first week of therapy in susceptible patients. Airway obstruction may lead to death. The mechanism of the disorder seems to be related to accumulation of bradykinin produced by these drugs. In fact, when serum levels of C1-INH (a serum alpha-2 globulin molecule and a member of the serpin family of protease inhibitors) falls below 30% of the reference range, whether secondary to decreased production, dysfunction, or destruction, a domino effect occurs, leading to angioedema. C1-INH is a major inhibitor of kallikrein, which converts high molecular weight kininogen to bradykinin. The plasma bradykinin level rises substantially during acute attacks of hereditary, acquired, and ACE inhibitor–induced angioedema. Therefore bradykinin has been proposed as the primary mediator involved in ACE inhibitor–induced angioedema.

Theoretically, angiotensin II receptor antagonists should be less likely than ACE inhibitors to precipitate angioedema because angiotensin II receptor antagonists do not cause accumulation of kinins. However, angioedema has been rarely reported in patients receiving angiotensin II receptor antagonists. Although angiotensin II receptor antagonists have been suggested as potential alternatives to ACE inhibitors for patients at risk of angioedema, the safety of angiotensin II receptor antagonists in patients with a prior history of angioedema has not been definitively established. Therefore some authors have recommended that angiotensin II receptor antagonists should be avoided in patients with a history of angioedema.

A, C, D All these listed disorders do not contraindicate the use of ACE inhibitors.

13. Answer: A

The antihypertensive effect of clonidine is mediated by an action on the CNS. The drug activates presynaptic α_2-adrenoceptors located in the nucleus tractus solitarius and in the rostral ventrolateral medulla. It also activates nonadrenergic binding sites (called imidazoline receptors) located in the rostral ventrolateral medulla. Both actions decrease the firing from the reticulospinal tract, leading to a decreased central adrenergic tone.

B, C Clonidine has negligible effects on these functions.

D, E Clonidine can slightly decrease heart contractility and can dilate the veins, but these actions are consequences of the decreased central sympathetic outflow and play a minor role in clonidine-induced decrease in blood pressure, which is mainly due to arteriolar vasodilation.

▶ *Learning objective:* Describe the most common adverse effects of clonidine.

14. Answer: D

The adverse effects that induced the patient to stop all antihypertensive medications were most likely caused by clonidine, because hydrochlorothiazide and amlodipine were previously used without a problem. Daytime sedation and drowsiness are common adverse effects of clonidine, occurring in up to 50% of patients. The effects are probably related to the CNS depressant action of the drug, which is most likely mediated by the activation of central α_2-adrenoceptors.

A Clonidine can cause hypersensitivity reactions, including angioedema, but the incidence is very rare.

B Clonidine tends to cause xerostomia, not sialorrhea.

C Clonidine tends to cause bradycardia, hence tachypalpitations are unlikely.

E Clonidine can cause fluid retention and edema, but this is a very rare effect of the drug.

▶ *Learning objective:* Identify the drug used to manage the patient's hypertensive crisis.

15. Answer: C

The high blood pressure and signs of heart failure (shortness of breath, increased pulse and respiratory rates, the gallop rhythm) indicate that blood pressure can be immediately life-threatening and must be lowered within a matter of minutes to hours. Fenoldopam is a parenteral, rapid-acting drug used to treat hypertensive emergencies. The half-life of the drug is 5 to 10 minutes, and therefore it should be given by IV infusion.

Other drugs used for the same purpose include nitroprusside, labetalol, and esmolol. However, in this patient the following must be considered:

A Esmolol is contraindicated because of COPD.

B Nitroprusside is contraindicated because of toxic amblyopia.

D, **E**, **F** These drugs are not used to treat hypertensive emergencies.

▶ *Learning objective:* Describe the molecular mechanism of action of the most common drugs used to manage the hypertensive crisis.

16. Answer: E

The two drugs most frequently used for treating hypertensive emergencies in patients with signs of heart failure are nitroprusside and fenoldopam. Given that nitroprusside was contraindicated because of toxic amblyopia, A.B. most likely received fenoldopam, a selective D_1-adrenoceptor agonist. D_1-adrenoceptors are mainly located in the mesenteric and renal vascular beds, and activation of these receptors causes vasodilation, decreased blood pres-

sure, and increased diuresis. The half-life of the drug is 5 to 10 minutes, and therefore it is given by IV infusion.

A This would be the mechanism of action of α_1-adrenoceptors antagonists.

B This would be the mechanism of action of minoxidil.

C This would be the mechanism of action of nitroprusside.

D This would be the mechanism of action of Ca^{2+} channel blockers.

▶ *Learning objective:* Identify the specific reason for the choice of drug used to treat the patient's hypertensive crisis.

17. Answer: E

A.B. most likely received fenoldopam, a selective D_1-adrenoceptor agonist. D_1-adrenoceptors are mainly located in the mesenteric and renal vascular beds, and activation of these receptors causes vasodilation and decreased blood pressure. By activating D_1-adrenoceptors in the kidney, the drug causes kidney vasodilation and increases diuresis. Therefore it may be particularly advantageous in patients with impaired renal function.

A Heart failure is not a specific reason for the choice of fenoldopam because both nitroprusside and fenoldopam, are preferred in patients with hypertensive emergencies accompanied by heart failure.

B Fenoldopam has a very short half-life, but this was not the reason for the choice of the drug.

C The patient's hypertension was refractory, but this was not the reason for the choice of the drug.

D The patient's prostatic hyperplasia was not the reason for the choice of fenoldopam.

Case 14

General Anesthesia

E.G, a 58-year-old man, was admitted to the surgery department for the removal of a newly diagnosed colon cancer. Physical examination revealed a moderately obese patient with a body mass index of 31 and the following vital signs: blood pressure 145/88 mm Hg, pulse 90 bpm, respirations 15/min, temperature 97.9°F (36.6°C). The patient admitted he was quite afraid of the imminent operation.

E.G.'s past medical history was unremarkable except that he had been suffering from severe motion sickness since childhood. One week ago he felt a vague abdominal discomfort in the right lower abdominal quadrant. Two days later he experienced extreme abdominal pain and was admitted to the emergency department. A computed tomographic (CT) scan showed a large tumor mass involving the colon.

The anesthesiologist gave an oral dose of midazolam to control the patient's pain-anticipatory anxiety, and 30 minutes later an intravenous (IV) catheter was inserted. General anesthesia was induced with propofol IV, and E.G. lost consciousness within 30 seconds. Succinylcholine was given IV to facilitate endotracheal intubation, and E.G. was placed on artificial respiration. General anesthesia was maintained by a mixture of inhaled general anesthetics (2% sevoflurane, 50% nitrous oxide, and 48% oxygen) and supplemented by vecuronium. After surgery, sevoflurane and nitrous oxide were discontinued, 100% of pure oxygen was given for a few minutes, and then glycopyrrolate was given IV followed by an IV dose of neostigmine. A few minutes later, E.G. was able to breathe spontaneously and to respond to questions, even if he was still somewhat groggy. After surgery the patient complained of postsurgical pain that was controlled by ketorolac. He did not suffer from nausea and vomiting.

Two days later E.G. showed sudden muscle rigidity, tachypnea, and profuse sweating. His vital signs were as follows: blood pressure 175/95 mm Hg, pulse 125 bpm and irregular, respirations 30/min, temperature 104°F (40°C). Lab tests showed hyperkalemia, hypocalcemia, myoglobinemia, venous blood pH of 4.28, and creatine-kinase of 682 U/L (normal 38–170). A diagnosis of malignant hyperthermia was made, and an emergency therapy was started that included the immediate IV administration of dantrolene.

Questions

1. E.G. underwent general anesthesia that is traditionally subdivided in different stages. Which of the following stages is characterized by disturbed consciousness, mydriasis, irregular respiration, retching, and vomiting?

A. Stage I

B. Stage II

C. Stage III

D. Stage IV

2. Midazolam was given to E.G. Which of the following molecular actions most likely mediated the antianxiety effect of the drug in the patient's disease?

A. Decrease in glutamate-activated Ca^{2+} current

B. Increase in γ-aminobutyric acid (GABA)-activated Cl^- current

C. Decrease in norepinephrine-activated Na^+ current

D. Increase in GABA-activated K^+ current

E. Decrease in acetylcholine-activated Na^+ current

3. Propofol was given to E.G. Which of the following actions on ion channels most likely mediated the anesthetic effect of this drug?

A. Cl^- channel opening

B. Na^+ channel opening

C. K^+ channel blockade

D. Ca^{2+} channel opening

4. Which of the following adverse effects could occur shortly after the administration of propofol?

A. Hyperpnea

B. Increased intracranial pressure

C. Skeletal muscle spasms

D. Urinary incontinence

E. Hypotension

5. Propofol was given to E.G. to induce general anesthesia. Which of the following statements best explains why today IV anesthetics are extensively used for induction of general anesthesia?

A. IV anesthetics prevent postoperative nausea and vomiting.

B. Stages I and II of anesthesia are practically avoided.

C. IV anesthetics cause quick and complete muscle relaxation.

D. All IV anesthetics have pronounced analgesic properties.

E. Stage IV of anesthesia induced by inhalational anesthetics is prevented.

6. Succinylcholine was given to E.G. to facilitate endotracheal intubation. Which of the following phrases best explains the mechanism of muscle relaxant action of succinylcholine?

A. Blockade of acetylcholine release from motor neuron terminals

B. Long-lasting activation of nicotinic muscular (Nm) receptors

C. Competitive blockade of Nm receptors

D. Long-lasting activation of nicotinic neuronal (Nn) receptors

E. Competitive blockade of Nn receptors

7. Sevoflurane was given by inhalatory route to E.G. The drug has a minimum alveolar concentration (MAC) of about 1.8. Which of the following phrases best describes the MAC of an inhalational anesthetic?

A. The blood/gas partition coefficient of the anesthetic

B. The maximal efficacy of the anesthetic

C. The median effective dose (ED50) on a conventional quantal dose–response curve

D. The concentration of anesthetic in the blood

E. The concentration of anesthetic in the inspired air

8. Nitrous oxide was given by inhalatory route to E.G. Which of the following is the MAC of this inhalational anesthetic?

A. 2

B. 4

C. 10

D. 40

E. 80

F. > 100

9. Which of the following actions most likely occurred during E.G.'s surgical anesthesia?

A. Increased cardiac output

B. Bronchoconstriction

C. Decreased pulmonary dead space

D. Decreased systemic vascular resistance

E. Decreased heart rate

F. Coronary vasoconstriction

10. E.G.'s general anesthesia was supplemented by vecuronium. The inhibition of which of the following ion currents most likely mediated the muscle relaxant effect of this drug?

A. K^+ current

B. Na^+ current

C. Cl^- current

D. Ca^{2+} current

E. Mg^{2+} current

11. Vecuronium caused a progressive paralysis of all skeletal muscles. Which of the following pairs of skeletal muscles were most likely the last to be paralyzed?

A. Extraocular muscles–diaphragm

B. Extraocular muscles–pharyngeal muscles

C. Extraocular muscles–intercostal muscles

D. Intercostal muscles–diaphragm

E. Laryngeal muscles–intercostal muscles

F. Laryngeal muscles–diaphragm

12. When sevoflurane and nitrous oxide were discontinued, E.G. regained consciousness in a few minutes. Which of the following properties best explains why anesthetic recovery was so rapid when inhalational administration of both drugs was stopped?

A. Rapid redistribution into lipid tissue

B. Very fast biotransformation

C. Low MAC values of both drugs

D. Low blood/gas partition coefficient of both drugs

E. Preferential concentration of both drugs in the cerebral cortex

13. Neostigmine was given to E.G. after surgery. Which of the following phrases best explains the reason for this treatment?

A. Prevent postoperative adynamic ileus

B. Stimulate the brain respiratory center

C. Speed up the recovery from neuromuscular blockade

D. Restore normal consciousness

E. Counteract postsurgical pain

14. Glycopyrrolate was given a few seconds before neostigmine. Which of the following phrases best explains the reason for this treatment?

A. Counteract some unwanted effects of vecuronium

B. Speed up the elimination of sevoflurane

C. Counteract some unwanted effects of neostigmine

D. Control postsurgical pain

E. Speed up the elimination of nitrous oxide

15. Ketorolac was given to E.G. The analgesic effect of the drug was most likely mediated by a decreased abnormal sensitivity of which of the following neuronal structures?

A. Autonomic neurons

B. Naked nerve terminals

C. Spinal motor neurons

D. Periaqueductal gray area

E. Brain cortex

16. E.G. did not suffer from nausea and vomiting after surgery. Which of the following drugs given to the patient could have prevented this adverse effect?

A. Midazolam

B. Propofol

C. Sevoflurane

D. Nitrous oxide

E. Vecuronium

F. Neostigmine

17. E.G. was diagnosed with malignant hyperthermia. Which of the following pairs of drugs received by the patient most likely triggered this disorder?

A. Sevoflurane–succinylcholine

B. Sevoflurane–neostigmine

C. Propofol–midazolam

D. Propofol–vecuronium

E. Succinylcholine–midazolam

F. Succinylcholine–neostigmine

18. Which of the following ions most likely mediates the symptoms and signs of malignant hyperthermia?

A. Na^+

B. K^+

C. Ca^{2+}

D. Cl^-

E. Mg^{2+}

19. E.G. was treated with IV dantrolene. Which of the following molecular actions most likely mediated the therapeutic effect of the drug in the patient's disorder?

A. Blockade of Ca^{2+} channels in skeletal muscle cell membrane

B. Blockade of excitatory neurotransmitter release in the brain

C. Activation of $GABA_B$ receptors in the spinal cord

D. Activation of $GABA_A$ receptors in the spinal cord

E. Decreased Ca^{2+} current from skeletal muscle sarcoplasmic reticulum

Answers and Explanations

▶ *Learning objective:* Identify the signs that characterize stage II of general anesthesia.

1. Answer: B

The subdivision of general anesthesia in different stages is based on the observation of the patient's overt signs with diethyl ether, an anesthetic no longer used routinely but still employed worldwide in some emergency situations. The progression of these signs is related to the increasing concentration of the anesthetic in the central nervous system (CNS). Stage II (also named the stage of excitement) is characterized by many excitatory symptoms and signs, including delirium and combative behavior. This stage is most likely due to a depression of the brain cortex that removes the inhibitory control of the cortex over several subcortical excitatory structures.

A Stage I includes analgesia (depending on the agent), amnesia, unaltered consciousness, and euphoria.

C Stage III (also named surgical anesthesia) includes unconsciousness, muscle relaxation (depending on the agent), regular respiration, miosis, and decreasing eye movements.

D Stage IV (also named medullary depression) includes mydriasis, no eye movements, respiratory arrest, and cardiovascular collapse.

▶ *Learning objective:* Describe the molecular action that most likely mediates the antianxiety effect of midazolam.

2. Answer: B

Benzodiazepines bind to receptors located at the interface between alpha and gamma subunits of the $GABA_A$ receptor–chloride ion channel macromolecular complex. The binding increases the affinity of the $GABA_A$ receptor for GABA, which in turn causes an increased frequency of chloride channel opening. Because the extracellular chloride concentration is about 120 mM and the intracellular chloride concentration is about 20 mM, chloride channel opening will increase the inward Cl⁻ current. This in turn will increase the negative charges inside the cell, causing hyperpolarization of the cell membrane.

A This would be the mechanism of action of nitrous oxide.

C This would be the mechanism of action of central presynaptic adrenergic agonists (e.g., clonidine).

D This would be the mechanism of action of baclofen.

E This would be the mechanism of action of central cholinergic antagonists (e.g., scopolamine).

▶ *Learning objective:* Identify the ion channel action that most likely mediates the anesthetic effect of propofol.

3. Answer: A

Propofol is the short-acting IV general anesthetic most frequently used for anesthesia induction in the United States. Its mechanism of action is thought to be very close to that of barbiturates. It increases the affinity of the GABA$_A$ receptors for GABA, which in turn causes an increased frequency of Cl⁻ channel opening. At high doses it can cause direct opening of Cl⁻ channels in the absence of GABA.

B Na⁺ channel opening would cause depolarization of cell membranes, and therefore an excitatory, not a depressive, effect on the CNS.

C K⁺ channel blockade would cause depolarization of cell membranes, and therefore an excitatory, not a depressive, effect on the CNS.

D Ca²⁺ channel opening would cause depolarization of cell membranes, and therefore an excitatory, not a depressive, effect on the CNS.

▶ *Learning objective:* Describe an adverse effect that could occur shortly after the administration of propofol.

4. Answer: E

Propofol produces a dose-dependent decrease in blood pressure that is significantly greater than that induced by all the other IV anesthetics. This decrease is a result of profound vasodilation in both arterial and venous circulation.

A IV anesthetics like propofol tend to cause a dose-dependent decrease of respiratory rate. Apnea, not hyperpnea, can occur in up to 40% of cases, requiring assisted ventilation.

B Intracranial pressure is usually decreased, not increased.

C A dose-dependent decrease in skeletal muscle tone is an action common to most general anesthetics.

D Propofol tends to cause urinary retention, not urinary incontinence.

▶ *Learning objective:* Explain the main reason for the extensive use of IV anesthetic in general anesthesia.

5. Answer: B

Most IV anesthetics cause unconsciousness in 10 to 40 seconds. The loss of consciousness is the most important sign that starts stage III of general anesthesia; therefore this stage is reached almost immediately after the IV injection. Thus stage I and II are practically avoided, and, because stage II is very disturbing for the patient, IV anesthetics represent a significant advancement in the procedure of general anesthesia. Today IV anesthetics are almost always used for induction when long general anesthesia is needed or as the sole anesthetic for short anesthetic procedures.

A All IV anesthetics, except propofol, can cause nausea and vomiting.

C Most IV anesthetics cause incomplete muscle relaxation. Even inhalational anesthetics rarely cause complete muscular relaxation, which explains the concomitant use of neuromuscular blocking drugs to provide additional insurance of immobility.

D With the exception of ketamine neither parenteral nor currently available fluorinated inhalational anesthetics are effective analgesics.

E IV anesthetics cannot prevent stage IV of general anesthesia, which can be induced by an excessive dose of inhalational anesthetics.

▶ *Learning objective:* Explain the molecular mechanism of action of succinylcholine.

6. Answer: B

Succinylcholine is a depolarizing neuromuscular blocking drug. It acts as a cholinergic agonist at Nm receptors. Therefore, the cation channels open and cause depolarization of the motor end plate, but because the drug is not metabolized as fast as acetylcholine, the activation of Nm receptors is long lasting. This long-lasting activation causes a long-lasting depolarization of the motor end plate, which remains unresponsive to subsequent stimuli (depolarizing blockade). Because the end plate membrane requires repolarization and repetitive firing to maintain muscle tension, a flaccid paralysis results.

A Blockade of acetylcholine release from motor neuron terminals would be the mechanism of action of botulinum toxin.

C Competitive blockade of Nm receptors would be the mechanism of action of nondepolarizing neuromuscular blocking drugs (e.g., tubocurarine).

D Long-lasting activation of Nn receptors would be the mechanism of action of high doses of nicotine.

E Competitive blockade of Nn receptors would be the mechanism of action of ganglionic blockers (e.g., mecamylamine).

▶ *Learning objective:* Explain the meaning of the MAC of an inhalational anesthetic.

7. Answer: C

The MAC is defined as the alveolar concentration of an inhaled anesthetic that results in the immobility of 50% of patients when exposed to a supramaximal noxious stimulus. Thus MAC represents the ED_{50} on a conventional quantal dose–response curve and is therefore a measure of the potency of the inhaled anesthetic.

A The blood/gas partition coefficient of the anesthetic is not the MAC. However, this coefficient is usually inversely proportional to the MAC.

B The MAC is a measure of the potency, not the efficacy, of inhaled anesthetics.

D The MAC is not a measure of the concentration of anesthetic in the blood.

E The MAC is not a measure of the concentration of anesthetic in the inspired air.

▶ *Learning objective:* Identify the MAC of nitrous oxide.

8. Answer: F

Nitrous oxide has an MAC > 100. This means that even when all the molecules of the inspired gas are molecules of the anesthetic, the concentration is not able to cause immobility in 50% of patients. The fact that, in spite of the very poor anesthetic potency, nitrous oxide is extensively used in combination with halogenated inhalational anesthetics can be explained by the following properties:

▶ The drug has a low toxicity and can cause very good analgesia even with 20% concentration.
▶ The MACs of all inhalational anesthetics are additive. Because the MAC reflects an adequate dose for only 50% of patients, successful clinical anesthesia may require 0.5 to 2.0 MAC for individual patients. More than 90% of all patients become anesthetized following the administration of 1.3 MAC, and, presumably, 1.5 to 2.0 MAC is required to ensure anesthesia in all patients. This means that, for example, 0.5 MAC of nitrous oxide plus 1.2 MAC of sevoflurane can provide general anesthesia in most patients.

A, B, C, D, E See correct answer explanation.

▶ *Learning objective:* Identify a physiological effect that most likely occurs during general anesthesia maintained with sevoflurane and nitrous oxide.

9. Answer: D

E.G.'s surgical anesthesia was maintained by sevoflurane and nitrous oxide. All fluorinated inhalational anesthetics like sevoflurane cause vasodilation in most vascular beds. Nitrous oxide causes little effect on systemic vascular resistance, because it causes an activation of the sympathetic nervous system that counteracts its direct depressant effect.

A Cardiac output is decreased by sevoflurane and not much affected by nitrous oxide.

B, C All halogenated anesthetics, as well as nitrous oxide, cause bronchodilation, not bronchoconstriction, and therefore the pulmonary dead space is increased, not decreased.

E, F Sevoflurane does not cause bradycardia and does not affect coronary vessel tone. Nitrous oxide causes an activation of the sympathetic nervous system causing, if anything, effects opposite to those listed.

▶ *Learning objective:* Identify the inhibition of the ion current that most likely mediated the muscle relaxant effect of vecuronium.

10. Answer: B

Vecuronium is a nondepolarizing skeletal muscle relaxant. These drugs block competitively Nm acetylcholine receptors. The Nm receptors are ionotropic (i.e., they form part of a ligand-gated cation channel). Binding of acetylcholine to these receptors causes opening of the channel, which is permeable to both Na^+ and K^+. Because the resting potential of the muscle plasma membrane is near the potassium equilibrium potential, opening of acetylcholine receptor channels causes little increase in the efflux of K^+ ions. Na^+ ions, on the other hand, flow into the muscle cell, producing a net depolarization to about −15 mV from the muscle resting potential of −85 to −90 mV. This depolarization of the muscle membrane generates an action potential, which is conducted along the membrane surface via voltage-gated Na^+ channels, initiating the signal transduction pathway leading to skeletal muscle contraction. By blocking Nm receptors, the drug primarily inhibits Na^+ current through ligand-gated cation channels, leading to muscle relaxation.

A, C, D, E All these currents are not involved in the mechanism of action of nondepolarizing neuromuscular blockers.

▶ *Learning objective:* Identify the pairs of skeletal muscles that are the last to be paralyzed by vecuronium.

11. Answer: D

The action of nondepolarizing skeletal blocking agents progresses from motor weakness to a total flaccid paralysis. Small, rapidly moving muscles, such as those of the eye, jaw, and larynx, relax before those of the limbs and trunk. Ultimately the intercostal muscles and finally the diaphragm are paralyzed. Recovery of muscle function usually occurs in the reverse order to that of their paralysis, and the diaphragm ordinarily is the first muscle to regain function.

A, B, C, E, F Extraocular muscles and laryngeal muscles are the first, not the last, to be paralyzed.

▶ *Learning objective:* Explain the main reason for the rapid recovery from general anesthesia maintained by sevoflurane and nitrous oxide.

12. Answer: D

One of the most important factors impacting both the rate of induction and the recovery from anesthesia is the blood/gas partition coefficient of the anesthetic agent, which indicates the solubility of the anesthetic in blood. The reason for this importance can be explained by the following facts:

▶ The partial pressure of a gas in a gas mixture is the portion of the total pressure that is supplied by that gas.
▶ A gas moves from one compartment to another within the body according to its partial pressure gradient.
▶ The more soluble an anesthetic is in blood, the more of it must be dissolved in blood to raise its partial pressure. In other words, the blood acts as an inactive reservoir that is bigger for more soluble anesthetics and smaller for less soluble anesthetics.
▶ Induction of inhalation anesthesia depends on the time needed to achieve an optimal partial pressure of the anesthetic in the brain.

- ▶ Recovery from inhalation anesthesia depends on the rate of elimination of the anesthetic from the brain.
- ▶ When the administration of the anesthetic gas is discontinued, the drug must go from the brain into the blood and from the blood into the expired air. This transfer is longer for more soluble drugs (it takes more time to fill the blood reservoir) and shorter for less soluble drugs. Therefore, the higher the blood/gas partition coefficient, the slower the induction and recovery from anesthesia.

The blood/gas partition coefficient of sevoflurane is 0.65, whereas that of nitrous oxide is 0.47. Since both coefficients are low, both anesthetics cause a rapid anesthetic recovery.

A Redistribution can be a factor that speeds up the recovery from anesthesia, but both anesthetics have a low lipid solubility, and therefore redistribution into lipid tissue is minimal.

B Biotransformation of sevoflurane is very low (~ 3%), and that of nitrous oxide is zero.

C The MAC of an inhalational anesthetic is a measure of the potency of the drug; namely, it is a pharmacodynamic variable. The speed of induction is dependent upon pharmacokinetic variables.

E Inhalational anesthetics distribute uniformly into the brain. They are not concentrated in a specific region of the brain, even if different parts of the brain have different sensitivity to the action of inhalational anesthetics

- ▶ *Learning objective:* Explain the reason for the administration of neostigmine after general anesthesia supplemented by vecuronium.

13.   Answer: C

Reversible cholinesterase inhibitors, such as neostigmine, can reverse the paralysis induced by nondepolarizing neuromuscular blocking drugs, such as vecuronium. The drug blocks Nm receptors at the motor end plate, whereas acetylcholine activates these receptors. The two drugs competitively antagonize each other, and the increased concentration of acetylcholine brought about by cholinesterase inhibitors can therefore reverse the muscle paralysis induced by vecuronium. This antagonism is exploited clinically, and reversible cholinesterase inhibitors are often used to speed up the recovery from the neuromuscular blockade remaining after completion of surgery. Neostigmine is the preferred drug, because it does not enter the brain and is therefore free of central adverse effects.

A Cholinesterase inhibitors are sometimes used to prevent postoperative ileus, but they are given 2 to 4 days after the operation when abdominal peristalsis is not resumed.

B, D Neostigmine cannot cross the blood–brain barrier and therefore is devoid of central effects.

E Neostigmine has no analgesic action.

- ▶ *Learning objective:* Explain the reason for glycopyrrolate administration after surgery.

14.   Answer: C

Neostigmine is a reversible cholinesterase inhibitor. These drugs will increase acetylcholine at all peripheral cholinergic synapses, causing several unwanted muscarinic effects. These effects can be counteracted by the administration of an antimuscarinic drug that is given routinely just before the neostigmine administration. Glycopyrrolate is a quaternary compound that effectively antagonizes muscarinic effects of acetylcholine and, to a lesser extent, nicotinic effects. It is usually preferred to atropine in the postsurgical setting because its onset and duration of action are shorter than those of atropine and quite close to those of neostigmine.

A Neostigmine, not glycopyrrolate, is given to counteract some unwanted effects of vecuronium.

B Sevoflurane elimination depends on the physicochemical features of the drug and cannot be increased by glycopyrrolate administration.

D Glycopyrrolate has no analgesic effects and cannot control postsurgical pain.

E Nitrous oxide elimination depends on the physicochemical features of the drug and cannot be increased by glycopyrrolate administration.

15. Answer: B

Ketorolac is a nonsteroidal anti-inflammatory drug (NSAID) that inhibits prostaglandin biosynthesis. Prostaglandins are endogenous compounds that are released from the damaged tissues and can sensitize nociceptors, causing pain.

Nociceptors are naked nerve endings found in almost every tissue of the body. By inhibiting prostaglandin biosynthesis in the damaged area, NSAIDs cause a decrease in the abnormal hypersensitivity of these nerve endings, leading to an analgesic effect. Ketorolac is an effective analgesic but only a moderately effective anti-inflammatory drug. Its analgesic efficacy seems greater than that of most other NSAIDs and is thought to be equivalent to a standard dose of opioids when the pain is acute and not excruciating.

A, C Autonomic and motor neurons are efferent neurons and therefore are not involved in pain sensation.

D, E Periaqueductal gray area and brain cortex are involved in pain sensation, but their sensitivity is not altered by prostaglandins.

16. Answer: B

All inhalational and most IV anesthetics can cause postoperative nausea and vomiting in about 15 to 30% of patients. E.G. was at increased risk of this adverse effect because of his history of motion sickness. Propofol is the only IV anesthetic that has antiemetic properties. Several studies have showed that the median plasma concentration of the drug associated with an antiemetic response was much lower than the one associated with general anesthesia, allowing the drug to have antiemetic properties even in the subhypnotic dose range. A very large meta-analysis has shown that propofol, when compared to thiopental for induction of anesthesia, resulted in an

18% reduction in postoperative nausea and vomiting.

A Midazolam is a benzodiazepine drug. These drugs can have mild antiemetic activity, but midazolam was not the primary drug that prevented the patient's nausea and vomiting.

C, D, E, F All these agents can cause, not prevent, postoperative nausea and vomiting.

17. Answer: A

Malignant hyperthermia is a life-threatening elevation of body temperature that can result from a hypermetabolic response to concurrent use of succinylcholine and a halogenated inhalational anesthetic. The syndrome is very rare (the incidence during general anesthesia is estimated to range from 1/5,000 to 1/50,000 individuals) but has a mortality rate of more than 60%, if untreated. Malignant hyperthermia susceptibility is inherited as an autosomal dominant disorder due to a mutation in the gene encoding the skeletal muscle ryanodine receptor. The syndrome may develop during anesthesia or in the early postoperative period, as in the present case.

B, C, D, E, F These drugs (midazolam, neostigmine, vecuronium, propofol) do not cause malignant hyperthermia.

18. Answer: C

The pathogenesis of malignant hyperthermia is thought to involve a mutation in the gene encoding the skeletal muscle ryanodine receptor, which is a ligand-gated Ca^{2+} channel responsible for the regulation of Ca^{2+} release from the sarcoplasmic reticulum. This mutation would result in an excessive release of Ca^{2+}, which would be the main cause of the symptoms and signs of the disorder.

A, B, D, E See correct answer explanation.

19.   Answer: E

Malignant hyperthermia is thought to result from an excessive release of Ca^{2+} through skeletal muscle sarcoplasmic Ca^{2+} channels (named ryanodine receptors). This causes massive muscle contraction, hyperthermia, and lactic acidosis. Dantrolene is a drug of choice in this disorder, because it blocks Ca^{2+} channels in skeletal muscle sarcoplasmic reticulum, thus preventing the massive release of the ion. Cardiac and smooth muscle are minimally affected by dantrolene, because they have a different type of Ca^{2+} channel in their sarcoplasmic reticulum.

A Dantrolene blocks Ca^{2+} channels in the sarcoplasmic reticulum, not in the cell membrane of skeletal muscle.

B Dantrolene can enter the brain and has mild sedative activity, but this is not the mechanism of its therapeutic effect in malignant hyperthermia.

C Activation of $GABA_B$ receptors in the spinal cord would be the mechanism of action of baclofen, a centrally acting spasmolytic drug.

D Activation of $GABA_A$ receptors in the spinal cord would be the mechanism of action of benzodiazepines.

Case 15

Glaucoma

O.P., a 72-year-old African American woman, visited her ophthalmologist's office for a routine ophthalmic examination. The patient had a history of heavy smoking, hypertension for 8 years, type 2 diabetes mellitus for 12 years, and chronic obstructive pulmonary disease (COPD) for 10 hears. Recently she developed urinary incontinence due to an overactive bladder syndrome. Family history indicated that both parents suffered from open-angle glaucoma.

O.P.'s medications included hydrochlorothiazide and losartan for hypertension, glyburide for diabetes, ipratropium and albuterol for COPD, and darifenacin for urinary incontinence.

Pertinent eye exam results were as follows:

Tonometry

▸ Intraocular pressure in the right eye: 28 mm Hg (normal < 20)
▸ Intraocular pressure in the left eye: 32 mm Hg

Ophthalmoscopy

Enlarged cupping of the optic disc in both eyes and loss of vision in the superior portion of the visual field. Pupils were normal in both eyes, and gonioscopy indicated that the anterior chambers were open in both eyes. There were no signs of cataract formation.

A diagnosis of open-angle glaucoma was made, and the ophthalmologist prescribed eye drops of latanoprost once daily. He also suggested discontinuing a drug the patient was taking because it could have contributed to the increased intraocular pressure.

Three weeks later O.P. returned to the ophthalmologist's office for another visit. Her intraocular pressure measured 24 mm Hg in the right eye and 28 mm Hg in the left eye. The patient denied noncompliance and side effects. The ophthalmologist decided to add a second drug to the therapy and prescribed apraclonidine eye drops. One week later O.P. complained to her ophthalmologist that apraclonidine caused red eyes, ocular pruritus, lacrimation, and foreign body sensation. The doctor substituted apraclonidine with dorzolamide eye drops. The new therapy worked well, and O.P.'s intraocular pressure went back to 18 mm Hg in both eyes.

However, 2 months later O.P. presented to the ophthalmologist's office complaining of haloes around lights, loss of vision, nausea, and extreme eye pain. Eye examination showed an intensely red left eye, corneal edema, and a mildly dilated pupil that reacted poorly to light. Tonometry measured an intraocular pressure of 24 mm Hg in the right eye and 40 mm Hg in the left eye.

A diagnosis of acute angle-closure glaucoma was made and an emergency therapy was started. O.P. was given eye drops of apraclonidine and pilocarpine to the affected eye and an intravenous (IV) injection of mannitol.

Questions

1. O.P. was diagnosed with open-angle glaucoma. Which of the following is the most common initial symptom of this disease?

A. Miosis

B. Visual field loss

C. Myopia

D. Presbyopia

E. Astigmatism

F. Color blindness

2. The elevated IOP in glaucoma is primarily related to increased aqueous humor production and/or decreased outflow. Which of the following eye structures is the site of the production of aqueous humor?

A. Ciliary muscle

B. Radial muscle of iris

C. Sphincter muscle of iris

D. Ciliary epithelium

E. Trabecular meshwork

F. Zonula fibers

3. Aqueous humor production is under the control of the autonomic nervous system. Activation of which of the following autonomic receptors in the eye most likely decreases the production of aqueous humor?

A. Nicotinic neuronal receptors

B. β_2-adrenoceptors

C. α_2-adrenoceptors

D. Muscarinic M_3 receptors

E. β_1-adrenoceptors

4. In the eye, aqueous humor outflow can occur through two different pathways. Which of the following represents the primary route for this outflow?

A. Posterior chamber → trabecular meshwork → pupil → choroidal vessels

B. Posterior chamber → pupil → anterior chamber → Schlemm's canal

C. Posterior chamber → pupil→ choroidal vessels → Schlemm's canal

D. Anterior chamber → pupil → choroidal vessels → trabecular meshwork

E. Anterior chamber → trabecular meshwork → Schlemm's canal → choroidal vessels

F. Anterior chamber→ choroidal vessels→ trabecular meshwork → Schlemm's canal

5. In the eye which of the following is the secondary route of aqueous humor outflow?

A. The trabecular meshwork route

B. The posterior chamber route

C. The iris route

D. The uveoscleral route

E. The retinal route

6. The intrinsic eye muscles that regulate the pupil diameter and the lens curvature are under the control of autonomic receptors. Which of the following correctly pairs the intrinsic eye muscle with the primary receptor that controls it?

A. Sphincter muscle of iris–α_1-adrenoceptors

B. Radial muscle of iris–muscarinic M_3 receptors

C. Ciliary muscle-α_1-adrenoceptors

D. Sphincter muscle of iris–β_1-adrenoceptors

E. Radial muscle of iris–β_1-adrenoceptors

F. Ciliary muscle–muscarinic M_3 receptors

7. During the first visit, latanoprost was prescribed to O.P. Which of the following molecular actions most likely mediated the therapeutic effect of the drug in the patient's disease?

A. β-adrenoceptor blockade

B. α_2-adrenoceptor blockade

C. Prostaglandin receptor activation

D. Inhibition of cholinesterase

E. Muscarinic M_3-receptor activation

F. Inhibition of carbonic anhydrase

8. Which of the following actions on aqueous humor most likely mediated the therapeutic effect of latanoprost in the patient's disease?

A. Increased outflow through the Schlemm's canal

B. Decreased production by the ciliary epithelium

C. Increased outflow through the uveoscleral route

D. Decreased production by eye vessel constriction

E. Increased outflow through the trabecular meshwork

9. The ophthalmologist suggested discontinuing a drug the patient was taking because it could have contributed to the increased IOP. Which of the following drugs taken by O.P. could have contributed to her IOP?

A. Ipratropium

B. Hydrochlorothiazide

C. Losartan

D. Darifenacin

E. Glyburide

F. Albuterol

10. O.P. was prescribed brimonidine. Which of the following molecular actions most likely mediated the therapeutic effect of the drug in the patient's disease?

A. Activation of muscarinic M_3 receptors

B. Activation of β_2-adrenoceptors

C. Activation of α_2-adrenoceptors

D. Blockade of muscarinic M_3 receptors

E. Blockade of β_2-adrenoceptors

F. Blockade of α_2-adrenoceptors

11. O.P. was prescribed dorzolamide. Which of the following molecular actions most likely mediated the therapeutic effect of the drug in the patient's disease?

A. Decreased diffusion of CO_2 across the ciliary epithelium

B. Decreased HCO_3^- synthesis in the ciliary epithelium

C. Dilation of conjunctival vessels

D. Increased outflow of HCO_3^- through the uveoscleral route

E. Increased outflow of HCO_3^- through the Schlemm's canal

F. Contraction of the radial muscle of the iris

12. During the emergency therapy, O.P. was given eyedrops of apraclonidine. Which of the following is most likely the primary site of action of this drug?

A. Ciliary epithelium

B. Radial muscle of the iris

C. Sphincter muscle of the iris

D. Trabecular meshwork

E. Schlemm's canal

F. Ciliary muscle

13. During the emergency therapy, O.P. was given eyedrops of pilocarpine. Which of the following molecular actions most likely mediated the therapeutic effect of the drug in the patient's disease?

A. Activation of muscarinic M_3 receptors

B. Activation of β_2-adrenoceptors

C. Activation of α_2-adrenoceptors

D. Blockade of muscarinic M_3 receptors

E. Blockade of β_2-adrenoceptors

F. Blockade of α_2-adrenoceptors

14. O.P. was given an IV injection of mannitol. Which of the following actions most likely mediated the therapeutic effect of the drug in the patient's disease?

A. Dilation of Schlemm's canal

B. Constriction of the conjunctival vessels

C. Increased plasma osmolarity

D. Decreased aqueous humor production

E. Increased iris-corneal angle

Answers and Explanations

▶ *Learning objective:* Identify the most common initial symptom of open-angle glaucoma.

---

1. Answer: B

Glaucomas are a group of eye disorders characterized by progressive optical nerve damage at least partly due to elevated intraocular pressure (IOP). Glaucoma is more accurately defined as an optic neuropathy with progressive loss of retinal ganglion cells, which is manifested initially as visual field loss and, ultimately, irreversible blindness if left untreated.

Glaucomas are categorized as open-angle and closed-angle (angle-closure). The "angles" referred to are the angles formed by the junction of the iris and cornea at the periphery of the anterior chamber. The normal anterior chamber angle provides drainage for the aqueous humor. When this drainage pathway is narrowed or closed, inadequate drainage leads to elevated intraocular pressure and damage to the optic nerve.

▶ **Open-angle glaucoma** is a syndrome characterized by progressive peripheral visual field loss followed by central field loss associated with an open anterior chamber angle and often, but not always, accompanied by an elevated IOP. In fact approximately 15% of patients with open-angle glaucoma have a consistently normal IOP (i.e., < 20 mm Hg). Open-angle glaucoma accounts for about 90% of glaucomas in the United States.

▶ **Angle-closure glaucoma** is associated with narrowing or closure of the anterior chamber angle that may be chronic or, rarely, acute. In people with narrow angles, the distance between the pupillary iris and the lens is also very narrow. When the iris dilates, forces pull it centripetally and posteriorly, causing iris–lens contact, which prevents aqueous from passing between the lens and iris into the anterior chamber (this mechanism is termed pupillary block). Angle-closure glaucoma has a higher incidence in individuals of Inuit and Chinese descent. Because of the higher frequency in populous Asia, angle-closure glaucoma accounts for about 30% of glaucomas worldwide.

Glaucoma is the third most common cause of blindness worldwide. It can occur at any age but is six times more common among people over 60. In addition to older age, the main risk factors for glaucoma include elevated IOP, black race, family history, diabetes, and hypertension. All these risk factors occurred in the present case.

A Miosis is not a symptom of glaucoma, but drug-induced miosis can decrease the IOP in glaucoma patients.

C Myopia is not a symptom of glaucoma, but it can be a risk factor for glaucoma.

D Presbyopia is a condition associated with aging of the eye that results in progressively worsening ability to focus clearly on close objects. The cause is lens hardening that prevents increases in lens curvature. Presbyopia is not a symptom of glaucoma.

E Astigmatism is a type of refractive error in which the eye does not focus light evenly on the retina. This results in distorted or blurred vision at all distances. Astigmatism is not a symptom of glaucoma.

F Color blindness is the decreased ability to see color or differences in color. It is not a symptom of glaucoma.

▶ *Learning objective:* Describe the eye structure that is the site of the production of aqueous humor.

2. Answer: D

The ciliary body is the part of the eye that includes the ciliary muscle and the ciliary epithelium. This epithelium extends forward from the anterior end of the choroid to the root of the iris (~ 6 mm). It consists of a corrugated anterior zone, the pars plicata (2 mm), and a flattened posterior zone, the pars plana (4 mm). The ciliary processes arise from the pars plicata. They are composed mainly of capillaries and veins that drain through the vortex veins. The capillaries are large and fenestrated. The ciliary epithelium covering the ciliary processes is responsible for the formation of aqueous humor.

A The ciliary muscle is the intrinsic eye muscle that control the lens curvature. It is part of the ciliary body.

B The radial muscle of iris (also called the iris dilator muscle, pupil dilator muscle, pupillary dilator), is a smooth muscle of the eye, running radially in the iris. It consists of contractile cells called myoepithelial cells. When stimulated, these cells contract, widening the pupil.

C The sphincter muscle of the iris (also called the pupillary sphincter, pupillary constrictor, circular muscle of the iris) is a smooth muscle of the eye that runs circularly around the iris. It encircles the pupil of the iris, and its contraction constricts of the pupil.

E The trabecular meshwork is an area of tissue in the eye located around the base of the cornea, near the ciliary body, and is responsible for draining the aqueous humor from the eye via the anterior chamber

F The zonula fibers are a ring of fibrous strands connecting the ciliary body with the lens of the eye. These fibers are sometimes collectively referred to as the suspensory ligaments of the lens.

▶ *Learning objective:* Identify the eye autonomic receptors that mediate the decreased production of aqueous humor.

3. Answer: C

In the eye aqueous humor production by ciliary epithelium is primarily under the control of the sympathetic nervous system. The activation of α_2-adrenoceptors decreases the production of aqueous humor, whereas the activation of β_2-adrenoceptors (and to a lesser extent activation of β1-adrenoceptors) increases it.

A Nicotinic neuronal receptors are located in the autonomic ganglia. They do not control the production of aqueous humor.

B Activation of β_2-adrenoceptors increases, not decreases, the production of aqueous humor.

D Muscarinic M_3 receptors in the eye are located primarily on sphincter muscle of the iris and control the pupillary diameter.

E Activation of β_1-adrenoceptors increases, not decreases, the production of aqueous humor.

▶ *Learning objective:* Describe the primary pathway for eye aqueous humor outflow.

4. Answer: B

The aqueous humor is secreted by the ciliary epithelium into the posterior chamber of the eye. From there it flows through the pupil to reach the anterior chamber, and then it outflows through the trabecular meshwork and the Schlemm's canal.

A, C, D, E, F See correct answer explanation.

▶ *Learning objective:* Identify the secondary route for eye aqueous humor outflow.

5. Answer: D

About 5 to 20% of the aqueous humor drains through the uveoscleral route. Unlike the trabecular outflow route, the uveoscleral outflow route is not a distinctive pathway with pores and channels. Rather, it is a route whereby aqueous humor seeps through, around, and between tissues, including the supraciliary space, ciliary muscle, suprachoroidal space, choroidal vessels, emissarial canals, sclera, and lymphatic vessels.

A The trabecular meshwork route is the primary, not secondary, route of aqueous humor outflow.

B, C, E The aqueous humor cannot outflow through these routes.

▶ *Learning objective:* Identify the intrinsic eye muscle and the primary receptor that controls it.

6. Answer: F

The autonomic control of the eye intrinsic muscle is the following:

The sphincter muscle of iris is primarily controlled by muscarinic M_3 receptors. The activation of these receptors causes miosis.

The radial muscle of iris is primarily controlled by α_1-adrenoceptors. The activation of these receptors causes mydriasis.

The ciliary muscle is primarily controlled by muscarinic M_3 receptors. The activation of these receptors causes increased lens curvature, which accommodates the eyes for near vision.

A, B, C, D, E See correct answer explanation.

▶ *Learning objective:* Identify the molecular mechanism of action of latanoprost in glaucoma.

7. Answer: C

Latanoprost is a prostaglandin $F_{2\alpha}$ analogue. Prostaglandins have largely replaced β-blockers as first-line agents for the therapy of glaucoma, because they are at least as effective as β-blockers and are associated with minimal systemic adverse effects. They have additive effects when administered with carbonic anhydrase inhibitors and α_2-adrenoceptor agonists.

Moreover, β-blockers are contraindicated in the present case because of COPD. Systemic absorption after topical administration does occur and can worsen bronchoconstriction by blocking bronchial β_2-adrenoceptors.

A The β-adrenoceptor blockade would be the mechanism of antiglaucoma action of beta-blockers.

B The α_2-adrenoceptor blockade would increase, not decrease, the production of aqueous humor.

D By increasing acetylcholine availability, cholinesterase inhibitors were used in the past to increase aqueous humor outflow in glaucoma patients.

E Muscarinic M_3 receptor activation is the mechanism of action of cholinergic drugs (e.g., pilocarpine), sometimes used to increase aqueous humor outflow in glaucoma patients.

F Inhibition of carbonic anhydrase is the mechanism of action of carbonic anhydrase inhibitors (e.g., dorzolamide), used to decrease aqueous humor production in glaucoma patients.

▶ *Learning objective:* Identify the action on aqueous humor that is mediated by latanoprost.

8. Answer: C

Latanoprost is a prostaglandin $F_{2\alpha}$ analogue. Prostaglandins lower the IOP primarily by increasing the outflow of the aqueous humor through the uveoscleral route.

A, E This would be the mechanism of action of cholinergic drugs.

B This would be the mechanism of action of β-blockers or alphaα_2-agonists.

D This would be the mechanism of action of α-agonists (e.g., epinephrine or phenylephrine).

▶ *Learning objective:* Identify a drug that can increase the IOP.

9. Answer: D

Darifenacin is an antimuscarinic drug that blocks mainly M3 receptors. By blocking these receptors in the ciliary muscle, the drug can cause relaxation of the muscle, which in turn squeezes the pores of the trabecular meshwork, thereby hindering the outflow of the aqueous humor into the Schlemm's canal. The decreased outflow raises the IOP.

A Ipratropium is an antimuscarinic drug but it is given by inhalatory route and has very low lipid solubility. Therefore systemic absorption is negligible.

B Thiazide diuretics like hydrochlorothiazide do not affect IOP. The two diuretic subclasses that can decrease, not increase, IOP are carbonic anhydrase inhibitors and osmotic diuretics.

C Losartan is an angiotensin receptor antagonist. It does not affect IOP.

E Glyburide is a sulfonylurea derivative used as an oral antidiabetic agent. It does not affect IOP.

F Albuterol is a β2-adrenoceptor agonist. Even if β2-adrenoceptor activation could increase the production of aqueous humor, the drug is not contraindicated in glaucoma.

▶ *Learning objective:* Describe the molecular mechanism of action of brimonidine in glaucoma.

10. Answer: C

Brimonidine is an α_2-adrenoceptor agonist. Activation of α_2-adrenoceptors in the ciliary epithelium causes a decreased production of aqueous humor, and α_2-adrenoceptor agonists are used in glaucoma as alternative agents or as an adjunctive therapy. They have additive effects when given concomitantly with prostaglandins, as in the present case.

A, B, D, E, F See correct answer explanation.

▶ *Learning objective:* Describe the molecular mechanism of action of dorzolamide in glaucoma.

11. Answer: B

Dorzolamide is a carbonic anhydrase inhibitor used as a second-line agent in open-angle glaucoma. The rationale for the use of carbonic anhydrase inhibitors in open-angle glaucoma is based on the fact that aqueous humor is rich in bicarbonate. By inhibiting carbonic anhydrase in ciliary epithelium, bicarbonate synthesis is decreased.

A CO_2 can diffuse freely through most tissues.

C, F Dorzolamide has no action on conjunctival vessels or the iris muscle.

D, E Dorzolamide has no direct action on bicarbonate outflow. Because production is decreased, outflow, if any, should be decreased, not increased.

▶ *Learning objective:* Identify the site of action of apraclonidine in the eye.

12. Answer: A

Acute angle-closure glaucoma is a medical emergency. Treatment must be initiated immediately, because vision can be lost quickly and permanently. The emergency therapy involves the use of several drugs with different mechanisms of action in order to achieve additive effects. Apraclonidine is the α_2-adrenoceptor agonist most frequently used in the acute treatment of angle-closure glaucoma. Activation of α_2-adrenoceptors in ciliary epithelium causes a decreased production of aqueous humor.

B, D, E, F See correct answer explanation.

▶ *Learning objective:* Describe the molecular mechanism of action of pilocarpine in glaucoma.

13. Answer: A

Pilocarpine is a muscarinic agonist. Activation of M_3 receptors causes contraction of the sphincter muscle of the iris and the ciliary muscle. With pilocarpine-induced miosis, the iris is pulled away from the trabecular meshwork, thereby widening the anterior chamber, which in turn increases aqueous humor outflow. Activation of M_3 receptors in the ciliary muscle causes contraction of the muscle, which also helps widen the anterior chamber.

B, C, D, E, F See correct answer explanation.

▶ *Learning objective:* Identify the action mediating the therapeutic effect of mannitol in glaucoma.

14. Answer: C

Mannitol is a hyperosmotic agent used mainly as a diuretic. Because mannitol is a polar drug, when given parenterally it is confined to the extracellular fluid space. This creates an osmotic gradient between plasma and ocular fluids that withdraws water from the eye. Because hyperosmotic drugs like mannitol can quickly reduce the IOP, they are first-line agents in the treatment of acute angle-closure glaucoma.

A Dilation of Schlemm's canal would be the mechanism of action of pilocarpine.

B Constriction of the conjunctival vessels cannot affect the production or the outflow of aqueous humor.

D Decreased aqueous humor production would be the mechanism of action of β-blocker or α_2-agonists.

E Increased iris–corneal angle would be the action of miotic agents (e.g., pilocarpine).

Case 16

Gout

I.L., a 62-year-old man, presented to the emergency department complaining of extreme pain in his right knee. He awoke in the early hours of the morning with a sore and stiff knee, which he self-medicated with acetaminophen before trying to go back to sleep. When his pain became excruciating, he came to the hospital.

The patient's medical history included essential hypertension, chronic constipation, and heartburn. Drugs taken by the patient on admission were chlorthalidone and losartan for hypertension, lactulose for constipation, and ranitidine for heartburn.

I.L. had no known drug or food allergies and denied the use of illicit drugs, but admitted that he drinks two or three cans of beer daily.

Physical examination showed an obese man in acute distress with the following vital signs: blood pressure 130/78 mm Hg, pulse 106 bpm, respirations 22/min, temperature 97.8°F (36.6°C). The patient's right knee was exquisitely tender and erythematous, warm to the touch, and swollen. The rest of physical examination was normal.

The patient was admitted to the hospital with the presumptive diagnosis of acute arthritis, likely due to gout.

Pertinent laboratory results on admission were:

Blood hematology

- ► Red blood cell count (RBC): $4.4 \times 10^6/\mu L$ (normal 4.0–6.0)
- ► Hemoglobin (Hb): 12.2 g/dL (normal 12–16)
- ► Hematocrit (Hct): 46% (normal 36–48)
- ► White blood cell count (WBC): $13 \times 10^3/\mu L$ (normal 4–10)
- ► Platelets: $320 \times 10^3/\mu L$ (normal 130–400)
- ► Erythrocyte sedimentation rate (ESR): 45 mm/h (normal < 20)

Blood chemistry

- ► Blood pH: 7.38 (normal 7.35–7.45)
- ► Bicarbonate: 22 mEq/L (normal 22–28)
- ► Creatinine: 3.7 mg/dL (normal 0.6–1.2)
- ► Blood urea nitrogen (BUN): 45 mg/dL (normal 8–25)
- ► Uric acid: 14 mg/dL (normal 3.4–8.2)
- ► Na^+: 138 mEq/L (normal 135–146)
- ► K^+: 3.2 mEq/L (normal 3.6–5.3)
- ► Total calcium: 11.5 mg/dL (normal 8.5–10.5)
- ► Total cholesterol: 230 mg/dL (normal < 200)
- ► Low-density lipoprotein (LDL): 110 mg/dL (normal < 100)
- ► High-density lipoprotein (HDL): 42 mg/dL (normal > 40)
- ► Triglycerides: 140 mg/dL (normal < 150)

Synovial fluid analysis

50 WBC/HPF (high-power field) (normal < 5). Negatively birefringent crystals were found, both free in the fluid and engulfed by white blood cells.

The diagnosis of acute gouty arthritis was confirmed, and the patient received an intra-articular injection of betamethasone. The pain started decreasing and disappeared completely 6 hours later. The following day I.L. started a treatment with oral triamcinolone, and 2 days later he was dismissed from the hospital with the following postdischarge therapy:

▶ Oral betamethasone, to be tapered over 2 weeks
▶ Oral allopurinol, to be initiated after betamethasone discontinuation

Three weeks later I.L. presented to his family physician complaining of a pruritic rash on the distal extremities and thorax. The physician discontinued allopurinol and prescribed febuxostat.

At his 3-month follow-up appointment, I.L.'s uric acid levels were still 10.2 mg/dL, and probenecid was added to the current treatment. The therapy was able to normalize uric acid levels, but 1 month later I.L. was admitted to the emergency department with excruciating pain in his right flank that radiated into the genital region. A diagnosis of renal colic was made and an appropriate therapy was started. His pain subsided, and later he was dismissed from the hospital.

One year later I.L.'s gout was found substantially worsened in spite of the ongoing therapy. The patient reported he had frequent gout attacks affecting more than one joint. The attacks were only partially controlled by betamethasone, and his serum uric acid level was found to be 11.8 mg/dL. Further exams led to the diagnosis of chronic refractory gout. The patient's therapy was updated, and pegloticase was added to the current regimen.

Questions

1. I.L. was diagnosed with acute gouty arthritis. The pathophysiology of this disease is primarily related to abnormal uric acid metabolism. Which of the following is one of the enzymes involved in the formation of uric acid?

A. Phosphoribosyltransferase

B. Adenosine deaminase

C. Nucleoside diphosphate kinase

D. Formyltransferase

E. Dihydrofolate reductase

2. Uric acid is the product of degradation of purines. Which of the following pairs of nucleosides are progenitors of purines?

A. Cytidine–adenosine

B. Adenosine–guanosine

C. Uridine–adenosine

D. Guanosine–cytidine

E. Guanosine–uridine

F. Cytidine–uridine

3. I.L. was found to have high serum levels of uric acid. The results of which of the following pairs of the patient's blood exams could explain the reason for his hyperuricemia?

A. ESR–LDL

B. ESR–creatinine

C. ESR–BUN

D. LDL–BUN

E. LDL–creatinine

F. Creatinine–BUN

4. I.L. was suffering from acute arthritis. The results of which of the following pairs of blood exams were most indicative of an inflammatory cause of his arthritis?

A. ESR–BUN

B. ESR–uric acid

C. ESR–WBC

D. BUN–uric acid

E. BUN–WBC

F. Uric acid–WBC

5. The analysis of the patient's synovial fluid showed negatively birefringent crystals. Which of the following was most likely the chemical nature of those crystals?

A. Calcium pyrophosphate

B. Calcium oxalate

C. Monosodium urate

D. Iron oxalate

E. Ammonium acid urate

6. Which of the following drugs taken by the patient could have contributed to his hyperuricemia?

A. Acetaminophen

B. Chlorthalidone

C. Losartan

D. Lactulose

E. Ranitidine

7. The treatment of an acute gout attack can be performed either with a nonsteroidal anti-inflammatory drug (NSAID), a glucocorticoid, or colchicine. Which of the following molecular actions most likely mediates the therapeutic effect of colchicine in gout?

A. Inhibition of cyclooxygenase

B. Blockade of tumor necrosis factor alpha

C. Inhibition of tubulin polymerization

D. Blockade of interleukin 1 receptors

E. Inhibition of tubulin depolymerization

8. Allopurinol was prescribed to I.L. Which of the following was most likely the primary goal of this prescription?

A. Decrease the formation of urate precursors

B. Block the crystals-induced inflammatory reaction

C. Inhibit renal urate excretion

D. Maintain subsaturating serum urate levels

E. Inhibit renal urate reabsorption

9. Plasma levels of which of the following pairs of endogenous compounds most likely increased after a few days of allopurinol therapy?

A. Guanine–xanthine
B. Xanthine–hypoxanthine
C. Inosine–guanine
D. Adenine–inosine
E. Adenine–hypoxanthine

10. I.L.'s family physician decided to substitute allopurinol with febuxostat. Which of the following statements best explains the reason for this decision?

A. Febuxostat is by far more effective than allopurinol.
B. The patient had been receiving a thiazide-like diuretic.
C. The patient was at risk of a serious hypersensitivity reaction.
D. Allopurinol can precipitate an acute gout attack.
E. The patient had been receiving losartan.

11. Febuxostat was prescribed to I.L. Which of the following molecular actions most likely mediated the therapeutic effect of the drug in the patient's disease?

A. Inhibition of adenosine formation
B. Conversion of uric acid to allantoin
C. Activation of purine phosphorylase
D. Inhibition of xanthine oxidase
E. Inhibition of renal urate reabsorption

12. Probenecid was prescribed to I.L. Which of the following regions of the kidney most likely represents the primary site of action of this drug?

A. Early distal tubule
B. Thick ascending limb of Henle
C. Proximal tubule
D. Collecting duct
E. Thin descending limb of Henle
F. Bowman's capsule

13. I.L. suffered from a renal colic. Which of the following was the most likely cause of the patient's disorder?

A. Polycystic kidney disease
B. Benign prostatic hyperplasia
C. Acute renal artery occlusion
D. Urolithiasis
E. Urinary tract infection

14. I.L. received an acute therapy for his renal colic. Which of the following analgesic treatments would be most appropriate to reduce the patient's pain?

A. Oral ibuprofen
B. Intravenous acetaminophen
C. Intravenous tramadol
D. Intravenous ketorolac
E. Oral piroxicam

15. Pegloticase was prescribed to I.L. Which of the following actions most likely mediated the therapeutic effect of the drug in the patient's disease?

A. Inhibition of adenosine formation
B. Conversion of uric acid to allantoin
C. Activation of purine phosphorylase
D. Inhibition of xanthine oxidase
E. Inhibition of renal urate reabsorption

Answers and Explanations

▶ *Learning objective:* Identify an enzyme involved in the formation of uric acid.

1.   Answer: B

The production of uric acid starts from the degradation of purine nucleotides that yields the formation of nucleosides, including adenosine. Adenosine deaminase is the enzyme that converts adenosine into inosine. Inosine is further metabolized by phosphorylation into the corresponding free base hypoxanthine.

A, C, D, E All these enzymes are involved in the synthesis, not in the degradation, of purines.

▶ *Learning objective:* Identify the nucleosides that are progenitors of purines.

2. Answer: B

Purines can result from the normal turnover of cellular nucleic acids or can be obtained from the diet. Dietary purines are not used to a large extent for the synthesis of tissue nucleic acids. Instead they are generally converted into uric acid by intestinal mucosal cells. Most of the uric acid enters the blood and is eventually excreted in the urine.

Adenine and guanine are the two purines that result from the breakdown of their precursors, adenosine and guanosine.

A, D, F Cytidine is the nucleoside of cytosine.

C, E, F Uridine is the nucleoside of uracil.

Cytosine and uracil are pyrimidines, not purines.

▶ *Learning objective:* Identify the lab exams that can explain the patient's hyperuricemia.

3. Answer: F

Hyperuricemia is the hallmark of gouty arthritis. Even if hyperuricemia does not always lead to gout—and rare cases of gout with normal uric acid levels have been described—the greater the degree and duration of hyperuricemia the greater the likelihood of gout and the more severe the symptoms. Urate levels can be elevated because of decreased excretion, increased production, or a combination of these. Decreased renal excretion of uric acid is the main cause of gout in about 90% of patients. The high creatinine and BUN levels indicate that I.L. was most likely suffering from renal insufficiency. Because approximately 70% of uric acid is excreted by the kidneys, hyperuricemia occurs when renal function deteriorates. Therefore the high creatinine and BUN levels best explain the reason for his hyperuricemia.

A, B, C, D, E See correct answer explanation.

▶ *Learning objective:* Identify the two exam results that are most indicative of an inflammatory cause of the patient's arthritis.

4. Answer: C

I.L.'s clinical symptoms and signs were already consistent with the diagnosis of inflammatory arthritis. Both the increase in ESR and the WBC indicate that the patient was affected by an acute inflammatory disorder.

A, D, E Increased blood urea nitrogen (BUN) is not a sign of inflammatory arthritis.

B, D, F Increased blood uric acid is not a sign of inflammatory arthritis.

▶ *Learning objective:* Identify the chemical nature of crystals found in the synovial fluid of a patient with gout.

5. Answer: C

The presence of monosodium urate crystals in the synovial fluid is a diagnostic sign of gout, a disease that can be defined as a crystal-induced arthritis. Urate crystals are deposited in several tissues, including cartilage, tendons, and skin around cooler distal joints and tissues. The characteristic pain and inflammation of gout develop when white blood cells in the joint start surrounding and digesting urate crystal deposits. These cells recognize crystals as foreign material and release cytokines that contribute to the pain, swelling, and redness associated with a gout attack.

A, B These salts can cause joint deposition of crystals leading to intermittent attacks of acute arthritis similar to gouty arthritis (referred to as pseudogout).

D This salt cannot cause acute gout arthritis. However, it appears to play a role in gout, in the nucleation and growth of the otherwise extremely soluble monosodium urate. This could explain why gout usually appears after age 40, when ferritin levels in blood exceed 100 ng/dL. Beer is rich in oxalate and iron, and ethanol increases iron absorption. This could explain why beer intake can increase the risk of a gout attack.

E This salt can cause, albeit very rarely, urolithiasis. It does not cause acute arthritis.

► *Learning objective:* Identify a drug that can trigger hyperuricemia in a patient at risk.

6. Answer: B

Chlorthalidone is a thiazide-like diuretic. Hyperuricemia can occur in up to 40% of patients after chronic treatment with thiazides or thiazide-like diuretics, as in the present case.

It is thought that these drugs can cause hyperuricemia by two primary mechanisms:

They selectively enhance urate reabsorption by acting as a counter-ion for urate transport. First, the thiazide enters the proximal tubule cell from the peritubular capillary blood through an anion exchanger on the basolateral membrane. The diuretic is then released into the tubular fluid from the cell by the urate anion exchanger on the luminal membrane, driving reabsorption of urate.

Volume depletion appears to play an important role in diuretic-induced hyperuricemia, because urate retention does not occur if the diuretic-induced fluid losses are replaced. How volume depletion increases net urate reabsorption is still uncertain, but volume depletion increases Na⁺ reabsorption in the proximal tubule, and there is a parallel relationship between Na⁺ reabsorption and urate reabsorption in the proximal tubule.

A, C, D, E These drugs cannot cause hyperuricemia.

► *Learning objective:* Identify the mechanism of action of colchicine in gout.

7. Answer: C

Colchicine has been successfully used to treat acute gout for centuries, despite little published research supporting its efficacy. The drug binds to the intracellular protein tubulin, thereby preventing its polymerization into microtubules, thus blocking mitosis in metaphase. Cells with the highest rate of division are affected early. Granulocyte migration into the inflamed area and phagocytosis of urate crystals by macrophages are inhibited, thus relieving the pain and inflammation of gouty arthritis. These actions are specific, and the drug is devoid of general analgesic or anti-inflammatory effects.

A Inhibition of cyclooxygenase would be the mechanism of action of NSAIDs.

B Blockade of tumor necrosis factor α would be the mechanism of action of several monoclonal antibodies used as immunosuppressants.

D Blockade of interleukin 1 receptors would be the mechanism of action of anakinra, a recombinant version of the interleukin 1 receptor antagonist, rarely used in rheumatoid arthritis.

E Colchicine inhibits tubulin polymerization, not depolymerization.

► *Learning objective:* Identify the primary goal of allopurinol treatment in gout.

8. Answer: D

Allopurinol is a urate-lowering drug. Gout is a disease caused by crystal deposition of monosodium urate. In the absence of urate saturation of extracellular fluids (reflected by hyperuricemia) urate crystal deposition and symptoms and signs of gout do not occur. Therefore, the long-term goal of gout therapy is to achieve and maintain subsaturating serum urate concentrations. Hyperuricemia is typically defined as occurring above the saturation point of monosodium urate, at which point the risk of crystallization increases. In practice, the most widely recommended goal range of urate-lowering therapy is serum urate < 6 mg/dL, which is substantially below the urate solubility limit.

Urate-lowering medications lower urate levels in one of three ways:

► Increase uric acid elimination by the kidney
► Decrease production of urate
► Convert urate to the more readily excreted allantoin

A The formation of urate precursor is increased, not decreased, by allopurinol.

B Allopurinol is not an anti-inflammatory drug.

C, E Allopurinol does not affect renal urate handling.

▶ *Learning objective:* Identify the two endogenous compounds that are most likely increased after a few days of allopurinol therapy.

9. Answer: B

Allopurinol is a purine drug that is biotransformed into alloxanthine. Both allopurinol and alloxanthine are noncompetitive inhibitors of xanthine oxidase. By inhibiting the enzyme the drug inhibits the transformation of hypoxanthine into xanthine and of xanthine into uric acid. Therefore, the plasma level of uric acid will decrease with a small, concomitant rise of hypoxanthine and xanthine.

A, C Guanine is biotransformed into xanthine by guanine deaminase. This enzyme is not inhibited by allopurinol.

D, E Adenine and inosine are precursors of hypoxanthine. Because hypoxanthine is increased, its precursors, if anything, should be decreased by negative feedback.

▶ *Learning objective:* Identify a reason for the substitution of allopurinol with febuxostat.

10. Answer: C

Allopurinol has been associated with a number of hypersensitivity reactions, including life-threatening reactions, such as Stevens–Johnson's syndrome, exfoliative dermatitis, and toxic epidermal necrolysis. For this reason, the drug must be immediately discontinued if a patient develops a cutaneous reaction while taking the drug, as in the present case.

A Febuxostat is a urate-lowering drug more effective than allopurinol, but this was not the reason for substituting allopurinol.

B Allopurinol hypersensitivity has been rarely associated with the combined use of thiazide diuretics, but the cause–effect relationship is poorly defined, and this was not the reason for suspending the drug.

D All urate-lowering drugs can precipitate an acute gout attack, but this was not the reason for suspending the drug.

E There are no adverse interactions between allopurinol and losartan.

▶ *Learning objective:* Explain the mechanism of action of febuxostat.

11. Answer: D

Febuxostat is a nonpurine xanthine oxidase inhibitor. The drug is a selective inhibitor of the enzyme, thereby reducing the formation of uric acid without affecting other enzymes in the purine metabolic pathway. The drug is well tolerated in patients with allopurinol intolerance, and this explains the physician's choice.

A Adenosine is the precursor of adenine. Febuxostat does not inhibit adenosine formation.

B Conversion of uric acid to allantoin would be the mechanism of antiuric action of pegloticase.

C Purine nucleoside phosphorylase is an enzyme that metabolizes inosine into hypoxanthine and guanosine into guanine. Activation of this enzyme would increase, not decrease, the formation of uric acid.

E Inhibition of renal urate reabsorption would be the mechanism of action of uricosuric drugs like probenecid.

▶ *Learning objective:* Identify the site of action of probenecid.

12. Answer: C

Probenecid is a uricosuric agent. These drugs interfere with the uric acid transport in the proximal kidney tubule. In humans all uric acid is freely filtered by the glomerulus and then eliminated by the following three active transport mechanisms located in subsequent segments of the proximal tubule:

1. Tubular reabsorption: 98% is actively reabsorbed by the organic anion transporters (OATs) in the basolateral cell membranes of the proximal tubule.
2. Tubular secretion: 50% is actively secreted.
3. Postsecretory tubular reabsorption: 40% is actively reabsorbed.

Therefore, about 10% of filtered uric acid load is finally eliminated by the kidney.

Uricosuric drugs like probenecid compete with uric acid for these transport mechanisms. They have a paradoxical effect because, depending on dosage, they may either decrease or increase the elimination of uric acid. It seems that the secretory mechanism is more sensitive to the blocking action of uricosuric drugs, so low doses can block uric acid secretion only. Higher doses are able to block both mechanisms; therefore, because most uric acid is reabsorbed, the net result is an increased elimination.

A The early distal tubule is the site of action of thiazide diuretics.

B The thick ascending limb of Henle is a site of action of loop diuretics.

D The collecting duct is the site of action of potassium-sparing diuretics.

E The thin descending limb of Henle is the site of action of osmotic diuretics.

F Uric acid is freely filtered by the glomerulus. Bowman's capsule does not regulate the excretion of uric acid.

▶ *Learning objective:* Identify the most likely reason for a renal colic in a patient suffering from gout.

13. Answer: D

The patient was most likely suffering from urolithiasis due to uric acid stones. Even large calculi remaining in the renal parenchyma or renal pelvis are usually asymptomatic unless they cause obstruction. Symptoms such as severe pain usually occur when calculi pass into the ureter. The pain from renal colic typically begins in the flank and often radiates to the anterior abdominal wall below the costal margins or to the groin. It is typically colicky (comes in waves) due to ureteric peristalsis, but it may be constant. It is often described as one of the strongest pain sensations known. About 20% of patients with gout develop urolithiasis. This percentage can increase in patients receiving uricosuric agents, such as probenecid, because these drugs increase the renal elimination of uric acid.

A Pain from polycystic kidney disease is usually located in the abdomen or lower back. It can be severe but is usually short-lived.

B Pain from benign prostatic hyperplasia is usually located in the lower abdomen and is mainly related to urinary urgency.

C Acute renal artery occlusion can cause steady, aching flank or abdominal pain that can be similar to pain from renal colic. However, the gouty arthritis of the patient suggests that urolithiasis is the most likely cause of his pain.

E Pain from urinary tract infection is usually located on the lower abdomen and is burning pain on urination.

▶ *Learning objective:* Identify the most appropriate analgesic treatment for a patient suffering from renal colic.

14. Answer: D

Both NSAIDs and opioids have traditionally been used for pain control in patients with acute renal colic, and prospective randomized controlled studies suggest that some NSAIDs are at least as effective as opiates. NSAIDs have the possible advantage of decreasing ureteral smooth muscle tone (prostaglandins cause smooth muscle contraction), thereby directly treating the mechanism by which pain is thought to occur.

Ketorolac is an NSAID whose analgesic efficacy seems greater than that of most other NSAIDs, and the drug has been used successfully to replace morphine in acute pain.

A, E When the pain is excruciating, a parenteral, not an oral, analgesic treatment is needed.

B Acetaminophen is a mild analgesic.

C Tramadol is a centrally acting analgesic structurally related to opioids. However, it is a mild analgesic and is not appropriate for the treatment of very severe pain.

▶ *Learning objective:* Explain the mechanism of action of pegloticase.

15. Answer: B

Pegloticase is a recombinant mammalian uricase. This enzyme, absent in humans, converts uric acid to allantoin, a product very soluble and easily eliminated by the kidney. The drug has been shown to maintain low urate levels for up to 21 days after a single dose, allowing intravenous administration every 2 weeks. Pegloticase, which has been recently approved for treatment of refractory gout, can cause infusion-related reactions and anaphylactoid reactions in > 10% of patients receiving the drug. Therefore, it is used only as a last resort in patients with severe, refractory gout, as in the present case.

A Adenosine is the precursor of adenine. Pegloticase does not inhibit adenosine formation.

C Purine nucleoside phosphorylase is an enzyme that metabolizes inosine into hypoxanthine and guanosine into guanine. Activation of this enzyme would increase, not decrease, the formation of uric acid.

D Inhibition of xanthine oxidase would be the mechanism of action of allopurinol and febuxostat.

E Inhibition of renal urate reabsorption would be the mechanism of action of uricosuric drugs like probenecid.

Case 17

Graves' Disease

H.T., a 50-year-old woman, presented to her physician complaining of nervousness, profuse perspiration, and palpitation. She had lost 10 pounds in the past 2 months, despite having an increased appetite. She also complained of muscle weakness, and reported that her menses had been scant and irregular for the past five or six periods.

Physical examination revealed a thin, flushed, hyperkinetic, and nervous woman.

Her vital signs were as follows:

- Blood pressure: 180/90 mm Hg
- Pulse: 128 beats/min, irregularly irregular
- Respirations: 30/min
- Temperature: 99.5°F (37.5°C)

Further examination revealed the following:

- Lid lag with stare
- Eye proptosis
- Decreased visual acuity
- A diffusely enlarged thyroid gland without nodules
- A bruit in the left lobe of the thyroid
- Warm, moist skin
- A fine tremor
- Proximal muscle weakness

Pertinent laboratory results were as follows:

Blood hematology

- Red blood cell count (RBC): $4.1 \times 10^6/\mu L$ (normal 4.0–6.0)
- Hemoglobin (Hb): 13 g/dL (normal 12–16 g/dL)
- White blood cell count (WBC): $9.5 \times 10^3/\mu L$ (normal 4–10)
  - Neutrophils: 56% (normal 55–70%)
  - Lymphocytes: 40% (normal 20–40%)
  - Eosinophils 2% (1–4%)
  - Basophils 0% (0.5–1%)
  - Monocytes 2% (2–8%)

Blood chemistry

- Fasting blood glucose: 75 mg/dL (normal 70–110)
- Total bilirubin: 1.0 mg/dL (normal 0.3–1)
- Aspartame aminotransferase (AST): 50 U/L (normal 10–35)
- Alkaline phosphatase (ALP): 200 IU/mL (normal 30–120)
- Free T4: 3 ng/dL (normal 0.7–1.9)

► Thyroid-stimulating hormone (TSH): 0.1 µU/mL (normal 0.4–4.0)
► Thyroid peroxidase antibody (TPA): 200 IU/mL (normal < 0.8)

Radioactive iodine uptake (RAIU) test

24 hours: 80%

A diagnosis of Graves's disease was made. The physician discussed therapeutic options with her and prescribed methimazole for her treatment.

After 3 weeks into therapy, the patient developed a sore throat and high fever. Some blood tests were ordered, and results indicated the development of a serious adverse effect of methimazole, so the drug was stopped immediately. She recovered well from the adverse effect in 2 weeks. After stabilization of her condition, her physician informed her about other treatment options, such a radioactive iodine (RAI) and surgery. She preferred RAI over surgery.

Her thyroid function was evaluated every 6 to 8 weeks. After 6 months of radioiodine therapy, signs and symptoms of hypothyroidism developed. She was started on a levothyroxine replacement therapy for the treatment of hypothyroidism.

Over the years H.T. did well, until one winter evening, at age 62, her daughter visited her and found her very sluggish. Her daughter noticed her slurring while talking to her. Later in the evening, H.T. became unconscious and was brought to the emergency department. Physical examination revealed dehydration, dry skin, bradycardia, and edema around her ankles. Her body temperature was 90°F (32.2°C), and lab results revealed hyponatremia and hypoglycemia. An emergency therapy was started with appropriate intravenous (IV) fluids and thyroid hormones.

Questions

1. H.T. was diagnosed with Graves' disease, which is caused by production of autoantibodies. Which of the following is the primary mechanism by which these autoantibodies act to increase the thyroid function?

A. Cause inflammation of thyroid follicular cells

B. Stimulate TSH receptors on the thyroid follicular cells

C. Inhibit the activity of adenylyl cyclase

D. Inhibit the function of sodium-iodide symporter

E. Inhibit the activity of thyroid dual oxidase

2. H.T.'s lab results showed that her TSH was below the normal range, and her free thyroid hormone levels were elevated. Which of the following is the most likely cause of decreased TSH levels in this patient?

A. Rapid weight loss

B. Thyroid peroxidase antibodies

C. Elevated serum thyroid hormone levels

D. Pituitary adenoma

E. Hypertension

3. H.T.'s 24-hour RAIU by the thyroid gland was found to be 80%. What range of radioactive iodine uptake would indicate a normal thyroid function?

A. 1–3%

B. 5–35%

C. 18–58%

D. 25–68%

E. 28–75%

4. H.T. was initially started on treatment with methimazole. The inhibition of activity of which of the following molecules most likely mediated the therapeutic effect of methimazole in the patient's disease?

A. Sodium-iodide symporter

B. Tyrosine kinase

C. 5'-deiodinase

D. Thyroid peroxidase

E. Thyroid dual oxidase

5. How much time would it most likely take to achieve biochemical euthyroidism in the patient in response to methimazole?

A. 1–5 days

B. 14–20 days

C. 1–3 months

D. 6–8 months

E. 12 months

6. It will take a long time before the levels of thyroid hormones in H.T.'s circulation reach the normal range. Meanwhile, which of the following drugs would be appropriate to add to her therapy to provide rapid clinical relief of her cardiac symptoms?

A. Dobutamine

B. Atenolol

C. Propylthiouracil

D. Phentolamine

E. Atropine

7. After 3 weeks into therapy, H.T. developed a serious adverse effect of methimazole. Which of the following was most likely this adverse effect?

A. Thyroid storm

B. Hypothyroidism

C. Agranulocytosis

D. Myxedema coma

E. Myocardial infarction

8. Which of the following drugs could facilitate H.T.'s recovery from agranulocytosis?

A. Olanzapine

B. Filgrastim

C. Epoetin alfa

D. Levothyroxine

E. Propylthiouracil

9. H.T. was given RAI for the treatment of her Graves' disease. Which of the following actions most likely mediated the therapeutic effect of this drug in the patient's disease?

A. Enhancement of iodine uptake by the thyroid follicular cells

B. Inhibition of iodine absorption from the gastrointestinal tract

C. Depletion of the thyroid glandular tissue

D. Increased metabolism of thyroid hormones

E. Inhibition of the synthesis of thyrotropin autoantibodies

10. Which of the following drugs would be appropriate to give to H.T. immediately after RAI therapy in order to correct her eye symptoms and signs?

A. Iodine salts

B. Propylthiouracil

C. Propranolol

D. Levothyroxine

E. Prednisone

11. H.T. was started on lifelong replacement therapy with levothyroxine to treat her hypothyroidism. What is the location of thyroid receptors to which levothyroxine binds to exert its therapeutic effects?

A. Plasma membrane

B. Nucleus

C. Reticulum endothelium

D. Mitochondria

E. Lysosomal membrane

12. One evening, H.T. became unconscious and was brought to the emergency department. Which of the following was most likely the disorder the patient was suffering from?

A. Thyroid storm

B. Myxedema coma

C. Hyperosmolar hyperglycemic syndrome

D. Subarachnoid hemorrhage

E. Heat stroke

13. H.T. had hypothermia when she was brought to the emergency department. Which of the following would most likely be the best method to facilitate normalization of her body temperature?

A. External heating by electric blankets

B. Administration of thyroid hormones

C. Administration of β-blockers

D. Administration of epinephrine

E. Transfusing packed red cells

Answers and Explanations

▶ *Learning objective:* Explain the pathophysiology of Graves' disease.

1. Answer: B

Graves' disease is an autoimmune disorder in which different types of autoantibodies are found in the circulation. These include antibodies against TSH receptors, thyroid peroxidase, and thyroglobulin. The following three types of anti-TSH autoantibodies are identified in these patients, and all are involved in increasing thyroid function:

▶ ***Thyroid-stimulating immunoglobulin (TSI):*** Almost all patients with Graves' disease have detectable levels of this autoantibody, which is relatively specific to the disease. TSI is an immunoglobulin G (IgG) antibody that binds to TSH receptors and mimics the action of TSH to stimulate thyroid hormone synthesis and their release into the circulation.

▶ ***Thyroid growth-stimulating immunoglobulin (TGI):*** This autoantibody is also directed against TSH receptors and is involved in stimulating proliferation of thyroid follicular epithelium.

▶ ***TSH-binding inhibitor immunoglobulin (TBII):*** These antibodies prevent TSH from binding to TSH receptors normally. By doing so, some forms of TBII stimulate TSH receptors, whereas other forms inhibit thyroid function.

It is clear that autoantibodies to TSH receptors, especially TSI, are central to disease pathogenesis in Graves' disease. Usually a lab test to measure TSH antibodies is not necessary to make a diagnosis of Graves' disease. Clinical signs and symptoms, and thyroid function tests along with thyroid peroxidase antibody (TPA) titers (which is comparatively a cheaper test compared to tests to measure anti-TSH antibodies), are sufficient to make a diagnosis of Graves' disease. TPA is more specific in Hashimoto's disease, but about 60 to 70% of patients with Graves' disease have TPAs, which, along with signs and symptoms and other lab tests, would indicate the autoimmune cause of the disease.

A This occurs in Hashimoto's thyroiditis, in which an initial damage to the follicular cells cause leakage of thyroid hormones to increase their levels in the circulation before, eventually, hypothyroidism develops.

C Binding of TSH or TSI to the TSH receptor increases, not inhibits, adenylyl cyclase activity, resulting in the increased synthesis of thyroid hormones.

D Function of sodium-iodide symporter is increased, not inhibited, to uptake iodide required for the increased synthesis of thyroid hormones.

E Dual oxidase function is required, not inhibited, to provide hydrogen peroxidase for the adequate function of thyroid peroxidase to synthesize thyroid hormones.

▶ *Learning objective:* Describe the hypothalamus–pituitary–thyroid axis in Graves' disease.

2. Answer: C

Normally TSH from the anterior pituitary acts on TSH receptors on the cell surface of thyroid follicular cells to stimulate thyroid hormone synthesis, the process that is controlled by feedback regulation. Increased thyroid hormone levels would decrease TSH release, and decreased thyroid hormone levels would increase TSH release so as to stimulate thyroid hormone synthesis.

In Graves' disease autoantibodies against the TSH receptors, especially the TSI, mimic the action of TSH and increase the synthesis of thyroid hormones. Increased levels of thyroid hormones suppress TSH release from the anterior pituitary through feedback control. Because of these pathophysiological changes, increased levels of thyroid hormones and low or undetectable levels of TSH are found.

A Rapid weight loss can affect anterior pituitary function, but it is not the cause of decreased TSH in Graves' disease. Moreover the patient's weight loss is not voluntary but rather was caused by the increased metabolic rate in response to high levels of thyroid hormones.

B This is seen in Hashimoto's thyroiditis, which eventually causes hypothyroidism. TSH levels are elevated in this condition.

D In case of a pituitary adenoma, the pressure effects of the tumor could cause suppression of thyrotrope function and decreased TSH release, which would result in decreased serum thyroid hormone levels. In the present case, TSH is low and thyroid hormone levels are high.

E Increased blood pressure in the patient is not the cause of Graves' disease, but it is a consequence of increased levels of thyroid hormones in the circulation.

► *Learning objective:* Describe the radioiodine uptake test.

3. Answer: B

Normal 24-hour RAIU is between 5 and 35%. The RAIU test provides a useful assessment of thyroid function and is done by using ^{123}I or trace amounts of ^{131}I. The test is helpful in confirming hyperthyroidism, determining the cause of hyperthyroidism, and calculating the dose of radioactive iodine therapy for the treatment of Graves' disease. RAIU is a measure of iodine utilization by the thyroid gland, which is an indirect measure of thyroid hormone synthesis. In hyperthyroidism conditions, such as Graves' disease, the RAIU is elevated. In hypothyroidism, RAIU will be below normal or undetectable, depending on the stage of hypothyroidism and damage to the thyroid gland.

A, C, D, E See correct answer explanation.

► *Learning objective:* Describe the mechanism of action of methimazole.

4. Answer: D

Thioamide drugs, methimazole and propylthiouracil, inhibit thyroid hormone synthesis by inhibiting the activity of thyroid peroxidase. Thyroid peroxidase catalyzes the following:

► Oxidation of iodide to iodine
► Transfer of iodine to tyrosine residues of thyroglobulin, leading to monoiodotyrosine (MIT) and diiodotyrosine (DIT)

Coupling of two DIT residues to synthesize T4 (tetraiodothyronine) or one MIT with one DIT to synthesize T3 (triiodothyronine) Thioamides have been found to induce remission in about 30 to 50% of patients after 1 or 2 years of therapy. However, this remission may not be lifelong in the majority of patients. Remission seems to result from suppression of autoantibody synthesis due to a possible immunosuppressive effect of thioamides.

Thioamides are usually preferred for children, pregnant women, and young adults with uncomplicated Graves' disease, with mild-to-moderate symptoms.

A Thyroid sodium-iodide symporter is present on the basolateral membrane of the thyroid follicular cells and carries out the function of uptake of iodide. It is not inhibited by methimazole.

B The intracellular part of the insulin receptor has tyrosine kinase activity. This is not inhibited by methimazole.

C 5'-deiodinase catalyzes deiodination of T4 to T3. Methimazole does not inhibit this reaction, but another thioamide agent, propylthiouracil, can inhibit this enzyme. This is because propylthiouracil is used in the management of thyroid storm.

E Thyroid dual oxidase (DUOX) is present on the apical membrane of thyroid follicular cells. DUOX catalyzes the generation of hydrogen peroxide that is required by thyroid peroxidase to oxidize iodide to iodine. It is not inhibited by methimazole.

► *Learning objective:* Identify the time needed for thioamide agents to achieve biochemical and clinical euthyroidism in patients suffering from hyperthyroidism.

5. Answer: C

The therapeutic response and reduction in thyroid hormone levels in the circulation in response to an effective thioamide therapy invariably occurs after a latency period. This is because the thioamide agents act by inhibiting the synthesis of thyroid hormones. These agents do not inhibit the release of already synthesized thyroid hormones present as a reservoir (in the form of colloid) in the thyroid gland. Usually the reservoir has sufficient hormone content to supply hormones for 1 to 3 months, even if the new synthesis is shut down. So the release of thyroid hormones from the thyroid gland continues until the glandular hormone stores are depleted. That is why, even when the synthesis of new thyroid hormones is inhibited by thioamides, it would usually take 1 to 3 months before achieving a biochemical euthyroid state, provided the patient responds to the drugs. Response to thioamides is monitored by measuring serum free T4 levels. TSH levels are not valuable, because in the first several months, TSH remains suppressed even if the thyroid hormone levels decrease.

A, B, D, E See correct answer explanation.

▶ *Learning objectives:* Identify a drug to be used for rapid management of cardiac symptoms in a patient with Graves' disease.

6. Answer: B

Elevated levels of thyroid hormones in Graves' disease enhance the expression of β-receptors in the cardiac tissue. This causes an increased response to endogenous catecholamines, resulting in sinus tachycardia, as in the present case. Elderly patients with thyrotoxicosis can develop cardiac arrhythmias. This is the reason why H.T. presented with palpitations as one of her symptoms. As explained earlier, it takes about 1 to 3 months before a euthyroid state is achieved in response to thioamides. It would mean that a symptomatic patient with Graves's disease would continue to experience cardiac symptoms for a considerable period of time before noticing any response to sole therapy with thioamides. In order to control cardiac symptoms rapidly, much before the response to thioamides is produced, β-adrenoceptor blockers (preferably a β_1 selective adrenoceptor blocker, such as atenolol) are prescribed along with thioamides. Atenolol would decrease the cardiac rate and would prevent development of cardiac arrhythmias in these patients. The drug can be stopped after the adequate therapeutic effects of thioamides become evident and the condition is well controlled.

A Dobutamine is a β_1-adrenoceptor agonist that is used in the treatment of acute heart failure and cardiogenic shock.

C Propylthiouracil is another thioamide agent that would take a similar amount of time as methimazole before its therapeutic effects become discernible.

D Phentolamine is an α-adrenoceptor antagonist and does not act as a β-adrenoceptor blocker.

E Atropine is a muscarinic receptor antagonist that would increase the heart rate.

▶ *Learning objective:* Describe the adverse effects of thioamide agents.

7. Answer: C

Adverse effects occur in a small number of patients taking thioamides. Serious adverse effects include agranulocytosis and hepatitis. Baseline values of WBC with differentials and liver function test are obtained before starting therapy with thioamide agents, as was done for H.T. The baseline values assist in differentiating these adverse effects from other causes. The level of liver enzymes may be slightly raised at baseline (as seen in H.T.) because of an increased metabolic rate and increased liver enzymatic activity. Agranulocytosis is seen in 0.1 to 0.5% of patients, and it usually occurs in the first 3 months of starting therapy with thioamides. Usually the patient presents with a sudden high-grade fever and sore throat, and the lab tests reveal agranulocytosis. When agranulocytosis develops, therapy with thioamides is stopped immediately, and after resolution of the condition, an alternative therapeutic option is considered for the treatment of Graves' disease.

Hepatitis is a rare (0.1–0.2%) but serious adverse effect of propylthiouracil, sometimes requiring liver transplantation. Because of this, in 2009 the U.S. Food and Drug Administration issued an advisory that propylthiouracil should not be used as the first-line drug for hyperthyroidism in adults or children. Hyperthyroidism situations in which propylthiouracil is preferred over methimazole include the following:

First trimester of pregnancy: Both thioamides can cross the placenta to reach fetal circulation, but methimazole has been shown to cause developmental defects when used during the first trimester.

Thyroid storm: Propylthiouracil, and not methimazole, has the additional mechanism to inhibit peripheral conversion of T4 to T3, the effect of which would be highly advantageous in controlling thyroid storm. Free T3 levels can drop by 30 to 40% with 1 day's therapy with propylthiouracil.

Patient intolerance of methimazole: If the patient develops adverse effects other than agranulocytosis or hepatitis, both agents are contraindicated for further use.

A Thyroid storm is a consequence of untreated hyperthyroidism.

B Hypothyroidism can occur as a result of overtreatment with thioamides, but it can be avoided by regularly evaluating the patient's condition and measuring the thyroid hormone levels. Also, the development of hypothyroidism is not life-threatening, and the patient would not present with sudden development of a high fever.

D Myxedema coma is an emergency condition that develops in untreated hypothyroidism, usually in elderly hypothyroid patients in the presence of some precipitating factors, such as a cold or acute infection.

E Thioamides do not cause myocardial infarction as their direct adverse effect.

▶ *Learning objective:* Describe the therapeutic uses of recombinant granulocyte-colony stimulating factor (G-CSF).

8. Answer: B

Filgrastim is a recombinant G-CSF, which can be administered to stimulate proliferation and differentiation of progenitor cells of the granulocyte lineage. It can decrease the time to recovery from agranulocytosis.

A Olanzapine is an antipsychotic drug that has agranulocytosis as one of its adverse effects.

C Epoetin alfa is a recombinant human erythropoietin that is administered primarily to stimulate red blood cell generation in certain types of anemia, such as in chronic renal failure.

D Levothyroxine is T4, which is used as a replacement therapy in hypothyroidism.

E Once a patient develops agranulocytosis or hepatitis in response to one thioamide agent, none of the thioamides is reintroduced for therapy due to cross reactivity.

▶ *Learning objective:* Describe the mechanism of action of radioactive iodine in the treatment of Graves' disease.

9. Answer: C

^{131}I is the only iodine isotope that is used in the treatment of thyrotoxicosis, whereas others are used in the diagno-

sis. It is the preferred treatment for most patients over age 21. An adequate dose of ^{131}I is given orally, and the drug is rapidly absorbed by the gastrointestinal (GI) tract and concentrated by the thyroid follicular cells. The emission of beta rays by the ^{131}I causes destruction of the thyroid gland from within. Gradually the glandular tissue is depleted, and the patient usually becomes euthyroid over a period of 2 to 6 months.

A patient is usually treated with thioamides before administering ^{131}I. The goal is to decrease thyroid hormone synthesis and decrease the hormone pool in the colloid. This is done to decrease the chances of acute thyrotoxicosis or thyroid storm in response to high amounts of thyroid hormones leaking into the circulation as a result of glandular destruction caused by radioiodine. The thioamide therapy is withdrawn 3 to 7 days before the treatment to prevent inadequate response to ^{131}I.

A Actually uptake of ^{131}I by the thyroid gland is reduced if iodides are given before ^{131}I administration. This is the reason that iodide salts are not recommended before the radioiodine therapy.

B ^{131}I does not interfere with GI absorption of normal iodine.

D ^{131}I is not an enzyme inducer and does not increase the metabolism of thyroid hormones.

E This is an additional effect of thioamides.

▶ *Learning objective:* Identify a drug to be given to hyperthyroid patients with exophthalmos.

10. Answer: E

The patient most likely received prednisone. It has been shown that a treatment with a glucocorticoid agent, such as prednisone, immediately after the administration of ^{131}I to a hyperthyroid patient who also has an ophthalmopathy, prevents exacerbation of the ophthalmopathy. H.T. had ophthalmopathy (see lid lag with stare, eye proptosis, and decreased visual acuity) so she was a candidate for receiving glucocorticoid therapy after treatment with radioactive iodine.

A The main effect of iodine salts is to inhibit thyroid inhibition of hormone release (the main mechanism), likely through blockade of thyroglobulin proteolysis. Because of this, they are mainly used in cases of thyroid storm.

B Propylthiouracil is an antithyroid drug used to treat hyperthyroidism.

C Propranolol is a β-adrenoceptor antagonist used to treat the cardiovascular symptoms of hyperthyroidism.

D Levothyroxine is used as replacement therapy for managing hypothyroidism resulting from RAI therapy, and not to correct eye symptoms and signs of Graves' disease.

▶ *Learning objective:* Describe the mechanism of action of levothyroxine.

11. Answer: B

In response to an adequate therapy with radioiodine, a patient with Graves' disease would usually become euthyroid over a period of 2 to 6 months. Eventually, > 80% of the patients who are adequately treated with radioiodine would develop hypothyroidism, usually within the first 2 years after therapy. The development of hypothyroidism is the best assurance that the patient will not have a recurrence of hyperthyroidism. Serum free T4 and TSH levels are monitored every 6 to 8 weeks, and when hypothyroidism develops (low serum thyroid hormone levels and elevated TSH), replacement therapy with T4 is started promptly.

Given T4's long half-life, it is administered once a day. The drug is well absorbed orally (bioavailability ~ 70%). Some fraction of T4 is converted to its active form, triiodothyronine (T3) by the action of 5'-deiodinases in the periphery. In the bloodstream, T4 and T3 circulate, bound extensively to thyroid-binding proteins (TBPs). These hormones dissociate from TBPs before entering into the cells through membrane-bound active transporters.

Inside the cells, T4 is converted to T3 by the action of intracellular 5'-deiodinases; then T3 moves into the nucleus. Thyroid receptors (TR) are present in the nucleus bound to the thyroid response elements (TREs) of the DNA. In the absence of T3, corepressors are bound to the TR. Binding of T3 to TR monomer promotes disruption of TR homodimer, and one TR monomer is replaced with one retinoid X receptor (RXR) monomer. The formation of heterodimer of RXR-TR, which is bound to the TRE, promotes displacement of corepressors and binding of coactivators. The TR–coactivator complex activates gene transcription, leading to alteration in protein synthesis.

A, C, D Thyroid receptors are not located on these cell structures.

▶ *Learning objective:* Describe the life-threatening complication of untreated hypothyroidism.

12. Answer: B

The patient was most likely suffering from myxedema coma, a rare but life-threatening complication of untreated hypothyroidism, which is treated as an acute medical emergency. It carries a high mortality rate (> 50%) even when the treatment is initiated promptly. The disorder is characterized by stupor, progressive weakness, hypothermia, hypoventilation, hypoglycemia, and hyponatremia, and may ultimately result in shock and death. It usually occurs in the winter in older patients with hypothyroidism who encounter some precipitating factors, such as acute infection, or have an underlying pulmonary or vascular disorder. Elderly patients, especially those who live alone, may forget to take their medicines regularly and appropriately. H.T. might not have been taking levothyroxine for quite some time, resulting in uncontrolled hypothyroidism. The patient's signs and symptoms, the lab results, and the history of hypothyroidism fit with the diagnosis of myxedema coma. Emergency therapy included a loading dose of T4 given by IV, followed by a daily IV maintenance dose. The T4 loading dose is given to saturate the thyroid hormone binding sites before the adequate levels of free T4 can be achieved. T3 is also added to the treatment for the initial few days. This is because initially, the patient has low metabolism and may not be able to convert T4 to the active form, T3, due to low enzymatic activity. After a couple of days of treatment, once the patient shows signs of reviving body metabolism, T3 can be stopped.

The IV route is used for administering thyroid hormones because all body functions, including GI function, are low in myxedema coma; thus oral absorption of drugs (which could be administered through a nasogastric tube) would be poor. Once the condition is stabilized, the patient can be discharged on oral levothyroxine to be taken lifelong.

A Thyroid storm is a complication of untreated hyperthyroidism.

C The patient did not have a history of diabetes mellitus, or of chronic therapy with glucocorticoids, that could cause chronic hyperglycemia as an adverse effect. Moreover, her blood tests revealed hypoglycemia.

D Subarachnoid hemorrhage results in a severe thunderclap headache and usually occurs in patients with a history of hypertension. The patient's condition and constellation of signs and symptoms do not fit with the diagnosis of subarachnoid hemorrhage.

E H.T. developed the condition during the winter. The circumstances in which she developed unconsciousness and her other signs and symptoms do not match with heat stroke.

▶ *Learning objective:* Describe the management of myxedema coma.

13. Answer: B

Myxedema coma is treated as an acute medical emergency, usually in an intensive care unit. The patient is administered appropriate IV fluids and thyroid hormones. Despite the starting of prompt treatment, the condition carries a high mortality rate. One important clinical sign that would indicate that the patient is responding to thyroid hormone therapy is a rise in body temperature.

A External heating can be lethal in these patients, because it would cause cutaneous vasodilation and diversion of blood from the body core to the outside, in an existing hypotensive situation. Thus external heating can precipitate shock and cause death. Therefore, external heating is contraindicated in patients with myxedema coma.

C Administration of β-blockers can further deteriorate the condition by worsening bradycardia.

D Epinephrine will not be able to elevate body temperature. The patient needed replacement with thyroid hormones. Once the patient starts responding to thyroid hormone therapy, the body temperature would increase to return to normal.

E The patient might need transfusion of blood for indications other than hypothermia, but this is not indicated to raised body temperature.

Growth Retardation and Hypogonadism

R.D., A 10-year-old boy, was brought to the pediatric endocrinologist because his parents were concerned that he was not gaining height like his peers. R.D. was feeling weak, was not able to keep up with the school demands, would not show interest in outdoor games, and lacked concentration.

He had a normal vaginal delivery and was fully vaccinated. His past medical history was not significant for any major medical condition.

Physical examination showed a thin boy, looking younger than his age.

Pertinent exam results were as follows:

Blood hematology

▶ Hemoglobin (Hb): 11 g/dL (normal 12–16)
▶ White blood cell count (WBC): 5 × 10³/μL (normal 4–10)
▶ Red blood cell count (RBC): 3.5 × 10⁶/μL (normal 4.0–6.0)
▶ Growth hormone (GH) stimulation test: GH 0.6 ng/mL (normal > 10.0)
▶ Insulin-like growth factor-1 (IGF-1): 30 ng/mL (normal, males aged 9-10, 110–565 ng/mL)
▶ Thyroid-stimulating hormone (TSH): 3.0 μU/mL (normal, school-aged children, 0.4-5.5.0)
▶ Ca^{2+}: 9.5 mg/dL (normal 8.4–10.2)
▶ Na^+ 137 mEq/dL (normal 136–145)
▶ K^+ 4.0 mEq/dL (normal 3.5–5.0)

Karyotype test

Karyotype: 46, XY

R.D. was diagnosed with growth retardation due to GH deficiency. He was prescribed daily injections of an appropriate drug for the treatment.

R.D. responded well to the therapy, and his school performance also improved dramatically.

At age 14, although R.D. had gained normal height, he complained that he had not started developing facial hair, which his friends had developed. There was no family history of constitutional delay in pubertal development. There was no history of trauma, mumps orchitis, radiation therapy, or chemotherapy. He was examined and was found to lack pubic and axillary hair growth, and the size of his penis and testes did not show any signs of starting puberty. His sense of smell was normal.

Pertinent blood tests revealed the following results:

▶ Total testosterone: 3.0 ng/dL (normal for boys aged 14–15, 33–585)
▶ Free testosterone: 0.1 ng/dL (normal for boys aged 14–15, 0.5–15.3)
▶ Luteinizing hormone (LH): 1.2 U/L (normal 6–23)
▶ Follicle-stimulating hormone (FSH): 0.5 U/L (normal 4–25)
▶ Prolactin: 3.0 μg/L (normal < 20.0)

A diagnosis of hypogonadotropic hypogonadism was established, and an appropriate therapy was started. The patient responded well and achieved normal male adult features as he grew.

At age 28, R.D. married his longtime girlfriend. The couple desired to have children. His ejaculate was examined and was found to be lacking mature spermatozoa. He was advised that he needed to undergo an additional hormonal treatment to enable him to produce adequate amounts of mature sperm. An appropriate therapy was started, and within 1 year he was found to produce an adequate amount of semen with an adequate amount of sperm having normal morphology. The couple conceived, and his therapy with the drugs to stimulate spermatogenesis were discontinued.

Questions

1. R.D. was diagnosed with GH deficiency. Which of the following drugs was most likely prescribed to him for the treatment of his short stature?

A. Octreotide

B. Bromocriptine

C. Somatropin

D. Levothyroxine

E. Hydrocortisone

2. R.D. was prescribed a replacement therapy with somatropin, a recombinant HG hormone. Which of the following targets is activated by somatropin to mediate its therapeutic effects in short stature due to GH deficiency?

A. Jak2 tyrosine-protein kinase

B. Calcineurin

C. Mitogen-activated protein kinase

D. Epidermal growth factor receptor (EGFR)

E. IGF-1 receptors

3. R.D. was diagnosed with hypogonadotropic hypogonadism. Which of the following terms best describes this disorder?

A. Primary hypogonadism

B. Secondary hypogonadism

C. Drug-induced hypogonadism

D. Age-related hypogonadism

E. Hypogonadism due to hyperprolactinemia

4. Which of the following therapeutic agents was most likely prescribed to R.D. for the treatment of hypogonadism?

A. Testosterone cypionate

B. Oxandrolone

C. Gn-RH

D. FSH and LH

E. Testosterone gel

F. Finasteride

5. Which of the following cell structures is the location of the androgen receptors with which testosterone would bind to bring about therapeutic effects in R.D.?

A. Centrioles

B. Cytoplasm

C. Endoplasmic reticulum

D. Plasma membrane

E. Mitochondria

6. R.D. had responded well to testosterone therapy for the normal development of secondary sexual characteristics but still was not able to produce adequate amounts of mature sperm. What was the most likely reason for failure of his spermatogenesis?

A. External testosterone is degraded faster in the body.

B. Testosterone does not affect sperm production.

C. Testosterone levels in the spermatic tubules were inadequate.

D. Testosterone receptors were mutated.

7. Testosterone can increase bone mass during sexual maturation. Which of the following hormones is testosterone converted to in order to affect bone mass?

A. Dehydroepiandrosterone (DHEA)

B. Estradiol

C. Cortisol

D. Progesterone

E. Calcitriol

8. When R.D. visited his physician after getting married, he was examined and was found to have a normal sense of smell. His sense of smell was examined to rule out which of the following syndromes?

A. Kallmann's syndrome

B. Klinefelter's syndrome

C. Sheehan's syndrome

D. Prader–Willis's syndrome

E. Turner's syndrome

9. Which of the following drugs was most likely administered to achieve normal sperm production in R.D.?

A. Human chorionic gonadotropin (HCG)

B. Clomiphene

C. Oxandrolone

D. Anastrozole

E. Flutamide

10. R.D. was also administered recombinant FSH (rFSH). Which of the following actions most likely mediates the effectiveness of the drug in treating infertility in men?

A. Activation of Sertoli cells

B. Decreased synthesis of ABP

C. Apoptosis of spermatogonia

D. Stimulation of ejaculation

11. R.D. continued using testosterone replacement by using the gel formulation. At age 45, however, he started experiencing difficulties in achieving and maintaining penile erection. Which of the following drugs could be appropriate to treat his disorder?

A. Tadalafil

B. Increased testosterone dose

C. FSH

D. Oxandrolone

E. Alprostadil

12. R.D. was examined to rule out which of the following disorders before prescribing treatment for his erectile dysfunction?

A. Cardiovascular disorders

B. Liver dysfunction

C. Renal dysfunction

D. Retinopathy

E. Peptic ulcer disease

Answers and Explanations

▶ *Learning objective:* Describe the pharmacotherapy of GH deficiency.

1. Answer: C

Somatropin is a recombinant human growth hormone (rhGH), a peptide with 191 amino acids. A replacement therapy with somatropin is started for a child with growth retardation due to GH deficiency. The drug is administered daily as subcutaneous injections. The response is evaluated by measuring gain in height to inform dose modifications. The usual acceptable response is considered to be 5 to 7 cm linear growth per year. The treatment is continued until the desired height is achieved, bone age is advanced to between 13 to 15 years for girls and 15 to 16 years for boys, or linear growth velocity decreases to < 2.5 cm per year. Dose adjustment is guided by monitoring serum insulin-like growth factor-1 (IGF-1) levels specific to age and gender, and Tanner staging. After attaining appropriate height and bone maturation, during the teenage years and thereafter, GH replacement is indicated under the guidelines of adult GH deficiency. If the peak GH levels are < 5.0 ng/mL in response to a GH stimulation test, the patient would qualify for continued GH replacement. If left untreated, adult patients with GH deficiency experience a low quality of life, reduced muscle mass and bone density, high blood cholesterol, and increased body fat.

A Octreotide is a somatostatin analogue that is used to suppress GH release from the anterior pituitary.

B Bromocriptine is a dopamine agonist that can be used to suppress prolactin secretion.

D Levothyroxine is used for replacement therapy for hypothyroidism.

E Hydrocortisone is a glucocorticoid that can be used for replacement therapy for adrenal insufficiency, or for anti-inflammatory indications.

▶ *Learning objective:* Describe the mechanism of action of somatropin.

2. Answer: A

Somatropin acts similarly to endogenous GH. The drug binds to the extracellular domain of GH receptors, which induces receptor dimerization and activates the intracellular domain of the receptor. Activated domain associates with Jak2 tyrosine-protein kinase and phosphorylates relevant proteins that activate downstream signaling pathways, including signal transducer and activator of transcription (STAT), which ultimately modulate gene expression.

Most of the anabolic actions of GH are mediated by somatomedins (IGF, particularly type 1 [IGF-1]), the peptides produced mainly in the liver and cartilage in response to the action of GH. GH is released in a pulsatile manner and accordingly its blood levels fluctuate. Therefore a single measurement of GH levels is not sufficient in establishing the diagnosis of GH deficiency. This is the reason for doing a GH suppression test to evaluate GH deficiency. In contrast to the pattern of GH release and its fluctuating plasma levels, IGF-1 levels remain stable throughout the day. Therefore, levels of IGF-1 act as a useful indicator of average GH levels. This is the reason why IGF-1 levels are also measured along with a GH stimulation test to help in evaluating GH deficiency, as was done for R.D.

Hypothyroidism can cause growth retardation, even in the presence of normal GH levels, and can also interfere with GH release. This is the reason for measuring TSH levels in R.D. to rule out thyroid dysfunction.

Effects of GH can be subdivided into the following:

▶ **Direct effects (short-term, *mainly catabolic*):** These effects include lipolysis, and hyperglycemia by stimulating gluconeogenesis and by decreasing insulin sensitivity of tissues.
▶ **Indirect effects (long-term, anabolic):** These effects are mediated by somatomedins whose synthesis is promoted by GH, including skeletal growth, muscle protein synthesis, nucleic acid synthesis, and cell proliferation.

B Calcineurin is a phosphatase enzyme that is a target for the action of immuno-suppressant drugs, such as cyclosporine and tacrolimus.

C Mitogen-activated protein kinases (MAP kinases) are the potential targets for cancer chemotherapy.

D Epidermal growth factor receptors are cell surface receptors that are used as targets for anticancer drugs. For example, trastuzumab, a monoclonal antibody against human epidermal growth factor receptor 2 (HER2), is used in the treatment of breast cancer.

E Growth hormone binds to growth hormone receptors to mediate its effects. GH binds to its receptors in the cartilage to stimulate IGF-1 synthesis. IGF-1 binds to insulin-like growth factor receptor (IGFR) to mediate its growth promoting effects.

▶ *Learning objective:* Differentiate between primary and secondary hypogonadism.

3. Answer: B

Hypogonadism is defined as diminished gonadal function resulting in diminished biosynthesis of sex hormones. It can be subdivided as follows:

▶ **Primary hypogonadism**, when gonadal function is diminished because of an anomaly (anatomical or functional) of the gonads themselves.
▶ **Secondary hypogonadism**, when the gonads are normal but their function is diminished due to deficiency of gonadotropin secretion due to abnormality of the gonadotropes in the anterior pituitary.
▶ **Tertiary hypogonadism**, when the gonads are normal but their function is diminished due to deficiency of gonadotropin-releasing hormone (GnRH) in the hypothalamus.

In the present case, the patient's testes responded to gonadotropins to increase testosterone synthesis, so he had secondary hypogonadism. However, regardless of the site of abnormality (testes, pituitary, or hypothalamus) that causes hypogonadism

157

in a boy, replacement therapy is started with testosterone with the goal of achieving normal pubertal growth. Hyperprolactinemia can suppress the release of Gn-RH to cause hypogonadotropic hypogonadism. This is the reason for testing prolactin levels in R.D., which were found to be normal.

A See correct answer explanation.

C Certain drugs, such as ketoconazole and anticancer drugs, can interfere with gonadal function, but in the present case, this was not the causative factor.

D Serum testosterone levels decrease with age. Usually the levels start declining after age 30. However, this was not the case with R.D., who had not yet achieved even puberty.

E Hyperprolactinemia can suppress gonadotropin release, resulting in diminished gonadal function. However, R.D. did not have hyperprolactinemia.

▶ *Learning objective:* Identify the appropriate formulations of testosterone for replacement therapy in a boy with hypogonadism.

4. Answer: A

Replacement therapy in boys with hypogonadism of any etiology is typically initiated with testosterone. Although there are different methods of testosterone administration (gel, patch, injection, buccal tablet), the preferred formulation for boys is intramuscular administration of a testosterone ester (testosterone enanthate, testosterone cypionate) every 2 to 4 weeks, as in the present case. This route provides some advantages in this age group. One is that patients do not have to take the medicine daily, and also that continuous release from the injected site helps to achieve and maintain stable serum levels of testosterone in the normal range, which is critical for the normal development of secondary sexual characteristics.

Testosterone patches, gel, and buccal tablets are more suitable for adult males. Of these, testosterone gel is the most preferred formulation for testosterone replacement in adult males with hypogonadism. While using a gel formulation, the patient has to be cautious not to bring the part of the body where the drug is applied into contact with other people, to avoid having an impact on their normal reproductive function.

B Oxandrolone is an anabolic steroid. These drugs are used to increase muscle mass in cachectic patients. They are also abused as performance-enhancing agents by athletes and body builders, even though they are not approved for this purpose.

C, D Even though, theoretically, administration of either pulsatile Gn-RH (pump) or appropriate spacing and doses of FSH and LH could achieve the same outcome as long as their target tissues (anterior pituitary and gonads, respectively) are functional, these hormones are not used for boys' hypogonadism. Gonadotropin therapy is expensive, and antibodies against FSH and LH can develop after long-term use.

E Testosterone gel is more suitable for adult males.

F Finasteride is an inhibitor of 5α-reductase, the enzyme that catalyzes the transformation of testosterone into dihydrotestosterone. It would be absolutely contraindicated in this patient.

▶ *Learning objective:* Describe the mechanism of action of testosterone.

5. Answer: B

Androgen receptors belong to the intracellular receptor superfamily that includes steroid receptors, sterols (vitamin D), thyroid receptors, and retinoids. Androgen receptors are localized to the cytoplasm when they are bound to a protein called heat shock protein. Testosterone is a lipid soluble molecule, and free testosterone freely diffuses across the plasma membrane of target cells into the cytosol. Intracellular 5α-reductase enzyme converts testosterone (T) to dihydrotestosterone (DHT) in specific tissues. DHT is more potent than T and has a higher affinity for androgen receptors. After binding the heat shock protein is released, and the hormone-receptor complex is translocated from the cytoplasm to the nucleus, where it initiates transcription of androgen-dependent genes.

A, C, D, E These structures do not mediate the cell action of testosterone.

▶ *Learning objective:* Describe the reason why testosterone replacement therapy is not adequate to achieve fertility in a man with hypogonadism.

6. Answer: C

Adequate concentration of testosterone is required inside the spermatic tubules to initiate spermatogenesis. LH stimulates Leydig cells in the testicular interstitium to synthesize and secrete testosterone. Testosterone then enters into the closely situated spermatic tubules. FSH acts on the Sertoli cells in the spermatic tubules to stimulate the synthesis of androgen-binding protein (ABP) that is released into the lumen of spermatic tubules. ABP binds to testosterone and assists in maintaining adequate concentration of testosterone inside the tubules in order to stimulate spermatogenesis.

In a male patient with hypogonado-tropic hypogonadism under replacement therapy with testosterone, testosterone therapy can act in the peripheral tissues to produce the desired physiological effects on the development of secondary sexual characteristics, and effects on muscles, bones, and metabolism. However, in the absence of ABP, due to lack of FSH action on the Sertoli cells, testosterone would not be able to attain optimal concentration inside the spermatic tubules. Thus testosterone replacement alone would not be able to establish fertility in a man with hypogonadism.

A Metabolism of testosterone administered from outside is not different from that of endogenous testosterone.

B Adequate concentration inside the seminiferous tubules is critical for spermatogenesis.

D In case of androgen receptor mutation, the patient would not have responded to testosterone replacement to achieve features of puberty.

▶ *Learning objective:* Describe how androgens affect bone mineral density.

7. Answer: B

In men, both androgens and estrogens play a crucial role in gaining the cortical bone size during sexual maturation. Studies have shown that absence of estrogen receptors in males result in a decrease in cortical bone mass. In both men and women, estrogens are derived from androgen precursors. Androgens aromatization, a reaction catalyzed by aromatase, yields estrogens. Therefore testosterone must be converted to estradiol to affect bone growth.

A DHEA is itself an androgen that is produced in the adrenal cortex.

C Cortisol is synthesized by the adrenal cortex. Androgens are not its precursors.

D Synthesis of all steroid hormones requires cholesterol. Cholesterol is converted to pregnenolone, a rate-limiting step in steroid biosynthesis. Pregnenolone is then converted to progesterone.

E Calcitriol is 1,25-dihydroxycholecalciferol that is synthesized in the proximal renal tubules by the action of 1α-hydroxylase, a mitochondrial oxygenase, on 25-hydroxycholecalciferol.

▶ *Learning objective:* Describe various syndromes in which infertility is a constituent.

8. Answer: A

Kallmann's syndrome is a rare condition in which patients have hypogonadotropic hypogonadism and absent or diminished sense of smell. Impaired sense of smell distinguishes this form of hypogonadotropic hypogonadism from other conditions that cause hypogonadism. Other features of this syndrome are unilateral renal agenesis, impaired hearing, abnormalities of bones and teeth, and cleft lip.

B Klinefelter's syndrome is a genetic disorder due to a karyotype of 47, XXY and associated with hypogonadism and infertility. R.D. had a normal karyotype.

C Sheehan's syndrome is the development of panhypopituitarism caused by postpartum pituitary gland necrosis due to postpartum blood loss.

D Prader–Willis's syndrome is a genetic disorder due to loss of several genes on chromosome 15. Patients have weak muscles, a slow rate of growth, mild to moderate intellectual impairment, infertility, and a ravenous appetite that causes type 2 diabetes.

159

E Turner's syndrome is a genetic disorder in which a female is partly or completely missing one X chromosome to have a karyotype of 45, X. R.D. had a normal karyotype.

▶ *Learning objective:* Describe the appropriate therapy for treating infertility in men with hypogonadotropic hypogonadism.

9.   Answer: A

LH and HCG are glycoproteins. Because HCG and LH are structurally similar, and given that HCG can bind to LH receptors to bring about LH effects, HCG can be used to stimulate testosterone synthesis from the Leydig cells. These hormones bind to cell membrane–bound G-protein-coupled receptors on the Leydig cells and stimulate adenylyl cyclase activity (increased intracellular cyclic adenosine monophosphate [cAMP]) to promote testicular steroidogenesis.

B Clomiphene is a partial agonist for estrogen receptors. It is used as an ovulation inducer and is a first-line agent to treat infertility in women with polycystic ovarian disease.

C Oxandrolone is an anabolic androgen that has more anabolic than androgenic activity. It is usually used to increase muscle mass in cachectic patients. It is also abused as a performance-enhancing agent by athletes and body builders, even though it is not approved for this purpose.

D Anastrozole is an aromatase inhibitor that inhibits conversion of androgens to estrogens. It is indicated in the treatment of endometriosis and breast cancer and to induce ovulation.

E Flutamide is an androgen receptor antagonist that can be used to treat hyperandrogenism.

▶ *Learning objective:* Explain the role of FSH in stimulating spermatogenesis.

10.   Answer: A

FSH binds to cell membrane–bound FSH receptors to stimulate Sertoli cells. Sertoli cells secrete a variety of substances, including ABP, to support spermatogenesis. Failure of Sertoli cell function results

in infertility. LH stimulates Leydig cells to secrete testosterone that enters the closely situated seminiferous tubules, where it binds to ABP to achieve an optimal testosterone concentration to stimulate spermatogenesis. Initially the patient is treated with HCG, usually three times a week. The maturation of prepubertal testes, as indicated by growth in testicular size, typically occurs in more than 6 months, and the plasma testosterone levels indicate full induction of testicular steroidogenesis. At this point HCG doses are decreased and rFSH is injected three times a week along with HCG to stimulate spermatogenesis. In some patients, it may take up to 2 years for optimal spermatogenesis to establish.

B Synthesis of ABP is increased by the action of FSH.

C FSH acts on Sertoli cells to support spermatogenesis and to facilitate differentiation of spermatogonia to first-order spermatocytes that progresses stepwise, ending in the development of mature spermatids.

D Ejaculation of semen is a sympathetic system-mediated phenomenon.

▶ *Learning objective:* Describe the treatment of erectile dysfunction.

11.   Answer: A

Tadalafil and sildenafil are phosphodiesterase 5 (PDE5) inhibitors. PDE5 degrades cyclic guanosine monophosphate (cGMP). Inhibition of PDE5 results in increased amounts of intracellular cGMP levels in the vascular smooth muscles of the corpora cavernosa, causing their relaxation by dephosphorylation of the myosin-light chain. This relaxation yields increased blood flow inside the corpora cavernosa, which results in penile erection.

B R.D. is already on testosterone replacement therapy with age-specific doses. Increasing testosterone dose further would not be beneficial.

C FSH, along with LH, would stimulate testicular function to increase testicular testosterone production. However, R.D. is already on testosterone replacement therapy. Therapy with gonadotropins in a patient with hypogonadotropic hypogonadism is reserved only for the treatment of infertility.

D Oxandrolone is an anabolic androgen that has more anabolic than androgenic activity. It is usually used to increase muscle mass in cachectic patients. It is also abused as a performance-enhancing agent by athletes and body builders, even though it is not approved for this purpose.

E Alprostadil is a prostaglandin E_1 analogue that is used to treat erectile dysfunction. It is available as a penile suppository and for injection into the corpora cavernosa. It is not the first-line treatment and can be used when therapy with PDE5 inhibitors fails.

▶ *Learning objective:* Describe the contraindications of PDE5 inhibitors.

12. Answer: A

PDE5 inhibitors increase the amount of intracellular cGMP levels, causing vasodilation. Therefore they are contraindicated in patients with cardiovascular disorders. If a patient has a history of cardiac arrhythmias, PDE5 inhibitors can cause hypotension and compensatory tachycardia that can worsen the patient's tachyarrhythmias. PDE5 inhibitors potentiate the action of nitrates (which also cause a nitric oxide mediated increase in cGMP) and severe hypotension, and a few myocardial infarctions have been reported in men using both drugs. This is the reason why it is critical to rule out cardiovascular disorders and a history of treatment with vasodilator drugs, such as nitrates, in potential candidates for therapy with PDE5 inhibitors.

B, C, D, E PDE5 inhibitors are not contraindicated in patients with these disorders.

Case 19

Heart Failure

J.K., a 69-year-old Caucasian man, was admitted to the hospital because of increasing fatigue, increasing shortness of breath, and increased swelling in his lower extremities. Two months ago he had started feeling tired and weak, particularly at the end of the day. He also noted a productive cough and the need to urinate three to four times at night. He denied any recent chest pain or dizziness. One week before admission, he noted increased difficulty in breathing when in bed and since then, he had been able to sleep only in the sitting position. The medical history of the patient was significant for hypertension, apparently well controlled with hydrochlorothiazide and losartan.

J.K.'s vital signs on admission were as follows: blood pressure 102/88 mm Hg, pulse 96 bpm, respirations 26/min. Physical examination showed a dyspneic patient with cyanosis of the lips, fingers, and toes; distended neck veins; and pronounced pitting edema of the extremities. His liver was enlarged and tender to palpation and pulmonary crackles were heard on auscultation. On cardiac examination a third sound (S3) was heard. A chest X-ray showed cardiomegaly, some alveolar edema, and a small right pleural effusion. The electrocardiogram (ECG) showed left ventricular hypertrophy and a ventricular rate of 105 bpm. The echocardiogram showed a left ventricular ejection fraction of 35%.

A diagnosis of low-output systolic heart failure was made. The cardiovascular ongoing therapy was discontinued, and a new therapy was prescribed that included furosemide, carvedilol, captopril, spironolactone, and digoxin.

After 1 week of therapy, J.K.'s condition improved substantially. The patient's blood pressure was 115/80 mm Hg, dyspnea was substantially decreased, and he was able to sleep comfortably. The only complaints the patient now had were tinnitus, occurring two or three times daily, and some hearing loss. The patient also noted a small increase in his breast. The doses of his medications were adjusted, and after another week J.K. was discharged from the hospital with the same medical treatment.

Two weeks later J.K. was admitted to the emergency department in a confused state. His wife stated that J.K. had apparently taken several tablets of digoxin for a suicidal purpose. Physical examination showed a disoriented patient who exhibited hallucinatory behavior and complained of nausea, vomiting, abdominal pain, and snowy vision. His blood pressure was 110/70, and his heart rate was 40 to 60 bpm. An ECG revealed atrial fibrillation and a third-degree atrioventricular (AV) block. The ventricular rate did not exceed 45 bpm and an intravenous (IV) atropine injection was without effect. Lab results on admission showed serum potassium level of 8.7 mEq/L. A transvenous pacing catheter was inserted, with ventricular pacing instituted at 60 bpm. An antidote was administered together with supportive therapy. The patient's condition gradually improved, and 2 days later J.K. made a complete recovery from his poisoning.

Questions

1. J.K. was diagnosed with low-output systolic heart failure. Which of the following signs represents the most specific information indicating the patient's disease?

A. The S3 sound

B. Pitting edema of the extremities

C. Cyanosis of the lips

D. The X-ray cardiomegaly

E. The ejection fraction of 35%

2. J.K.'s blood pressure on admission was found to be 102/88 mm Hg. Which of the following cardiovascular actions was most likely the primary cause of this result?

A. Increased heart rate

B. Increased pulmonary venous pressure

C. Decreased stroke volume

D. Decreased preload

E. Decreased afterload

3. J.K. noticed that he needed to urinate three to four times at night. Which of the following phrases best explains the reason for the patient's symptom?

A. Decreased preload on lying

B. Redistribution of fluids back into the blood

C. Increased heart contractility on lying

D. Increased nocturnal sympathetic activity

E. Decreased bladder contractility on lying

4. J.K. said that recently he had been able to sleep only in the sitting position. Which of the following phrases best explains the reason for the patient's symptom?

A. Decreased afterload

B. Decreased pulmonary venous pressure

C. Increased diaphragm contractility

D. Increased diuresis

E. Less gravitational control of fluid balance

5. J.K. was diagnosed with low-output systolic heart failure. From the patient's symptoms and signs, which of the following was most likely his stage of heart failure, according to the American Heart Association and the American College of Cardiology?

A. Stage A

B. Stage B

C. Stage C

D. Stage D

6. Furosemide was prescribed to J.K. Which of the following parts of the nephron represents the primary site of action of furosemide?

A. Proximal convolute tubule

B. Proximal straight tubule

C. Thick ascending limb of Henle's loop

D. Thin descending limb of Henle's loop

E. Early distal tubule

F. Late distal tubule

G. Collecting duct

7. Which of the following cardiovascular actions was most likely the main contributor to the therapeutic effect of furosemide in J.K.'s heart failure?

A. Decreased cardiac output

B. Increased heart contractility

C. Increased heart rate

D. Decreased preload

E. Decreased afterload

8. Furosemide is able to decrease the concentrating ability of the kidney. Which of the following renal actions most likely mediated this drug effect?

A. Increased intracellular osmolality in the thick ascending limb of Henle

B. Blockade of apical Na^+ channels in the kidney cell membrane

C. Blockade of vasopressin receptors in the collecting tubule

D. Increased solute osmolality in the lumen of the proximal tubule

E. Decreased hypertonicity of medullary interstitium

9. J.K. was treated with hydrochlorothia-zide and later with furosemide, two diuret-ics that can cause hypokalemia. Which of the following statements best explains the main reason for this diuretic-induced adverse effect?

A. Increased urine flow through the collecting tubule

B. Blockade of K^+ reabsorption in the proximal tubule

C. Inhibition of renin secretion from juxtaglomerular cells

D. Blockade of Na^+ reabsorption in the late distal tubule

E. Inhibition of Na^+/K^+ adenosine triphosphatase (ATPase) in the late distal tubule

10. The postdischarge therapy for J. K. included a substitution of hydrochloro-thiazide with furosemide. Which of the fol-lowing statements best explains why loop diuretics are far more effective than thia-zide diuretics?

A. Loop diuretics increase renin secretion.

B. Loop diuretics are also weak inhibitors of carbonic anhydrase.

C. The diuretic effect of thiazides undergoes partial tolerance.

D. The antihypertensive action of thiazides may reduce the glomerular filtration rate (GFR).

E. More sodium is physiologically reabsorbed at the loop of Henle than at the distal convolute tubule.

11. Furosemide was given to J.K. also, because it is able to increase the exceed-ingly low glomerular filtration rate that usually occur when cardiac output is sharply reduced. Which of the follow-ing mechanisms most likely mediated the effect of this class of diuretics?

A. Dilation of the afferent glomerular arteriole

B. Inhibition of Na^+ sensing by macula densa

C. Activation of β_1-receptors of juxtaglomerular cells

D. Dilation of the efferent glomerular arteriole

E. Inhibition of adenosine release by the macula densa

12. J.K. complained of tinnitus, hear-ing loss, and vertigo. Which of the follow-ing drugs taken by the patient most likely caused these symptoms?

A. Furosemide

B. Carvedilol

C. Captopril

D. Spironolactone

E. Digoxin

13. J.K. noticed a small growth of his breast. Which of the following drugs most likely caused this adverse effect?

A. Furosemide

B. Carvedilol

C. Captopril

D. Spironolactone

E. Digoxin

14. Carvedilol was prescribed to J.K. The decreased activity of which of the follow-ing enzymes most likely mediated the ther-apeutic effect of the drug in the patient's disease?

A. Na^+/K^+ ATPase

B. Phospholipase C

C. Guanylate cyclase

D. Adenylate cyclase

E. Tyrosine kinase

15. Which of the following physiological actions most likely contributes to the therapeutic effect of carvedilol in J.K.'s disease?

A. Increased renin secretion

B. Decreased preload

C. Prevention of chronic sympathetic overactivity

D. Increased myocardial remodeling

E. Downregulation of cardiac β-receptors

16. Captopril was prescribed to J.K. The plasma levels of which of the following pairs of endogenous compounds were most likely increased after a few days of therapy?

A. Bradykinin–aldosterone

B. Angiotensin I–bradykinin

C. Aldosterone–angiotensin II

D. Angiotensin I–angiotensin II

E. Angiotensin I–aldosterone

F. Bradykinin–angiotensin II

17. ACE inhibitors are given indefinitely in patients with systolic heart failure. Which of the following actions most likely contributes to mortality reduction obtained by the long-term use of these drugs in systolic heart failure?

A. Increased cardiac contractility

B. Increased left ventricular filling pressure

C. Coronary vasodilation

D. Decreased ventricular automaticity

E. Decreased myocardial remodeling

18. Spironolactone was prescribed to J.K. Which of the following is most likely the main reason for the use of spironolactone in heart failure?

A. It counteracts the hypokalemia induced by loop diuretics.

B. It enhances the diuretic action of loop diuretics.

C. It can substantially decrease morbidity and mortality.

D. It counteracts the bradycardia induced by β-blockers.

E. It prolongs the action of ACE inhibitors given concomitantly.

19. A decreased synthesis of which of the following ion channels most likely occurred in J.K.'s kidney after a few days of spironolactone therapy?

A. K^+ channels

B. Na^+ channels

C. Ca^{2+} channels

D. Mg^{2+} channels

E. Cl^- channels

20. Digoxin was prescribed to J.K. The drug can exert other beneficial effects on heart failure, in addition to its inotropic action. Which of the following pharmacological actions most likely contributed to the efficacy of the drug in the patient's disease?

A. Increased sympathetic activity

B. Increased parasympathetic activity

C. Decreased abnormal heart automaticity

D. Decreased myocardial remodeling

E. Decreased sensitivity of carotid baroreceptors

21. Two weeks after hospital discharge J.K. was admitted to the emergency department because of digoxin poisoning. The patient complained of nausea and vomiting. Which of the following was the most likely cause of these symptoms?

A. Increased vestibular firing to the vomiting center

B. Direct stimulation of the chemoreceptor trigger zone

C. Increased cortical firing to the vomiting center

D. Facilitation of muscarinic transmission at the gastric muscle cells

E. Sensitization of carotid sinus baroreceptors

22. Upon admission to the emergency department after digoxin poisoning, J.K.'s ventricular rate did not exceed 45 bpm. Which of the following statements best explains the most likely reason for this low ventricular rate?

A. Digoxin-induced stimulation of the vagal nucleus

B. Direct depressant effect of digoxin upon the sinoatrial (SA) and AV nodes

C. Digoxin-induced depression of the vasomotor center

D. Digoxin-induced increase in intraventricular conduction

E. Digoxin-induced compensation of cardiac insufficiency

23. On admission to the emergency department, J.K. was found to have a serum K^+ level of 8.7 mEq/L. Which of the following statements best explains the reason for this lab result?

A. Digoxin blocked the renal elimination of K^+.

B. The inhibition of the Ca^{2+}/Na^+ exchanger increased K^+ exit from cells.

C. Captopril therapy favored K^+ retention.

D. The inhibition of Na^+/K^+ ATPase increased K^+ exit from cells.

E. Spironolactone therapy favored K^+ retention.

24. J.K.'s poisoning was treated with an effective antidote. Which of the following was most likely the mechanism of action of this antidote?

A. It increases the elimination of digoxin by the kidney.

B. It binds to Na^+/K^+ ATPase, preventing digoxin binding.

C. It binds to digoxin and neutralizes it.

D. It blocks the absorption of digoxin from the intestine.

E. It stimulates digoxin metabolism by the liver.

Answers and Explanations

▸ *Learning objective:* Identify the best cardiac sign indicating low-output systolic heart failure.

> **1. Answer: E**

In low-output heart failure, contractility is decreased (i.e., the force of contraction for any given end diastolic volume is decreased). The ejection fraction (i.e., the fraction of blood ejected during systole), is the best measure of heart contractility.

A The S3 sound is the most sensitive indicator of ventricular dysfunction, but it can also occur in high-output heart failure, where heart contractility is normal.

B, C, D All these listed signs are typical of systolic heart failure, but they are non-specific, because they can occur in several other cardiovascular disorders.

▸ *Learning objective:* Describe the main cardiovascular action that causes the decrease of mean blood pressure in systolic heart failure.

> **2. Answer: C**

The patient's blood pressure record indicates a decreased systolic pressure and an increased diastolic pressure. Therefore the pulse pressure is sharply decreased. Stroke volume is the major determinant of pulse pressure, because the blood volume ejected from the ventricle during systole causes arterial pressure to increase from its lowest value (diastolic pressure) to its highest value (systolic pressure). In systolic heart failure stroke volume is decreased because of a decrease in heart contractility.

A The heart rate is a determinant of blood pressure because in a normal patient an increase of heart rate usually causes an increase in mean blood pressure (BP = HR × SV × TPR), where SV refers to stroke volume and TPR refers to total peripheral resistance. In heart failure the activation of the sympathetic nervous system causes an increase in heart rate and in total peripheral resistance. However, in spite of this, the mean blood pressure is decreased because of the decrease in stroke volume.

B In systolic heart failure the pulmonary venous pressure can be sharply increased. However, the increased pulmonary venous pressure is not the cause for the decreased pulse pressure, because both are due to the decreased contractility of the left ventricle.

D, E In heart failure both preload and afterload are increased, not decreased.

▶ *Learning objective:* Explain why there is an increased need to urinate during the night in patients with heart failure.

3.   Answer: B

The need to get up more frequently at night to urinate, "nocturia," is a common symptom in heart failure and is caused by the redistribution of fluids from areas such as the ankle back into the blood after lying down. This increased fluid is filtered by the kidney, and the increased diuresis distends the bladder and wakes the person up.

A When the patient is lying down preload is increased, not decreased.

C In systolic heart failure myocardial contractility is always decreased. It does not change by changing the body position.

D Parasympathetic, not sympathetic, activity is predominant during night sleep. Even if in heart failure sympathetic activity is increased, it is less prominent during the night.

E Bladder contractility does not change by changing the body position.

▶ *Learning objective:* Explain the reason for orthopnea in heart failure.

4.   Answer: E

Shortness of breath that occurs when the patient is lying flat is termed orthopnea. In heart failure, during the day gravitational effects may favor a loss of intravascular fluid into the interstitial space. When the patient is in a horizontal position, the edema fluid may be redistributed and return to the vascular system, augmenting the venous return. The failing left ventricle is not able to cope with the extra volume of blood delivered to it, resulting in an increase in pulmonary venous and capillary pressure. This pulmonary congestion leads to pulmonary interstitial edema and decreased airway compliance. This factor, along with the elevated diaphragm in the lying posture, decreases the vital capacity of the lung. The patient is unable to breathe easily when lying down and must elevate his or her head on pillows to breathe comfortably.

A In heart failure afterload is usually increased, not decreased.

B In heart failure pulmonary venous pressure is increased, not decreased.

C The diaphragm is a striated muscle. Contractility of striated muscles is usually decreased, not increased, in heart failure because of muscle underperfusion.

D Diuresis is increased in heart failure when the patient is lying flat, but both the increased diuresis and the orthopnea are due to the same cause—redistribution of fluids back into the blood after lying down.

▶ *Learning objective:* Identify the stage of heart failure from the patient's symptoms and signs.

5.   Answer: C

According to the American Heart Association and the American College of Cardiology, heart failure can be subdivided into the following four stages:

▶ *Stage A (high risk heart failure):* Patients have one or more risk factors for developing heart failure but have no structural heart disease, no symptoms, and no limitation of physical activity.
▶ *Stage B (asymptomatic heart failure):* Patients have structural heart disease (i.e., enlarged or dysfunctional left ventricle from any cause) but no symptoms at rest and slight limitation of physical activity.
▶ *Stage C (symptomatic heart failure):* Patients have structural heart disease, previous or current symptoms, and marked limitation of physical activity.
▶ *Stage D (refractory heart failure):* Patients have structural heart disease and symptoms at rest in spite of medical treatment.

J.K. had a symptomatic heart failure that improved substantially after therapy. This disease is classified as stage C heart failure.

A, B, D See correct answer explanation.

▶ *Learning objective:* Identify the primary site of action of furosemide.

6. Answer: C

Furosemide is a loop diuretic. These drugs block the Na⁺/K⁺/2Cl⁻ symport located in the thick ascending limb of Henle's loop. The blockade increased the NaCl content in the tubular lumen, which in turn increases diuresis.

A, B, D, E, F, G See correct answer explanation.

▶ *Learning objective:* Describe the main action underlying the therapeutic effect of furosemide in heart failure.

7. Answer: D

Loop diuretics like furosemide are usually necessary to restore and maintain euvolemia in heart failure. They reduce extracellular fluid volume and increase venous capacitance. In this way they reduce preload, leading to a lower ventricular filling pressure. This reduces the workload of the heart. However, despite the efficacy of loop diuretics in controlling congestive symptoms and improving exercise capacity, their use does not reduce mortality in heart failure.

A Because patients with heart failure often operate on the plateau phase of Starling's curve, preload reduction can occur without a concomitant reduction of cardiac output.

B, C Loop diuretics do not affect cardiac contractility and rate.

E Loop diuretics can increase venous capacitance, but they have little effect on systemic vascular resistance (i.e., afterload).

▶ *Learning objective:* Describe the action mediating the furosemide-induced decrease of kidney concentrating ability.

8. Answer: E

Furosemide is a loop diuretic. These drugs act by blocking the Na⁺/K⁺/2Cl⁻ symport in the thick ascending limb of the loop of Henle. A consequence of this blockade is that the hypertonicity of medullary interstitium is decreased because fewer ions are reabsorbed. This action causes a decreased concentrating ability of the kidney, which is a specific feature of loop diuretics.

A Osmolality is the total concentration of all osmotically active solutes. By blocking the Na⁺/K⁺/2Cl⁻ symport, loop diuretics actually decrease, not increase, the intracellular osmolarity.

B Apical Na⁺ channels are located in the collecting tubule. These channels are blocked by some potassium-sparing diuretics like triamterene. Loop diuretics do not affect these channels.

C Loop diuretics have no effect on vasopressin receptors.

D This action results from diuretics that act in the proximal tubule, such as carbonic anhydrase inhibitors. By causing volume depletion, loop diuretics can indirectly increase ion reabsorption in the proximal tubule. This would decrease, not increase, solute osmolality in the lumen of the proximal tubule.

▶ *Learning objective:* Explain the primary reason for diuretic-induced hypokalemia.

9. Answer: A

All diuretics (except potassium-sparing diuretics) can cause hypokalemia, which is due to several factors. The following are the three most important, in order of decreasing relevance:

▶ The increased urine flow along the collecting tubule. Under almost all circumstances, an increase in luminal flow increases K⁺ excretion. This is a consequence of the high apical permeability of the principal cells of the collecting tubule to K⁺. The high luminal flow sweeps the newly secreted K⁺ downstream, thereby maintaining the K⁺ gradient across the apical membrane.
▶ The high Na⁺ load in the collecting tubule. The higher the Na⁺ concentration in the collecting tubule, the higher the reabsorption of Na⁺ through epithelial Na⁺ channels. This creates a luminal negative potential, which favors K⁺ and H⁺ excretion.

▶ The diuretic-induced hypovolemia, which in turn triggers aldosterone secretion.

B The reabsorption of K^+ in the proximal tubule is not affected by diuretics.

C Furosemide actually stimulates renin secretion.

D The blockade of Na^+ reabsorption in the late distal tubule would cause K^+ sparing. This is the mechanism of action of triamterene and amiloride.

E Na^+/K^+ ATPase is not affected by diuretics.

▶ *Learning objective:* Explain why loop diuretics are far more effective than thiazide diuretics.

10.   Answer: E

The $Na^+/K^+/2Cl^-$ symport in the thick ascending limb of the loop of Henle is responsible for the reabsorption of about 25% of the Na^+ filtered by the glomerulus, whereas the Na^+/Cl^- symport in the distal convolute tubule is responsible for about 10% of Na^+ reabsorption. Loop diuretics inhibit $Na^+/K^+/2Cl^-$ symporter, whereas thiazide diuretics inhibit Na^+/Cl^- symporter. Therefore the diuresis induced by loop diuretics is by far more effective than that induced by thiazides.

A The increased renin secretion has nothing to do with the effectiveness of loop diuretics.

B Both sulfonamide loop diuretics and thiazides are weak inhibitors of carbonic anhydrase, and, moreover, this action contributes very little to the diuretic effect of these drugs.

C The effect of thiazides does not undergo tolerance. In fact the antihypertensive effect of these drugs (which is also related to the depletion of Na^+ body stores) remains the same after years of treatment.

D The antihypertensive effect of thiazides is mild and is not accompanied by a decrease in GFR.

▶ *Learning objective:* Explain why loop diuretics can increase an abnormally low GFR.

11.   Answer: B

J.K. was suffering from heart failure. Essentially all patients with clinically evi-dent heart failure require loop diuretics, because they are the most effective and are the only diuretics able to increase an excessively low GFR. By blocking the $Na^+/K^+/2Cl^-$ symporter they inhibit Na+ transport into the macula densa. In this way the macula densa can no longer detect Na^+ concentration in tubular fluid. This initiates a signal that stimulates renin release from juxtaglomerular cells, thereby increasing the synthesis of angiotensin II. Angiotensin II constricts the efferent arterioles more than the afferent, increasing GFR.

A, D By activating the renin angiotensin system, loop diuretics cause (indirectly) actions opposite to those listed.

C Activation of β_1-adrenoceptors of juxtaglomerular cells can increase angiotensin synthesis, but loop diuretics do not activate β_1-adrenoceptors.

E This is a second feedback mechanism mediated by juxtaglomerular cells but is activated by an increased Na^+ concentration into tubular fluid and leads to a decrease, not an increase, of renin release.

▶ *Learning objective:* Identify the drug that can cause tinnitus, hearing loss, and vertigo.

12.   Answer: A

The adverse effects reported by J.K. were most likely due to furosemide. Loop diuretics can cause tinnitus, vertigo, and hearing loss; few cases of deafness have been reported. This ototoxicity is dose related, reversible, and likely due to alteration in the electrolyte composition of the endolymph.

B Carvedilol does not cause tinnitus and hearing loss. It causes vertigo in 2 to 3% of patients, likely due to drug-induced postural hypotension.

C, D, E These drugs do not cause tinnitus, hearing loss, and vertigo.

▶ *Learning objective:* Identify the drug that can cause gynecomastia.

13.   Answer: D

Gynecomastia is a common adverse effect of spironolactone, occurring in about 10% of patients taking the drug. Owing to its affinity for other steroid receptors, spironolactone may act by displacing androgen from the androgen receptors and sex hormone–binding globulin. The drug can also increase the metabolic clearance of testosterone. All these actions can contribute to the drug-induced gynecomastia.

A, B, C The risk of gynecomastia with these drugs is negligible or absent.

E Gynecomastia can occur with digoxin, likely because of the steroid nucleus of the drug, but its frequency is < 1%.

▸ *Learning objective:* Explain the molecular mechanism of action of carvedilol.

14. Answer: D

Carvedilol is a αβ-adrenoceptor blocker. Activation of all β-receptors increases the synthesis of cyclic adenosine monophosphate through an increased activity of the adenylate cyclase enzyme. By blocking these receptors, all β-blockers do the opposite (i.e., the activity of adenylate cyclase is decreased).

A A decreased activity Na^+/K^+ ATPase mediates the action of digoxin.

B A decreased activity of phospholipase C can inhibit several physiological actions, including α_1-adrenoceptor-mediated contraction of vascular smooth muscle.

C A decreased activity of guanylate cyclase can inhibit some cyclic guanosine monophosphate–mediated actions, including the relaxation of vascular smooth muscle.

E A decreased activity of tyrosine kinase can inhibit the action of several drugs, including insulin and many other trophic hormones.

▸ *Learning objective:* Describe the action mediating the therapeutic effect of carvedilol in heart failure.

15. Answer: C

Carvedilol is a nonselective αβ-adrenoceptor blocker. Today β-blockers are first-line agents for systolic heart failure. Guidelines suggest early use, low dose, gradual titration, and selected agents. There is fairly strong evidence that the benefits of β-blockers in systolic heart failure are not a class effect. Metoprolol, bisoprolol, and carvedilol are

the β-blockers shown to reduce mortality in large heart failure trials.

Beneficial effects of β-blockers in systolic heart failure include the following:

▸ Prevention of chronic overactivity of the sympathetic nervous system, which leads to decreased heart rate and reduced myocardial remodeling through inhibition of the mitogenic activity of catecholamines
▸ Inhibition of renin secretion by blocking β_1-receptors in juxtaglomerular cells, which in turn decreases the activity of the renin–angiotensin system
▸ Upregulation of β_1-receptors (in heart failure, β_1-receptors are downregulated, due to the chronic activation of the sympathetic nervous system)

A By blocking β_1-adrenoceptors carvedilol decreases, not increases, renin secretion.

B By increasing the duration of the diastole, β-blockers tend to increase, not decrease, preload.

D By inhibiting the renin–angiotensin system, β-blockers tend to decrease, not to increase, myocardial remodeling.

E Cardiac β-adrenoceptors are upregulated, not downregulated, by β-blockers.

▸ *Learning objective:* Recognize the two endogenous compounds whose plasma levels are increased by angiotensin-converting enzyme (ACE) inhibitors.

16. Answer: B

ACE inhibitors, such as captopril, reduce the synthesis of angiotensin II (by inhibiting the conversion of angiotensin I to angiotensin II), which in turn increases plasma levels of angiotensin I. ACE inhibitors also inhibit the metabolism of bradykinin; therefore plasma levels of this compound are also increased.

C, D, F Angiotensin II is decreased because of inhibition of the ACE.

A, C, E Aldosterone is decreased, due to the decrease activity of angiotensin II.

▶ *Learning objective:* Describe a long-term action of ACE inhibitors that can reduce mortality in heart failure.

17. Answer: E

ACE inhibitors decrease the synthesis of angiotensin II. This decrease attenuates many of the deleterious effects of this peptide hormone that drive heart failure progression. This includes reduction of norepinephrine release, sodium and water retention, myocardial fibrosis, myocyte apoptosis, and myocardial remodeling. Over time this remodeling causes a pathological increase of ventricular mass that adversely affects heart function. Decrease of myocardial remodeling by ACE inhibitors is a main factor mediating the mortality reduction achieved with long-term use of these drugs.

A ACE inhibitors do not appreciably affect cardiac contractility. The increased pumping performance of the heart after treatment with these drugs is mediated by Starling's law, not by an increase in cardiac contractility.

B Left ventricular filling pressure is increased in heart failure. By decreasing preload ACE inhibitors decrease, not increase, left ventricular filling pressure.

C By decreasing the workload of the heart, ACE inhibitors can indirectly cause coronary vasoconstriction.

D ACE inhibitors have negligible effects on ventricular automaticity.

▶ *Learning objective:* Explain the reason for spironolactone use in systolic cardiac failure.

18. Answer: C

Two recent clinical trials have shown that spironolactone significantly reduces (~30%) mortality and hospitalization for heart failure due to left ventricular systolic dysfunction. This reduction was achieved in the absence of a demonstrable diuretic effect, supporting the hypothesis that aldosterone antagonists attenuate the deleterious effects of aldosterone on the heart, which may include promoting the development of cardiac hypertrophy and fibrosis.

A Spironolactone is a K⁺-sparing diuretic and can counteract the loop diuretic–

induced hypokalemia. However, this is not at all the main reason for the therapeutic effect of this drug in systolic heart failure.

B Spironolactone is a mild diuretic; therefore it can enhance very little the diuretic action of loop diuretics.

D Spironolactone has no direct effect on heart rate.

E Spironolactone can enhance the beneficial effects of ACE inhibitors, but this is a pharmacodynamic interaction. The drug has no effect on the metabolism of ACE inhibitors; therefore it cannot prolong the action of these drugs.

▶ *Learning objective:* Describe the ion channels whose synthesis was inhibited by spironolactone.

19. Answer: B

Aldosterone increases the synthesis of aldosterone-controlled channels in the distal tubule and collecting duct. This in turn increases Na^+ and water reabsorption in these segments of the nephron. By blocking aldosterone receptors spironolactone decreases the synthesis of these channels, which can account for the diuretic action of the drug.

A, C, D, E The synthesis of these channels is not affected by aldosterone.

▶ *Learning objective:* Identify the physiological action that can contribute to the therapeutic effect of digoxin in heart failure.

20. Answer: B

Digoxin has beneficial autonomic effects caused by reduced sympathetic tone and increased parasympathetic activity at serum concentrations below those associated with positive inotropism. The parasympathetic activation is likely due to different actions, including the following:

▶ Stimulation of the nucleus ambiguus of the vagus nerve
▶ Facilitation of muscarinic transmission in heart muscle cells
▶ Sensitization of carotid sinus baroreceptors, due to the inhibition of Na+/K+ ATPase, which reduces the sympathetic outflow from the central nervous system

A Digoxin decreases, not increases, sympathetic activity due to actions not related to the increase in cardiac output produced by the drug. These include both the reduction of sympathetic outflow from the central nervous system mentioned above and a direct sympathoinhibitory effect. Only very high doses of digoxin can increase sympathetic activity.

C Digoxin is an arrhythmogenic drug that increases, not decreases, abnormal heart automaticity in both the normal and the failing heart.

D Digoxin does not prevent progressive myocardial remodeling that occurs in chronic heart failure.

E Sensitivity of carotid baroreceptors is increased, not decreased, by digoxin.

▸ *Learning objective:* Explain the mechanism of digoxin-induced nausea and vomiting.

21. Answer: B

Nausea, vomiting, and diarrhea can occur after digoxin administration, even if their incidence is decreased substantially as a consequence of increased understanding of digoxin pharmacokinetics. Digoxin-induced nausea and vomiting are primarily due to direct stimulation of the chemoreceptor trigger zone.

A Digoxin does not stimulate vestibular nuclei.

C Increased cortical firing from the brain cortex to the vomiting center can occur and can explain why some bad thoughts can cause nausea and vomiting, but this is not the emetic mechanism of digoxin.

D Digoxin can cause facilitation of muscarinic transmission, but this action is mild and is not the primary mechanism of the emetic action of the drug.

E Digoxin can cause sensitization of carotid sinus baroreceptors, but this sensitization does not cause nausea and vomiting.

▸ *Learning objective:* Explain the reason for atropine-resistant bradycardia in digoxin poisoning.

22. Answer: B

Digoxin-induced decrease in heart rate results primarily from the following actions:

▸ A vagal activation
▸ A direct depressive action upon the SA and AV node

In the present case, however, the decrease in heart rate was resistant to atropine treatment, suggesting that it was due mainly to the direct depressant effect upon SA and AV nodes.

A See correct answer explanation.

C Toxic doses of digoxin usually increase sympathetic nervous system activity.

D This action would have caused ventricular arrhythmias.

E Therapeutic doses of digoxin can decrease the heart rate in patients with heart failure, because the compensation of cardiac insufficiency offsets the activation of the sympathetic nervous system, but toxic doses usually increase sympathetic nervous system activity.

▸ *Learning objective:* Explain the reason for the severe hyperkalemia found in this case of digoxin poisoning.

23. Answer: D

The main cause of the dramatic rise in serum potassium was the blockade of Na^+/K^+ ATPase all over the body. This blockade increases K^+ levels in the extracellular space, especially that of skeletal muscle, because of the large mass of this tissue.

A Digoxin does not affect renal potassium elimination.

B A consequence of digoxin action is the inhibition of the Ca^{2+}/Na^+ exchanger, but this has nothing to do with the hyperkalemia found in this case of digoxin poisoning.

C, E Both captopril and spironolactone can cause a mild K^+ retention, but this retention cannot explain the high hyperkalemia found in the present case.

▸ *Learning objective:* Explain the mechanism of action of digoxin antidote.

24. Answer: C

The antidote used in cases of life-threatening poisoning by digoxin, as in the present case, is available in the form of antibodies (purified Fab [fragment antigen binding] fragments from ovine antidigoxin antisera).

These antibodies bind to most digitalis glycosides and neutralize them. They are extremely effective in reversing digitalis poisoning.

A Digoxin is primarily excreted as such by the kidney, but digoxin antibodies do not increase this excretion.

B Digoxin antibodies bind to digoxin, not to Na^+/K^+ ATPase.

D Absorption of digoxin is not affected by digoxin antibodies.

E Metabolism of digoxin is not affected by digoxin antibodies.

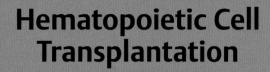

Hematopoietic Cell Transplantation

Q.T., a 42-year-old man, was found to have the following blood exam results during an insurance checkup:

Blood hematology

- ▶ Red blood cell count (RBC): $3.8 \times 10^6/\mu L$ (normal, 4.0–6.0)
- ▶ Hemoglobin (Hb): 10.1 g/dL (normal 12–16)
- ▶ Hematocrit (Hct): 30.7% (normal 36–48)
- ▶ White blood cell count (WBC): $70 \times 10^3/uL$ (normal 4–10) with some metamyelocytes and myelocytes
- ▶ Platelet: $1{,}200 \times 10^3/\mu L$ (normal 130–400)

The patient was asymptomatic, and the only pertinent finding from physical examination was a palpable spleen 8 cm below the left costal margin. A bone marrow aspirate showed a hypercellular marrow with 4% blasts. Cytogenetic analysis of bone marrow confirmed the diagnosis of Philadelphia chromosome-positive chronic myelogenous leukemia (CML).

Q.T. started a therapy with imatinib that induced a normalization of the WBC count and the disappearance of Philadelphia chromosome-positive cells.

On routine follow-up at 6 months, cytogenetic analysis of Q.T.'s bone marrow demonstrated 10% Philadelphia chromosome-positive cells. The oncologist decided to substitute imatinib with nilotinib, and the new drug treatment was able to induce a complete clinical and cytogenetic remission.

One year later Q.T. was readmitted to the hospital because of increasing tiredness, fever (100.4°F [38.2°C]), night sweats, and a 20-pound weight loss over the last 4 months. A blood exam gave the following results:

- ▶ RBC: $2.8 \times 10^6/\mu L$ (normal, men 4.5–5.5)
- ▶ Hb: 8.5 g/dL (normal, 12–16)
- ▶ Hct: 32% (normal 36–48)
- ▶ WBC: $40 \times 10^3/\mu L$ (normal 4–10) with 18% blasts
- ▶ Platelet: $1{,}100 \times 10^3/\mu L$ (normal 130–400)
- ▶ Ferritin: 28 ng/mL (normal 30–300)
- ▶ Iron 50 µg/dL (normal, men 65–170)

A diagnosis of accelerated phase of CML was made, and the patient was scheduled for hematopoietic stem cell transplantation. A search for a related allogeneic donor identified a partially human leukocyte antigen (HLA)-matched sibling donor. QT. was admitted to the transplantation unit and underwent a high-dose myeloablative regimen with busulfan and fludarabine. Then the donor bone marrow was given intravenously.

After transplantation the patient received immunosuppressive therapy that included cyclosporine and methotrexate.

Twenty days later Q.T. presented with a maculopapular rash involving the nape of the neck, ears, shoulders, and palms of the hands, persistent nausea, and abdominal cramps with diarrhea. Blood exams showed a rise in the serum levels of conjugated bilirubin and alkaline phosphatase. A skin biopsy confirmed the presumptive diagnosis of acute graft-versus-host disease.

Questions

1. Q.T. was diagnosed with chronic myelogenous leukemia. Which of the following sets of differential white blood cell count most likely occurred in his blood exam result?

Set	Neutrophils (%)	Eosinophils (%)	Basophils (%)	Lymphocytes (%)
A.	64	4	2	30
B.	58	3	2	35
C.	84	8	4	4
D.	70	2	1	27
E.	62	2	1	35

2. Q.T. was diagnosed with Philadelphia chromosome-positive chronic myelogenous leukemia. Which of the following is the specific oncogene of this chromosome that is most important in the pathogenesis of chronic myelogenous leukemia?

A. *DBL*

B. *ALK-NPM*

C. *AKT-2*

D. *BCR-ABL*

E. *GSP*

3. Q.T. started a therapy with imatinib. Which of the following molecular actions most likely mediated the therapeutic effect of the drug in the patient's disease?

A. Alkylation of DNA strands

B. Inhibition of tyrosine kinase

C. Inhibition of thymidylate synthetase

D. Intercalation of DNA paired bases

E. Inhibition of dihydrofolate reductase

F. Inhibition microtubule assembly

4. Which of the following adverse effects most likely occurred during the imatinib therapy?

A. Gastroesophageal reflux

B. Angina

C. Fluid retention

D. Alopecia

E. Bone pain

5. Q.T. underwent a complete remission when imatinib was substituted with nilotinib. Which of the following statements best explains the reason for this remission?

A. Nilotinib is much more potent than imatinib.

B. Nilotinib acts as an alkylating agent.

C. The *BCR-ABL* oncogene underwent a new mutation.

D. Imatinib can undergo pharmacokinetic tolerance.

E. Imatinib works poorly when bone marrow shows > 2% myeloblasts.

6. Q.T. was diagnosed with an accelerated phase of chronic myelogenous leukemia. Which of the following symptoms and signs best explains this diagnosis?

A. Platelet: $1100 \times 10^3/\mu L$

B. WBC $40 \times 10^3/\mu L$

C. 20-pound weight loss

D. 18% myeloblasts

E. Hb: 8.5 g/dL

F. Fever

7. Q.T. underwent a myeloablative regimen that included busulfan. Which of the following molecular actions most likely mediated the therapeutic effect of the drug in the patient's disease?

A. Formation of covalent bonds with DNA bases
B. Prevention of DNA chain elongation
C. Inhibition of thymidylate synthase
D. Prevention of DNA resealing
E. Inhibition of microtubule assembly

8. Q.T.'s myeloablative regimen included fludarabine. Which of the following molecular actions most likely mediated the anticancer effect of this drug?

A. Alkylation of DNA strands
B. Inhibition of dihydrofolate reductase
C. Inhibition of thymidylate synthetase
D. Inhibition of microtubule polymerization
E. Inhibition of DNA polymerase
F. Inhibition of topoisomerase enzymes

9. After transplantation Q.T. received an immunosuppressive therapy that included cyclosporine. Which of the following actions most likely mediated the prophylactic effect of the drug in the patient's disease?

A. Induction of the recipient's thymus involution
B. Reduction of the recipient's secretion of immunoglobulin G antibodies
C. Decreased proliferation of transplanted bone marrow T cells
D. Increased proliferation of the recipient's macrophages
E. Decreased proliferation of the recipient's bone marrow T cells

10. Because of the cyclosporine treatment, Q.T. was most likely at risk for which of the following adverse drug effects?

A. Alopecia
B. Hypotension
C. Nephrotoxicity
D. Hypokalemia
E. Hypoglycemia

11. Q.T. was diagnosed with acute graft-versus-host disease. Which of the following drugs most likely represents the initial standard treatment of this disease?

A. Infliximab
B. Azathioprine
C. Methylprednisolone
D. Cyclophosphamide
E. Aldesleukin
F. Thalidomide

Answers and Explanations

▶ *Learning objective:* Identify the most likely differential white blood cell count in a patient with chronic myelogenous leukemia.

1. Answer: C

Chronic myelogenous leukemia is a myeloproliferative disorder that affects primarily the granulocytic lineage. Therefore the white blood cells are predominantly neutrophils and immature granulocytes with < 10% myeloblasts. Eosinophilia and basophilia are also common, and up to 50% of patients have pronounced thrombocytosis, as in the present case.

A, B, D, E All these differential blood cell counts are within normal ranges.

▶ *Learning objective:* Identify the specific oncogene of Philadelphia chromosome that is most important in the pathogenesis of chronic myelogenous leukemia.

2. Answer: D

The chronic phase of myelogenous leukemia is characterized by < 10% blasts in the blood and bone marrow, which explains the diagnosis in the present case.

Most chronic myelogenous leukemias appear to be induced by a translocation known as Philadelphia chromosome, which is present in up to 95% of patients. This chromosome results from a reciprocal translocation in which a piece of chromosome 9 containing the oncogene *ABL* is translocated to chromosome 22 and fused

177

to the gene *BCR*. The fusion *BCR-ABL* onco-gene mediates the synthesis of a specific tyrosine kinase that promotes unregulated white blood cell growth, leading to marked elevation of the white blood cell count and an increase (often massive) in the size of the spleen.

A This oncogene mediates the diffuse B-cell lymphoma.

B This oncogene mediates large-cell lymphomas.

C This oncogene mediates ovarian cancer.

E This oncogene mediates thyroid carcinoma.

▶ *Learning objective:* Explain the mechanism of action of imatinib.

3.   Answer: B

Imatinib is a tyrosine kinase inhibitor. These drugs have substantially changed the prognosis of chronic myelogenous leu-kemia. Before imatinib 10% of patients died within 2 years of diagnosis; with imatinib survival is > 90% at 5 years. Tyrosine kinase inhibitors inhibit the specific *BCR-ABL* tyro-sine kinase that results from the oncogene expression of cells characterized by the presence of Philadelphia chromosome. The inhibition of the enzyme blocks the down-stream activation of abnormal myeloid cell proliferation. Therefore imatinib is currently approved as a standard initial treatment for patients with chronic-phase chronic myelogenous leukemia.

A This would be the mechanism of action of alkylating drugs.

C This would be the mechanism of action of fluorouracil.

D This would be the mechanism of action of anthracyclines.

E This would be the mechanism of action of methotrexate.

F This would be the mechanism of action of vinca alkaloids.

▶ *Learning objective:* Identify the most frequent adverse effect of imatinib therapy.

4.   Answer: C

Fluid retention (up to 76%) and edema (up to 86%) are among the most frequently

reported adverse reactions to imatinib. Severe fluid retention including anasarca, pleural effusion, pericardial effusion, asci-tes, and/or pulmonary edema has occurred in up to 10% of patients with chronic myelogenous leukemia. The mechanism of this drug-induced edema is still unclear.

A, B, D, E The incidence of these ima-tinib-induced adverse effects is < 10%.

▶ *Learning objective:* Identify the most likely reason for failure of imatinib therapy.

5.   Answer: C

Despite the positive effect of imatinib, nearly 20% of patients who take the drug do not have a complete cytogenetic response. This is most often due to the development of a new mutation in the *BCR-ABL* oncogene, which allows the dis-ease to become resistant to treatment. Nilotinib is a second-generation tyrosine kinase inhibitor that has a higher bind-ing affinity (up to 50-fold higher) for the *ABL* kinase when compared with imatinib and overcomes imatinib resistance due to *BCR-ABL* oncogene mutations. The drug is approved both as a first-line therapy and as therapy for chronic phase resistant to ima-tinib. This explains the oncologist's choice of nilotinib.

A Potency refers to the dose needed to achieve the therapeutic effect. Since the standard dose for imatinib is 600 mg daily and the one for nilotinib is 300 mg daily, nilotinib is more potent than imatinib, but drug potency is by no means related to drug efficacy, which refers to the maxi-mum effect a drug can give, irrespective of the dose used. Because nilotinib achieved an effect no longer obtained by imatinib, it could be concluded that a reason for the drug's success could be that nilotinib is more effective, not more potent, than imatinib.

B Nilotinib is a tyrosine kinase inhibi-tor, not an alkylating agent.

D Pharmacokinetic tolerance refers to a tolerance due to a pharmacokinetic mechanism (e.g., increased metabolism, increased elimination). Imatinib does not undergo pharmacokinetic tolerance.

E Imatinib works well, not poorly, when bone marrow shows 5 to 10% myeloblasts.

▸ *Learning objective:* Identify the symptom/sign that best explains the diagnosis of accelerated phase of chronic myelogenous leukemia.

6. Answer: D

Chronic myelogenous leukemia is classically subdivided into the following phases:

▸ **Chronic stable phase:** myeloblasts fewer than 10% in the blood and/or bone marrow
▸ **Accelerated phase:** myeloblasts 10 to 19% in the blood and/or bone marrow, persistent thrombocytosis (> 1,000 × 10^3/μL) unresponsive to therapy, increasing spleen size unresponsive to therapy, cytogenetic evidence of clonal evolution
▸ **Blast phase** (also called blast crisis): myeloblasts ≥ 20% in the blood and/or bone marrow, extramedullary myeloblast proliferation, large foci or clusters of blasts on bone marrow biopsy

Therefore the percent myeloblast in the blood and/or bone marrow is the best indicator of the phase of chronic myelogenous leukemia. Because Q.T.'s blood exams showed 18% myeloblasts the diagnosis of accelerated phase was appropriate.

A Persistent thrombocytosis unresponsive to therapy can be a sign of the accelerated phase, but the percent of myeloblasts is by far a more specific sign.

B This result can occur also in the chronic stable phase of the disease.

C, E, F These signs and lab exams can occur in many severe chronic diseases.

▸ *Learning objective:* Explain the mechanism of action of busulfan.

7. Answer: A

The primary goal of a myeloablative preparative regimen is to eradicate residual malignancy. Combination chemotherapy with near-lethal doses of anticancer drugs with or without concomitant radiotherapy is the most common myeloablative regimen. Busulfan is an alkylating anticancer drug. These agents act by intermolecular cyclization to form either an ethyleneimonium or a carbonium ion, which is strongly electrophilic (i.e., electron attracting). These intermediates can alkylate; that is, they can transfer alkyl groups to various cellular constituents by formation of covalent bonds with nucleophile (i.e., electron donor) groups of these constituents. Alkylation of guanine of a single strand of the DNA molecule results in miscoding or in depurination by excision of guanine residues. Alkylation of guanine of both strands of the DNA molecule results in cross-linking. Busulfan forms DNA–DNA intrastrand crosslinks between the DNA bases guanine and adenine and between guanine and guanine. DNA crosslinking prevents DNA replication. Because the intrastrand DNA crosslinks cannot be repaired by cellular machinery, the cell undergoes apoptosis.

B This would be the mechanism of action of cytarabine.

C This would be the mechanism of action of fluorouracil.

D This would be the mechanism of action of topoisomerase inhibitors.

E This would be the mechanism of action of vinca alkaloids.

▸ *Learning objective:* Identify the anticancer subclass that includes fludarabine.

8. Answer: E

Fludarabine is a purine analogue that is rapidly biotransformed intracellularly to the active fludarabine triphosphate. This false nucleotide inhibits DNA-polymerase and can also be directly incorporated into DNA, resulting in inhibition of DNA synthesis and function.

A Alkylation of DNA strands would be the mechanism of action of alkylating agents like cyclophosphamide, cisplatin, and nitrosoureas.

B Inhibition of dihydrofolate reductase would be the mechanism of action of antifolate drugs like methotrexate.

C Inhibition of thymidylate synthetase would be the mechanism of action of fluoropyrimidines like fluorouracil.

D Inhibition of microtubule polymerization would be the mechanism of action of vinca alkaloids.

F Inhibition of topoisomerase enzymes would be the mechanism of action of topoisomerase inhibitors like topotecan and etoposide.

▸ *Learning objective:* Identify the cyclosporine action that mediates its prophylactic effect after hematopoietic cell transplantation.

9. Answer: C

Because the tissue transplanted in allogeneic hematopoietic cell transplantation is immunologically active, there is potential for the following bidirectional graft rejection.

▸ *Host-versus-graft disease:* where cytotoxic T cells and natural killer cells belonging to the host (recipient) recognize antigens of the graft (donor hematopoietic stem cells) and elicit a rejection response
▸ *Graft-versus-host disease:* where immunologically active T cells in the graft recognize host antigens and elicit an immune response

Host-versus-graft effects are more common in solid organ transplantation, whereas graft-versus-host effects are more common in hematopoietic cell transplantation. In order to prevent the bidirectional graft rejection, an immunosuppressive therapy is commonly given after bone marrow transplantation. Without postgrafting immunosuppression, serious acute graft-versus-host disease would occur in almost every allogeneic recipient. The most common prophylaxis regimen is the combination of cyclosporine and methotrexate, as in the present case.

Cyclosporine inhibits calcineurin, an enzyme that is necessary for the activation of a T cell–specific transcription factor involved in the synthesis of interleukin 2. The decreased production of interleukin 2 in turn causes a decreased T cell proliferation in the transplanted bone marrow.

A Induction of the recipient's thymus involution has already occurred in an adult person.

B Secretion of immunoglobulin antibodies is controlled by plasma cells that are derived from B lymphocytes. Interleukin 2 does not affect proliferation of B lymphocytes.

D By decreasing the production of interleukin 2, cyclosporine can inhibit, not activate, the proliferation of macrophages.

E By decreasing the production of interleukin 2, cyclosporine inhibits T cell proliferation, both in the transplanted bone marrow and in the recipient bone marrow. However, the recipient bone marrow was already profoundly inhibited by the myeloablative preparative regimen. Therefore cyclosporine is given to prevent graft-versus-host disease, not host-versus-graft disease.

▸ *Learning objective:* Identify a common adverse effect of cyclosporine.

10. Answer: C

Nephrotoxicity is a serious, dose-dependent, and frequent adverse effect of cyclosporine, affecting > 30% of patients receiving the drug. Cyclosporine causes vasoconstriction of the afferent and efferent glomerular arterioles and reduction in renal blood flow and glomerular filtration rate. The exact mechanism of vasoconstriction is unclear, but there appears to be substantial impairment of endothelial cell function, leading to reduced production of vasodilators (prostaglandins and nitric oxide) and enhanced release of vasoconstrictors (endothelin and thromboxanes). In addition renal biopsy reveals an obliterative arteriolopathy, suggesting primary endothelial damage.

A, B, D, E Cyclosporine tends to cause effects opposite to those listed.

▸ *Learning objective:* Identify the drug used as initial standard therapy in acute graft-versus-host disease.

11. Answer: C

Acute graft-versus-host disease is a common complication of allogeneic hematopoietic cell transplantation that classically presents within 100 days after transplantation. It is thought to be primarily a T cell–mediated disease that occurs when immune cells transplanted from a nonidentical donor (the graft) recognize the transplant recipient (the host) as foreign, thereby initiating an immune reaction that causes disease in the transplant recipient. The disease can occur in spite of the strong immunosuppressive therapy that is commonly used to prevent it. The skin, gastrointestinal tract, and liver are the principal target organs, as in the present case. Corticosteroids are the first-line treatment for established acute graft-versus-host disease. A complete response occurs in 25 to 40% of patients, with a lower likelihood of response in more severe cases. Patients who do not respond to therapy or have ongoing severe acute graft-versus-host disease usually die from a combination of the disease and infectious complications.

A, B, D These drugs are immunosuppressive agents, but they are minimally or not at all effective for the therapy of acute graft-versus-host disease.

E, F These drugs are immunostimulant, not immunosuppressive, agents.

Case 21

Hodgkin's Lymphoma

R.U., a 36-year-old man, was admitted to the hospital with malaise, night sweats, loss of weight, and intermittent fever dating from a flulike illness 2 months previously. His past medical history indicated that last year he suffered from infection with mononucleosis. The patient did not smoke, and denied the use of alcohol or illicit drugs. He had a brother and a sister, both in good health. None of his relatives had any history of malignancy.

Physical examination showed bilateral cervical and axillary lymphadenopathy. The glands were 2 to 5 cm in diameter, firm, rubbery, discrete, and fairly mobile. His liver and spleen were not enlarged. The rest of the physical examination was unremarkable.

Pertinent laboratory results on admission were as follows:

Blood hematology

- ► Erythrocyte sedimentation rate (ESR): 78 mm/h (normal < 20)
- ► Red blood cell count (RBC): $4.8 \times 10^6/\mu L$ (normal, 4.0–6.0)
- ► White blood cell count (WBC): $8 \times 10^3/\mu L$ (normal 4–10)
- ► Hemoglobin (Hb): 10.5 g/dL (normal 12–16)
- ► Hematocrit (Hct): 34% (normal 36–48)
- ► Platelet: $320 \times 10^3/\mu L$ (normal 130–400)
- ► Ferritin: 250 ng/mL (normal 30–300)
- ► Iron: 120 µg/dL (normal, men 50–140)
- ► Creatinine: 1.1 mg/dL (normal 0.6–1.2)
- ► Blood urea nitrogen (BUN): 22 mg/dL (normal 8–25)
- ► Alkaline phosphatase: 220 U/L (normal 25–100)

Positron emission tomography scan

Abnormal high fluorodeoxyglucose (FDG) uptake on cervical and axillary lymph nodes

Bone marrow histology

Normal

Cervical lymph node histology

The gross architecture of the node was destroyed. The tissue consisted of a large amount of histiocytes, eosinophils, lymphocytes, plasma cells, and several Reed–Sternberg's cells with some degree of collagen sclerosis.

A diagnosis of Hodgkin's lymphoma was made, and R.U. underwent four cycles of combination therapy with the ABVD regimen (Adriamycin [doxorubicin], bleomycin, vinblastine, and dacarbazine). Three antiemetic drugs were also given in order to prevent chemotherapy-induced nausea and vomiting.

Questions

1. R.U. was diagnosed with Hodgkin's lymphoma. Which of the following histopathology features of the patient's lymph node was most likely the best index of his disease?

A. Large amount of lymphocytes
B. Collagen necrosis
C. Destruction of the normal architecture
D. Sternberg's cells
E. Large amount of plasma cells

2. Hodgkin's lymphoma is usually subdivided into four stages. From R.U.'s symptoms and signs, which of the following was most likely the stage of the patient's lymphoma?

A. Stage I
B. Stage II
C. Stage III
D. Stage IV

3. R.U. started a combination therapy with an ABVD regimen. Which of the following pairs of adverse effects did the patient most likely experience soon after starting this therapy?

A. Anemia–hair loss
B. Hyperkalemia–anemia
C. Neutropenia–anemia
D. Neutropenia–hair loss
E. Hyperkalemia–hair loss
F. Hyperkalemia–neutropenia

4. R.U. received a multidrug therapy in order to prevent chemotherapy-induced nausea and vomiting. Which of the following pairs of brain regions are most likely primarily involved in the chemotherapy-induced emesis?

A. Amygdala–locus ceruleus
B. Locus ceruleus–nucleus tractus solitarius
C. Locus ceruleus–chemoreceptor trigger zone
D. Amygdala–nucleus tractus solitarius
E. Amygdala–chemoreceptor trigger zone
F. Chemoreceptor trigger zone–nucleus tractus solitarius

5. R.U.'s antiemetic therapy included ondansetron. Blockade of which of the following receptors most likely mediated the therapeutic effect the drug in the patient's disease?

A. H_1 histamine receptors
B. M_1 muscarinic receptors
C. $5\text{-}HT_3$ serotonin receptors
D. NK_1 neurokinin receptors
E. D_2 dopamine receptors
F. CB_1 cannabinoid receptors

6. R.U.'s antiemetic therapy included aprepitant. Blockade of which of the following receptors most likely mediated the antiemetic effect the drug in the patient's disease?

A. H_1 histamine receptors
B. M_1 muscarinic receptors
C. $5\text{-}HT_3$ serotonin receptors
D. NK_1 neurokinin receptors
E. D_2 dopamine receptors
F. CB_1 cannabinoid receptors

7. In addition to ondansetron and aprepitant, R.U. was given a third drug in order to prevent chemotherapy-induced emesis. Which of the following was most likely the third drug?

A. Scopolamine
B. Diphenhydramine
C. Haloperidol
D. Dexamethasone
E. Promethazine

8. R.U.'s anticancer therapy included doxorubicin. Which of the following molecular actions most likely contributed to the therapeutic effect of the drug in the patient's disease?

A. Intercalation between DNA strands
B. Inhibition of microtubule disassembly
C. Inhibition of microtubule assembly
D. Alkylation of nucleophilic groups on DNA bases
E. Inhibition of tyrosine kinases

9. Which of the following is a life-threatening adverse effect of doxorubicin?

A. Pulmonary fibrosis

B. Acute heart failure

C. Ischemic stroke

D. Acute kidney failure

E. Acute liver failure

10. R.U.'s anticancer therapy included bleomycin. Which of the following molecular actions most likely mediated the therapeutic effect of the drug in the patient's disease?

A. Intercalation between DNA strands

B. Inhibition of DNA polymerase

C. Cleavage of single- and double-strand DNA

D. Inhibition of topoisomerase I

E. Inhibition of thymidylate synthase

11. Which of the following is a life-threatening adverse effect of bleomycin?

A. Pulmonary fibrosis

B. Myocardial infarction

C. Pulmonary thromboembolism

D. Acute liver failure

E. Neurogenic shock

12. R.U.'s anticancer therapy included vinblastine. This drug most likely acts in which of the following phases of the cell cycle?

A. G_0

B. G_1

C. S

D. G_2

E. M

13. R.U.'s anticancer therapy included dacarbazine. Which of the following molecular actions most likely contributed to the therapeutic effect of the drug in the patient's disease?

A. Intercalation between DNA strands

B. Inhibition of microtubule disassembly

C. Inhibition of microtubule assembly

D. Alkylation of nucleophilic groups on DNA bases

E. Inhibition of tyrosine kinase

Answers and Explanations

▶ *Learning objective:* Identify the best histopathology index of Hodgkin's lymphoma.

1. Answer: D

Hodgkin's lymphoma is a lymphoid tumor characterized by the presence of large, binucleated, malignant cells called Stenberg's cells surrounded by a large amount of inflammatory cells, including lymphocytes, eosinophils, and plasma cells. Even if Stenberg's cells can be (rarely) found in other disorders (such as infectious mononucleosis, non-Hodgkin's lymphomas, carcinomas, and sarcomas) their presence is highly suggestive of Hodgkin's lymphoma.

A, B, C, E All these histopathology results can be found in several inflammatory or tumor disorders.

▶ *Learning objective:* Identify the stage of Hodgkin's lymphoma from the patient's symptoms and signs.

2. Answer: B

Hodgkin's lymphoma is usually subdivided in the following stages:

▶ *Stage I:* There is Hodgkin's lymphoma in only one group of lymph nodes or lymphoma in only one body organ.

▶ *Stage II:* There is Hodgkin's lymphoma in two or more groups of lymph nodes, or in an organ and one or more groups of lymph nodes. In both cases, the two sites of lymphoma must be on the same side of the diaphragm.

▸ **Stage III:** There is Hodgkin's lymphoma on both sides of the diaphragm.

▸ **Stage IV:** There are many groups of lymph nodes containing Hodgkin's lymphoma, and the disease has spread to body organs, such as the liver, bones, or lungs.

Because R.U. has only two groups of abnormal lymph nodes on the same side of the diaphragm (cervical and axillary), his lymphoma should be classified as stage II.

A, C, D See correct answer explanation.

▸ *Learning objective:* Identify two early adverse effects caused by the ABVD anticancer regimen.

3. Answer: D

Because anticancer drugs are cytotoxic, certain adverse effects are common to most agents. These toxicities occur as a result of inhibition of host cell division, mainly in those tissues with rapid renewal of cell population, including bone marrow; therefore myelosuppression is a common adverse effect. Because of the life span of the blood cells, myelosuppression first results in neutropenia (the peripheral life span of neutrophils is 1–3 days) followed by thrombocytopenia (the peripheral life span of platelets is 8–10 days) and then by lymphocytopenia. Myelosuppression is dose dependent and is therefore a dose-limiting adverse effect.

Because hair bulb cells replicate every 12 to 24 hours, they are quite susceptible to various chemotherapeutic agents. Hair loss usually begins about 5 to 10 days after starting chemotherapy and may be prominent after 1 month. Alopecia is reversible and usually hair regeneration occurs 1 to 2 months after discontinuation of the treatment.

A, B, C Anemia is not common but can occur during anticancer chemotherapy. However, it usually occurs later, because of the long life span of erythrocytes.

B, E, F Hyperkalemia is related to kidney toxicity. This adverse effect is not common and usually occurs several weeks after starting the treatment.

▸ *Learning objective:* Identify the two brain regions most likely involved in the pathophysiology of chemotherapy-induced emesis.

4. Answer: F

Chemotherapy-induced emesis results from stimulation of a multistep reflex pathway that is controlled by the brain and triggered by afferent impulses to the vomiting center from the chemoreceptor trigger zone, gastrointestinal tract (by way of vagal afferent fibers), and, possibly, the cerebral cortex. The mechanism that is best supported by research involves an effect of chemotherapy on the upper small intestine. Local generation of free radicals leads to localized exocytotic release of serotonin from the enterochromaffin cells. Serotonin then interacts with 5-HT$_3$ receptors on vagal afferent terminals in the wall of the bowel. This stimulates vagal afferent fibers, which project to the dorsal brain stem, primarily to the nucleus tractus solitarius (NTS), and, to a lesser extent, to the chemoreceptor trigger zone (CTZ). Neural fibers project from these areas to the final effector of the emetic reflex, the vomiting center, an anatomically indistinct area occupying a more ventral location in the medulla. Antineoplastic agents may also induce emesis through a direct activation of the chemo neurons of the CTZ.

A, B, C, D, E Other potential sources of afferent input to the vomiting center that result in emesis after chemotherapy include a number of structures, such as the amygdala and locus ceruleus, but evidence for this pathways is less well established.

▸ *Learning objective:* Identify the receptors blocked by ondansetron.

5. Answer: C

About 70 to 80% of patients will experience nausea and vomiting during chemotherapy. Chemotherapy-induced emesis can occur in two different patterns:

▸ **Acute emesis** that occurs during the first 24 hours after chemotherapy. In the absence of effective prophylaxis, it most commonly begins within 1 to

2 hours of chemotherapy and usually peaks in the first 4 to 6 hours.

▶ **Delayed emesis** that occurs more than 24 hours after chemotherapy. In the absence of antiemetic prophylaxis, delayed emesis peaks at approximately 48 to 72 hours after therapy, then gradually subsides over the next 2 to 3 days. While the frequency and number of episodes of emesis may be less during the delayed period compared with acute emesis, the delayed form is less well controlled with current antiemetic medications.

It is thought that the pathophysiology of nausea and vomiting involves both central and peripheral mechanisms mediated by various neurotransmitters. The two most important neurotransmitters seem to be serotonin and substance P. It has been postulated that chemotherapy-induced local irritation and damage of the gastrointestinal (GI) mucosa causes a release of serotonin from enterochromaffin cells of the GI tract. Serotonin in turn will activate peripheral 5-HT receptors located in the gut (afferent fibers of the vagus nerve) as well as central receptors in the CTZ.

Ondansetron is a $5-HT_3$ antagonist. These agents inhibit the action of serotonin in the GI tract and CTZ, thereby blocking the transmission of emetic signals to the vomiting center. They are effective mainly against the acute phase symptoms.

A, B, D, E, F The blockade of histamine (H_1), acetylcholine (M_1), neurokinin (NK_1), dopamine (D_2), and cannabinoid (CB_1) receptors can inhibit nausea and vomiting from various causes, but ondansetron does not block these receptors.

▶ *Learning objective:* Identify the receptors blocked by aprepitant.

6. Answer: D

Substance P (also released from the GI mucosa) is thought to activate NK_1 receptors located in the gut as well as in the NTS and the CTZ. Activation of these receptors can cause nausea and vomiting. Aprepitant is the first NK_1 receptor antagonist that was shown to inhibit both the acute and the delayed emesis induced by cytotoxic

chemotherapeutic drugs. NK_1 antagonists appear to be more effective than $5-HT_3$ antagonists in reducing chemotherapy-induced emesis.

A Blockade of H_1 histamine receptors would mediate the antiemetic effect of the first generation of some antihistaminic drugs, like diphenhydramine.

B Blockade M_1 muscarinic receptors would mediate the antiemetic effect of scopolamine.

C Blockade $5-HT_3$ serotonin receptors would mediate the antiemetic effect of ondansetron.

E Blockade D_2 dopamine receptors would mediate the antiemetic effect of dopamine antagonists like metoclopramide.

F Blockade CB_1 cannabinoid receptors would mediate the antiemetic effect of cannabinoids, like dronabinol.

▶ *Learning objective:* Identify the drug that is commonly associated with ondansetron and aprepitant for prevention of chemotherapy-induced emesis.

7. Answer: D

Glucocorticoids are commonly given together with $5-HT_3$ antagonists and NK_1 antagonists for prevention of chemotherapy-induced emesis. They are very effective in preventing both acute and delayed emesis and improve the antiemetic control of serotonin antagonists by about 15 to 20%. The exact mechanism of antiemetic action of glucocorticoids is still unknown.

A, B, C, E All these drugs have antiemetic properties, but they are minimally or not at all effective for prevention of chemotherapy-induced nausea and vomiting.

▶ *Learning objective:* Identify one of the mechanisms of anticancer action of doxorubicin.

8. Answer: A

Doxorubicin is an anthracycline antibiotic. These anticancer drugs likely act with multiple mechanisms, including the following:

▶ Intercalation between adjacent base pairs of DNA, causing blockade of DNA replication

▶ Inhibition of topoisomerase II, one of the enzymes that catalyzes DNA repair (it breaks and then reseals DNA strands)
▶ Generation of free radicals that can oxidize DNA bases
▶ Inhibition of membrane fluidity and ion transport

The end result of these multiple mechanisms is cell apoptosis.

B Inhibition of microtubule disassembly would be the mechanism of action of taxanes (paclitaxel, docetaxel).

C Inhibition of microtubule assembly would be the mechanism of action of vinca alkaloids.

D Alkylation of nucleophilic groups on DNA bases would be the mechanism of action of alkylating drugs (cyclophosphamide, nitrosoureas).

E Inhibition of tyrosine kinases would be the mechanism of action of tyrosine kinase inhibitors (imatinib, erlotinib).

▶ *Learning objective:* Identify a potentially lethal effect of doxorubicin.

9. Answer: B

Doxorubicin is an anticancer anthracycline antibiotic. Anthracyclines (doxorubicin, daunorubicin, etc.) are the anticancer drugs with the highest risk of cardiac toxicity, which is dose-dependent and cumulative. They can cause a dilated cardiomyopathy associated with cardiac failure. When heart failure develops, mortality is approximately 50%. Doxorubicin cardiotoxicity can be acute, occurring within 2 to 3 days of its administration. The incidence of acute cardiotoxicity is approximately 11%. The incidence of chronic doxorubicin cardiotoxicity is much lower, with an estimated incidence of about 1.7%. It is usually evident within 30 days of administration of its last dose, but it may occur even 6 to 10 years after its administration.

The proposed mechanisms of doxorubicin cardiotoxicity include increased oxidative stress, inhibition of nucleic acid and protein synthesis, increased production of free radical within the myocardium, and decreased expression of cardiac-specific genes. The importance of many of the proposed mechanisms remains to be established.

A Pulmonary fibrosis would be a life-threatening adverse effect of bleomycin, an anticancer antibiotic.

C Ischemic stroke can occur in cancer patients under chemotherapy, but association with doxorubicin is very rare.

D Acute kidney failure can occur in cancer patients under chemotherapy but is associated primarily with cisplatin.

E Acute liver failure is a rare drug-induced disorder. Half of the cases in the United States are due to acetaminophen.

▶ *Learning objective:* Identify the most likely mechanisms of anticancer action of bleomycin.

10. Answer: C

Bleomycin is an anticancer antibiotic. Although the exact mechanism of action of bleomycin is unknown, available evidence seems to indicate that the main mode of action is the single- and double-strand DNA breaks. It is believed that bleomycin chelates metal ions (primarily iron), which in turn react with oxygen to produce superoxide and hydroxide free radicals that cleave DNA. The effects of bleomycin are cell cycle–specific, with its main effects occurring during the G2 and M phases of the cell cycle.

A This would be the mechanism of action of anthracyclines.

B This would be the mechanism of action of fludarabine.

D This would be the mechanism of action of topotecan.

E This would be the mechanism of action of fluorouracil.

▶ *Learning objective:* Identify a potentially lethal effect of bleomycin.

11. Answer: A

Several distinct pulmonary syndromes have been linked to the use of bleomycin, including bronchiolitis obliterans with organizing pneumonia, eosinophilic hypersensitivity, and, most commonly, interstitial pneumonitis, which may ultimately progress to pulmonary fibrosis. Bleomycin-induced interstitial pneumonitis occurs in about 10% of patients treated with the drug. The mortality of patients with bleomycin-induced interstitial pneumonitis is very high (about 50%). Although normally bleomycin-induced pneumonitis develops gradually during treatment, the development of the disease up to 2 years after discontinuation of bleomycin therapy has also been reported.

B, C, D, E All these adverse effects are exceedingly rare, or absent, in patients receiving bleomycin.

▸ *Learning objective:* Identify the phase of the cell cycle most affected by the action of vinblastine.

12. Answer: D

The cell cycle is subdivided into the following phases:

- ▸ G_0, the resting phase, where the cell has left the cycle and has stopped dividing
- ▸ G_1 (also called the growth phase), where the cell synthesizes cellular components
- ▸ S, the synthesis phase, where the cell replicates DNA
- ▸ G_2, where the cell synthesizes cellular component for mitosis
- ▸ M, mitotic phase, where the cell undergoes nuclear division

Anticancer drugs can be subdivided into two groups:

- ▸ **Cell-cycle nonspecific** drugs are able to kill a cell during any phase of the cycle

(even if the cells in the nonresting phases are more sensitive).
- ▸ **Cell-cycle specific** drugs are able to kill a cell only during a specific phase and are unable to work in the resting phase.

Vinblastine is a cell cycle–specific anticancer drug. It acts by inhibiting the assembly of microtubules, an important part of the mitotic spindle. Therefore it acts in the G_2 phase of the cell cycle.

A, B, C, E See correct answer explanation.

▸ *Learning objective:* Identify the mechanism of anticancer action of dacarbazine.

13. Answer: D

Dacarbazine is a prodrug that must be metabolically activated in the liver. The active metabolite functions as an alkylating agent.

A Intercalation between DNA strands would be the mechanism of action of anthracyclines (daunorubicin, doxorubicin).

B Inhibition of microtubule disassembly would be the mechanism of action of taxanes (paclitaxel, docetaxel).

C Inhibition of microtubule assembly would be the mechanism of action of vinca alkaloids (vincristine, vinblastine).

E Inhibition of tyrosine kinase would be the mechanism of action of tyrosine kinase inhibitors (imatinib, erlotinib).

Case 22

Hormonal Contraception

H.C., a 36-year-old woman, visited her physician for consultation on using a contraceptive method for continuous contraception. She wanted to use a nonoral hormonal method. She had a history of using different types of hormonal contraceptives since the age of 21, including an oral combination hormonal contraceptive (CHC) and the hormonal patch.

Past history revealed that, at age 21, she had had unprotected sexual intercourse with her boyfriend, and for the first time she had used an emergency contraceptive pill to prevent an unwanted pregnancy. After that incident she had consulted her physician about starting an appropriate hormonal contraceptive for continuous contraception. She had a history of acne that would flare up just before her menses. She had tried 8 months of different treatments for acne, including benzoyl peroxide and doxycycline, to which she had not responded well. She was a nonsmoker at that time, and her family history was not significant for any cardiovascular disorder. Her menstrual periods were painful with cramps, for which she would take naproxen, on as-needed basis, during her periods. Noting that there was nothing abnormal on her physical examination and her vitals were normal, she was prescribed a formulation of an oral CHC containing ethinyl estradiol and norgestimate. She selected the quick-start method for using the CHC. Her acne resolved after a few cycles of CHC use. She reported that she was overall satisfied using the CHC for both acne as well as contraception.

She also revealed that she had many times missed taking her CHC doses but had never missed for two consecutive days. Her physician had given her appropriate instructions on how to cover for the missed dose so as to continue the contraceptive effect in such cases.

H.C. gave a history of anemia that she had developed while being on the CHC. She was given iron supplements for 3 to 4 months, and her physician switched her to an extended-cycle CHC.

At age 23, when she and her partner decided to have a child, she discontinued taking the CHC. After 4 months of discontinuation of contraceptives, she conceived. Her pregnancy was normal, and she gave birth to a baby boy after a normal vaginal delivery. She chose to breastfeed her child. Because she wanted a contraceptive method immediately after delivery, her gynecologist gave her an appropriate contraceptive. After a year of using hormonal contraceptives, she stopped using them.

A year after the baby's birth, H.C. started a demanding job. She started smoking to deal with the stress and would smoke more than 15 cigarettes a day. She now smokes one pack a day.

Her son is 11 years old and in good health.

Physical examination revealed a white woman (height 162 cm, weight 55 kg) who looked in normal body shape with no pallor or cyanosis. Her vital signs were as follows: blood pressure 122/86 mm Hg, pulse 72 bpm, respirations 16/min. The rest of the physical examination was unremarkable.

Questions

1. H.C. had a history of using an emergency contraceptive pill. Which of the following drugs did she most likely take to prevent pregnancy after having unprotected sexual intercourse?

A. Misoprostol

B. Norethindrone

C. Levonorgestrel

D. Clomiphene

E. Leuprolide

2. H.C. was prescribed an oral CHC containing ethinyl estradiol and norgestimate. Which of the following is most likely the primary mechanism of action of oral CHCs to prevent pregnancy?

A. Increased fallopian tube motility

B. Inhibition of fertilization

C. Suppression of ovarian estrogen synthesis

D. Increased gonadotropin release

E. Inhibition of ovulation

3. The patient responded well to an oral CHC in resolving her acne after a few cycles of CHC use. Which of the following effects of estrogen in CHC is associated with improvement in acne?

A. Suppression of estrogen production from the ovaries

B. Inhibition of androgen binding to androgen receptors

C. Increased estrogen production from the ovaries

D. Suppression of adrenal androgen synthesis

E. Increased production of sex hormone–binding globulin in the liver

4. One of the adverse effects of norethindrone, a progestin that is present in conventional oral combination hormonal contraceptive preparations, is acne. Which of the following receptors does this agent interact with to cause this adverse effect?

A. Glucocorticoid

B. Mineralocorticoid

C. Estrogen

D. Androgen

E. Gonadotropin

5. H.C.'s physician prescribed an oral CHC preparation that contained ethinyl estradiol and norgestimate. Taking into account H.C.'s medical history, which of the following properties made norgestimate an appropriate progestin for this patient?

A. Less estrogenic

B. Less glucocorticoid

C. Less progestational

D. Less androgenic

E. Less mineralocorticoid

6. H.C. revealed that she had also used a hormonal patch for contraception. Which of the following is the most likely mechanism of action by which the patch exerts its contraceptive effects?

A. Inhibition of fertilization

B. Changes in fallopian tube motility

C. Increased viscosity of cervical mucus

D. Histological changes in the endometrium

E. Inhibition of ovulation

7. Some new preparations of CHCs have drospirenone as the progestin constituent. Women, especially those who have mild–moderate renal insufficiency or are on medications such as angiotensin-converting enzyme (ACE) inhibitors, need to be monitored for which of the following adverse effects while using drospirenone-containing CHCs?

A. Hypernatremia

B. Acne

C. Hirsutism

D. Hyperkalemia

E. Breakthrough bleeding

8. H.C. used the "quick-start" method to start taking her oral combination contraceptive pills. Which of the following best explains this method?

A. Take the first pill of CHC on the first day of menstruation.

B. Take the first pill of CHC on the first Sunday after the beginning of menstruation.

C. Take two pills of CHC after each unprotected sexual intercourse.

D. Take the first pill of CHC as soon as possible regardless of the cycle day.

9. The patient reported having missed a CHC dose and having remembered it the next day. What advice did she most likely receive from her physician to cover for the missed dose?

A. Take two pills together and continue with the usual dose for rest of the cycle.

B. Start a new cycle of pills.

C. Use condoms for the next 28 days.

D. Take the usual dose the next day and for the rest of the cycle.

E. Stop the CHC pills and switch to progestin-only pills.

10. H.C. had a history of anemia and had taken iron supplements for the treatment. Her physician had also switched her to an extended-cycle contraceptive. Which of the following events best explains extended-cycle contraceptives?

A. No menses occur on these preparations.

B. Menstrual cycles extend to 45-day cycles.

C. They allow less frequent menses.

D. They need to be taken lifelong.

E. Only oral formulations achieve the goals of this preparation.

11. H.C. chose to use a hormonal contraceptive method immediately after the delivery of her baby. Which hormonal agent would be most appropriate for her?

A. Transdermal patch

B. Vaginal ring

C. Oral combination hormonal contraceptive

D. Ulipristal

E. Progestin-only pill

12. Which of the following instructions did the patient need to follow while using the progestin-only pill for achieving its best possible contraceptive effect?

A. Take the pills at the same time every day.

B. Do not smoke while on these pills.

C. Take the pills just after having sexual intercourse.

D. Do not drive while on these pills.

13. There are some noncontraceptive benefits of using combination hormonal contraceptives. Which of the following diseases does the use of CHCs help to prevent?

A. Thromboembolism

B. Breast cancer

C. Ovarian cancer

D. Pancreatitis

E. Myocardial infarction

14. H.C. visited her physician at the age of 36 for consultation on restarting an appropriate hormonal contraceptive. Which of the following preparations would be most appropriate for her?

A. Transdermal patch

B. Vaginal ring

C. Combination hormonal contraceptive pills

D. Levonorgestrel-releasing IUD

E. Progestin-only pill

Answers and Explanations

▶ *Learning objective:* Describe emergency contraception.

1. Answer: C

Levonorgestrel is a widely recommended agent for an emergency contraception. When a woman is not on any hormonal contraceptive for continuous contraception and the couple is not using any physical barrier method (such as condoms) or when the contraceptive method fails (such as condom rupture), emergency contraceptives are useful in preventing unwanted pregnancy. Plan B-One Step is one of the emergency contraceptive preparations that contains 1.5 mg of levonorgestrel. It is recommended that the drug be taken within 72 hours of unprotected sexual intercourse for it to be successful. The sooner it is taken, the better the efficacy. This is available over the counter, and no age restrictions apply to obtain the drug. This preparation should not be used for regular contraception, because it is not as effective for that purpose, and also it is not an abortifacient for terminating an established pregnancy. Other contraceptive methods that could be used as emergency contraception are ulipristal pill (can be taken within 5 days after the unprotected sexual intercourse) and an intrauterine device (IUD).

A Misoprostol is a prostaglandin analogue. In obstetrics, it is used in medical termination of pregnancy. The drug acts by stimulating uterine contractions and facilitates expulsion of uterine contents resulting from conception.

B Norethindrone is a progestin agent that is present in traditional oral CHCs, but it is not used for emergency contraception.

D Clomiphene is a partial estrogen receptor agonist and is used for inducing ovulation in patients with polycystic ovary disease.

E Leuprolide is a gonadotropin-releasing hormone agonist. It is used for the treatment of infertility when administered in a pulsatile manner.

▶ *Learning objective:* Describe the mechanism of contraceptive action of combination hormonal contraceptives.

2. Answer: E

The overall effect of CHCs is inhibition of ovulation, which is considered the primary mechanism of CHCs to achieve contraception. The estrogen component decreases follicle-stimulating hormone (FSH) release and thereby prevents the development of a dominant graafian follicle in the ovaries. The estrogen component also acts to stabilize the endometrial lining, thus preventing breakthrough bleeding. The progestin agent inhibits ovulation by suppressing the luteinizing hormone (LH) release and the LH surge required for ovulation.

Other possible effects of CHCs might include the following:

▶ Thickening of cervical mucus that interferes with sperm travel

▶ Deciduation of the endometrium, making it nonreceptive for implantation

▶ Possibly decreased fallopian tube motility

A combination hormonal contraceptive is a preparation that contains both an estrogen and a progestin. There are different oral CHCs available. In most of them the estrogen component is ethinyl estradiol. Progestin agents can be different; for example, there are oral CHC preparations containing norethindrone, levonorgestrel, norgestimate, or drospirenone.

Oral CHCs can also be classified based on the content of estrogen. High-dose oral CHCs have 50 µg estrogen, low-dose CHCs have 25 to 35 µg of estrogen, and very low dose CHCs have 10 to 25 µg of estrogen. High-dose oral CHCs were found to be associated with a high incidence of cardiovascular disorders in women taking these preparations. Low-dose and very low dose CHCs seem to have less chance of causing these adverse effects as long as the patient does not have any risk factor. This is the reason why H.C.'s physician obtained her personal and family history and conducted a physical examination to rule out any risk factor that would otherwise preclude the use of CHCs.

Based on the type of formulation, there are different types of CHCs, such as oral (which are also called combined oral contraceptives [COCs]), vaginal ring, and patch.

Some common adverse effects of CHCs are nausea and breast tenderness, which are related to the estrogen component and usually subside within a few cycles of CHC use. Other adverse effects, such as mood changes and water retention, are associated with the progestin component. Usually if the symptoms persist and are distressful, an alternative CHC that contains a lower amount of estrogen or a different progestin agent can be tried, depending on the type of adverse effects.

A CHCs cause a reduction, not an increase, in fallopian tubule motility, thus impairing ovum transit through it.

B Inhibition of fertilization is just a consequence, not the primary mechanism of action, of CHCs.

C CHCs inhibit the development of a dominant graafian follicle and thus suppress hormone synthesis (steroidogenesis) by the different cells of the graafian follicle. Inhibition of steroidogenesis is not the cause of inhibition of ovulation; rather it is the result of inhibition of graafian follicle growth.

D Gonadotropin release is suppressed, not increased, by the hormones in CHC preparations by a feedback mechanism.

▶ *Learning objective:* Describe the mechanism by which combination hormonal contraceptives act to show therapeutic effects in acne.

3. Answer: E

Acne is the result of overactive sebaceous glands in response to many factors. Important ones are high androgen levels or overreactivity to androgens. Therefore, a therapeutic approach used to treat acne is to decrease the androgenic activity in these patients. This can be achieved by doing the following:

▶ Decreasing androgen production
▶ Decreasing the availability of free form of androgens
▶ Antagonizing androgen actions

The estrogen component in the combined preparation can have therapeutic effects in acne by multiple mechanisms including the following:

▶ Decreased sex hormone-binding globulin (SHBG) levels
▶ Decreased sebaceous gland activity (effect opposite of androgens)
▶ Decreased androgen synthesis from the ovaries

The free form of androgens in the bloodstream is the form that can enter the cells and interact with its intracellular receptors to exert its androgenic effects. The plasma protein–bound form is largely nonbioavailable for biological effects. Increased synthesis of SHBG in the liver, in response to the estrogen component of oral CHCs, results in increased binding of plasma androgens to SHBG and decreased levels of bioavailable free plasma androgen. Estrogens also act to decrease sebaceous gland activity. Through feedback regulation, the estrogen component of CHCs decreases FSH release from the anterior pituitary, which, in addition to suppressing the development of a dominant graafian follicle, also suppresses the ovarian steroidogenesis. Suppression of steroidogenesis results in decreased synthesis of both ovarian androgens and estrogens, thus resulting in a decrease in plasma androgen levels.

A Ovarian estrogen synthesis is also suppressed by CHCs, but a decrease in ovarian estrogen levels is not related to the CHC's therapeutic effects in acne.

B Hormonal components in CHCs do not act as androgen receptor antagonists.

C Ovarian steroidogenesis, including synthesis of estrogens, progestins, and androgens, is suppressed, not increased, by CHCs.

D The adrenal gland is not under the control of the hypothalamus–pituitary–ovary axis.

▶ *Learning objective:* Describe the characteristics of different types of synthetic progestins.

4. Answer: D

Synthetic progestins are derived from either C-21 or 19-nortestosterone substrates. While all of these agents are "progestins," they have slightly different spectra of activities, which may be considered either adverse effects or advantageous effects, arising from their basic structural differences.

Traditional oral CHCs contain original 19-nor derivatives, such as norethindrone. These progestins have some androgenic actions that manifest as adverse effects, such as acne, hirsutism, and weight gain.

A, B, C, E Progestins do not interact with these receptors to cause acne.

▶ *Learning objective:* Describe the clinical application of different types of progestin agents.

5. Answer: D

Synthetic progestins are derived from either C-21 or 19-nortestosterone substrates.

Traditional oral CHCs contain original 19-nor derivatives, such as norethindrone. These progestins have some androgenic actions that manifest as adverse effects. Newer 19-nor derivatives, called gonanes, including norgestimate and levonorgestrel, have less androgenic activity. Most of the newer CHC preparations contain proges-

tins from the gonane class, so as to decrease the risk of androgenic adverse effects. The patient's physician made a good decision to prescribe an oral CHC that contained norgestimate so as to avoid aggravation of her acne.

A, B, E Of course norgestimate also has negligible estrogenic, glucocorticoid, and mineralocorticoid activities, but these properties do not explain why this drug is an appropriate contraceptive for a patient with acne.

C Norgestimate has progestational, not less progestational, activity.

▶ *Learning objective:* Describe different formulations of combined hormonal contraceptives.

6. Answer: E

CHCs are available in a variety of formulations—oral, vaginal ring, and the patch. All these formulations are combination hormonal contraceptives that contain an estrogen and a progestin agent. The mechanism of contraceptive action of all these formulations is the same—inhibition of ovulation. The estrogen component decreases FSH release and so prevents the development of a dominant graafian follicle in the ovaries. It also acts to stabilize the endometrial lining, thus preventing breakthrough bleeding. The progestin agent inhibits ovulation by suppressing the LH release and the LH surge required for ovulation.

The patch is usually changed every week for 3 weeks. The fourth week is used as a patch-free week to allow withdrawal bleeding to occur. However, depending on the indication, the patch can be used as an extended-cycle contraceptive when the patch is applied every week for a longer duration of time without providing a patch-free period.

A Hormonal contraceptives do not inhibit fertilization of an egg already in the tube.

B, C, D All these can be additional mechanisms of the action of hormonal contraceptives, but they are not the primary mechanism.

▶ *Learning objective:* Describe the characteristics of newer synthetic progestin agents.

▶ *Learning objective:* Describe different methods of starting combination hormone. contraceptives.

7. Answer: D

Drospirenone is a new synthetic progestin. It is structurally related to spironolactone (a potassium-sparing diuretic) and has antiandrogenic and antimineralocorticoid activities. Due to antimineralocorticoid activity, this agent has potassium-sparing effects and can cause hyperkalemia in women who have preexisting conditions, such as renal insufficiency that causes potassium retention or who are taking drugs such as ACE inhibitors that have the potential to elevate serum potassium levels.

However, because drospirenone has antiandrogenic activity, it does not cause androgenic adverse effects, such as acne or hirsutism. Also, women who experience water retention or edema with the use of CHCs containing progestins that are derivatives of 19-nortestosterone, drospirenone-containing CHCs might be more suitable.

One of the significant adverse effects of drospirenone that has been reported is increased risk of thromboembolism compared to CHCs containing other progestins. Although all CHC preparations can increase the risk of thromboembolism, some studies have shown that the risk is greater with drospirenone-containing CHCs. Further studies are needed to evaluate this risk.

A Hypernatremia does not occur with drospirenone. Drospirenone acts as an aldosterone antagonist, so it would facilitate excretion of sodium in the urine while retaining potassium in exchange.

B, C These effects are androgenic effects that do not occur with drospirenone.

E Breakthrough bleeding can occur as an adverse effect of CHCs, even if it is seen more commonly with the use of progestin-only preparations. When this happens, a CHC preparation containing higher amounts of estrogens can be prescribed to stabilize the endometrial lining.

8. Answer: D

The quick-start method allows the CHC to be taken immediately after it is prescribed, regardless of the menstrual cycle day. This method is believed to minimize the confusion about when to take the first pill and has the potential to increase adherence. The method is also believed to provide contraception sooner and prevent unwanted pregnancy.

A This fits with the "day 1 start" method.

B This explains the "Sunday start" method.

C This does not explain a method for starting the first cycle of a CHC; this rather fits more with the Yuzpe method of "emergency contraception" in which CHC pills that contain levonorgestrel or norgestrel as the progestin component are taken after unprotected intercourse, as two separate doses 12 hours apart.

▶ *Learning objective:* Describe the guidelines for providing backup contraception for a missed dose of an oral combination hormone contraceptive.

9. Answer: A

The packet insert for CHC preparations provides specific instructions for covering one or multiple missed CHC doses. For the traditional 21-day active pill preparation, if a woman misses one single dose of her oral CHC, according to the "US selected practice recommendations for contraceptive use," it is recommended that she take the missed dose as soon as possible and continue to take the remaining pills at the usual time, even if it means taking two pills on the same day. In the present case, the patient's physician followed the guidelines in advising her to take two pills together (one for the missed dose of the previous day and one for the usual daily dose) and continue with her usual single pill for the rest of the cycle. According to the guidelines, no additional contraceptive is needed as a backup in such a scenario.

B, C, D, E None of these answer choices conforms to the guidelines.

▶ *Learning objective:* Explain extended-cycle contraceptive formulations.

10.   Answer: C

Extended–cycle contraceptives allow less frequent menses. These are available as oral, transdermal patch, and vaginal ring. The dose of hormones in these preparation is the same as in 21- or 24-day-cycle CHCs. When used as extended-cycle contraceptives, these formulations are used continuously for a longer than usual period (21 days in the 21-day pill pack, 24 days in the 24-day pill pack), and allow less frequent hormone-free periods for withdrawal bleeding to occur. For example, consider preparations such as Seasonale (brand name), an oral CHC, which comes as an 84-day active hormone pill pack. The pill is taken as one pill a day continuously for 84 days, and the following 7 days are pill free (or nonhormonal inactive pills) to allow withdrawal bleeding. A woman on this preparation would have only four menstrual periods a year. A similar approach is used for the transdermal patch and the vaginal ring, in which the patch-free or the vaginal ring-free period is provided less frequently. The extended-cycle contraceptive approach is used for decreasing blood loss in menses, especially in women with menorrhagia and anemia, and is also useful in the treatment of dysmenorrhea and endometriosis. In the present case, the patient had developed anemia. Although the regular 21-day cycle CHCs (3 weeks of active hormone with 1 week a hormone-free period) also decrease menstrual blood loss with chronic use, considering the patient's anemia, having fewer menses would be therapeutically more reasonable. This was the reason her physician switched her to extended-cycle contraception. Because there was no history of menorrhagia, most likely her iron deficiency anemia was due to dietary deficiency; still, it was reasonable to use an extended-cycle CHC in order to decrease the contribution of menstrual blood loss to anemia. The extended-cycle contraceptive methods are also used purely for lifestyle preferences (useful for women who want convenience for their menstruation, including women who travel, are on deployment in the military, or seek more control regarding the timing of menstruation and wish to have fewer restrictions in their sexual life due to menstruation).

A progestin-containing IUD (Levonorgestrel-IUD), once inserted, is effective for 5 years to provide continuous contraception. It is also used for the management of menorrhagia as well as purely as a preference. A few months after its insertion, monthly menses become lighter.

A, B, D, E As already explained, all these statements do not define extended-cycle contraception.

▶ *Learning objective:* Describe appropriate contraceptive methods in the immediate postpartum period.

11.   Answer: E

The risk of venous thromboembolism (VTE) is elevated during the postpartum period; the risk declines rapidly in the first 21 days postpartum and returns to baseline levels after 42 days (6 weeks) postpartum.

Estrogen-containing contraceptives (CHCs) are associated with an increased risk of VTE. Due to this, CHCs are not recommended during the first 21 days (3 weeks) of the postpartum period. During the time 21 to 42 days postpartum, women without risk factors for VTE generally can initiate CHCs, but women with risk factors for VTE (e.g., previous VTE, postpartum hemorrhage, recent cesarean delivery) generally should not use these methods. After 42 days (6 weeks) postpartum, no restrictions on the use of CHCs, based on postpartum status, apply. Earlier it was believed that the estrogen component of CHCs would decrease the quality and quantity of breast milk, but current studies have failed to find such an association. Nevertheless, some physicians avoid using CHCs for this reason.

Progestin-only contraceptives do not augment the risk of VTE, nor do they seem to interfere with lactation. Updated Centers for Disease Control and Prevention recommendations state that progestin-only contraceptives (mini-pill, IUD, implant) may be initiated immediately postpartum.

Therefore, choice E, progestin-only pill, is the most appropriate choice of hormonal contraceptive for this patient. Other appropriate options for her could be an IUD, either a copper-containing IUD or a levonorgestrel-releasing IUD.

A, B, C These are all CHCs so they are not recommended for H.C.

D Ulipristal is a selective progestin receptor modulator used only as an emergency contraceptive within 5 days of unprotected sexual intercourse.

▶ *Learning objective:* Describe the pharmacokinetics of progestins and its clinical applicability.

12. Answer: A

Due to clearance of progestin agents from the circulation, the contraceptive action of oral progestin agents persists for about 24 hours. It is therefore important to take the next dose exactly at the same time in order to avoid a decline in plasma levels of progestins below the minimal required levels for achieving the contraceptive effects. If a dose is delayed, but not more than 3 hours, the missed dose should be taken immediately, and no backup birth control method is needed. If the pill is taken more than 3 hours later than the usual time, it is advised to exercise abstinence or use a backup birth control method (usually a male condom) for at least 2 days, while continuing taking the remaining pills at the usual time. Mechanisms by which progestin-only contraceptive pills exhibit contraceptive effect include (1) thickening of the cervical mucus, thus making it impermeable to sperms; (2) thinning of endometrial lining, making it unfavorable for implantation; and (3) inhibition of ovulation. But unlike CHCs, inhibition of ovulation is not the primary mechanism for their contraceptive effect.

B Women who smoke can take progestin-only contraceptives.

C This statement explains how emergency contraceptives are administered. Levonorgestrel (1.5. mg dose) is used for emergency contraception and is taken as soon as possible within 72 hours after the unprotected intercourse.

D No hormonal contraceptive has been shown to interfere with driving.

▶ *Learning objective:* Identify the disease whose risk is decreased with the use of combination hormonal contraceptives.

13. Answer: C

Most of the available studies are on the effects of oral CHCs. Meta-analysis of various studies has shown that the use of oral CHCs significantly decreases the risk for ovarian cancer. Protection seems to increase with longer use of CHCs. Studies have suggested that risk is decreased by 10 to 12% after 1 year of use and by approximately 50% after 5 years of use. All types of oral CHCs, irrespective of the type or amount of estrogen and progestin in the pills, seems to provide same degree of protection against ovarian cancer.

Some other conditions in which CHCs have been found to be of therapeutic value are acne, hirsutism, premenstrual syndrome, menorrhagia, dysmenorrhea, endometriosis, and functional ovarian cysts.

A, E Hormonal constituents in CHCs affect the synthesis of clotting factors, which increases the chances of blood clots. Chances of this are greater in women who are above the age of 35 and are smokers. CHCs are thus contraindicated in women over 35 who are smokers. In these women there is a multifold greater risk of myocardial infarction and stroke.

B Older studies indicated a possible link between CHC use and breast cancer, but recent students suggest that CHC use does not increase the risk of breast cancer. It has not been found that CHC use could provide any protection against breast cancer.

D An association between development of pancreatitis and CHC has not been found.

▶ *Learning objective:* Identify the most appropriate hormonal contraceptive for women who are over the age of 35 and are smokers.

14. Answer: D

CHCs greatly increase their risk of developing serious cardiovascular problems, such as myocardial infarction, thromboembolism, and stroke. The estrogen component of the CHCs is associated with causing these adverse effects. The risk increases with age and the number of cigarettes smoked. Progestin-only contraceptives (pill, IUD, or depot injection) are considered safe in these women. Therefore, a levonorgestrel-releasing IUD would be most appropriate for her. This IUD is effective for 5 years to prevent pregnancy. Initial problems after insertion of an IUD are abdominal pain, cramps, and heavy bleeding, which subside in 3 to 4 months in most users. In fact, the levonorgestrel IUD is also indicated for the treatment of menorrhagia (heavy menstrual periods). Levonorgestrel-releasing IUDs act by multiple mechanisms to prevent pregnancy, including the following (in decreasing order of importance):

▶ Thickening the cervical mucus, which prevents transport of sperms from the vagina to the uterus
▶ Transforming the endometrial lining so it is unfavorable for implantation
▶ Inhibiting ovulation

A, B, C These are combined hormonal contraceptives, so they are contraindicated for H.C.

E This contraceptive is an oral progestin-only preparation. Because the patient wanted to take a nonoral contraceptive, this choice is not appropriate for her.

Case 23

Human Immunodeficiency Virus Infection

F.M., a 25-year-old man, presented to the local hospital with new complaints of fever, night sweats, weight loss, and a white exudate in his mouth. He stated that these symptoms had been present for the past 4 weeks. Medical history of the patient indicated that he had used heroin in the past, but he stated that he had successfully completed a rehabilitation program and had been "clean" for the last 8 months. Six months ago the patient received a blood transfusion after a trauma due to a car accident. He recovered completely in 3 weeks.

F.M. was unmarried and lived at home with his parents. The patient was circumcised ad admitted he had had sexual intercourse (always protected) with different women over the past 6 months.

Physical examination showed a healthy-looking man with the following vital signs: blood pressure 122/74 mm Hg, heart rate 76 bpm, respirations 14/min, temperature 98°F (36.6°C). Oral examination disclosed white patches on the tongue and on other areas of the mouth and throat. The rest of the physical examination was noncontributory.

A diagnosis of oral candidiasis was made, and a local therapy with miconazole mucoadhesive buccal tablets was prescribed. Infection with human immunodeficiency virus (HIV) was also suspected, and several lab exams were ordered with the following results:

Blood hematology

- ▶ Red blood cell count (RBC): $3.1 \times 10^6/\mu L$ (normal, 4.0–6.0)
- ▶ Hemoglobin (Hb): 10.2 g/dL (normal, men 12–16)
- ▶ Hematocrit (Hct): 37% (normal 36–48)
- ▶ White blood cell count (WBC): $11 \times 10^3/\mu L$ (normal 4–10)
- ▶ Platelet: $250 \times 10^3/\mu L$ (normal 130–400)
- ▶ Creatinine: 1.3 mg/dL (normal 0.6–1.2)
- ▶ Blood urea nitrogen (BUN): 30 mg/dL (normal 8–25)
- ▶ Sodium: 140 mEq/L (normal 135–146)
- ▶ Potassium: 4.5 mEq/L (normal 3.6–5.3)
- ▶ Glucose: 92 mg/dL (normal 60–110)

Antigen/antibody immunoassay

Positive for both HIV-1 and HIV-2 infection
F.M. was informed that he was HIV seropositive and was referred to the HIV clinic for further evaluation. Pertinent laboratory exam results on admission were as follows:

- ▶ CD4 lymphocytes: 170 cells/mm³
- ▶ Viral load: 120,000 copies/mL

A diagnosis of acquired immunodeficiency syndrome (AIDS) was made. The therapy of oral candidiasis was changed and miconazole was substituted with oral fluconazole. After a careful discussion with the physicians, the patient agreed to undergo a highly active antiretroviral therapy (HAART) and was dismissed from the clinic with a postdischarge therapy that included the following four-drug combination: emtricitabine, tenofovir, lopinavir, and rito-navir. He was also instructed to come back to the clinic every 2 months for routine follow-up.

At his first checkup F.M. stated that his night sweats and fevers had disappeared, he "felt great" and had had no drug-related problems. His viral load values were < 50 copies/mL (undetectable) and his CD4+ T cell count had increased from 120 to 425 cells/mm^3. Given the response to date, no changes were required, and the current regimen was confirmed.

Six months later a routine follow-up showed that the patient was still asymptomatic but that the CD4+ T cell count was 180 cells/mm^3. The antiretroviral therapy was changed, discontinuing emtricitabine and tenofovir and adding raltegravir.

One year later F.M. was admitted to the HIV clinic because of worsening of his disease. He admitted he had recently disregarded the antiviral therapy because he felt quite well. He complained of a low-grade fever, fatigue, cough with blood-streaked sputum, and excessive night sweating over the last month. He also complained of floating spots, light flashes, and difficulty with far vision. Further exams led to the diagnosis of pulmonary tuberculosis and cytomegalovirus (CMV) retinitis. The antiretroviral treatment (lopinavir, ritonavir, and raltegravir) was maintained, and an appropriate therapy was started that included a multi-drug tuberculosis treatment (isoniazid, rifampin, pyrazinamide, ethambutol, pyridoxine) and intravenous ganciclovir for CMV retinitis.

Questions

1. A local miconazole therapy and later an oral fluconazole therapy was prescribed to treat F.M.'s oral candidiasis. Which of the following molecular actions most likely mediated the therapeutic effect of both drugs in the patient's disease?

A. Inhibition of conversion of squalene to lanosterol

B. Formation of artificial pores in the fungal membrane

C. Inhibition of fungal mitosis

D. Inhibition of squalene synthesis

E. Inhibition of conversion of lanosterol to ergosterol

2. Which of the following two facts from F.M.'s medical history most likely suggested the presence of HIV infection?

A. Oral candidiasis–sex with different partners

B. Heroin addiction–sex with different partners

C. Previous blood transfusion–oral candidiasis

D. Sex with different partners–previous blood transfusion

E. Oral candidiasis–heroin addiction

F. Heroin addiction–previous blood transfusion

3. F.M. was infected by HIV. Which of the following sets of blood cells represents the main target of this virus?

A. Neutrophils–monocytes–B lymphocytes

B. T helper lymphocytes–monocytes–macrophages

C. Neutrophils–monocytes–T-helper lymphocytes

D. Macrophages–B lymphocytes–T-helper lymphocytes

E. B lymphocytes–neutrophils–macrophages

4. F.M. was diagnosed with AIDS. Which of the following lab results or disorders is diagnostic for his disease?

A. Oral candidiasis

B. CD4 lymphocytes

C. Heroin addiction

D. HIV infection

E. Viral load

5. F.M. agreed to start a HAART therapy. How long should the patient continue to take this multidrug therapy?

A. For 6 months

B. For 1 year

C. For 2 years

D. For 5 years

E. Indefinitely

6. F.M.'s HAART therapy included emtricitabine and tenofovir. Both drugs most likely act by inhibiting which of the following enzymes or virion action?

A. Integrase strand transfer

B. Neuraminidase

C. Reverse transcriptase

D. Protease

E. Virion entry

7. Which of the following steps of the viral growth cycle is specifically inhibited by emtricitabine and tenofovir?

A. Virion entry

B. Uncoating

C. Viral DNA growing

D. Proteolytic cleavage

E. Assembly

F. Release

8. Which of the following is a rare but life-threatening adverse effect that can be caused by emtricitabine and tenofovir?

A. Stroke

B. Pulmonary embolism

C. Ulcerative colitis

D. Lactic acidosis

E. Acute renal failure

9. F.M.'s HAART therapy included lopinavir and ritonavir. Which of the following steps of the viral cycle is specifically inhibited by this drug combination?

A. Virion entry

B. Uncoating

C. Viral DNA growing

D. Proteolytic cleavage

E. Assembly

F. Release

10. Which of the following was most likely the main reason for the association of ritonavir with the other antiretroviral drugs?

A. To increase lopinavir plasma levels

B. To decrease tenofovir toxicity

C. To increase emtricitabine oral bioavailability

D. To prolong tenofovir half-life

E. To decrease emtricitabine toxicity

11. Since F.M.'s initial antiretroviral therapy was no longer effective, the treatment was changed and raltegravir was added. The inhibition of which of the following viral enzymes most likely mediated the therapeutic effect of the drug in the patient's disease?

A. Neuraminidase

B. DNA polymerase

C. Reverse transcriptase

D. Protease

E. Integrase strand transfer

12. F.M.'s tuberculosis therapy included isoniazid. The synthesis of which of the following mycobacterial cell components was most likely inhibited by this drug?

A. Plasmids

B. Ribosomes

C. Cell wall

D. Cytoplasmic membrane

E. Nucleoid

F. Capsule

13. F.M.'s tuberculosis therapy included rifampin. The inhibition of which of the following enzymes most likely mediated the therapeutic efficacy of rifampin in the patient's disease?

A. DNA dependent RNA-polymerase

B. Arabinosyl transferase

C. Transpeptidase

D. Topoisomerase II

E. RNA-dependent DNA-polymerase

14. F.M.'s tuberculosis therapy included ethambutol. Which of the following statements best explains why ethambutol was added to the therapeutic regimen?

A. To enhance the antibacterial activity of pyrazinamide

B. To provide antibacterial activity against atypical mycobacteria

C. To prevent the neurotoxic effects of isoniazid

D. To prevent Pneumocystis jiroveci pneumonia

E. To delay the emergence of drug resistance

15. Pyridoxine was added to F.M.'s tuberculosis therapy. The addition of this vitamin was done to prevent which of the following drug-induced adverse effects?

A. Lactic acidosis

B. Liver steatosis

C. Peripheral neuropathy

D. Pseudomembranous colitis

E. Kidney failure

F. Hyperglycemia

16. Ganciclovir was prescribed to F.M. to treat his CMV retinitis. The inhibition of which of the following enzymes most likely mediated the therapeutic effect of the drug in the patient's disease?

A. Neuraminidase

B. DNA polymerase

C. Reverse transcriptase

D. RNA polymerase

E. Arabinosyl transferase

F. Transpeptidase

Answers and Explanations

▶ *Learning objective:* Explain the mechanism of action of azoles.

1. Answer: E

Both miconazole and fluconazole belong to the antifungal azole subclass. Azoles inhibit fungal cytochrome P450 enzymes. The inhibition impairs the activity of a P-450-dependent lanosterol demethylase that converts lanosterol to ergosterol. The ultimate effect is an inhibition of ergosterol synthesis in fungal cells, which leads to disruption of the fungal cell membrane. The ultimate effect may be fungicidal or fungistatic, depending on the organism and on drug concentration. The specificity of azole drugs results from their greater affinity for fungal than for mammalian cytochrome P-450 enzymes.

A Inhibition of conversion of squalene to lanosterol would be the mechanism of action of terbinafine.

B Formation of artificial pores in the fungal membrane would be the mechanism of action of amphotericin B.

C Inhibition of fungal mitosis would be the mechanism of action of griseofulvin.

D No antifungal drugs can inhibit the synthesis of squalene. In mammalian cells this synthesis can be inhibited by 3-hydroxy-3-methylglutaryl–coenzyme A (HMG-CoA) reductase inhibitors through an inhibition of the synthesis of mevalonate.

▶ *Learning objective:* Identify the two events of the patient's history that most likely suggested HIV infection.

2. Answer: E

Oral candidiasis and heroin addiction are the facts that most likely arose the suspicion of HIV infection in the present patient. In otherwise healthy, immunocompetent individuals, the appearance of opportunistic infections, such as oral candidiasis, is rare. This is because an intact cell-mediated immunity protects against infection. In immunosuppressed individuals, such as those infected with HIV, the immune system is significantly damaged and places patients at risk for opportunistic infections. A subject that used illicit drug injection is at risk of HIV infection because there are three primary modes of HIV transmission: sexual, parenteral, and perinatal. The patient stated that he had been "clean" over the least 8 months, but HIV infection can be asymptomatic for years.

A, B, D Of course sexual intercourse with different partners increases the risk of HIV infection, but condom use reduces the risk of transmission by approximately 20-fold. Moreover the patient was circumcised, which is estimated to reduce the risk of acquisition of HIV infection during heterosexual intercourse by 60%. Therefore sex with different partners is not the primary risk factor for HIV infection acquisition in the present case.

C, D, F Even if HIV infection from contaminated blood or blood products is well known, it is extremely rare today, because these products are tested for HIV antibodies.

▶ *Learning objective:* Identify the blood cells that are the main target of HIV.

3. Answer: B

Once the HIV enters the human body the outer glycoprotein on its surface (gp160) has affinity for CD4 receptors located mainly on the surface of T-helper lymphocytes, monocytes, macrophages, and dendritic cells. Once initial binding occurs the association of HIV with the cell is enhanced by further binding to chemokine coreceptors. CD4 and coreceptor attachment of HIV to the cell promotes membrane fusion and finally internalization of the viral genetic material and enzymes necessary for replication.

A, C, D, E Neutrophils and B lymphocytes are devoid of CD4 receptors and therefore are not the target of HIV.

▶ *Learning objective:* Identify the sign that is diagnostic for AIDS in a patient with HIV infection.

4. Answer: B

HIV infection and AIDS are not synonyms. HIV infection is a prerequisite for developing AIDS, but many patients with HIV infection do not have AIDS for years. According to the US Centers for Disease Control and Prevention (CDC), a person has AIDS if he/she is infected with HIV and presents one of the following:

▶ A CD4+ T cell count below 200 cells/mm^3

▶ One or more diseases included in a long list of defining illnesses, which comprises several disseminated fungal infections, some neoplasms, and most mycobacterial infections

▶ The present patient is HIV seropositive and has a CD4+ T cell count of 170 cells/mm^3, a diagnostic sign of AIDS.

A Candidiasis is included in the illness list when it involves either the esophagus, bronchi, trachea, or lungs. Oral candidiasis can be a sign of HIV infection but not of AIDS.

C Heroin addiction is not included in the list of illnesses that can be diagnostic for AIDS in a patient with HIV infection.

D HIV infection alone is not diagnostic for AIDS.

E Viral load is associated with the progression of HIV infection but is not included in the definition of AIDS, according to the US CDC.

▶ *Learning objective:* Identify the appropriate duration of HAART therapy in a patient diagnosed with AIDS.

5. Answer: E

Once therapy is initiated, antiretroviral therapy is a lifetime commitment. Eradication of HIV is not possible at this time. Therefore the goals of HAART therapy are to decrease morbidity and mortality, improve quality of life, restore and preserve immune function, and prevent further transmission. The best way to achieve these goals is maximal and durable suppression of HIV replication, which is interpreted as undetectable plasma viral load.
A, B, C, D See correct answer explanation.

▶ *Learning objective:* Identify the antiviral drug class that includes both emtricitabine and tenofovir.

6. Answer: C

Reverse transcriptase inhibitors are considered the main support of antiretroviral therapy and are generally used in combination with other classes of agents like protease inhibitors or integrase strand transfer inhibitors. Reverse transcriptase inhibitors block the enzyme specific to retroviruses (also called RNA-dependent DNA polymerase), which uses viral RNA to make a complementary single-stranded DNA copy. Reverse transcriptase inhibitors can be subdivided into two subclasses:

Nucleoside or nucleotide reverse transcriptase inhibitors (NRTIs)

Nucleoside analogues (zidovudine, abacavir, didanosine, emtricitabine, lamivudine, stavudine) require phosphorylation by host cell kinases to become active.

Nucleotide analogues only include tenofovir. The active nucleotide analogue acts by inhibiting reverse transcriptase of HIV-1 and HIV-2. Differences in the mechanism of phosphorylation and different specificity for viral versus host cell polymerases explain the variation among different drugs of this group.

Nonnucleoside reverse transcriptase inhibitors (NNRTIs)

Nonnucleoside analogues (delavirdine, nevirapine, efavirenz) do not require phosphorylation to be active. They act by inhibiting the reverse transcriptase of HIV-1 only. There is no cross resistance between NRTIs and NNRTIs.

A Integrase strand transfer would be inhibited by antiretroviral integrase inhibitors (raltegravir, elvitegravir).

B Neuraminidase would be inhibited by anti-influenza neuraminidase inhibitors (oseltamivir and zanamivir).

D Protease would be inhibited by antiretroviral protease inhibitors (atazanavir, indinavir, nelfinavir, lopinavir).

E Virion entry would be inhibited by antiretroviral entry inhibitors (maraviroc, enfuvirtide).

▸ *Learning objective:* Identify the step of the viral cycle specifically inhibited by emtricitabine and tenofovir.

7. Answer: C

Emtricitabine and tenofovir are nucleoside/nucleotide reverse transcriptase inhibitors. The reverse transcriptase is an enzyme that makes a complementary single-stranded DNA copy. The copy is then duplicated to form the double-stranded proviral DNA, which migrates into the nucleus and becomes integrated with the genetic material of the host cell. By blocking the enzyme these drugs prevent viral DNA from growing.

A Virion entry would be inhibited by antiretroviral entry inhibitors (maraviroc, enfuvirtide).

B Uncoating would be inhibited by drugs like interferons and amantadine.

D Proteolytic cleavage would be inhibited by antiretroviral protease inhibitors (atazanavir, indinavir, nelfinavir, lopinavir).

E Assembly would be inhibited by drugs like interferons and rifampin.

F Release would be inhibited by anti-influenza neuraminidase inhibitors (oseltamivir and zanamivir).

▸ *Learning objective:* Identify a rare but potentially lethal adverse effect that can be caused by nucleoside/nucleotide reverse transcriptase inhibitors.

8. Answer: D

Emtricitabine is a nucleoside, and tenofovir is a nucleotide reverse transcriptase inhibitor. All nucleoside/nucleotide reverse transcriptase inhibitors can cause lactic acidosis, presumably as a consequence of inhibition of human DNA polymerase, which in turn can lead to mitochondrial toxicity. The disorder is quite rare but is lethal in up to 50% of cases.

A, B, C, E These adverse effects are not associated with the use of nucleoside/nucleotide reverse transcriptase inhibitors.

▸ *Learning objective:* Identify the step of the viral cycle specifically inhibited by lopinavir and ritonavir.

9. Answer: D

Lopinavir and ritonavir are protease inhibitors. During the later stages of the HIV growth cycle, synthesis of polyproteins occurs, and these become immature budding particles. A viral protease is responsible for cleaving these precursor molecules to produce the final structural proteins of the mature virion core. By inhibiting the protease enzyme, these drugs prevent the processing of viral polyproteins into functional proteins, resulting in the production of immature, noninfectious viral particles.

A Virion entry would be inhibited by antiretroviral entry inhibitors (maraviroc, enfuvirtide).

B Uncoating would be inhibited by drugs like interferons and amantadine.

C Viral DNA growing would be inhibited by antiretroviral reverse transcriptase inhibitors.

E Assembly would be inhibited by drugs like interferons and rifampin.

F Release would be inhibited by anti-influenza neuraminidase inhibitors (oseltamivir and zanamivir).

▸ *Learning objective:* Explain the reason for the association of ritonavir with other protease inhibitors.

10. Answer: A

Ritonavir is a drug with a pronounced inhibitory action on CYP3A4. When used in combination with any other protease inhibitor agents ritonavir can substantially increase their plasma levels, permitting lower and less frequent dosing.

B, C, D, E Ritonavir does not display these actions.

▶ *Learning objective:* Identify the enzyme specifically inhibited by raltegravir.

11.   Answer: E

When the initial HAART therapy is not effective, most likely because resistance has emerged, an alternative treatment is started. Many patients who have failed the initial regimen still have virus that is fully sensitive to protease inhibitors, because these agents have a high barrier to resistance. Therefore a treatment with the previously used protease inhibitors plus an integrase strand transfer inhibitor like raltegravir is a commonly used strategy, as in the present case.

Integrase strand transfer is the viral enzyme that transfers the reverse transcribed HIV DNA into the chromosomes of host cells. Integrase inhibitors bind the enzyme while it is in a specific complex with viral DNA. As a result, viral DNA cannot become incorporated into the human genome, and cellular enzymes degrade unincorporated viral DNA.

A Neuraminidase would be inhibited by anti-influenza neuraminidase inhibitors.

B Viral DNA polymerase would be inhibited by anti-herpes DNA polymerase Inhibitors.

C Reverse transcriptase would be inhibited by antiretroviral reverse transcriptase inhibitors.

D Protease would be inhibited by antiretroviral protease inhibitors.

▶ *Learning objective:* Identify the bacterial cell component whose synthesis is specifically inhibited by isoniazid.

12.   Answer: C

Isoniazid enter bacilli by passive diffusion. Inside the cell, the drug is not toxic by itself (it is in fact a prodrug) but is activated to an isonicotinoyl radical that is able to inhibit the synthesis of mycolic acid, an essential component of the mycobacterial cell wall. The synthesis of the cell wall is inhibited, leading to bacterial cell death.

A, B, D, E, F The synthesis of all these cell components is not inhibited by isoniazid.

▶ *Learning objective:* Explain the mechanism of action of rifampin.

13.   Answer: A

Rifampin inhibits DNA-dependent RNA-polymerase in mycobacteria and other sensitive microorganisms by binding to the beta subunit of the enzyme to form a stable drug–enzyme complex. This leads to suppression of initiation of chain formation in RNA synthesis. The ultimate effect is bactericidal.

B This enzyme would be inhibited by ethambutol.

C This enzyme would be inhibited by β-lactam antibiotics.

D This enzyme would be inhibited by fluoroquinolones.

E This enzyme would be inhibited by reverse transcriptase inhibitors.

▶ *Learning objective:* Explain the main reason for the use of ethambutol in the pharmacotherapy of tuberculosis.

14.   Answer: E

The main reason for the use of any drug combination in the therapy of tuberculosis is to delay the emergence of resistance. In the case of ethambutol, this is by far the primary reason, since the drug has only weak bacteriostatic activity against *M. tuberculosis* and so cannot add any significant antibacterial effect to a given therapeutic regimen.

A, B, C, D Ethambutol does not display these actions.

▶ *Learning objective:* Identify the drug-induced adverse effect that can be prevented by the concomitant administration of pyridoxine.

15.   Answer: C

Pyridoxine was added to prevent some isoniazid-induced adverse effects. Isoniazid can cause neurotoxicity, including peripheral neuropathy (the most common), optic neuritis insomnia, restlessness, tinnitus, vertigo, muscle twitching, and (with high doses) ataxia, transient loss of memory, confusion, hallucinations, and seizures. This neurotoxicity stems from several causes, but pyridoxine deficiency seems the most common. Isoniazid induces a state of functional pyridoxine deficiency by at least the two following mechanisms: Isoniazid metabolites directly attach and inactivate pyridoxine.

▶ Isoniazid inhibits pyridoxine phosphokinase, the enzyme necessary to activate pyridoxine to pyridoxal 5'-phosphate, the cofactor in many pyridoxine-dependent reactions.
▶ Most neurotoxic effects of isoniazid can be corrected (without losing the antibacterial effect) by pyridoxine supplementation.

A, B, D, E, F All these adverse effects can be drug-induced, but they are not caused by isoniazid and cannot be prevented by pyridoxine administration.

▶ *Learning objective:* Identify the enzyme specifically inhibited by ganciclovir.

16. Answer: B

Ganciclovir is a nucleoside analogue that must be phosphorylated first by a specific CMV phosphotransferase and then by host cell enzymes to become active. The activated compound competitively inhibits viral DNA polymerase, thereby blocking DNA elongation. This explains why ganciclovir is a first-line agent for CMV infection.

A Neuraminidase would be inhibited by anti-influenza neuraminidase inhibitors.

C Reverse transcriptase would be inhibited by antiretroviral reverse transcriptase inhibitors.

D Ganciclovir inhibits DNA, not RNA polymerase.

E Arabinosyl transferase would be inhibited by ethambutol

F Transpeptidase would be inhibited by β-lactam antibiotics.

Case 24

Infective Endocarditis

T.M., a 64-year-old man, was admitted to the hospital with complaints of fatigue, remittent low-grade fever, night sweats, chest pain, shortness of breath, and an unintentional weight loss of 16 pounds.

T.M.'s past medical history indicated that 5 years earlier he had had prostate cancer, which was surgically removed. Three years ago he had been diagnosed with mitral valve prolapse, and 1 year later with hypercholesterolemia, presently treated with atorvastatin. Two weeks ago the patient had undergone dental surgery for an endosseous implant.

T.M. had been smoking 5 to 10 cigarettes daily for several years and was drinking 2 to 3 glasses of wine daily, but he denied use of illicit drugs. He was retired from work as a plumber and lived at home with his wife.

Physical examination showed an ill-appearing man in no acute distress, with the following vital signs: blood pressure 114/80 mm Hg, heart rate 96 bpm, respirations 22/min, temperature 100.2°F (37.8°C). Inspection revealed petechial skin lesions on the upper trunk, subungual splinter hemorrhages, and nontender hemorrhagic macules on the hand palms and soles of both feet. Heart examination disclosed a holosystolic murmur, heard loudest over the apex and left lower sternal border. The rest of the physical examination was unremarkable.

Pertinent laboratory results on admission were as follows:

Blood hematology:

- Erythrocyte sedimentation rate: 60 mm/h (normal < 20)
- Red blood cell count (RBC): $4.19 \times 10^6/\mu L$ (normal, 4.0–6.0)
- Hemoglobin (Hgb): 11 g/dL (normal 12–16)
- Hematocrit (Hct): 32% (normal 36–48)
- White blood cell count (WBC): $8 \times 10^3/\mu L$ (normal 4–10)
- Platelets: $280 \times 10^3/\mu L$ (normal 130–400)
- Creatinine: 1.2 mg/dL (normal 0.6–1.2)
- Blood urea nitrogen (BUN): 22 mg/dL (normal 8–25)
- Sodium: 140 mEq/L (normal 135–146)
- Potassium: 4.3 mEq/L (normal 3.5–5.5)
- Glucose: 102 mg/dL (normal 60–110)

Echocardiography

A transesophageal echocardiography showed mitral valve prolapse with regurgitation and several large vegetations on the orifice of the valve.

Blood cultures

Three blood cultures were obtained over 24 hours, and all were growing viridans streptococci.

A diagnosis of subacute infective endocarditis was made, and an initial therapy was started with penicillin G and gentamicin, pending antimicrobial susceptibility test results.

Two days later the fever had not disappeared, and the results of susceptibility tests indicated that the bacteria were resistant to penicillin G, ampicillin, and third-generation cephalosporins but sensitive to vancomycin, clindamycin, and gentamicin. A therapy with vancomycin and gentamicin was started and continued for 4 weeks. After this period T.M. had no symptoms and signs of disease, blood culture was negative, and he was dismissed from the hospital.

Questions

1. T.M. was diagnosed with subacute infective endocarditis. Which of the following sets of bacteria is most commonly involved in the pathogenesis of this disease?

A. Viridans streptococci–Pseudomonas–Proteus

B. Pseudomonas–Serratia–staphylococci

C. Enterococci–Escherichia–Klebsiella

D. Proteus–Salmonella–Serratia

E. Viridans streptococci–staphylococci–enterococci

F. Escherichia–Salmonella–Klebsiella

2. Which of the following risk factors from T.M.'s history was most likely involved in the development of his endocarditis?

A. Smoking

B. Previous prostate cancer

C. Previous dental surgery

D. Alcohol use

E. Hypercholesterolemia

3. Which of the following hemodynamic factors most likely predisposed T.M. to the development of his endocarditis?

A. Blood flow from a high- to a low-pressure heart chamber

B. High systemic blood pressure

C. Low velocity laminar blood flow through heart valves

D. Low heart rate

4. Taking into account T.M.'s symptoms and signs, the patient was most likely at risk for which of the following complications of his disease?

A. Vertebral osteomyelitis

B. Cerebral abscess

C. Ventricular tachycardia

D. Meningitis

E. Heart failure

F. Pulmonary embolism

5. T.M. started a therapy that included penicillin G. Which of the following molecular actions most likely contributed to the therapeutic effect of the drug in the patient's disease?

A. Activation of autolytic enzymes in the bacterial cell wall

B. Activation of bacterial acetyl-transferase

C. Activation of the efflux pump in the bacterial cell membrane

D. Inhibition of transglycosylase in the bacterial cell wall

E. Inhibition of DNA-dependent RNA polymerase

6. Penicillin G is a narrow-spectrum β-lactam antibiotic. Which of the following sets of activity spectrum is correct for penicillin G?

Set	Klebsiella pneumoniae	Chlamydia trachomatis	Neisseria meningitidis	Treponema pallidum	Actinomyces israelii
A.	Sensitive	Resistant	Sensitive	Resistant	Sensitive
B.	Resistant	Sensitive	Sensitive	Sensitive	Sensitive
C.	Resistant	Resistant	Sensitive	Sensitive	Sensitive
D.	Sensitive	Sensitive	Sensitive	Resistant	Sensitive

7. T.M. started a therapy with vancomycin. Which of the following bacterial structures represents the site of action of this drug?

A. Ribosome

B. Capsule

C. Outer membrane

D. Peptidoglycan layer

E. DNA

8. The inhibition of which of the following molecular actions most likely mediated the therapeutic effect of vancomycin in the patient's disease?

A. Elongation of peptidoglycan chains

B. Relaxation of supercoiled DNA

C. Binding to 30S ribosomal subunit

D. Translocation of peptidyl transfer RNA (tRNA)

E. Synthesis of mycolic acid

9. Vancomycin is an antibiotic with a narrow activity spectrum. Which of the following sets of activity spectrum is correct for vancomycin?

Set	*Pseudomonas aeruginosa*	*Chlamydia trachomatis*	*Clostridium difficile*	*Treponema pallidum*	*Enterococcus faecalis*
A.	Sensitive	Resistant	Resistant	Sensitive	Sensitive
B.	Sensitive	Sensitive	Resistant	Resistant	Sensitive
C.	Resistant	Sensitive	Resistant	Sensitive	Resistant
D.	Resistant	Resistant	Sensitive	Resistant	Sensitive

10. Which of the following adverse reactions to vancomycin could T.M. have had shortly after his first intravenous (IV) administration?

A. Stabbing limb pain

B. Hypertension and bradycardia

C. Generalized itching and facial flushing

D. Hearing loss and tinnitus

E. Severe headache

11. Viridans streptococci from T.M.'s blood cultures were found to be sensitive to clindamycin, an antibiotic that acts by inhibiting bacterial protein synthesis. Which of the following steps of protein synthesis is primarily inhibited by this antibiotic?

A. Binding of initiator RNA to site P of the ribosome

B. Transfer of the peptide chain from site P to site A of the ribosome

C. Transfer of peptidyl tRNA from site A to site P of the ribosome

D. Binding of aminoacyl tRNA to the site A of the ribosome

Answers and Explanations

▸ *Learning objective:* Identify the set of bacteria that are most commonly involved in the pathogenesis of infective endocarditis.

1. Answer: E

Endocarditis is predominantly a gram-positive bacterial infection. Viridans streptococci, staphylococci (*S. aureus*), and enterococci (*E. faecalis*) are the bacteria most commonly involved.

A, B, C, D, F Endocarditis caused by gram-negative bacteria (including Pseudomonas, Proteus, Serratia, Escherichia, and Klebsiella) is relatively uncommon but has increased significantly over the years, especially in intravenous drug users and in patients with prosthetic heart valves. These infections are very difficult to treat and have a poor prognosis, with mortality rates as high as 60 to 80%.

▶ *Learning objective:* Identify a predisposing factor for infective endocarditis.

2. Answer: C

Numerous studies have demonstrated that dental surgery, and even minor oral trauma like tooth brushing and dental plaque cleaning, may be associated with a low-grade bacteremia due to viridans streptococci, which are normal mouth flora. This most likely occurred in the present case.

A, B, D, E None of these disorders are risk factors for infective endocarditis. Risk factors for this disorder include history of prior infective endocarditis, presence of a prosthetic valve or cardiac device, history of valvular or congenital heart disease, intravenous drug use, indwelling intravenous catheter, immunosuppression, or a recent dental or surgical procedure.

▶ *Learning objective:* Identify a hemodynamic factor that can predispose to infective endocarditis.

3. Answer: A

Subacute infective endocarditis occurs mainly because of the concomitant presence of the following factors:

▶ Bacteremia
▶ An abnormal heart valve

The patient had a mitral valve prolapse. Because of the incompetent valve, regurgitation can occur (see the presence of a holosystolic murmur and the echocardiography report). The regurgitant blood flow from the high-pressure left ventricle into the low-pressure left atrium allows formation of platelet-fibrin thrombi on the atrial surface of the mitral valve. Bacteria can be deposited on these thrombi, forming a vegetation. This consists of bacteria encased

in a meshwork of platelets and fibrin. Once infected, the vegetation continues to grow through further deposition of platelet and fibrin. The vegetation serves as a barrier to host defenses. It is not vascularized and is therefore not easily sterilized by host factors or antimicrobials. It is for this reason that cure requires prolonged administration of antibiotics and sometimes operative intervention.

B Hypertension per se is not a risk factor for endocarditis, and the patient was not hypertensive.

C High-velocity turbulent blood flow, not low-velocity laminar blood flow, is a hemodynamic factor predisposing to endocarditis.

D Heart rate per se is not a risk factor for endocarditis, and the patient had no low heart rate.

▶ *Learning objective:* Identify the most common complication of infective endocarditis.

4. Answer: E

Patients with infective endocarditis can develop a vast array of complications that can be explained on the basis of the following four pathogenetic processes, which can occur during the course of the disease:

▶ Valvular destruction and local intracardiac complications
▶ Septic embolization of vegetations to other organs
▶ Sustained bacteremia, which contributes to metastatic seeding
▶ Immunopathological phenomena

Cardiac complications are the most common complications seen in infective endocarditis, occurring in about one-third of patients. Heart failure is the most common cause of death. Moreover, cardiac examination of the patient showed the presence of a holosystolic murmur. The development of a regurgitant murmur leads to congestive heart failure in > 90% of cases.

A, B, C, D, F All these can be complications of infective endocarditis, but their risk is substantially lower than that of heart failure in the present case.

▶ *Learning objective:* Explain the mechanism of action of penicillin.

5. Answer: A

Streptococci of the viridans group are found to be the cause of infective endocarditis in the present patient. Several viridans streptococci strains are still sensitive to penicillins, which explains the choice of penicillin G as the initial therapy. Penicillin G is a β-lactam antibiotic. The mechanism of action of β-lactam antibiotics includes the following two actions:

▶ They bind to specific β-lactam receptors, called penicillin-binding proteins, located on the cytoplasmic membrane. These proteins are enzymes endowed with various catalytic functions, which are inhibited by binding with the antibiotic. The most important enzymes inhibited are transpeptidases, which catalyze the final cross-link step in the synthesis of murein (also called peptidoglycan). Because peptidoglycan layers are constituents of the bacterial cell wall, the synthesis of this wall is blocked.

▶ Autolytic enzymes (called autolysins or murein hydrolases) are present in the cell wall and degrade the peptidoglycan. β-Lactam antibiotics can activate these autolysins (apparently by blocking an autolysin inhibitor), thereby promoting the lysis of bacteria.

B, C These are mechanisms of resistance to antibiotics.

D This would be the mechanism of action of vancomycin.

E This would be the mechanism of action of rifampin.

▶ *Learning objective:* Identify the activity spectrum of penicillin G.

6. Answer: C

Penicillin G is effective against the following bacteria:

▶ Some gram-positive bacteria (including *Actinomyces israelii*)

▶ Some gram-negative bacteria (including *Neisseria meningitidis*)
▶ Spirochetes (including *Treponema pallidum*)

Penicillin G is not effective against most gram-negative bacteria (e.g., *Klebsiella pneumoniae*) and atypical bacteria (e.g., *Chlamydia trachomatis*).

A This would be a correct antibacterial spectrum for aminoglycosides.

B This would be a correct antibacterial spectrum for macrolides.

D This would be a correct antibacterial spectrum for fluoroquinolones.

▶ *Learning objective:* Identify the site of action of vancomycin.

7. Answer: D

Vancomycin is a cell wall synthesis inhibitor. The drug binds to the nascent peptidoglycan layer, inhibiting its synthesis. Since peptidoglycan is much more abundant in gram-positive bacteria, vancomycin is mainly active against these bacteria.

A This would be the site of action of protein synthesis inhibitors.

B No antibiotic acts on bacteria capsule.

C Gram-negative bacteria have an outer membrane. Vancomycin is not active against gram-negative bacteria.

E This would be the site of action of nucleic acid function inhibitors like fluoroquinolones.

▶ *Learning objective:* Explain the mechanism of action of vancomycin.

8. Answer: A

Vancomycin inhibits cell wall synthesis by binding to the terminus of the nascent peptidoglycan peptide. The binding inhibits transglycosylase (also named glucosyltransferase), the enzyme that catalyzes the elongation of the peptidoglycan chain by linking together the peptidoglycan monomers. This prevents the elongation of linear peptidoglycan chains. The binding also inhibits transpeptidase, but since transglycosylation precedes transpeptidation, inhibition of transglycosylase is the primary mechanism of action of the drug.

B Relaxation of supercoiled DNA would be inhibited by fluoroquinolones.

C Binding to the 30S ribosomal subunit would be inhibited by aminoglycosides.

D Translocation of peptidyl tRNA would be inhibited by macrolides.

E Synthesis of mycolic acid would be inhibited by some antimycobacterial antibiotics, such as isoniazid.

▶ *Learning objective:* Identify the activity spectrum of vancomycin.

9. Answer: D

Vancomycin is an antibiotic active primarily against gram-positive cocci, including methicillin-resistant staphylococci and enterococci. It is also active against many gram-positive anaerobes, including *Clostridium difficile*. Most gram-negative bacteria are intrinsically resistant to vancomycin, because their outer membranes are impermeable to large glycopeptide molecules.

A This would be a correct antibacterial spectrum for carbapenems.

B This would be a correct antibacterial spectrum for fluoroquinolones.

C This would be a correct antibacterial spectrum for macrolides.

▶ *Learning objective:* Describe the adverse effects of vancomycin.

10. Answer: C

A common reaction to vancomycin is the so-called red man syndrome, which can occur after IV infusion of the antibiotic and includes hypotension, tachycardia, generalized pruritus, and facial flushing, as in the present case. The syndrome is caused by histamine release.

A Stabbing limb pain is a symptom of paresthesia. Vancomycin-induced paresthesias are very rare.

B Hypotension and tachycardia, not hypertension and bradycardia, can occur shortly after vancomycin injection.

D Vancomycin can cause, rarely, ototoxicity (hearing loss and tinnitus), but this adverse effect usually appears after a few days of therapy, not shortly after the first injection.

E Headache is reported in 5 to 7% of cases after chronic treatment but not soon after the first injection.

▶ *Learning objective:* Explain the mechanism of action of clindamycin.

11. Answer: C

Clindamycin is a lincosamide antibiotic with a mechanism of action quite close to that of macrolides. The drug binds to the 50S subunit of bacterial ribosome and inhibits bacterial protein synthesis, primarily by blocking the translocation of the newly synthesized peptidyl-tRNA from the acceptor site (A) to the donor site (P) of the ribosome.

A. This would be part of the mechanism of action of aminoglycosides.

B. This would be the mechanism of action of chloramphenicol.

D. This would be the mechanism of action of tetracyclines.

Case 25

Iron Deficiency Anemia

J.M., a 62-year-old woman, was admitted to her local hospital because of an abdominal pain, dizziness, and severe tiredness most of the day. She said these symptoms had started about 1 month ago and had gotten progressively worse over the past 2 weeks.

The patient's medical history was remarkable for hyperthyroidism, diagnosed 10 years ago. She was treated with radioactive iodine to destroy the gland, and she had been taking levothyroxine since. Further questioning revealed that about 2 months ago J.M. had started having bilateral joint pain in her knees and ankles and had started self-medicating with naproxen, four to five tablets daily. Other drugs taken by the patient on admission included magnesium hydroxide for occasional constipation and lovastatin for hypercholesterolemia. The patient never smoked and denied the use of alcohol or illicit drugs.

Physical examination showed a pale Caucasian woman with the following vital signs: blood pressure 128/76 mm Hg, pulse 108 bpm, respirations 24/min, body temperature 97.7°F (36.5°C). The patient's conjunctiva, oral mucosa, and nail beds were pale, and her tongue was pale and swollen. The rest of the physical examination was unremarkable.

Pertinent laboratory results on admission were as follows:

Blood hematology

- ▶ Red blood cell count (RBC): $2.8 \times 10^6/\mu L$ (normal, 4.0–6.0)
- ▶ White blood cell count (WBC): $8 \times 10^3/\mu L$ (normal 4–10)
- ▶ Platelets: $320 \times 10^3/\mu L$ (normal 130–400)
- ▶ Mean corpuscular volume (MCV): 70 fL (normal 80–100)
- ▶ Hemoglobin (Hgb): 5.5 g/dL (normal 12–16)
- ▶ Hematocrit (Hct): 26% (normal 36–48)
- ▶ Ferritin: 6 ng/mL (normal 30–300)
- ▶ Iron: 8 µg/dL (normal, women 50–140)
- ▶ Transferrin: 520 mg/dL (normal 250–425)

Blood chemistry

- ▶ pH: 7.42 (normal 7.35–7.45)
- ▶ Creatinine: 1.1 mg/dL (normal 0.6–1.2)
- ▶ Blood urea nitrogen (BUN): 30 mg/dL (normal 8–25)
- ▶ Uric acid: 6.2 mg/dL (normal 4-8.5)
- ▶ Sodium: 132 mEq/L (normal 135–146)
- ▶ Potassium: 3.4 mEq/L (normal 3.6–5.3)
- ▶ Total cholesterol: 210 mg/dL (normal < 200)

Stool occult blood test

Positive

Gastroscopy

Severe gastritis with multiple bleeding lesions

Biopsy test for *Helicobacter pylori*

Negative

J.M. was diagnosed with severe iron deficiency anemia due to bleeding erosive gastritis, most likely secondary to nonsteroidal anti-inflammatory (NSAID) therapy.

The patient was treated with omeprazole and received a packed red blood cell transfusion that was repeated the following 2 days. One day later J.M.'s hemoglobin increased to 8.2 g/dL and hematocrit to 38%. At that time the patient was discharged from the hospital with a postdischarge therapy of omeprazole and oral ferrous gluconate.

J.M. was also advised to carefully avoid all NSAIDs, including those available over the counter.

Questions

1. Laboratory exams indicate that J.M.'s hemoglobin was low. Hemoglobin is a globular hemoprotein. Which of the following sets correctly defines the number of polypeptide chains and heme moiety of the hemoglobin molecule?

Set	Polypeptide chains	Heme moiety
A.	1	1
B.	4	4
C.	2	1
D.	4	2
E.	2	2

2. Hemoglobin is the main carrier of oxygen to the tissues. Which of the following is the number of oxygen molecules carried by one hemoglobin molecule?

A. 1

B. 2

C. 3

D. 4

E. 5

F. 6

3. The ability of hemoglobin to reversibly bind oxygen is affected by several factors. Which of the following factors can vastly increase the affinity of hemoglobin for oxygen?

A. Low pH of the environment

B. High concentration of dissolved carbon dioxide

C. Low concentration of dissolved oxygen

D. Oxygen already combined with heme

E. High temperature

4. Hemoglobin carries oxygen to different organs/tissues and releases oxygen to those tissues. Which of the following are the two most important tissue factors that can increase this release?

A. $[K^+]$–pH

B. $[K^+]$–temperature

C. Temperature–pH

D. $[Na^+]$–temperature

E. $[Na^+]$–pH

F. $[Na^+]$–$[K+]$

5. J.M. was diagnosed with iron deficiency anemia. Which of the following lab test results is most indicative of this type of anemia?

A. RBC count

B. Iron

C. Hemoglobin

D. Ferritin

E. Transferrin

6. J.M. was diagnosed with iron deficiency anemia, most likely secondary to NSAID overuse. Which of the following pairs of drug properties best explains the reasons for NSAID-induced gastric damage?

A. Drug pK_a–inhibition of lipoxygenase

B. Inhibition of cyclooxygenase-1 (COX-1)–antiplatelet action

C. Drug pK_a–antiplatelet action

D. Inhibition of lipoxygenase–antiplatelet action

E. Drug pK_a–inhibition of COX-1

F. Inhibition of COX-1–inhibition of lipoxygenase

7. Which of the following physiological actions most likely indicates the body's attempt to compensate for the patient's anemia?

A. Decreased cardiac output

B. Decreased body temperature

C. Increased kidney renin production

D. Decreased tissue oxygen extraction

E. Increased heart rate

8. Iron is available in a variety of foods but is especially abundant in meat. Which of the following ranges most likely indicates the average amount of iron (in mg) absorbed daily by a normal individual?

A. 8–10

B. 2–3

C. 5–6

D. 0.5–1

E. 11–12

F. > 12

9. An oral iron preparation of ferrous gluconate was prescribed to J.M. Which of the following transport systems was most likely involved in the patient's intestinal absorption of the drug?

A. Aqueous diffusion

B. Lipid diffusion

C. Facilitated diffusion

D. Active transport

E. Exocytosis

10. J.M. was found to have elevated serum transferrin levels. Which of the following phrases best explains the most likely reason for this increase?

A. Decreased binding capacity of the transferrin molecule

B. Iron stores depletion

C. Decreased availability of ferroportin

D. Increased availability of ferritin

E. Decreased heme iron absorption

11. Iron is transported in plasma as ferric iron bound to transferrin. Which of the following pairs of cells are most likely the primary targets of this transport?

A. Erythroblasts–erythrocytes

B. Erythrocytes–hepatocytes

C. Enterocytes–erythroblasts

D. Erythroblasts–hepatocytes

E. Erythrocytes–enterocytes

F. Enterocytes–hepatocytes

12. Iron therapy is needed for iron deficiency anemia, and treatment can be done with oral or parenteral iron preparations. Which of the following is, albeit rare, a life-threatening adverse effect of intravenous iron preparations?

A. Myocardial infarction

B. Pulmonary thromboembolism

C. Anaphylaxis

D. Ventricular arrhythmia

E. Stroke

13. An oral iron preparation of ferrous gluconate was prescribed to J.M. Which of the following should be the duration of her oral iron therapy?

A. 1–2 weeks

B. 3–4 weeks

C. 3–6 months

D. 7–10 months

E. 1 year

14. Which of the following adverse effects could be most likely expected from J.M.'s oral iron therapy?

A. Headache

B. Abdominal cramps

C. Palpitations

D. Urinary frequency

E. Joint pain

F. Shortness of breath

Answers and Explanations

▶ *Learning objective:* Identify the correct number of polypeptide chains and heme moiety of the hemoglobin molecule.

1. Answer: B

Hemoglobin belongs to a group of specialized proteins that contain heme as a tightly bound molecule. Hemoglobin A, the major hemoglobin in adults, is composed of four polypeptide chains. Each chain has a heme-binding pocket; therefore the hemoglobin molecule has four polypeptide chains and four heme moieties.

A, C, D, E See correct answer explanation.

▶ *Learning objective:* Identify the number of oxygen molecules carried by one hemoglobin molecule.

2. Answer: D

One hemoglobin molecule contains four heme moieties. Heme is a porphyrin ring complex that includes one atom of ferrous ion. Each of the four iron atoms can reversibly bind one oxygen molecule. The iron stays in the ferrous state, so that the reaction is *oxygenation*, not oxidation.

A, B, C, E, F See correct answer explanation.

▸ *Learning objective:* Explain the factor that can vastly increase the affinity of hemoglobin for oxygen.

3. Answer: D

The quaternary structure of hemoglobin determines its affinity for oxygen. In deoxyhemoglobin, the globin units are tightly bound in a *tense (T) configuration*, which reduces the affinity of the molecule for oxygen. The binding of first oxygen molecule to hemoglobin produces a *relaxed (R) configuration*, where the affinity for oxygen is increased. In other words, the oxygenation of the first heme increases the oxygen affinity of the second heme, the oxygenation of the second heme increases the affinity of the third heme, and so on. The net result is that oxyhemoglobin has a > 300-fold increase in oxygen affinity.

A, B, C, E All these factors actually decrease, not increase, the oxygen affinity of hemoglobin.

▸ *Learning objective:* Identify the two most important tissue factors that can increase hemoglobin release of oxygen to the tissues.

4. Answer: C

In the capillaries of metabolically active tissues, there is a higher temperature and a higher production of carbon dioxide, both of which make the local pH more acidic. Both factors can decrease the oxygen affinity of hemoglobin, thus favoring the release of oxygen to the tissues. Of course blood cannot unload oxygen unless blood gets into the tissues, but in most systemic arterioles, local higher temperature and acidosis are also powerful stimuli for vasodilation.

A, B, F Local concentration of K^+ does not affect the oxygen affinity of hemoglobin.

D, E, F Local concentration of Na^+ does not affect the oxygen affinity of hemoglobin.

▸ *Learning objective:* Identify the most indicative lab result for the diagnosis of iron deficiency anemia.

5. Answer: D

Iron is stored as ferritin in reticulum endothelial tissues, but ferritin is also present in serum. Because stored ferritin is in equilibrium with serum ferritin, the latter reflects the body iron stores and is the most reliable indicator of total body iron status. Ferritin represents the more specific and more sensitive test for diagnosing iron deficiency. A ferritin level of < 10 ng/mL is diagnostic for iron deficiency anemia.

A By definition anemia is a condition where there is a reduction of circulating RBCs. Therefore a low RBC count cannot define a specific type of anemia.

B Iron can be low in many chronic diseases.

C Hemoglobin can be low in many types of anemia.

E Transferrin is usually increased in iron deficiency anemia but can also be increased in some nonanemic states, including pregnancy and after estrogen therapy.

▸ *Learning objective:* Describe the two NSAID properties that can explain the drug-induced gastric damage.

6. Answer: E

The patient's stool occult blood test and gastroscopy results indicate that her iron deficiency anemia was due to chronic blood loss, which is the most common cause of the disease. In the present case the loss was most likely caused by overuse of naproxen. The prevalence of endoscopically confirmed gastrointestinal ulcers in chronic NSAID users is 15 to 30%, and long-term use of these drugs is the most frequent cause of anemia due to chronic blood loss. NSAIDS cause gastric damage by two actions:

▸ *Local action:* NSAIDs are weak acids with a pK_a < 5 and therefore are mainly nonionized (i.e., lipid soluble) in the stomach lumen. Being mainly lipid-soluble, they can cross the cell membrane by lipid diffusion.

In the alkaline environment of the cytoplasm, however, they become ionized (i.e., water-soluble) and are trapped inside the gastric epithelial cells, causing death of these cells. The dead cells are digested by the gastric juice, leading to gastric ulcerations.

▶ **Systemic action:** By blocking COX-1, these drugs impair the cytoprotective effect of prostaglandins on gastrointestinal mucosa, brought about by maintaining blood flow and stimulating bicarbonate and mucus production.

A, D, F NSAIDs have negligible inhibitory activity on lipoxygenase enzyme.

B, C, D The antiplatelet action of NSAIDs can contribute to the chronic blood loss but is by no means the main cause of this effect.

▶ *Learning objective:* Describe a physiological action that tries to compensate for the consequences of the patient's anemia.

7. Answer: E

Anemia occurs when there is a decrease in the number of red blood cells or in hemoglobin content. In both cases not enough oxygen is provided to the tissues. The body can compensate for this decrease in two ways:

▶ It can increase cardiac output.
▶ It can increase oxygen extraction.

The patient's increased heart rate indicates that the increased cardiac output was trying to compensate for the ongoing anemia.

A In patients with anemia, cardiac output, if anything, is increased, not decreased.

B, C These actions have nothing to do with compensation for the effects of anemia.

D In patients with anemia tissue oxygen extraction is increased, not decreased.

▶ *Learning objective:* Identify the average milligrams of iron absorbed daily by a normal individual.

8. Answer: D

About 0.5 to 1 mg of ferrous iron is absorbed daily and can replace the 1 mg of iron lost daily through feces, urine, and sweat. The utilization of iron by the body is designed to maintain body stores, so very little physiological loss of iron occurs once it is in the body. Because the ability of the body to excrete iron is so limited, regulation of iron balance must be achieved by changing intestinal absorption, which is actually tightly regulated by the size of existing iron stores.

A, B, C, E, F See correct answer explanation.

▶ *Learning objective:* Describe the transport systems most likely involved in the intestinal absorption of iron.

9. Answer: D

Iron is absorbed primarily by duodenal epithelial cells. It crosses the luminal membrane of these cells by two active transport systems:

▶ **The inorganic iron** is transported via the divalent metal transporter. As its name suggests, this transporter is a protein that can bind a variety of divalent metals, including, copper, zinc, and manganese. However, its major role is active transport of ferrous iron. The expression of this transporter is regulated by body iron stores, and its synthesis can be increased in response to increased iron requirements, to maintain iron homeostasis.
▶ **The heme iron** (from meat hemoglobin and myoglobin) is transported intact via the heme carrier protein or through endocytosis. Inside the enterocytes, heme oxygenase splits the heme to release free iron.

Because the patient received ferrous gluconate, the drug was actively absorbed by the divalent metal transporter.

A Aqueous diffusion is a passive transport system that can transport small (molecular weight < 100 daltons) water-soluble molecules. Iron is a small, water-soluble molecule but is not transported through cell membranes by aqueous diffusion.

B Lipid diffusion is a passive transport system that can transport lipid-soluble molecules. Iron is not lipid-soluble.

C Facilitated diffusion is a passive transport system that uses a carrier. Iron is actively, not passively, transported by a carrier.

E Endocytosis, not exocytosis, is the transport system that can transport heme iron.

▶ *Learning objective:* Identify the most likely cause of the anemia-induced increase in serum transferrin.

---

10. Answer: B

When serum iron falls and iron stores are depleted, the body tries to restore iron homeostasis by increasing both intestinal iron absorption and serum transferrin levels.

A The binding capacity of transferrin molecules is not changed. One molecule of transferrin can bind two molecules of ferric iron.

C Ferroportin is a transporter that carries the iron through the basolateral membrane of enterocytes. Its availability has nothing to do with the increased transferrin.

D Ferritin is decreased, not increased, when transferrin is increased.

E When iron stores are depleted, intestinal absorption of both inorganic iron and heme iron are increased, not decreased.

▶ *Learning objective:* Identify the two cell types that represent the main targets of iron transport.

---

11. Answer: D

The iron carried by transferrin is ultimately deposited in most body tissues, given that all cells require iron to maintain normal function, but the bone marrow and the liver are the main target organs.

In the bone marrow, transferrin receptors are present in large numbers on erythroblasts and other proliferating erythroid cells. These receptors bind and internalize the transferrin–iron complex through the process of receptor-mediated endocytosis. The ferric iron is then released, reduced to ferrous iron, and used for hemoglobin synthesis or stored as ferritin.

In the liver a similar process stores iron as ferritin, making that organ the most abundant iron store.

A, B, E Red blood cells do not have transferrin receptors and cannot get the iron transported by transferrin.

C, E, F Duodenal epithelial cells (i.e., enterocytes) do not have transferrin receptors and cannot get the iron transported by transferrin.

▶ *Learning objective:* Describe a rare but life-threatening adverse effect of intravenous iron administration.

---

12. Answer: C

Use of intravenous iron allows administration of nearly full-replacement doses in one or two infusions, depending on the product. However, this therapy should be reserved for special patient populations, because severe adverse effects, including life-threatening infusion or anaphylactic reactions, have been reported in patients receiving intravenous iron preparations.

A Cardiac arrest has been very rarely associated with intravenous iron administration, but myocardial infarction has not been reported.

B Pulmonary edema and respiratory arrest have been very rarely associated with intravenous iron administration, but pulmonary thromboembolism has not been reported.

D There are no reports of cardiac arrhythmias following intravenous iron administration.

E There are no reports of strokes following intravenous iron administration.

▶ *Learning objective:* Describe the optimal duration of an oral iron therapy for iron-deficiency anemia.

---

13. Answer: C

Hematologic response to oral iron therapy is usually seen in 2 to 3 weeks with 1 to 2 g/dL increase in hemoglobin. Therefore the patient's anemia was expected to resolve in 1 to 2 months. However, iron therapy should be continued for 3 to 6 months to replace iron stores.

A, B, D, E See correct answer explanation.

▶ *Learning objective:* Describe a common adverse effect of oral iron preparations.

14. Answer: B

Gastrointestinal adverse effects are extremely common (up to 30%) with oral iron administration. These include a metallic taste, flatulence, abdominal cramps, constipation, diarrhea, nausea, and vomiting. These effects are usually dose-related and can be overcome by lowering the dose and taking the drug with meals. Sometimes changing the preparation can help.

A, C, D, E, F There are no reports of these adverse effects following oral iron administration.

Liver Cirrhosis

U.V., a 52-year-old man, was admitted to the hospital with a 1-week history of nausea, two episodes of vomiting blood, and lower abdominal cramps without diarrhea. Recently he had noted an increased daily drowsiness, an increased tenseness and girth of his abdomen, and a yellow color on his skin and eyes.

The patient had a long history of alcohol abuse, with multiple hospital admissions for alcoholic gastritis and alcohol withdrawal. He reported that, in spite of his disease, he was unable to stop drinking and often drank three or four glasses of whisky almost daily.

Physical examination revealed an afebrile and cachectic male in moderate distress. He was drowsy and minimally oriented to person, place, and time. Vital signs were as follows: blood pressure 100/50 mm Hg, pulse 110 bpm, respiration 22/min. The patient's skin and sclerae were slightly jaundiced, and multiple spider angiomas were found on his face and upper chest. A flapping tremor of the patient's hands was noted when the wrist was extended. Bilateral gynecomastia was present. Abdominal examination revealed prominent veins on a very tense abdomen. Palpation of the abdomen revealed that his liver measured 14 cm in the midclavicular line, and his spleen was palpable 3 cm below the left costal margin. Ascites was noted by shifting dullness and a fluid wave. During a proctoscopy examination internal hemorrhoids were observed. On questioning, U.V. said that he sometimes saw blood in his stools.

Pertinent laboratory results on admission were as follows:

Blood hematology

- Red blood cell count (RBC): $3.2 \times 10^6/mm^3$ (normal 4.0–6.0)
- White blood cell count (WBC): $6 \times 10^3/mm^3$ (normal 5–10)
- Platelets: $90/mm^3$ (normal 140–400)
- Hemoglobin (Hgb): 11 g/dL (normal 12–16)
- Hematocrit (Hct): 33% (normal 36–48)
- International normalized ratio (INR): 2.2 (normal 0.8–1.2)

Blood chemistry

- Sodium (Na^+): 132 mEq/L (normal 136–145)
- Chloride (Cl^-): 95 mEq/L (normal 96–106)
- Potassium (K^+): 3.3 mEq/L (normal 3.5–5.5)
- Bicarbonate (HCO_3^-): 24 mEq/L (normal 19–25)
- Blood urea nitrogen (BUN): 30 mg/dL (normal 6–20)
- Albumin: 2.2 g/dL (normal 3.5–4.0)
- Creatinine: 2.1 mg/dL (normal 0.6–1.2)
- Glucose: 136 mg/dL (normal 70–110)
- Aspartate transaminase (AST): 202 IU (normal, women 10–35)
- Alanine transaminase (ALT): 95 IU (normal, women 7–35)
- Alkaline phosphatase (ALP): 254 IU (normal 30–120)

▶ Unconjugated bilirubin: 8 mg/dL (normal 0.3–1.0)
▶ Conjugated bilirubin: 4 mg/dL (normal < 0.5)

Guaiac stool test

Positive

Abdominal paracentesis

▶ 500 mL of clear ascitic fluid with the following pertinent lab results:
▶ WBC: 600 cells/μL (normal < 300). More than 80% of these cells were neutrophils.
▶ RBC: absent

Microscopic analysis of the sediment showed numerous gram-negative bacteria, numerous leukocytes, and no abnormal cells.

A diagnosis of advanced alcoholic cirrhosis was made, and an appropriate therapy was started, which included the following drugs: spironolactone, furosemide, meropenem, propranolol, and lactulose.

Questions

1. U.V. was diagnosed with alcoholic cirrhosis. Which of the following morphological changes in the liver best characterizes this disorder?

A. Excessive amount of fat inside liver cells
B. Progressive fibrosis with hepatocyte regeneration
C. Generalized necrosis of hepatocytes
D. Diffuse liver inflammation
E. Progressive destruction of intrahepatic bile ducts

2. Liver cirrhosis is related to the unique anatomical structure of the liver where the venous blood of the portal vein is mixed with the arterial blood of the hepatic artery. In which of the following does this mixture occur?

A. Terminal portal venules
B. Portal vein branches
C. Liver sinusoids
D. Terminal hepatic arterioles
E. Hepatic artery branches

3. Alcoholic cirrhosis includes more than 50% of liver cirrhosis in the developed world. Which of the following disorders is most likely the second most prevalent cause of cirrhosis in the developed world, and the first one worldwide?

A. Portal vein thrombosis
B. Chronic hepatitis B
C. Glycogen storage diseases
D. Hemochromatosis
E. Wilson's disease

4. U.V. was found to be drowsy and minimally oriented to person, place, and time, and he exhibited a flapping hand tremor when his wrists were extended. These signs most likely indicate which of the following disorders?

A. Wernicke's encephalopathy
B. Hepatic encephalopathy
C. Korsakoff's psychosis
D. Alcohol withdrawal syndrome
E. Alcoholic hallucinosis

5. U.V. reported occasional vomiting of blood. Which of the following was the most likely cause of this patient's symptom?

A. Concomitant alcoholic gastritis
B. Concomitant renal insufficiency
C. Thrombocytopenia
D. Portal hypertension
E. Essential hypertension

6. U.V.'s skin and sclerae were slightly jaundiced. Which of the following was most likely a cause of these findings?

A. Increased bile production
B. Bile duct obstruction
C. Increased red blood cell hemolysis
D. Pancreatic cyst
E. Impairment of liver glucuronidation

7. Multiple spider angiomas were seen on U.V.'s chest. An increased level of which of the following hormones is thought to be a cause of these signs?

A. Estradiol
B. Serum testosterone
C. Aldosterone
D. Levothyroxine
E. Epinephrine

8. U.V.'s lab exams showed a serum K$^+$ level of 3.3 mEq/L. Which of the following disorders best accounts for this finding?

A. Chronic kidney disease

B. Necrosis of liver cells

C. Vomiting

D. Secondary hyperaldosteronism

E. Chronic metabolic alkalosis

9. Which of the following lab results best explains that U.V.'s liver cell injury is due to chronic alcoholism?

A. Increased INR

B. AST higher than ALT

C. Decreased albumin

D. Increased creatinine

E. Decreased hemoglobin

F. Decreased hematocrit

10. Which of the following lab results best indicates an impairment in a specific synthetic function of U.V.'s liver?

A. Increased INR

B. Increased ALP

C. Increased AST

D. Decreased hematocrit

E. Decreased Hemoglobin

F. Decreased HCO$_3^-$

11. The lab exam of U.V.'s ascitic fluid gave a neutrophil count of 600 cells/μL. This result suggests that the patient most likely suffered from which of the following disorders?

A. Abdominal carcinoma

B. Peritoneal tuberculosis

C. Acute heart failure

D. Spontaneous bacterial peritonitis

E. Acute pancreatitis

12. Spironolactone was administered to U.V. primarily to treat his ascites. Which of the following pathological conditions was most likely the main target of U.V.'s spironolactone treatment?

A. Chronic renal disease

B. Portal hypertension

C. Secondary hyperaldosteronism

D. Jaundice

E. Hypoalbuminemia

13. Which of the following is the primary renal site of action of spironolactone?

A. The proximal convolute tubule

B. The proximal straight tubule

C. The thick ascending limb of Henle

D. The thin descending limb of Henle

E. The early distal tubule

F. The collecting duct

14. Furosemide was prescribed for U.V. together with spironolactone. Which of the following renal transport systems was most likely blocked by furosemide?

A. Na$^+$/Ca^{2+} antiporter

B. Na$^+$/K$^+$/2Cl$^-$ symporter

C. Na$^+$/Cl$^-$ symporter

D. Na$^+$/K$^-$ antiporter

E. Na$^+$/H$^-$ antiporter

15. Meropenem was prescribed to U.V. Which of the following steps in the turnover of bacterial cell walls is specifically inhibited by meropenem?

A. Autolysin-mediated breaking of peptidoglycan chains

B. Elongation of linear amino sugar chains

C. Linking two amino sugars by glycosidic bond

D. Synthesis of N-acetylmuramic acid

E. Connection of two amino sugar chains by peptide bridges

16. Propranolol was prescribed for U.V. The drug was given primarily to prevent or counteract which of the following of his disorders?

A. Esophageal varices

B. Secondary hyperaldosteronism

C. Renal insufficiency

D. Hepatosplenomegaly

E. Ascites

17. Which of the following molecular actions most likely mediated the therapeutic effect of propranolol in the patient's disorder?

A. Opening of ligand-gated K^+ channels

B. Increased synthesis of diacylglycerol

C. Decreased activity of adenylate cyclase

D. Increased activity of tyrosine kinase

E. Opening of ligand-gated Na^+ channels

18. Lactulose was prescribed for U.V. Which of the following pathological conditions was most likely the main target of U.V.'s lactulose treatment?

A. Chronic kidney disease

B. Portal hypertension

C. Secondary hyperaldosteronism

D. Hepatic encephalopathy

E. Hypoalbuminemia

Answers and Explanations

▶ *Learning objective:* Describe the morphological changes of the liver that best characterize liver cirrhosis.

1. Answer: B

Cirrhosis is a progressive fibrosis of the liver that progresses to produce diffuse disorganization of normal hepatic structure. Regenerative nodules of hepatic parenchyma surrounded by fibrotic bands are the defining pathological feature in liver cirrhosis. In response to a vast array of hepatic injuries (including chronic infection and drugs), growth regulators induce hepato-

cellular hyperplasia that produces regenerating nodules surrounded by fibrotic tissue, and arterial growth. Regenerating nodules typically lack lobular organization, and cirrhosis can be subdivided into micronodular and macronodular, according to nodule size. Angiogenesis produces new vessels within the fibrous sheath that surrounds nodules, connecting the hepatic artery and the portal vein to the hepatic venules. Such interconnecting vessels cannot accommodate as much blood volume as normal. This leads to the pressure "backup" seen as portal hypertension.

A Fatty liver is the initial and most common consequence of alcohol ingestion. It can progress to cirrhosis, but fatty liver is potentially reversible and is not by itself true cirrhosis.

C, D Cell necrosis (often focal) and inflammation are features of alcoholic hepatitis. The disorder can progress to cirrhosis, but hepatitis is not cirrhosis.

E Progressive destruction of intrahepatic bile ducts characterizes the biliary, not the alcoholic, cirrhosis.

▶ *Learning objective:* Identify liver structures where the venous blood of the portal vein is mixed with the arterial blood of the hepatic artery.

2. Answer: C

The blood supply to the liver has two sources:

▶ The portal vein that contributes approximately 75% of the total liver circulation

▶ The hepatic artery that contributes approximately 25% of the total liver circulation

Blood from portal venules and hepatic arterioles combines in a complex network of liver sinusoids, which in turn converge to form the hepatic veins.

A Terminal portal venules are subdivisions of portal vein branches.

B Portal vein branches are subdivisions of the portal vein.

D Terminal hepatic arterioles are subdivisions of hepatic artery branches.

E Hepatic artery branches are three subdivisions of the common hepatic artery.

▶ *Learning objective:* Identify the first cause of liver cirrhosis worldwide.

3.   Answer: B

Chronic viral hepatitis B is likely the second most common cause of cirrhosis in the developed world and the first one worldwide. This seems primarily related to fact that vaccination is not a common preventive measure in the undeveloped world. Over the course of years, chronic viral hepatitis B can cause major damage to the liver, leading to cirrhosis.

A Portal vein thrombosis is frequently associated with liver cirrhosis, but thrombosis is an effect, rather than a cause, of cirrhosis.

C Glycogen storage diseases are primarily the result of genetic defects in the processing of glycogen synthesis or breakdown. Glycogen storage–induced liver cirrhosis can occur but is exceptionally rare.

D Hemochromatosis is a genetic condition that causes excess absorption of iron from the digestive tract. Over time, the excess iron accumulates in tissues throughout the body, leading to iron overload. Hemochromatosis can cause liver cirrhosis, but this is a rare disease; thus hemochromatosis-induced cirrhosis is very rare.

E Wilson's disease is a rare autosomal recessive inherited disorder of copper metabolism that is characterized by excessive deposition of copper in the liver. Cirrhosis is the most common initial presentation of the disease, but because Wilson's disease is rare, the induced cirrhosis is very rare.

▶ *Learning objective:* Identify the disorder of a cirrhotic patient characterized by disorientation and a flapping hand tremor.

4.   Answer: B

Hepatic encephalopathy is a frequent complication and one of the most debilitating manifestations of liver disease. The complication is due to a brain dysfunction caused by liver insufficiency; it manifests as a wide spectrum of neurological or psychiatric abnormalities ranging from subclinical alterations to coma. However, in a cirrhotic patient, symptoms like increased daily drowsiness, occasional disorientation in place and time, and flapping hand tremor (i.e., asterixis) are highly indicative of hepatic encephalopathy, as in the present case.

A Wernicke's encephalopathy is a disorder characterized by acute onset of confusion, nystagmus, and ataxia due to thiamin deficiency. Alcoholism is a common underlying condition. Even though the patient suffered from alcoholism, his symptoms and signs were not indicative of Wernicke's encephalopathy.

C Korsakoff's psychosis is a late complication of Wernicke's encephalopathy characterized by memory deficits, confusion, and prominent behavioral changes.

D The patient suffered from alcoholism, but his symptoms and signs were not indicative of alcohol withdrawal syndrome.

E Alcoholic hallucinosis is a rare complication of chronic alcohol abuse characterized primarily by auditory hallucinations that occur either during or after a period of heavy alcohol consumption.

▶ *Learning objective:* Explain the cause of blood vomiting in a cirrhotic patient.

5.   Answer: D

Symptoms of cirrhosis can be subdivided as follows:

▶ Symptoms and signs due to portal hypertension
▶ Symptoms and signs due to liver cell failure

The first group includes hematemesis and melena (because of esophageal varices), splenomegaly, dilated abdominal veins, hemorrhoids, and ascites, as in the present case.

A Alcoholic gastritis can cause melena, but hematemesis due to gastritis is much less common. The patient's clinical picture points out that vomiting of blood was most likely due to esophageal varices.

B The patient had renal insufficiency (see high creatinine levels), but the disorder does not cause hematemesis, even if it can increase the risk of hematemesis.

C The patient had thrombocytopenia (a common complication in liver disease), but the disorder does not cause hematemesis, even if it can favor hematemesis due to other causes.

E Essential hypertension is not a cause of hematemesis, and the patient had no hypertension.

▶ *Learning objective:* Explain the cause of jaundice in a cirrhotic patient.

---

6. Answer: E

Jaundice is yellowing of the skin, sclerae, and other tissues caused by excess circulating bilirubin. Bilirubin is formed in the reticuloendothelial system (also called the macrophage system) by the breakdown of hemoglobin. The sequence of events is hemoglobin → hematin → protoporphyrin → biliverdin → bilirubin. This form of bilirubin is often referred to as free or unconjugated bilirubin. After release into the circulation, the free bilirubin is bound to plasma albumin and is avidly removed from the plasma by hepatocytes. The liver converts bilirubin to the water-soluble form by conjugating it, primarily with glucuronic acid. In this respect the liver handles bilirubin as it handles a host of other compounds that it detoxifies or solubilizes by its conjugating mechanisms. The process of conjugation facilitates the bilirubin excretion into bile. When the hepatocytes are damaged, the liver is unable to excrete or conjugate bilirubin, and levels of both conjugated and unconjugated bilirubin increase. This is called hepatic jaundice, and it occurs in hepatitis and in cirrhosis, as in the present case.

A, C These findings would cause a prehepatic jaundice that is primarily associated with an increase in unconjugated bilirubin.

B, D These findings would cause a posthepatic jaundice that is primarily associated with an increase in conjugated bilirubin.

▶ *Learning objective:* Explain the most likely cause of spider angiomas that can be found in cirrhotic patients.

---

7. Answer: A

Spider angiomas are vascular lesions of the skin consisting of a central arteriole with slender projections resembling spider legs. Like other blood vessels, spider angiomas blanch when pressure is applied. Spider angiomas can be seen in healthy children and pregnant women. In such cases, angiomas are few in number and resolve with time or a normalization of estrogen levels. Numerous spider angiomas are more common in patients with chronic liver disease. Possible mechanisms of formation include neovascularization from angiogenic factors and direct effects of alcohol, but the most accepted mechanism is related to estrogen excess. It is well known that estrogens can cause vasodilation, likely through the release of nitric oxide. The failing liver is unable to metabolize estrogen normally, and plasma estrogens are increased. The same estrogen excess was also responsible for the gynecomastia found in this patient.

B Serum testosterone is reduced in up to 90% of men with liver cirrhosis.

C Hyperaldosteronism is common in liver cirrhosis, but spider angiomas are not a sign of aldosterone excess.

D Patients with hepatic cirrhosis have normal or raised plasma levothyroxine levels, but spider angiomas are not a sign of levothyroxine excess.

E Catecholamines are frequently raised in patients with liver cirrhosis, but spider angiomas are not a sign of epinephrine excess.

▶ *Learning objective:* Explain the most likely cause of hypokalemia in a cirrhotic patient.

---

8. Answer: D

Secondary hyperaldosteronism is common in patients with ascites because the decrease in extracellular fluid volume triggers the release of aldosterone. The hormone causes Na^+ retention by promoting its reabsorption in the distal renal tubule, where it increases the synthesis of apical Na^+ channels and basolateral N^+/K^+ adenosine triphosphatase. The enhanced Na^+ reabsorption increases the luminal negative potential of the distal tubule, which favors K^+ and H^+ excretion.

A, B The patient had chronic kidney disease (see high creatinine levels), and necrosis of hepatocytes can occur in cirrhosis, but these disorders are usually associated with hyperkalemia, not hypokalemia.

C Vomiting can cause K^+ loss when it is profuse and repeated. The patient reported only two episodes of vomiting.

E Chronic metabolic alkalosis can be the result, not the cause, of hypokalemia.

▶ *Learning objective:* Identify the lab result that best indicates a liver cell injury associated with alcoholic liver disease.

---

9. Answer: B

Both AST and ALT are good indicators of liver function because injury of hepatocytes results in the leakage of enzymes into the circulation. Most causes of liver cell injury are associated with an AST lower than the ALT. An exception is the alcoholic liver disease where AST is higher than ALT, often with a ratio higher than 2, as in the present case.

A, C, D, E, F All these lab results are present in U.V.'s exams, but they are not specific for alcoholic liver disease.

▶ *Learning objective:* Identify the lab exam result that best indicates an impairment in a specific synthetic function of the liver.

---

10. Answer: A

The INR is a standardized prothrombin time test. Prothrombin time depends on the synthesis of prothrombin in the liver along with other vitamin-dependent clotting factors. The increased prothrombin time means that this synthesis is impaired.

B, C, D, E, F All these lab results are indirectly related to an impairment of some liver functions, but they do not indicate a specific defect in the synthetic liver function.

▶ *Learning objective:* Describe the most likely diagnosis that is suggested by a high number of neutrophils in the ascitic fluid.

---

11. Answer: D

An ascitic fluid with a high neutrophil count suggests the diagnosis of spontaneous bacterial peritonitis, an acute bacterial infection of ascitic fluid with no easily identifiable source of the infecting agent. The most common bacteria causing the disorder are *Escherichia coli*, *Klebsiella pneumoniae*, and *Streptococcus pneumoniae*. Ascitic fluid cultures are negative in as many as 60% of patients with increased ascites neutrophil counts and clinical manifestations suggestive of spontaneous bacterial peritonitis.

A Fluid from an abdominal carcinoma usually has appositive cancer cytology that was absent in the present patient.

B Peritoneal tuberculosis is an uncommon site of extrapulmonary infection caused by *Mycobacterium tuberculosis*. The risk is increased in patients with cirrhosis, but U.V. had no symptoms suggesting tuberculosis infection.

C Acute heart failure can cause ascites, but the patient had no symptoms of acute heart failure, and the neutrophil count suggests that the ascites is infectious.

E Acute pancreatitis can cause ascites that is usually bloody. U.V.'s ascitic fluid was not bloody.

▶ *Learning objective:* Explain why spironolactone is the first-line agent in cirrhotic patients with ascites.

---

12. Answer: C

Spironolactone is the first-line diuretic for cirrhotic patients with ascites. The drug is an aldosterone receptor antagonist, and secondary hyperaldosteronism is common in advanced liver cirrhosis for the following reasons:

▶ Ascites-induced hypovolemia activates the renin–angiotensin–aldosterone system.
▶ Liver metabolism of aldosterone is reduced because of liver impairment.
▶ Hypoalbuminemia is a known consequence of liver cirrhosis. Because aldosterone is highly bound to albumin, cirrhotic patients have a higher concentration of free aldosterone (active aldosterone).

The aldosterone role in the pathophysiology of cirrhosis and the mechanism of action of spironolactone both explain why spironolactone is the best diuretic for the treatment of cirrhosis-induced ascites.

A The patient is suffering from chronic kidney disease (see lab values of creatinine and BUN), but spironolactone cannot improve the disease.

B Spironolactone cannot improve portal hypertension that is a hemodynamic consequence of liver cirrhosis.

D, E Both jaundice and hypoalbuminemia are signs of cirrhosis, but spironolactone cannot improve these signs.

▶ *Learning objective:* Identify the primary renal site of action of spironolactone.

13. Answer: F

Spironolactone is an aldosterone receptor antagonist. In the late distal tubule and the initial collecting duct, aldosterone increases the transcription (and therefore the synthesis) of several key proteins involved in Na^+ transport, including the basolateral Na^+/K^+ pump and the apical Na^+ channels. The net effect of these actions is to increase Na^+ reabsorption. By blocking aldosterone receptors, spironolactone does the opposite.

A, B, C, D, E See correct answer explanation.

▶ *Learning objective:* Identify the renal transport system that is specifically inhibited by furosemide.

14. Answer: B

Furosemide is a loop diuretic that blocks the $Na^+/K^+/2Cl^-$ symporter located in the thick ascending limb of Henle. The drug has little effect on ascites due to liver cirrhosis but can enhance the action of spironolactone when given concomitantly.

A Na^+/Ca^{2+} antiporter is located primarily in the basolateral membrane of the distal convoluted tubule. It is enhanced by the thiazide-induced blockade of NA^+ entry, increasing the overall absorption of Ca^{2+}.

C Na^+/Cl^- symporter is located in the early distal tubule. It is blocked by thiazides.

D Na^+/K^- antiporter is located in the basolateral membrane of all tubular cells.

E Na^+/H^- antiporter is located primarily in the apical membrane of the proximal tubule. It is indirectly affected by carbonic anhydrase inhibitors.

▶ *Learning objective:* Explain the mechanism of action of meropenem.

15. Answer: E

Meropenem is a β-lactam antibiotic of the carbapenem subclass. Carbapenems are broad-spectrum bactericidal antibiot-

ics active against most gram-positive and gram-negative, aerobic, and anaerobic bacteria (including methicillin-susceptible *Staphylococcus aureus, Bacteroides fragilis, Enterococcus faecalis, Pseudomonas aeruginosa*, and some atypical mycobacteria). Current guidelines recommend that cirrhotic patients with a neutrophil count of 500 cells/µL or greater in the ascitic fluid are most likely affected by spontaneous bacterial peritonitis and should receive empirical antibiotic therapy. A broad-spectrum bactericidal antibiotic is usually preferred.

The mechanism of action of all β-lactam antibiotics involves the inhibition of transpeptidase, the enzyme that catalyzes the final connection (cross-link) of two amino sugar chains by peptide bridges. In this way the synthesis of peptidoglycan is inhibited in the presence of meropenem.

A Activation, not inhibition, of autolysin-mediated breaking of peptidoglycan chains is an additional mechanism of action of β-lactam antibiotics.

B This would be the mechanism of action of vancomycin.

C A glycosidic bond does not link two amino sugars.

D This would be the mechanism of action of fosfomycin.

▶ *Learning objective:* Identify the disorder that indicates the use of propranolol in cirrhotic patients.

16. Answer: A

Esophageal varices that occur in advanced cirrhosis are a direct byproduct of portal hypertension. Since the esophageal veins are tributaries of the portal vein, portal hypertension causes the esophageal veins to dilate and become varicose. A primary cause of portal hypertension in cirrhosis is the formation of arteriovenous anastomoses, which allows the perfusion pressure of the hepatic artery to be partly transmitted to the portal vein. Propranolol is a nonselective β-blocker. By blocking $β_2$-adrenoceptors (particularly abundant in the liver vascular bed), liver arterial vessels are constricted, and the pressure transmitted into the portal vein decreases.

An additional effect of β-blockers may be the decreased systemic blood pressure that also contributes to the decreased portal hypertension. The incidence of bleeding from esophageal varices is 10 to 25%. Nonselective β-blockers prevent bleeding in more than half of patients with medium or large varices. However, they do not improve mortality and have the potential to reduce renal perfusion in patients who already have compromised renal perfusion. Therefore they must be used cautiously in the present case. Other drugs used to prevent bleeding include vasopressin and analogues, somatostatin analogues, and venodilators.

B Cirrhosis-induced secondary hyperaldosteronism is effectively counteracted by spironolactone.

C The patient is suffering from chronic kidney disease (see lab values for creatinine and BUN), but propranolol cannot improve the disease.

D, E Both jaundice and hypoalbuminemia are signs of cirrhosis, but propranolol cannot counteract these signs.

▶ *Learning objective:* Describe the molecular mechanism of action of propranolol.

17. Answer: C

Propranolol is a nonselective β-receptor blocker. Activation of all β-receptors increases the synthesis of cyclic adenosine monophosphate through an increased activity of the adenylate cyclase enzyme. By blocking these receptors, all β-blockers do the opposite (i.e., the activity of adenylate cyclase is decreased).

A Opening of ligand-gated K⁺ channels would be the mechanism of action of some antihypertensive drugs like minoxidil.

B Increased synthesis of diacylglycerol would be the signal transduction pathway of activation of some autonomic receptors, including $α_1$-adrenoceptors and muscarinic M_3 receptors.

D Increased activity of tyrosine kinase would be the signal transduction pathway of some hormones, such as insulin and atrial natriuretic peptide.

E Opening of ligand-gated Na⁺ channels would be the signal transduction pathway of activation of nicotinic muscular receptors.

▶ *Learning objective:* Identify the disorder appropriate for the use of lactulose in cirrhotic patients.

18. Answer: D

Eliminating toxic enteric products (mainly fecal ammonia) is a therapeutic goal in hepatic encephalopathy. Patients with severe liver disease have an impaired capacity to detoxify ammonia coming from the colon, where it is produced by bacterial metabolism of fecal urea. Ammonia is an important cause of brain toxicity. Lactulose is an osmotic laxative that, when given in high doses, can lower colonic pH. The low pH converts the ammonia into a polar ammonium ion that, being water-soluble, is poorly absorbed by the intestine. In other words, the decreased ammonia absorption occurs through an ion-trapping mechanism. Current guidelines state that lactulose should be given to all cirrhotic patients with symptoms and signs of hepatic encephalopathy, as in the present case.

A The patient is suffering from chronic kidney disease (see lab values for creatinine and BUN), but lactulose cannot improve the disease.

B Lactulose cannot improve portal hypertension that is a hemodynamic consequence of liver cirrhosis.

C, E Both secondary hyperaldosteronism and hypoalbuminemia are signs of cirrhosis, but lactulose cannot improve these signs.

T.Z., a 33-year-old man, was admitted to the hospital with a 2-month history of dry, non-productive cough, weight loss, increasing fatigue, and intermittent fever. Recently T.Z. also noted shortness of breath and coughing up blood-stained mucus. His past medical history was unremarkable. His social history indicated that T.Z. had been working as a psychiatrist in the local mental health unit and was married with two sons. The patient denied the use of alcohol or illicit drugs but had been smoking two packs of cigarettes daily for 15 years.

Physical examination showed a man in slight distress with the following vital signs: blood pressure 130/80 mm Hg, heart rate 65 bpm, respirations 26/min, body temperature 99.3°F (37.3°C).

Lung auscultation yielded wheezing in the right upper lobe; the remainder of lung fields were clear.

Pertinent laboratory results on admission were as follows:

Blood hematology

- Erythrocyte sedimentation rate (ESR): 35 mm/h (normal < 20)
- Red blood cell count (RBC): $3.8 \times 10^6/\mu L$ (normal 4.0–6.0)
- Hemoglobin (Hgb): 10.5 g/dL (normal 12–16)
- Hematocrit (Hct): 33% (normal 36–48)
- White blood cell count (WBC): $9 \times 10^3/\mu L$ (normal 4–10)
- Platelets: $85 \times 10^3/\mu L$ (normal 130–400)
- Creatinine: 1.1 mg/dL (normal 0.6–1.2)
- Potassium (K^+): 3.2 mEq/L (normal 3.6–5.3)
- Total calcium (Ca^{2+}): 12.8 mg/dL (normal 8.5–10.5)
- Blood urea nitrogen (BUN): 22 mg/dL (normal 8–25)
- Alkaline phosphatase: 160 U/L (normal 25–100)

Positron emission tomography scan

Lung: a solid nodule causing obstruction of the middle right lobe, and mediastinal lymphadenopathy

    No metastases in liver, bones, or brain

Transthoracic biopsy

Malignant squamous cells with keratin and intercellular bridges. An area of central necrosis was evident.

Cytogenetic analysis

Human epidermal growth factor receptor (HER) exon 21 mutation.

A diagnosis of lung cancer was made and surgical resection was offered, but the patient refused surgery. A course of chemoradiotherapy was started. Four chemotherapy cycles were prescribed with cisplatin and gemcitabine.

Two months later a positron emission tomography (PET) scan showed an extension of T.Z.'s tumor, and the oncologist decided to substitute gemcitabine with paclitaxel.

After four cycles of cisplatin and paclitaxel, tumor growth was not effectively controlled.

Taking into account the cytogenetic analysis, the oncologist chose to stop the ongoing regimen and to start an erlotinib treatment.

Questions

1. T.Z. had a long history of heavy smoking and was diagnosed with lung cancer, which is classically subdivided into non-small-cell cancers and small-cell cancers. Which of the following is the most likely current estimation of the percentage of small-cell cancers due to smoking?

A. 45–50%

B. 55–60%

C. 65–70%

D. 75–80%

E. 85–90%

F. 98–100%

2. From T.Z.'s symptoms and lab exams, which of the following is most likely the type of his cancer?

A. Small-cell cancer

B. Adenocarcinoma

C. Squamous cell cancer

D. Large-cell cancer

E. Carcinoid

3. T.Z. was diagnosed with lung cancer, a solid tumor. As a rule, a larger (and older) solid tumor is more difficult to remove by chemotherapy. Which of the following phrases best explains the reason for this chemotherapeutic weakness?

A. Higher tumor blood flow

B. Decreased P-glycoprotein activity

C. Decreased topoisomerase activity

D. Decreased growth fraction

E. Increased tumor metabolic rate

4. T.Z.'s chemotherapy included gemcitabine. The inhibition of which of the following pairs of enzymes most likely mediate the antitumor effect of this drug?

A. DNA polymerase–dihydrofolate reductase

B. Topoisomerase II–ribonucleotide reductase

C. Ribonucleotide reductase–DNA polymerase

D. Topoisomerase II–dihydrofolate reductase

E. Topoisomerase II–DNA polymerase

F. Dihydrofolate reductase–ribonucleotide reductase

5. T.Z.'s chemotherapy included cisplatin. Which of the following molecular actions most likely mediated the therapeutic effect of the drug in the patient's disease?

A. Cross-link formation on DNA strands

B. Inhibition of microtubule disassembly

C. Free radical–mediated breaking of DNA strands

D. Inhibition of thymidylate synthase

E. Inhibition of de novo pathway of purine biosynthesis

6. Owing to his cisplatin therapy, T.Z. was most likely at risk for which of the following drug-related adverse effects?

A. Hepatotoxicity

B. Nephrotoxicity

C. Myelosuppression

D. Opportunistic infections

E. Anaphylactoid reaction

7. T.Z.'s chemotherapy included paclitaxel. Which of the following molecular actions most likely mediated the therapeutic effect of this drug in the patient's disease?

A. Inhibition of topoisomerase I

B. Alkylation of DNA strands

C. Inhibition of purine biosynthesis

D. Enhancement of tubulin polymerization

E. Inhibition of DNA polymerase

F. Inhibition of tubulin polymerization

8. The patient was most likely at increased risk of which of the following adverse effects as a result of paclitaxel therapy?

A. Kidney failure

B. Liver failure

C. Peripheral neuropathy

D. Hallucinations

E. Urinary tract infection

F. Tuberculosis

9. T.Z.'s chemotherapy included erlotinib. The inhibition of which of the following tumor cell enzymes most likely mediated the therapeutic effect of this drug in the patient's disease?

A. Topoisomerase I

B. Tyrosine kinase

C. DNA polymerase

D. Dihydrofolate reductase

E. Topoisomerase II

F. Ribonucleotide reductase

10. Which of the following adverse effects could most likely occur during erlotinib treatment?

A. Blurred vision

B. Chest pain

C. Constipation

D. Seizures

E. Sweating

F. Skin rash

Answers and Explanations

▶ *Learning objective:* Identify the percentage of lung cancers that are due to smoking.

1. Answer: F

Today it is well known that most lung cancers are due to smoking. About 85 to 90% of non-small cell lung cancers are due to smoking, but practically all small-cell lung cancers are caused by smoking.

A, B, C, D, E See correct answer explanation.

▶ *Learning objective:* Identify the type of lung cancer from the patient's symptoms and lab exams.

2. Answer: C

The patient's transthoracic biopsy showed malignant squamous cells with keratin, intercellular bridges, and areas of central necrosis. These findings are typical of squamous cell cancer, which can produce keratin in the same way as normal squamous epithelial cells.

Moreover, lab exams showed hypercalcemia. The most common cause of hypercalcemia in patients with nonmetastatic solid tumors and in some patients with non-Hodgkin's lymphoma is a paraneoplastic syndrome caused by the secretion of parathyroid-related hormone. This condition, also called humoral hypercalcemia of malignancy (HHM), accounts for up to 80% of patients with hypercalcemia of malignancy. Patients with HHM most often have squamous cell carcinomas, as in the present case.

In patients with HHM, secretion of endogenous parathyroid hormone (PTH) itself is suppressed by the parathyroid-related hormone-mediated hypercalcemia. Thus serum intact PTH concentrations are typically suppressed or very low in patients with HHM.

A Small-cell lung cancer histology usually shows small cells with a high nucleo-cytoplasmic ratio.

B Lung adenocarcinoma histology usually shows glandular tumor cells producing mucus.

D Large-cell lung cancer histology usually shows sheets or nests of large polygonal or giant multinuclear cells.

E Lung carcinoid histology usually shows medium-sized polygonal cells with round to oval finely granular nuclei and scant vascular stroma.

▶ *Learning objective:* Explain why larger solid tumors are more difficult to eradicate by chemotherapy.

3. Answer: D

Several hematologic malignances follow the exponential growth (i.e., the proportion of cells in a tumor population that are actively dividing is constant). This is called the constant growth fraction.

For most other tumors (especially solid tumors), the growth rate is not constant but rather slows as a tumor increases in size (i.e., the growth fraction decreases). In other words, it takes longer for the tumor to double in size. This can be modeled using Gompertzian analysis (a plot of the log of the number of cancer cells in a tumor vs. time). The slower growth of the tumor is, in part, due to more cells entering the G0 (resting) phase of the cell cycle. One reason for this is related to the increased size of the tumor that is not supplemented by a parallel increase in blood flow. This reduces the delivery of oxygen and nutrients that the rapidly dividing cells need. This can explain why older and larger tumors are more difficult to eradicate by chemotherapy. Even if several anticancer drugs are not "cell cycle–specific," the responsiveness to most anticancer drugs is low when the cell is in the resting phase of the cell cycle. Moreover, the delivery of anticancer drugs to the tumor is reduced because of the reduced blood flow.

A The tumor blood flow is lower, not higher, when the tumor is larger.

B A decreased P-glycoprotein activity would increase responsiveness to the anticancer drug, because this protein normally pumps the drug out of cancer cells.

C Topoisomerase enhances the ability to self-repair DNA strand damage. A decreased topoisomerase activity would increase, not decrease, the effectiveness of anticancer drugs (of note some anticancer drugs are topoisomerase inhibitors).

E Since the tumor blood flow is lower when the tumor is larger, the tumor metabolic rate will be decreased, not increased.

▶ *Learning objective:* Identify the pairs of enzymes specifically inhibited by gemcitabine.

4. Answer: C

Gemcitabine is an antimetabolite anticancer drug. These drugs block specific steps of intermediary metabolism of proliferating cells. Even if these steps are similar for normal and for cancer cells, there are quan-

titative differences that render cancer cells more sensitive to antimetabolite actions. Gemcitabine is phosphorylated to the diphosphate and triphosphate nucleotide forms (i.e., to false nucleotides) that exert antitumor effect by several mechanisms:

▶ Inhibition of ribonucleotide reductase, which reduces the levels of deoxyribonucleotide triphosphates required for DNA synthesis
▶ Inhibition of DNA polymerase required for DNA synthesis
▶ Incorporation of the false nucleotide into DNA leading to termination of DNA synthesis

Gemcitabine has a broad spectrum of activity and is widely used to treat both hematologic cancers and solid tumors, including squamous cell lung cancer, as in the present case.

A, B, D, E, F Topoisomerase II and dihydrofolate reductase are not directly inhibited by gemcitabine.

▶ *Learning objective:* Explain the mechanism of action of cisplatin.

5. Answer: A

Cisplatin is the prototype of platinum analogues. These drugs have broad antineoplastic activity and are currently used for treatment of many solid tumors, including lung, ovarian, head and neck, bladder, esophageal, and colon cancer. Platinum analogues are activated inside the cells, yielding positively charged and highly reactive molecules. These molecules can react with various sites on DNA, forming both interstrand and intrastrand cross-links, which in turn block DNA.

B Inhibition of microtubule disassembly would be the mechanism of action of taxanes (paclitaxel, docetaxel).

C Free radical–mediated breaking of DNA strands would be the mechanism of action of bleomycin.

D Inhibition of thymidylate synthase would be the mechanism of action of fluorouracil.

E Inhibition of de novo pathway of purine biosynthesis would be the mechanism of action of several anticancer antimetabolite drugs.

► *Learning objective:* Identify the major adverse effect of cisplatin.

6. Answer: B

Cisplatin is the anticancer drugs with the highest risk of nephrotoxicity. The routine use of hydration and diuresis has reduced cisplatin-induced nephrotoxicity, but even with these procedures, renal insufficiency occurs in up to 30% of patients treated chronically with the drug. The mechanism of cisplatin-induced nephrotoxicity is most likely related to the concentration of the drug within the kidney, which exceeds that in blood, suggesting an active accumulation of drug by renal parenchymal cells. In vivo administration of nephrotoxic doses of cisplatin produces a large increase in both necrosis and apoptosis of renal cells, and there is a large body of evidence indicating that cisplatin activates the intrinsic mitochondrial pathway of apoptosis.

A, C, D, E The risk of all these adverse effects is low or negligible with cisplatin therapy.

► *Learning objective:* Describe the mechanism of action of paclitaxel.

7. Answer: D

Paclitaxel is the prototype of taxane derivatives. These drugs are alkaloids derived from plants of the genus *Taxus* (yews). They bind with high affinity to microtubules, enhancing tubulin polymerization. This prevents the microtubule disassembly and causes a mitotic arrest of cells in metaphase.

A Inhibition of topoisomerase II would be the mechanism of action of etoposide.

B Alkylation of DNA strands would be the mechanism of action of alkylating drugs.

C Inhibition of purine biosynthesis would be the mechanism of action of several anticancer antimetabolite drugs.

E Inhibition of DNA polymerase would be the mechanism of action of cytarabine.

► *Learning objective:* Describe the main adverse effects of paclitaxel.

8. Answer: C

Peripheral neuropathy is a common adverse effect of taxanes such as paclitaxel, affecting more than 50% of patients under treatment. The effect is dose-dependent and cumulative.

The exact pathophysiological mechanism of paclitaxel-induced peripheral neuropathy is not well understood, but the inhibition of tubulin depolymerization and the consequent microtubule dysfunction seems the most widely accepted mechanism. Intact microtubules are required for both anterograde and retrograde axonal transport, and neuronal survival and function depend on these transport processes. Increased axonal microtubule stability might alter axonal transport leading to a loss of axonal integrity, or axonal degeneration in more severe cases.

This phenomenon begins in the most vulnerable part of the nerve, the distal nerve endings of the longest nerves, where transport problems may manifest most quickly.

A, B The risk of these adverse effects is very low with paclitaxel therapy.

D Hallucinations are unlikely, because paclitaxel does not cross the blood–brain barrier.

E, F Paclitaxel causes a profound myelosuppression, which in turn increases the risk of opportunistic infections. These include candidiasis, cryptosporidiosis, cryptococcosis, and *M. Avium-cellulare* infection, but urinary tract infection and tuberculosis have not been reported.

► *Learning objective:* Describe the mechanism of action of erlotinib.

9. Answer: B

Erlotinib belongs to the drug class of human epidermal growth factor receptor (HER) inhibitors. Drugs that target HER2 belong to two subclasses:

▶ *Monoclonal antibodies* (cetuximab and panitumumab) that exert their activity through competitive inhibition of the binding of ligands to the extracellular region of the receptor
▶ *Tyrosine kinase inhibitors* that block the cytoplasmic-domain phosphorylation

Pharmacologically mediated blockade of HER2 results in growth arrest and apoptosis in cells that are dependent on HER2 for survival, through the inhibition of several downstream pathways.

Erlotinib is the prototype of the subclass of tyrosine kinase inhibitors approved for the treatment of non-small-cell lung cancers in patients whose tumors have epidermal growth factor exon 19 deletions or exon 21 mutations and are refractory to at least one prior chemotherapy regimen, as in the present case. This explains the oncologist's choice. Other drugs of this subclass include gefitinib, afatinib, and osimertinib. Tyrosine kinases are enzymes responsible for the activation of many proteins by signal transduction cascades. The proteins are activated by phosphorylation, a step counteracted by tyrosine kinase inhibitors. Disappointingly, their clinical efficacy is limited by the development of resistance, which is caused in more than 50% of the cases by the emergence of a secondary point mutation in the epidermal growth factor receptor.

A Topoisomerase I would be inhibited by topotecan and irinotecan.

C DNA polymerase would be inhibited by cytarabine.

D Dihydrofolate reductase would be inhibited by methotrexate.

E Topoisomerase II would be inhibited by etoposide.

F Ribonucleotide reductase would be inhibited by gemcitabine.

▶ *Learning objective:* Describe the main adverse effects of erlotinib.

10. Answer: F

Epidermal growth factor receptor (EGFR) inhibitors are thought to affect basal keratinocytes, and this leads to the development of cutaneous side effects. Inhibition of the EGFR-mediated signaling pathways affects keratinocytes by inducing growth arrest and apoptosis, increasing cell attachment and stimulating inflammation, all of which result in distinctive cutaneous manifestations. Skin rash is the most common, affecting > 50% of patients receiving the drug. In the majority of cases the rash is mild, although in 8 to 12% of cases the rash is severe enough that the treatment is stopped. The lesions are usually located in the skin areas rich with sebaceous glands (i.e., the face, neck, upper trunk area, and the scalp).

A, B, C, D, E All these adverse effects can occur during erlotinib therapy, but their incidence is < 10%.

Case 28

Megaloblastic Anemia

K.O., a 67-year-old man, presented to his family physician complaining that he had been feeling weak and lightheaded for the past 6 months. He also noted recently increased forgetfulness, emotional instability, some pain on his tongue, tingling and numbness of the fingers, and alternating constipation and diarrhea, but no weight loss.

K.O. had been suffering from atrophic gastritis diagnosed 8 years earlier and related to a *Helicobacter pylori* infection. In spite of the therapy, however, the disease did not improve, and a gastroscopy done 5 years ago indicated an extensive multifocal gastric atrophy. K.O. never smoked and denied the use of illicit drugs. He reported that his diet was balanced and that he was taking two to three glasses of wine daily during meals.

Physical examination showed an elderly, pleasant man with the following vital signs: blood pressure 132/80 mm Hg, pulse 84 bpm, respirations 16/min, body temperature 98.2°F (36.8°C). The patient's conjunctiva, oral mucosa, and nail beds were pale, and his tongue was red and painful. Neurological examination disclosed decreased cutaneous pain and vibratory sensation in both the upper and lower extremities.

Several laboratory exams were ordered, with the following results:

Blood hematology

▸ Red blood cell count (RBC): $3.8 \times 10^6/\mu L$ (normal, men 4.5–5.5)
▸ Hemoglobin (Hgb): 10.1 g/dL (normal 12–16)
▸ Hematocrit (Hct): 30% (normal 36–48)
▸ White blood cell count (WBC): $3.2 \times 10^3/\mu L$ (normal 4–10)
▸ Platelets: $125 \times 10^3/\mu L$ (normal 130–400)
▸ Mean corpuscular volume (MCV): 110 fL (normal 80–100)
▸ Ferritin: 300 ng/mL (normal, men 20–250)
▸ Iron: 70 µg/dL (normal, men 65–175)
▸ Serum vitamin B_{12}: 100 pg/mL (normal 200–900)
▸ RBC folate: 230 ng/mL (normal 140–400)

Blood chemistry

▸ Venous blood pH: 7.4 (normal 7.3–7.4)
▸ Creatinine: 1.4 mg/dL (normal 0.6–1.2)
▸ Blood urea nitrogen (BUN): 35 mg/dL (normal 8–25)
▸ Uric acid: 10.2 mg/dL (normal 4–8.5)
▸ Sodium (Na^+): 138 mEq/L (normal 135–146)
▸ Potassium (K^+): 3.9 mEq/L (normal 3.6–5.3)
▸ Total cholesterol: 220 mg/dL (normal < 200)

Gastric biopsy

Villiform aspect of the gastric mucosa with multifocal lymphoplasmacytic infiltration, including epithelial lymphocytosis. Oxyntic glands are replaced with metaplastic glands.

Urea breath test for *Helicobacter pylori*

Positive

K.O. was diagnosed with megaloblastic anemia, and a treatment was prescribed that included a parenteral drug administration for 1 month, followed by a daily oral dose of 1 mg of the same drug.

Questions

1. K.O. was diagnosed with megaloblastic anemia. Which of the following is the correct classification of his anemia?

A. Microcytic, hypochromic

B. Normocytic, normochromic

C. Macrocytic, hypochromic

D. Microcytic, normochromic

E. Macrocytic, normochromic

2. Which of the following was most likely the cause of the patient's anemia?

A. Concomitant folate-deficient diet

B. Lack of intrinsic factor

C. Vitamin B_{12}–deficient diet

D. Impaired folate absorption

E. Increased renal excretion of vitamin B_{12}

F. Increased renal excretion of folate

3. K.O.'s anemia was related to his atrophic gastritis. The patient's anemia symptoms and signs started only 5 years after the diagnosis of an extensive gastric atrophy, because the body has massive storages of cobalamin. Which of the following organs/tissues represents a huge reservoir of cobalamin?

A. The skeletal muscle

B. The liver

C. The kidney

D. The spleen

E. The bone marrow

4. Which of the following pairs of morphological findings would be most likely expected in K.O.'s peripheral blood smear?

A. Anisocytosis–reticulocytosis

B. Poikilocytosis–reticulocytosis

C. Neutrophil hypersegmentation–leukocytosis

D. Poikilocytosis–leukocytosis

E. Neutrophil hypersegmentation–poikilocytosis

F. Anisocytosis–leukocytosis

5. Which of the following patient's symptoms and signs can differentiate between anemia due to cobalamin deficiency and anemia due to folic acid deficiency?

A. Normal serum iron

B. Red and painful tongue

C. Decreased vibratory sensation

D. Low hematocrit

E. Increased serum ferritin

F. Pale conjunctiva

6. K.O.'s neurological examination showed a decreased cutaneous pain sensation in both upper and lower extremities. Which of the following was most likely the pathological basis of this symptom?

A. Insufficient blood flow to the extremities

B. Loss of cortical excitatory neurons

C. Increased activity of spinal inhibitory neurons

D. Myelin degeneration in the spinal cord

E. Compression of limb nerves

7. K.O. was diagnosed with megaloblastic anemia. The synthesis of which of the following endogenous compounds is impaired by both folic acid and cobalamin deficiency?

A. Dihydrofolate

B. Methionine

C. Tetrahydrofolate (THF)

D. Succinyl-CoA

E. Homocysteine

8. An appropriate antianemic drug treatment was prescribed for K.O. Which of the following molecular actions most likely mediated the effect of the prescribed drug?

A. Synthesis of succinyl-CoA

B. Isomerization of L-methylmalonyl-CoA

C. Demethylation of N5-methyltetrahydrofolate

D. Hydroxylation of dihydrofolic acid

E. Glycine formation from serine

9. How long should K.O. continue to take the antianemic drug?

A. 3 months

B. 6 months

C. 1 year

D. 2 years

E. Indefinitely

10. K.O.'s cobalamin treatment included parenteral cobalamin for 1 month, followed by a daily oral dose of 1 mg for life. Which of the following phrases best explains why high doses of oral cobalamin can be absorbed even when gastric intrinsic factor is absent?

A. Intrinsic factor is also secreted by the intestine.

B. About 0.5% of the given dose is absorbed by passive diffusion.

C. After a month of parenteral treatment cobalamin stores are fully refilled.

D. Intrinsic factor is needed for absorption of food-bound cobalamin only.

Answers and Explanations

▶ *Learning objective:* Identify the correct classification of megaloblastic anemias.

1. Answer: E

Megaloblastic anemias belong to the group of anemias due to deficient erythropoiesis. Megaloblastic states result from defective DNA synthesis. RNA synthesis continues, leading to large cells with a large nucleus. Cytoplasm maturity is greater than nuclear maturity, producing megaloblasts in the marrow before they appear in the peripheral blood. Deficient hematopoiesis results in intramedullary cell death, causing indirect hyperbilirubinemia and hyperuricemia. Because red blood cells are larger than normal, the anemia is called macrocytic. The terms *hypochromic* and *normochromic* (i.e., the "chromia" of red blood cells) do not refer to their content in hemoglobin (which is low in most anemias) but rather the percentage of cell volume occupied by hemoglobin (i.e., the mean corpuscular hemoglobin concentration [MCHC]). For these reasons, anemic conditions can be classified in terms of the hemoglobin content within red blood cells, just as normochromic or hypochromic. MCHC can be calculated as follows:

$$MCHC = Hgb \times 100/Hct$$
$$(\text{normal value } 32{-}36 \text{ g/dL}).$$

In pure megaloblastic anemia the MCHC is normal, as in the present case (10.1 g/dL × 100/30 = 33.6 g/dL). Therefore the patient's anemia is macrocytic and normochromic.

A Microcytic, hypochromic anemias are due to iron deficiency.

B Normocytic, normochromic anemias are due (at least initially) to RBC hypoproliferation.

C Macrocytic, hypochromic anemia occurs when macrocytic anemia is associated with iron deficiency anemia.

D Microcytic anemias are usually hypochromic, not normochromic.

▶ *Learning objective:* Identify the patient's cause of megaloblastic anemia.

2. Answer: B

The patient's symptoms and signs indicate that he was most likely suffering from megaloblastic anemia due to vitamin B_{12} deficiency. Vitamin B_{12} (also called cobalamin) is found in most animal products (meat, eggs, dairy products, etc.) and is conjugated in the stomach with the intrinsic factor, a glycoprotein secreted by the gastric parietal cells. The complex is subsequently absorbed in the distal ileum. The patient had been suffering from metaplastic atrophic gastritis, a disease that destroys the gastric parietal cells. When cobalamin absorption is blocked it takes about 4 to 5 years for the appearance of megaloblastic anemia, as in the present case.

A, D A decreased folate intake is unlikely since RBC folate is normal.

C A megaloblastic anemia due to a cobalamin deficient diet is exceedingly rare. Because of the size of the cobalamin storage pool and the existence of an enterohepatic cobalamin circulation, a very long time (as long as 20 years) is required for a clinically significant cobalamin deficiency to develop from a diet providing insufficient cobalamin (e.g., a strictly vegetarian diet).

E, F Renal excretion of cobalamin and folic acid is negligible in a normal person. It can be decreased in case of kidney failure and can be increased when in excess. However, both cases are not clinically relevant, due to the negligible overdose toxicity of both drugs.

▶ *Learning objective:* Identify the organ that represent a huge reservoir of cobalamin.

3. Answer: B

The liver represents a huge reservoir of cobalamin. In a normal adult, as much as 90% of the body stores of cobalamin is in the liver. Therefore the supply of cobalamin available to the tissues is directly related to the size of hepatic storage.

A, C, D, E See correct answer explanation.

▶ *Learning objective:* Identify two features that can be expected in a peripheral blood smear of a patient with megaloblastic anemia.

4. Answer: E

K.O. was diagnosed with megaloblastic anemia. Because this anemia is due to deficient hematopoiesis, the peripheral blood smear usually shows anisocytosis (i.e., the presence of red blood cells of unequal size) and poikilocytosis (i.e., the presence of abnormally shaped red blood cells). The presence of hypersegmented neutrophils (i.e., neutrophils with five or more nuclear segments) is also a common feature.

A, B, C, D, F In megaloblastic anemia, the deficient hematopoiesis can affect all cell lines. Therefore reticulocytopenia, not reticulocytosis, and later leukopenia, not leukocytosis, are the most likely findings.

▶ *Learning objective:* Identify the symptoms that can differentiate between folic acid anemia and cobalamin-deficiency anemia.

5. Answer: C

Anemias due to folic acid and to cobalamin deficiency are both megaloblastic and have identical peripheral symptoms and signs.

However, anemia due to folic acid deficiency lacks the neurological symptoms that are present in anemia due to cobalamin deficiency—namely, decreased vibratory and pain sensation, impaired memory, and emotional instability.

A, B, D, E, F All these symptoms and signs can occur in both folic acid and cobalamin deficiency anemias.

▶ *Learning objective:* Explain the most likely reason for anemia-induced loss of pain sensation.

6. Answer: D

A megaloblastic anemia associated with loss of pain sensation is most likely due to cobalamin deficiency. The exact mechanism of neurological damage in cobalamin deficiency is still not fully elucidated, but the leading hypothesis is that the impaired methionine synthesis may lead to depletion of S-adenosylmethionine, which is required for the synthesis of myelin phospholipids. The myelin degeneration in the spinal cord can in turn cause an impairment in sensory transmission that explains the loss of pain sensation.

A Insufficient blood flow to the extremities usually causes ischemic pain, not loss of pain sensation.

B Loss of cortical excitatory neurons usually causes loss of several motor and cognitive functions.

C Increased activity of spinal inhibitory neurons usually mediates neuropathic pain, not loss of pain sensation.

E Compression of limb nerves reduces flow in the vessels supplying the nerves with blood. This causes local ischemia, which in turn can cause ischemic pain, not loss of pain sensation.

▶ *Learning objective:* Identify the endogenous compound whose synthesis is impaired by both folic acid and cobalamin deficiency.

7. Answer: C

Both folic acid and cobalamin deficiency can impair the synthesis of THF. Folic acid is metabolized to dihydrofolate and then to THF. The lack of the parent compound (folic acid) impairs the synthesis of THF. Cobalamin catalyzes the conversion of N5-methyltetrahydrofolate to THF. This can explain why an increased supply of folic acid to a patient with cobalamin deficiency can still lead to a sufficient THF synthesis, thereby masking peripheral (but not neurological) symptoms of cobalamin deficiency.

A Dihydrofolate synthesis is decreased by folic acid deficiency but not by cobalamin deficiency.

B, D, E The synthesis of these compounds is affected by cobalamin deficiency but not by folic acid deficiency.

▶ *Learning objective:* Explain the mechanism of the antianemic action of cobalamin.

8. Answer: C

K.O.'s megaloblastic anemia was most likely due to cobalamin deficiency; therefore the patient most likely received cobalamin supplementation. Both folic acid and cobalamin deficiency lead to a decreased availability of THF. Cobalamin transfers a methyl group from N5-methyltetrahydrofolate to homocysteine, forming methionine and THF. In cobalamin deficiency, N5-methyltetrahydrofolate accumulates with associated depletion of THF (the so-called methylfolate trapping). The administration of cobalamin restores the demethylation of N5-methyltetrahydrofolate, correcting the megaloblastic anemia.

A, B These chemical reactions are also catalyzed by cobalamin, but they are not needed for the synthesis of THF.

B, D, E These reactions are not catalyzed by cobalamin.

▶ *Learning objective:* Identify the length of therapy for megaloblastic anemia due to lack of intrinsic factor.

9. Answer: E

Because K.O.'s megaloblastic anemia was most likely due to atrophic gastritis, and the lack of intrinsic factor was permanent, cobalamin supplementation must continue for life.

A, B, C, D See correct answer explanation.

▶ *Learning objective:* Explain why oral cobalamin is effective even when gastric intrinsic factor is absent.

10. Answer: B

It has been shown that a very high oral dose of cobalamin is as effective as parenteral therapy in patients with impaired intrinsic factor function. The reason is the presence of a second, much less efficient, transport system for cobalamin. Actually about 0.5% of the oral dose of the drug can be absorbed by passive diffusion. Because a normal person usually absorbs 1 to 5 µg of cobalamin daily, an oral dose of 1 mg can consistently produce adequate long-term cobalamin replacement.

A In humans, intrinsic factor is secreted only by parietal cells of the body and the fundus of the stomach.

C The fact that cobalamin stores are fully refilled has nothing to do with the intrinsic factor–mediated cobalamin absorption.

D Intrinsic factor is needed for absorption of both food-bound and free cobalamin.

Case 29

Migraine

I.J., a 36-year-old woman, presented to the neurologic clinic with a 2-month history of right-sided pulsatile head pain recurring on a weekly basis. The patient's history indicated that her headaches usually occurred in the morning and were preceded by lightheadedness, hand numbness, and unformed flashes of light or a band of absent vision with a shimmering or glittering zigzag border (scintillating scotomas). About 30 minutes later a throbbing headache would occur. It was always unilateral and was commonly associated with nausea, vomiting, and photophobia. The pain usually lasted all day unless she was able to lie in a dark room and avoid any noise. The headache was partially relieved by two tablets of either aspirin (500 mg tablet) or ketoprofen (50 mg tablet), but recently she avoided these drugs because of epigastric pain. Both I.J.'s mother and grandmother were also affected by a similar type of headache. Past medical history was unremarkable, and I.J. denied any other medical problem. General physical and neurologic examinations were within normal limits.

Current medications included only the analgesics for headache and a monophasic combination contraceptive (ethinyl estradiol 0.02 mg and norethindrone 1 mg).

A diagnosis of migraine was made, and I.J. was given a prescription for ergotamine tartrate (2 mg sublingual) and metoclopramide (10 mg oral). She was instructed to take both medications at the first sign of headache attack and was asked to record the number, frequency, severity, and duration of her headaches so that an accurate assessment of her abortive therapy could be made at her next clinic visit. I.J. was also instructed on how to predetermine her maximal tolerated dose of ergotamine so as to avoid its adverse effects. She was also instructed to avoid oral contraceptives and to use alternative birth control methods.

At her follow-up clinic visit 1 month later, I.J. reported only moderate relief from her headaches with ergotamine, in spite of an evident increased use of the drug. She admitted the occasional use of an over-the-counter preparation (Anacin, an aspirin–caffeine combination) trying to relieve her headache. She also reported a persistent tingling sensation in her legs, and pain occurring in her calf on walking. Inspection of her diary suggests that ergotamine did not improve her headache with respect to any of the parameters noted. I.J.'s physical examination reveals cold lower extremities and decreased distal pulses.

Ergotamine and metoclopramide were discontinued, and I.J. was given a prescription for acetaminophen (500 mg) and codeine (30 mg) combination. I.J. used the drug as directed for her next headache attacks. However, the headache continued to increase in intensity, and, 3 weeks later, the attacks were so frequent that she could no longer work. After vomiting twice during an attack I.J. was taken to the neurologic clinic by a friend. There she was treated with intramuscular sumatriptan. The dose was repeated 1 and 2 hours later, and the attack was abolished.

I.J. was discharged from the clinic with the following postdischarge therapy: oral sumatriptan at the first sign of the headache attack and oral propranolol for migraine prevention.

At her follow-up clinic visit 2 months later, I.J. reported that sumatriptan was quite effective in aborting an impending attack. However, the frequency of these attacks was not decreased in spite of a 300 mg daily dose of propranolol. The neurologist decided to discontinue propranolol and to substitute it with valproic acid. I.J. was also instructed to carefully avoid pregnancy while taking this drug.

Questions

1. I.J. was diagnosed with migraine. Which of the following is the prevalence of this disease for women in the United States?

A. 1–2%

B. 5–10%

C. 15–20%

D. 30–35%

E. 40–45%

2. Which of the following I.J.'s symptoms is practically diagnostic for her disease?

A. Throbbing pain

B. Nausea and vomiting

C. Photophobia

D. Scintillating scotomas

E. Lightheadedness

3. Which of the following pairs of pathophysiological actions most likely cause the pain of I.J.'s migraine attacks?

A. Vasoconstriction–fibrosis

B. Vasodilation–fibrosis

C. Vasoconstriction–necrosis

D. Vasodilation–necrosis

E. Vasoconstriction–inflammation

F. Vasodilation–inflammation

4. Which of the following cranial nerves seems primarily involved in the pathophysiology of I.J.'s migraine?

A. CN I

B. CN II

C. CN III

D. CN IV

E. CN V

F. CN XI

G. CN XII

5. Taking into account I.J.'s medical history, she was most likely at increased risk of which of the following neurologic disorders?

A. Chronic meningitis

B. Ischemic stroke

C. Epilepsy

D. Myasthenia gravis

E. Cerebellar ataxia

F. Alzheimer disease

6. Both aspirin and ketoprofen were effective in decreasing I.J.'s headache. Which of the following molecular actions most likely mediates the analgesic effect of both drugs in the patient's disorder?

A. Decreased synthesis of thromboxanes

B. Blockade of thromboxane receptors

C. Decreased synthesis of prostaglandins

D. Blockade of prostaglandin receptors

E. Decreased synthesis of leukotrienes

F. Blockade of leukotriene receptors

7. I.J. avoided aspirin and ketoprofen because of epigastric pain. Which of the following molecular actions most likely contributed to this adverse effect?

A. Increased prostaglandin activity

B. Increased ion-trapping activity

C. Inhibition of leukotriene synthesis

D. Activation of bradykinin synthesis

E. Increased nitric oxide activity

8. I.J. was started on a therapy with ergotamine tartrate. The activation of which of the following pairs of receptors most likely mediated the therapeutic effect of the drug in the patient's disorder?

A. α-adrenoceptors–5-HT receptors

B. β-adrenoceptors–5-HT receptors

C. Muscarinic M_3 receptors–α-adrenoceptors

D. Muscarinic M_3 receptors–β-adrenoceptors

E. Muscarinic M_3 receptors–5-HT receptors

F. α-adrenoceptors–β-adrenoceptors

9. I.J. started a therapy with metoclopramide. The blockade of which of the following receptors most likely mediates the antiemetic action of this drug?

A. Dopamine D_2-adrenoceptors

B. Muscarinic M_1 receptors

C. Histamine H_1 receptors

D. β-adrenoceptors

E. Nicotinic neuronal (Nn) acetylcholine receptors

10. At her follow-up clinic visit I.J. reported persistent tingling sensation in her legs and pain occurring in her calf on walking. Physical examination showed cold lower extremities and decreased distal pulses. Which of the following was most likely the primary cause of these symptoms and signs?

A. Excessive dosage of metoclopramide

B. Worsening of migraine disorder

C. Cluster headache superimposed to migraine

D. Excessive dosage of ergotamine

E. Excessive dosage of aspirin/caffeine combination

11. I.J. was given a prescription for an acetaminophen–codeine combination. Which of the following pairs of receptors/enzymes most likely mediates the analgesic effect of this combination?

A. κ-receptors–lipoxygenase

B. μ-receptors–cyclooxygenase

C. Glutamate receptors–phospholipase A

D. Muscarinic M_3 receptors–lipoxygenase

E. Thromboxane receptors–cyclooxygenase

12. I.J.'s postdischarge therapy included sumatriptan. Activation of which of the following receptors most likely mediated the therapeutic effect of the drug in the patient's disease?

A. α-adrenoceptors

B. β-adrenoceptors

C. Nn acetylcholine receptors

D. Muscarinic M3 receptors

E. $5-HT_{1D/1B}$ receptors

F. $5-HT_2$ receptors

13. I.J.'s postdischarge therapy included propranolol, a drug approved by the U.S. Food and Drug Administration (FDA) for the prophylactic treatment of migraine. In addition to propranolol, which of the following groups of drugs are the only agents approved at present by FDA for migraine prevention?

A. Timolol–valproate–topiramate

B. Verapamil–ketorolac–lamotrigine

C. Venlafaxine–lisinopril–valproate

D. Gabapentin–naproxen–topiramate

14. Valproate was prescribed to I.J. The drug most likely acts through an enhancement of which of the following central neurotransmitter systems?

A. Glutamatergic

B. Cholinergic

C. Noradrenergic

D. Serotoninergic

E. GABAergic

F. Dopaminergic

15. I.J. was instructed to avoid pregnancy while taking valproic acid since the drug has a well-known teratogenic effect. Which of the following is the most common malformation caused by this drug?

A. Tetralogy of Fallot

B. Hydrocephalus

C. Patent ductus arteriosus

D. Spina bifida

E. Phocomelia

F. Cleft lip

Answers and Explanations

▶ *Learning objective:* Identify the percent prevalence of migraine for women in the United States.

1. Answer: C

Migraine is the most common cause of recurrent moderate to severe headache. Its prevalence is 18% for women and 6% for men in the United States. The peak prevalence of the disorder is in the fourth to fifth decade of life and usually diminishes after age of 50. Studies show familial aggregation of migraine, and it is becoming increasingly clear that much of the vulnerability to migraine is inherited, as in the present case (as already described). The frequency of migraine attacks may vary from once in a lifetime to almost daily, indicating a pronounced individual variability of migraine predisposition. Attacks are initiated when internal or environmental triggers are of sufficient intensity to activate a series of events that culminate in the generation of migraine headache. Many patients experience vague vegetative or affective symptoms as much as 24 hours prior to the onset of a migraine attack. This phase is called the prodrome and should not be confused with the aura phase that occurs in up to 30% of patients and consists of focal neurological symptoms persisting up to 1 hour. Symptoms may include visual, or sensory disturbances, as in the present case. Within an hour of resolution of the aura symptoms, the typical migraine headache usually appears with its unilateral throbbing pain and associated nausea, vomiting, photophobia, and/or phonophobia. Without treatment, the headache may persist for up to 72 hours before ending in a resolution phase often characterized by deep sleep.

A, B, D, E See correct answer explanation.

► *Learning objective:* Describe the symptom that can be diagnostic for migraine when preceding a headache.

2. Answer: D

Migraine headache can be associated with a vast collection of symptoms, but scintillating scotomas preceding the headache are pathognomonic for this disease.

A Throbbing headache is a common symptom of migraine but can also occur with a variety of other conditions, including caffeine withdrawal, stress headache, cluster headache, sinusitis, and brain tumors.

B Nausea and vomiting can occur in other headache conditions, including idiopathic intracranial hypertension and brain tumors.

C, E These symptoms can occur in other headaches, including tension-type headache and cluster headache.

► *Learning objective:* Identify the pairs of pathophysiological actions that most likely cause the pain of a migraine attack.

3. Answer: F

Migraine is a form of neurovascular headache in which neural events result in dilation of blood vessels. The pain phase of migraine is thought to be caused by dilation of large arterial and venous meningeal vessels and a sterile neurogenic inflammation.

A, B, C, D Inflammation, not fibrosis or necrosis, is thought to mediate the migraine headache.

A, C, E Vasodilation, not vasoconstriction, is thought to mediate the migraine headache.

► *Learning objective:* Identify the cranial nerve that is most likely involved in the pathogenesis of migraine.

4. Answer: E

The pathophysiology of migraine remains unknown, but the current view is that a complex series of neural and vascular events initiates migraine. This is called the neurovascular theory and involves the following events:

A patient prone to migraine attack has a state of neuronal hyperexcitability in the cerebral cortex, especially the occipital cortex. The reason why these neurons in certain patients are more excitable is not clear, but a strong familial influence has long been apparent and has been demonstrated in twin studies.

A well-defined wave of neuronal activation followed by inactivation travels across the cortex. This cortical spreading depression (CSD) may be the cause of the aura preceding the migraine attack.

The CSD activates the trigeminal nerve, which innervates the meningeal circulation (the so-called trigeminovascular system). Several potent vasodilator neuropeptides are released by the trigeminal nerve endings, especially calcitonin gene–related peptide (the most powerful endogenous vasodilator known at present). Substance P and neurokinin A may also be involved.

These neuropeptides cause vasodilation of the meningeal vessels and a sterile neurogenic inflammation that sensitizes trigeminal afferents and is associated with further vasodilation. The mechanical stretching caused by vasodilation and perivascular edema resulting from inflammation may be the immediate cause of activation of pain nerve endings in the meninges.

Therefore, sensitization of the trigeminal afferents and dilation of meningeal blood vessels can be considered the final common pathways of the throbbing headache of the migraine attack.

A, B, C, D, F, G See correct answer explanation.

▶ *Learning objective:* Identify a risk factor in a woman with migraine taking oral contraceptives.

5. Answer: B

Migraine has been demonstrated to be a risk factor for ischemic stroke in both men and women. In addition, women who have migraine with aura appear to be at greater risk of ischemic stroke if they are concurrently taking oral contraceptives, as in the present case. The American College of Gynecology recommends that women who are > 35 or who have aura with their migraine attacks not take oral contraceptives; this was the reason why I.J. was instructed to avoid oral contraceptives.

A There is no evidence that migraine can increase the risk of chronic meningitis.

C Migraine can rarely trigger an epileptic seizure in a patient suffering from epilepsy, but there is no evidence that migraine can increase the risk of epilepsy.

D Myasthenia gravis patients frequently complain of headache, but there is no evidence that migraine can increase the risk of myasthenia gravis.

E Cerebellar ataxia can occur as a result of many diseases and presents with symptoms of an inability to coordinate balance, gait, extremity, and eye movements. There are many causes of cerebellar ataxia, but the disorder is not caused or triggered by migraine.

▶ *Learning objective:* Identify the molecular action that mediates the analgesic effect of both aspirin and ketoprofen in migraine.

6. Answer: C

Nonsteroidal anti-inflammatory drugs (NSAIDs), such as aspirin and ketoprofen, act by inhibiting cyclooxygenase enzymes involved in the synthesis of prostaglandins and thromboxanes. The analgesic effects of NSAIDs are primarily related to their inhibitory activity on prostaglandin biosynthesis. Prostaglandins are endogenous compounds that are released from damaged tissues and can sensitize nociceptors to cause pain. By inhibiting prostaglandin biosynthesis in the damaged area, NSAIDs cause an analgesic effect.

A, E NSAIDs decrease the synthesis of thromboxanes, and some of these drugs also decrease (to a lesser degree) the synthesis of leukotrienes, but these actions are not directly involved in the analgesic activity of these drugs.

B, D, F NSAIDs do not block prostaglandin, thromboxane, or leukotriene receptors.

▶ *Learning objective:* Identify an action that can contribute to aspirin- and ketoprofen-induced epigastric pain.

7. Answer: B

I.J. most likely suffered from a drug-induced gastric disorder. Erosive gastritis, bleeding, and peptic ulcer are well recognized adverse effects of NSAIDs, such as aspirin and ketoprofen. These effects are the consequence of both systemic and local actions.

▶ **Systemic actions** are related to inhibition of prostaglandin biosynthesis, which in turn leads to
- increased gastric acid secretion (prostaglandins decrease this secretion by inhibiting the cyclic adenosine monophosphate–mediated activation of the proton pump).
- decreased bicarbonate and mucus secretion by the gastric mucosa (which is increased by prostaglandins).

▶ *Local actions* occur via an ion-trapping mechanism. Most NSAIDs are weak acids with a pK_a < 5. Aspirin's pK_a is 3.5, ketoprofen's pK_a is 3.9. Therefore, these drugs are mainly nonionized (i.e., lipid-soluble) in the stomach lumen and can cross the cell membrane by lipid diffusion. In the alkaline environment of the cytoplasm they become ionized (i.e., water soluble) and are *trapped* inside the cell, causing cell damage.

A NSAIDs decrease, not increase, prostaglandin activity.

C NSAIDs do not inhibit leukotriene synthesis.

D Bradykinin synthesis is activated by angiotensin-converting enzyme inhibitors, not by NSAIDs.

E NSAIDs have no effect on nitric oxide activity.

▶ *Learning objective:* Identify the pair of receptors that are activated by ergotamine.

8. Answer: A

Ergotamine is an ergot alkaloid. These drugs act as agonists, partial agonists, or antagonists on α-adrenoceptors, dopamine receptors, and 5-HT receptors. The remarkably specific vasoconstricting action of these alkaloids on migraine was originally thought to be related to their partial agonist effects on brain vascular α-adrenoceptors and $5\text{-}HT_2$ receptors of meningeal vessels. However, current hypotheses emphasize their action on brain presynaptic 5-HT receptors.

B, C, D, E, F β-Adrenoceptors and muscarinic M_3 receptors are not involved in the pathogenesis of migraine.

▶ *Learning objective:* Identify the blockade of receptors that mediate the antiemetic action of metoclopramide.

9. Answer: A

Metoclopramide is a competitive D_2-adrenoceptor antagonist and a weak 5 HT receptor antagonist with antiemetic and prokinetic properties. The antiemetic action is primarily due to the blockade of D_2-adrenoceptors in the chemoreceptor trigger zone, whereas the prokinetic action is believed to be due to increased cholinergic smooth muscle stimulation, secondary to blockade of intestinal D_2-adrenoceptors. Metoclopramide is frequently coadministered with ergotamine to prevent ergotamine-induced nausea and vomiting, as in the present case.

B Blockade of muscarinic M_1 receptors in the chemoreceptor trigger zone can prevent nausea and vomiting, but metoclopramide does not block these receptors.

C Blockade of histamine H_1 receptors in the chemoreceptor trigger zone can prevent nausea and vomiting, but metoclopramide does not block these receptors.

D, E β-Adrenoceptors and Nn acetylcholine receptors are not involved in the control of nausea and vomiting.

▶ *Learning objective:* Explain the most likely cause of calf pain in a patient receiving antimigraine therapy.

10. Answer: D

I.J.'s symptoms and signs were most likely due to ergotamine-induced vasospasm. In humans, ergotamine and related compounds exert a powerful and long-lasting constricting action on most vessels. This is the reason for the patient's cold lower extremities and decreased distal pulses. The resulting ischemia most likely accounts for the tingling sensation in her legs and pain occurring in her calf on walking. Vasospasm due to ergot alkaloids is refractory to most vasodilators, but infusion of large doses of nitroprusside or nitroglycerin has been found to be effective in some cases.

A Excessive dosage of metoclopramide does not cause vasospasm.

B, C Migraine or cluster headache does not cause vasospasm.

E Caffeine tends to cause peripheral vasodilation, not vasospasm.

▶ *Learning objective:* Identify the pairs of endogenous compounds that most likely mediate the analgesic effect of the acetaminophen–codeine combination.

11. Answer: B

Acetaminophen–codeine is a commonly prescribed drug combination for treatment of moderate pain. This combination produces analgesia through two different mechanisms of action, leading to a synergistic analgesic effect.

Codeine is an opioid whose analgesic effect is mainly due to metabolism to morphine. Opioid analgesia is mediated through activation of central μ- and κ-receptors that leads to decreased perception of pain at the spinal cord and higher levels in the central nervous system (CNS).

Acetaminophen acts primarily in the CNS, where it increases the pain threshold by inhibiting both isoforms of central cyclooxygenase, COX-1 and COX-2, thus decreasing prostaglandin synthesis.

A κ-receptors in the spinal cord contribute to the analgesic effect of opioids, but acetaminophen does not affect lipoxygenase.

C Opioids decrease the release of many neurotransmitters, including glutamate, but acetaminophen does not affect phospholipase A.

D Opioids decrease the release of many neurotransmitters, including acetylcholine, but acetaminophen does not affect lipoxygenase.

E By inhibiting cyclooxygenase, acetaminophen affects (indirectly) the activity of thromboxane receptors, but these receptors do not mediate the analgesic effect of the drug.

▸ *Learning objective:* Identify the receptors that most likely mediate the antimigraine effect of sumatriptan.

12. Answer: E

Sumatriptan is the prototype of a new class of serotonin agonists (the so-called triptans). Unlike the ergot alkaloids that activate serotonergic, noradrenergic, and dopaminergic receptors, the triptans have selective agonistic activity at 5-HT_{1D} and 5-HT_{1B} subtype receptors. There are three proposed mechanisms for the effectiveness of triptans in acute migraine headache:

▸ Reducing the excitability of neurons in the trigeminovascular system via the activation of $5\text{-HT}_{1D/1B}$ receptors
▸ Attenuating the release of neuropeptides with inflammatory and vasodilating properties (e.g., calcitonin gene–related peptide, substance

P, neurokinin A) via activation of presynaptic 5-HT_{1D} receptors
▸ Vasoconstriction of cerebral and extracerebral vessels by activation of vascular 5-HT_{1B}

The efficacy of triptans in aborting a migraine attack is equivalent to or greater than that of other acute treatments. Therefore, these drugs represent today's first-line agents for abortive therapy of migraine attack, and they are also very effective in cluster headache. Their duration of action is often shorter than the duration of headache, and multiple doses may be required during a prolonged migraine attack, as in the present case. The coronary vessels also contain 5-HT_{1B} receptors, which explains the potential of triptans to cause coronary vasoconstriction.

A, B, C, D, F None of these receptors is activated by triptans.

▸ *Learning objective:* Identify the three drugs approved at present by FDA for migraine prevention.

13. Answer: A

When effective, prophylactic migraine treatment not only reduces the frequency of migraine attacks but also may reduce the severity of the ensuing headache. A vast array of drugs have been used for migraine prevention, including β-blockers, calcium channel blockers, tricyclic antidepressants, some antiepileptic drugs, some NSAIDs, and botulinum toxin. However, many prophylactic treatments are not so well grounded, and the only drugs presently approved by FDA for migraine prophylaxis are two β-blockers (propranolol and timolol) and two antiepileptic drugs (valproate and topiramate).

B Verapamil is a Ca^{2+} channel blocker frequently used off-label for migraine prevention.

B Lamotrigine is an antiseizure drug used in epilepsy and bipolar disorder, not for migraine prophylaxis.

B, D Ketorolac and naproxen are NSAIDs. These drugs are used frequently for migraine treatment, not for migraine prevention.

C Venlafaxine is an antidepressant drug sometimes used off-label for migraine prevention. Lisinopril is an angiotensin-converting enzyme inhibitor sometimes used off-label for migraine.

D Gabapentin is an antiseizure drug also used to treat some neuropathic pain. It is used off-label for migraine prevention.

▶ *Learning objective:* Identify the neurotransmitter system most likely involved in valproate-induced migraine prevention.

14. Answer: E

Valproic acid is an antiepileptic drug that most likely acts through multiple mechanisms. However, most antiepileptic drugs ultimately enhance, directly or indirectly, the central GABAergic system, which is the most important inhibitory system in the brain.

A Valproic acid inhibits, not enhances, the glutamatergic system.

B, C, D, F These systems are minimally involved in the mechanism of action of valproic acid.

▶ *Learning objective:* Identify the most common malformation caused by valproate given during pregnancy.

15. Answer: D

When given to a mother during pregnancy, valproic acid can increase the risk of neural tube defect to the developing baby by up to 20-fold. This defect can lead to a defective closure of the vertebral column, called spina bifida. The severity of the disorder ranges from spina bifida occulta (no apparent anomalies) to spina bifida cystica, a protruding sac that can contain meninges (meningocele), spinal cord (myelocele), or both (myelomeningocele).

A, B, C, E, F The risk of these valproate-induced malformations is very low or absent.

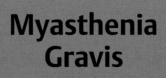

Myasthenia Gravis

B.D., a 72-year-old woman, complained to her physician of bilateral drooping eyelids (ptosis) and double vision (diplopia) for the past 2 weeks. These symptoms got worse when she was sewing, reading, or watching TV. Her ptosis was so severe at times that she held her eyes open to read. The woman also complained of slurring of speech that worsened when she continued to talk, trouble swallowing that deteriorated when she continued eating, and intermittent weakness in her arms that made it difficult to comb her hair. Her symptoms were generally not bothersome in the morning but would progress throughout the day.

Medical history of the patient was significant for hypercholesterolemia, gastroesophageal reflux disease, and chronic constipation. Three weeks earlier B.D. suffered from a urinary tract infection that resolved after a 10-day treatment with gentamicin. Drugs presently taken by the patient were lovastatin, omeprazole, lactulose, and bisacodyl. The rest of her medical history was unremarkable.

B.D. was admitted to the neurologic clinic for evaluation. Physical examination showed a well-nourished woman in no apparent distress with the following vital signs: blood pressure 132/75 mm Hg, heart rate 65 bpm, respirations 14/min. She had notable ptosis of both eyelids that got worse after repeated blinking exercises. When smiling, she appeared to be snarling. Electromyographic testing revealed progressive weakness and decreased amplitude of contraction of the distal arm muscles upon repeated mild shocks (five shocks per second) of the ulnar and median nerves. Both her symptoms and the electromyographic findings were reversed within 40 seconds of intravenous (IV) administration of edrophonium. A blood test revealed high levels of an antiacetylcholine receptor antibody in her plasma.

The diagnosis of myasthenia gravis was made, and an appropriate daily therapy was prescribed that included pyridostigmine and azathioprine. Atropine was also prescribed, to be taken "as needed" just before pyridostigmine.

Two weeks later B.D. was readmitted to the neurologic clinic because of exacerbation of her symptoms. She had extreme muscle weakness, ptosis, diplopia, and difficulty in swallowing, speaking, and breathing. An IV injection of edrophonium caused no improvement of her symptoms. A diagnosis of cholinergic crisis was made and an appropriate emergency therapy was started, which included temporary discontinuation of pyridostigmine treatment. B.D.'s symptoms disappeared rapidly, and a few days later she was dismissed from the clinic.

Questions

1. B.D. was diagnosed with myasthenia gravis, which is thought to be an autoimmune disease. Which of the following receptor molecules act as antigens in this disease?

A. Nicotinic neuronal receptors

B. β_1-adrenoceptors

C. Epidermal growth factor receptors

D. Interleukin-2 receptors

E. Nicotinic muscular receptors

2. Which of the following neuromuscular structures was most likely structurally damaged in B.D.'s disease?

A. Autonomic nerve endings

B. Motor nerve endings

C. Motor end plates

D. Pyramidal neuron endings

E. Striated muscle sarcomeres

3. Myasthenia gravis affects several body muscles. Impairment of which of the following pairs of eye muscles occurs most frequently in this disease?

A. Extraocular muscles–ciliary muscle

B. Extraocular muscles–radial muscle of the iris

C. Extraocular muscles–levator palpebrae

D. Ciliary muscle–radial muscle of the iris

E. Ciliary muscle–levator palpebrae

F. Radial muscle of the iris–levator palpebrae

4. It is known that subclinical myasthenia gravis can manifest after certain drug treatments. Which of the following drugs taken by the patient could have triggered her disease?

A. Lovastatin

B. Omeprazole

C. Gentamicin

D. Lactulose

E. Bisacodyl

5. B.D.'s ptosis of both eyelids got worse after repeated blinking, and her electromyographic testing revealed progressive decreased amplitude of contraction of the distal arm muscles upon repeated mild shocks. Which of the following phrases best explains why B.D.'s muscle contraction decreased after repeated stimulation?

A. Insufficient acetylcholine availability

B. More rapid acetylcholine metabolism

C. Sensitization of available acetylcholine receptors

D. Upregulation of acetylcholine receptors

E. Downregulation of acetylcholine receptors

6. B.D. had an impairment of her skeletal muscle contraction. Which of the following molecular actions most likely mediated the muscle contraction of a normal skeletal muscle fiber?

A. Closing Ca^{2+} channel in muscle cell membrane

B. Decreased Na^+ current in end plate membrane

C. Ca^{2+} release from sarcoplasmic reticulum

D. Binding Ca^{2+} to calmodulin

E. Cross-linking between actin and tropomyosin filaments

7. B.D.'s motor nerve endings continuously secrete single vesicles of acetylcholine (often named quanta) that cause miniature excitatory postsynaptic potentials (EPSPs). Which of the following statements best explains why EPSPs do not trigger muscle contraction in most cases?

A. They are all or none in nature.

B. They can summate.

C. They are caused by an insufficient depolarization of the cell membrane.

D. They are followed by an absolute refractory period.

E. They make the end plate less likely to fire an action potential.

8. A blood test revealed high levels of an antiacetylcholine receptor antibody in B.D.'s plasma. Which of the following antibodies was most likely increased in the patient's plasma?

A. IgA

B. IgE

C. IgG

D. IgM

E. IgD

9. Which of the following disorders was most likely associated with B.D.'s disease?

A. Rheumatoid arthritis

B. Thymus hyperplasia

C. Psoriasis

D. Hashimoto's thyroiditis

E. Guillain–Barré's syndrome

10. B.D.'s symptoms and electromyographic findings were reversed within 40 seconds of IV administration of edrophonium. Which of the following actions on acetylcholine turnover most likely mediated the effect of this drug?

A. Decreased metabolism

B. Increased biosynthesis

C. Increased release

D. Decreased reuptake

E. Decreased renal excretion

11. Pyridostigmine was prescribed for B.D. An increased opening of which of the following ion channels on the motor end plate most likely mediated the therapeutic effect of the drug in the patient's disease?

A. Ligand-gated Ca^{2+} channels

B. Ligand-gated K^+ channels

C. Ligand-gated Cl^- channels

D. Ligand-gated Na^+ channels

E. Voltage-gated K^+ channels

F. Voltage-gated Cl^- channels

12. Which of the following effects would have most likely occurred after pyridostigmine administration if an excessive dose was given?

A. Difficulty with near vision

B. Constipation

C. Decreased heart rate

D. Bronchodilation

E. Drowsiness

13. Atropine was prescribed for B.D. on an as needed basis in order to counteract some potential adverse effects of pyridostigmine. Which of the following adverse effects was most likely counteracted by atropine administration?

A. Diplopia

B. Swallowing difficulty

C. Increased salivation

D. Breathing difficulty

E. Overflow incontinence

F. Mydriasis

14. Azathioprine was prescribed for B.D. Which of the following endogenous molecules most likely represent the molecular target of this drug?

A. Calcineurin

B. Folinic acid

C. DNA

D. Tumor necrosis factor

E. RNA

15. Which of the following pairs of lab exams should be performed monthly after starting the azathioprine therapy?

A. Blood urea nitrogen–white blood cell count

B. Blood urea nitrogen–serum creatinine

C. Blood urea nitrogen–liver transaminases

D. Serum creatinine–liver transaminases

E. White blood cell count–liver transaminases

F. Serum creatinine–white blood cell count

261

16. B.D. was diagnosed with cholinergic crisis. Symptoms of this disorder usually include increased sweating, salivation, bronchial secretions, and miosis. Which of the following statements best explains why these symptoms were absent in B.D.?

A. The pyridostigmine dose was too low.

B. Atropine as needed was used frequently.

C. Azathioprine antagonized pyridostigmine effects.

D. Sympathetic tone is high in older patients.

E. The described symptoms do not occur in myasthenic patients.

17. Cholinergic crisis is related to an excess of acetylcholine at the neuromuscular junction, which causes flaccid skeletal muscle paralysis. Which of the following molecular actions most likely mediates this acetylcholine-induced effect?

A. Depolarizing blockade of nicotinic receptors

B. Autoimmune damage of nicotinic receptors

C. Increased acetylcholine release

D. Decreased acetylcholine reuptake

E. Decreased renal excretion of acetylcholine

Answers and Explanations

▶ *Learning objective:* Recognize the receptor molecule that acts as an antigen in myasthenia gravis.

1. Answer: E

Antigens are defined as an organism, a molecule, or part of a molecule that is recognized by the immune system. Myasthenia gravis is a relatively rare autoimmune disorder in which the immune system recognizes nicotinic muscular postsynaptic receptors as antigens and forms antibodies against them. The antibodies block and

destroy these receptors, causing an impairment in neuromuscular transmission.

A Nicotinic neuronal receptors can function as antigens in some diseases (dysautonomia).

B β_1-adrenoceptors can function as antigens in some diseases (chronic Chagas's disease, peritonitis), which can explain, in part, the impairment of cardiac function that can occur in these diseases.

C Epidermal growth factor receptors can be the antigens of some monoclonal antibodies such as cetuximab.

D Interleukin-2 receptors can be the antigens of some monoclonal antibodies, such as basiliximab.

▶ *Learning objective:* Identify the neuromuscular structure that is structurally damaged in myasthenia gravis.

2. Answer: C

Myasthenia gravis results from an autoimmune attack on end plate nicotinic muscular (Nm) acetylcholine receptors, which destroys these receptors, disrupting the neuromuscular transmission. A 70 to 90% decrease in the number of Nm receptors per end plate usually occurs in the affected muscle.

A, B, D Nerve endings are not affected by the disease, and synaptic vesicles are normal.

E Striated muscle sarcomeres are normal in myasthenic patients, even if muscle wasting can occur later in a long-lasting disease. Sarcomeres cannot contract normally because of an impairment of neuromuscular transmission and not because of structural damage.

▶ *Learning objective:* Describe the pairs of eye muscle most frequently impaired in myasthenic patients.

3. Answer: C

Diplopia (due to impairment of extraocular muscles) and ptosis (due to impairment of levator palpebrae) occur initially in 40% of myasthenic patients and eventually in 90%. The question of why the disease afflicts predominantly the extraocular muscles first remains unanswered, but extraocular muscles are 80% single-innervated twitch fibers with a high firing frequency. This increases their sensitivity to fatigue. Also the levator palpebrae, under constant activation during eye opening, may be more susceptible to fatigue.

A, B, D, E, F Myasthenia gravis affects striated muscles only. The ciliary muscle and the radial muscle of the iris are smooth muscles, not striated muscles.

▶ *Learning objective:* Identify the drug that can trigger myasthenia gravis in a predisposed patient.

4. Answer: C

Gentamicin is an aminoglycoside antibiotic. These drugs can cause neuromuscular blockade and therefore can worsen myasthenia gravis dramatically or trigger the disease in a predisposed patient, as probably happened in the present case. Other drugs that can worsen the disease include macrolides, tetracyclines, fluoroquinolones, and Ca^{2+} channel blockers.

A Lovastatin is a statin (i.e., an inhibitor of 3-hydroxy-3-methyl-glutaryl-coenzyme A reductase [HMG-CoA]) used for hypercholesterolemia.

B Omeprazole is a proton pump inhibitor used for gastrointestinal ulcers.

D Lactulose is an osmotic laxative used for constipation.

E Bisacodyl is a stimulant laxative used for constipation.

▶ *Learning objective:* Explain why the muscle contraction of a myasthenic patient decreases after repeated stimulation.

5. Answer: A

The release of acetylcholine from motor neuron endings decreases after repeated stimulation because of a temporary depletion of the presynaptic acetylcholine stores. The amount of neurotransmitter is always much more abundant than the number of receptors, but the proportion of activated receptors is related to the amount of neurotransmitter available (the law of mass action). Now let's say that after a repeated stimulation a lower amount of acetylcholine is released and this lower amount is still able to activate 20% of the 100 receptors available in a normal motor end plate. Assume that these 20 receptors are barely able to induce a normal contraction. Now assume that only 30 receptors are available in the myasthenic end plate. The same amount of acetylcholine will activate 20% of these receptors (i.e., 6 receptors). This number is too low to induce a normal contraction; therefore the amplitude of contraction will diminish. This explains the fatigability seen in myasthenic patients and also explains why drugs that increase acetylcholine availability are successfully used in myasthenic patients.

B Acetylcholine metabolism is normal in myasthenic patients.

C Available acetylcholine receptors are desensitized, not sensitized, by the autoimmune attack.

D, E Myasthenic patients' receptors are destroyed by the autoimmune attack, not up- or downregulated.

▶ *Learning objective:* Describe the molecular action that mediates the muscle contraction of a normal skeletal muscle fiber.

6. Answer: C

In a normal skeletal muscle fiber, binding of acetylcholine to Nm receptors causes an inward Na^+ current in the motor end plate that generates a depolarization sufficient for the production of an action potential. This potential spreads the depolarization along the T tubules of the muscle fibers, causing primarily a release of Ca^{2+} from the sarcoplasmic reticulum. Ca^{2+} binds to troponin C, uncovering myosin binding sites on actin. The formation of cross-linkages between actin and myosin and the sliding of thin on thick filaments causes contraction.

A Unlike smooth and cardiac muscle, the Ca^{2+} from the extracellular fluid is not the Ca^{2+} that is used for skeletal muscle contraction. Voltage-gated Ca^{2+} channels (also named dihydropyridine receptors) open, not close, during depolarization of T tubule membranes. This Ca^{2+} triggers the opening of only a ligand-gated Ca^{2+} channel (also named a ryanodine receptor), allowing the release of Ca^{2+} already stored in the sarcoplasmic reticulum. This is the Ca^{2+} used for skeletal muscle contraction.

B The Na+ current in the end plate membrane is increased, not decreased, after activation of end plate Nm receptors.

D In skeletal muscle, Ca^{2+} binds to troponin C, not to calmodulin.

E Cross-linking occurs between actin and myosin, not tropomyosin, filaments.

▶ *Learning objective:* Explain why miniature EPSPs cannot trigger muscle contraction.

7. Answer: C

Miniature EPSPs result from the opening of ligand-gated Na^+ channels that cause a depolarization of the motor end plate membrane. Because the number of open Na^+ channels is small, the voltage change of EPSPs is small and cannot reach the threshold for an action potential.

A Unlike the action potential, the EPSPs are not all or none in nature.

B The EPSPs can summate, but this is not the reason why they do not trigger muscle contraction.

D The presence of a refractory period cannot explain the absence of firing. Action potential is followed by an absolute refractory period and can nevertheless trigger muscle contraction.

E Because the EPSPs are the result of depolarization, they make the end plate more likely, not less likely, to fire an action potential.

▶ *Learning objective:* Identify the immunoglobulin antibody that is usually increased in myasthenic patients.

8. Answer: C

Antibodies that mediate autoimmune disorders are usually immunoglobulin G (IgG) or IgM. Autoantibodies against receptors are usually IgG. This immunoglobulin is the most common type of antibody found in the circulation, representing approximately 75% of serum antibodies in humans. IgG molecules are created and released by plasma B cells.

A IgA is an antibody located mainly in the gastrointestinal tract that provides protection against microbes that multiply in bodily secretions.

B IgE is an antibody involved in the type I hypersensitivity (allergic) responses.

D IgM is an antibody involved in type II hypersensitivity (allergic) responses.

E IgD is an antibody displayed almost exclusively on B-cell surfaces. Its main function is to signal the B cells to be activated.

▶ *Learning objective:* Identify the disorder that is frequently associated with myasthenia gravis.

9. Answer: B

Myasthenia gravis is an autoimmune disorder. The trigger for autoantibody production is unknown, but the thymus is most likely involved. More than 60% of myasthenic patients have thymus hyperplasia. In these patients, the thymus gland contains certain clusters of immune cells indicative of lymphoid hyperplasia, a condition usually found only in the spleen and lymph nodes during an active immune response. About 10% have a thymoma, a tumor of the thymus gland, that is generally benign, but can become malignant. The relationship between the thymus gland and myasthenia gravis is not yet fully understood, but it is believed that the thymus gland may give incorrect instructions to developing immune cells. This ultimately results in autoimmunity and the production of the acetylcholine receptor antibodies, thereby setting the stage for the attack on neuromuscular transmission.

A Rheumatoid arthritis is an autoimmune disorder due to an immune-mediated attack on the joints.

C Psoriasis is an autoimmune disorder due to immune-mediated overactivity of skin cells.

D Hashimoto's thyroiditis is an autoimmune disorder due to an immune-mediated attack on the thyroid cells.

E Guillain–Barré's syndrome is an autoimmune disorder due to an immune-mediated attack on the nerves controlling muscles in the legs.

▶ *Learning objective:* Explain the molecular mechanism of action of edrophonium.

Edrophonium is a short-acting competitive inhibitor of cholinesterases, the enzymes that metabolize acetylcholine. Cholinesterase enzymes are of two types:

▶ Acetylcholinesterase (AchE), found mainly in cholinergic neurons, the neuromuscular junction, and erythrocytes
▶ Butyrylcholinesterase (BuChE), found primarily in plasma and liver

These enzymes break the ester linkage of acetylcholine, resulting in the formation of choline and an acetylated enzyme. The acetylated enzyme is rapidly hydrolyzed, giving the regenerated free enzyme and acetic acid. The entire process takes about 150 microseconds.

Cholinesterase inhibitors can inhibit both enzymes, but their effects are primarily due to inhibition of acetylcholinesterase. The inhibition of acetylcholine metabolism increases the availability of the neurotransmitter at the neuromuscular junction, leading to improved neuromuscular transmission.

Edrophonium is a short-acting inhibitor (its distribution half-life is about 10 minutes); therefore its action is very brief. The drug is used as a test for diagnosis of myasthenia gravis. A rapid recovery of muscle function is a positive result, as in the present case.

B, C Biosynthesis and release of acetylcholine are not affected by cholinesterase inhibitors.

D Acetylcholine does not undergo reuptake into the cholinergic terminals.

E Acetylcholine is not excreted by the kidney.

▶ *Learning objective:* Identify the ion channels that mediated the therapeutic effect of pyridostigmine in myasthenic patients.

Pyridostigmine is a reversible cholinesterase inhibitor and is a first-line agent for the treatment of myasthenic patients. By inhibiting acetylcholinesterase, the drug increases the availability of acetylcholine, which in turn activates more Nm cholinergic receptors. This activation opens ligand-gated Na^+ channels on the motor end plate, triggering the signal transduction pathway that leads to neuromuscular contraction.

A Opening of the Ca^{2+} channels is included in the signal transduction pathway that follows activation of Nm acetylcholine receptors, but these channels are voltage-gated, not ligand-gated.

B, C, E, F K^+ and Cl^- channels are not directly involved in the therapeutic effect of pyridostigmine.

▶ *Learning objective:* Describe an effect that can occur after pyridostigmine administration.

Pyridostigmine is a cholinesterase inhibitor; therefore it increases the availability of acetylcholine at all peripheral cholinergic synapses. This can increase the activity of nicotinic neuronal receptors on both sympathetic and parasympathetic ganglia, of Nm receptors on the neuromuscular junction, and of muscarinic receptors on cardiac muscle, smooth muscle, and exocrine glands. Because both sympathetic and parasympathetic ganglia are stimulated the final effect depends on the predominant tone of the system. In our body the parasympathetic tone predominates in all systems except the vascular system, where the tone is mainly sympathetic. Therefore, in the heart, cholinesterase inhibitors decrease the heart rate, contractility, and atrioventricular conduction.

A Activation of muscarinic receptors in the ciliary muscle causes cyclospasm, which creates difficulty with far, not near vision.

B Activation of muscarinic receptors in the gastrointestinal tract causes diarrhea, not constipation.

D Activation of muscarinic receptors in the bronchial tree causes bronchoconstriction, not bronchodilation.

E Pyridostigmine crosses the blood–brain barrier very poorly; therefore drowsiness is unlikely.

▶ *Learning objective:* Recognize the potential adverse effect of pyridostigmine that can be counteracted by atropine treatment.

13. Answer: C

An antimuscarinic drug is sometimes used as needed to counteract unwanted muscarinic effects of cholinesterase inhibitors. These drugs can cause dose-related muscarinic effects, mainly in the gastrointestinal tract. Increased salivation is the most common adverse effect of pyridostigmine. Atropine can antagonize most muscarinic effects of acetylcholine, leaving the nicotinic effects untouched.

A, B, D These are effects due to depolarization blockade of Nm receptors. Atropine cannot affect these effects.

E Pyridostigmine would cause urge, not overflow, incontinence.

F Pyridostigmine would cause miosis, not mydriasis.

▶ *Learning objective:* Identify the endogenous molecule that represents the main molecular target for azathioprine.

14. Answer: C

The therapy of myasthenia gravis has two main goals:

▶ Enhancing cholinergic activity at the neuromuscular junction
▶ Reducing the potency of the immunologic attack

Azathioprine and glucocorticoids are the two immunosuppressive agents most commonly used in myasthenic patients. Azathioprine is a prodrug that is biotransformed into mercaptopurine and then into the corresponding false nucleotide. This false nucleotide is incorporated into replicating DNA, inhibiting the de novo pathway of purine synthesis and, in part, the salvage pathway for purine conservation. This cytotoxic action affects mainly cells with a high turnover rate and can explain the inhibition of the wave of lymphoid cell proliferation that follows antigenic stimulation, thereby causing an immunosuppressive effect.

A, B, D The synthesis of these molecules is not inhibited by azathioprine.

E Although continuous messenger RNA synthesis is necessary for sustained antibody synthesis by plasma cells, azathioprine appears to have less of an effect on this process than on DNA synthesis.

▶ *Learning objective:* Describe the two lab exams that should be performed monthly after starting the azathioprine therapy

15. Answer: E

Azathioprine is a cytotoxic drug that inhibits proliferation of cells with high turnover rate. Therefore, leukopenia is a potential serious adverse effect, and the drug should be stopped if the white cell count falls below 3,000 cells/mm^3.

Azathioprine has been associated with several forms of hepatotoxicity, including an acute cholestatic injury and a chronic hepatic injury marked by veno-occlusive disease or nodular regenerative hyperplasia. Actually azathioprine is the most common drug causing veno-occlusive disease, a nonthrombotic occlusion of the lumen of small intrahepatic veins. Azathioprine should be stopped if liver transaminases are more than three times greater than the upper limit of normal.

A, B, C, D, F Elevated blood urea nitrogen and serum creatinine are primarily indicative of kidney toxicity. Azathioprine-induced kidney toxicity is extremely rare.

▶ *Learning objective:* Explain the most likely reason why certain autonomic symptoms may be absent in a patient suffering from cholinergic crisis.

16. Answer: B

Cholinergic crisis is a pronounced muscular weakness and respiratory paralysis caused by excessive acetylcholine. In myasthenic patients it can occur mainly during the first weeks of therapy and is caused by a too high dose of a cholinesterase inhibitor, such as pyridostigmine. Increased sweating, salivation, bronchial secretions, and miosis are muscarinic effects of acetylcholine. When atropine is used frequently to counteract these effects, they can be masked during a cholinergic crisis. This most likely happened in the present case.

A The pyridostigmine dose was high, not low, given that cholinergic crisis occurred.

C Azathioprine does not affect pyridostigmine actions.

D Elderly people usually have an increased sympathetic tone, but B.D.'s symptoms are related to parasympathetic, not sympathetic, overactivity.

E The described symptoms do occur in myasthenic patients, unless counteracted by atropine treatment.

▶ *Learning objective:* Explain the reason for a flaccid skeletal muscle paralysis due to acetylcholine excess.

17. Answer: A

Acetylcholine activates the nicotinic receptors of the motor end plate, opening the ligand-gated Na⁺ channels. This causes depolarization of the end plate, which in turn spreads to adjacent membranes, causing contraction of the skeletal muscle. When acetylcholine is in excess on the synaptic cleft because of inhibition of its metabolism, Na⁺ channels remain open, and the end plate membrane remains depolarized and unresponsive to subsequent impulses. This is called depolarizing blockade (also called desensitization) of the nicotinic receptors. Furthermore, because excitation–contraction coupling requires end plate repolarization and repetitive firing to maintain muscle tension, a flaccid paralysis results.

B Extensive autoimmune damage of the nicotinic receptors can cause flaccid paralysis. This is referred to as myasthenic crisis but, in this case, edrophonium would have caused a transient improvement of symptoms.

C Acetylcholine release is normal during cholinergic crisis.

D, E Acetylcholine does not undergo reuptake into cholinergic terminals and is not excreted by the kidney.

Myocardial Infarction

M.G., a 58-year-old man, went to bed early one evening because he was not feeling well. He awakened in the middle of the night because of an excruciating chest pain and was taken by ambulance to the emergency department. M.G.'s past medical history was significant for exertional angina, relieved by nitroglycerin as needed, and for stage 1 essential hypertension treated with hydrochlorothiazide and losartan.

Physical examination on admission revealed an obese man (weight 90 kg, height 165 cm) in obvious distress who appeared diaphoretic and ashen. He complained of chest pain that was crushing and pressing (as a big stone sitting on his chest) and that radiated to his left arm and jaw. He was nauseated, and his skin was cold and clammy. His vital signs were blood pressure 130/100 mm Hg, pulse 110 bpm and regular, respirations 28/min and "noisy." Chest and neck examination were positive for bilateral rales at the lung bases and for distension of the jugular veins, respectively. An S3 gallop was heard on auscultation. The liver was slightly enlarged, and the extremities were without edema. Peripheral pulses were diminished. Urine output was 30 mL/h.

Pertinent laboratory results admission were as follows:

Blood hematology

▶ Potassium (K^+): 5.7 mEq/L (normal 3.5–5.5)
▶ Blood pH: 7.32 (normal 7.35–7.45)
▶ Troponin I: 60 ng/mL (normal < 2)
▶ Creatine kinase-MB (CK-MB) fraction: 12% (normal < 5%)

Electrocardiography

Acute ST elevation myocardial infarction (STEMI)

The patient was given a tablet of aspirin (325 mg to be chewed and swallowed immediately and was transferred to the intensive coronary unit (ICU), where an emergency therapy was started. The patient's pain did not respond to four sublingual nitroglycerin tablets and to an intravenous (IV) nitroglycerin bolus. The patient repeatedly complained that the pain was unbearable ("The worst pain I have ever experienced"), but the pain subsided after the intramuscular (IM) administration of an initial dose of 10 mg of morphine and an additional 5 mg dose 10 minutes later.

The patient was placed on a cardiac monitor, oxygen was given by nasal cannula, and a central venous catheter was inserted.

A percutaneous coronary intervention was started but had to be suspended because of excessive tortuosity of the proximal coronary segment.

An IV bolus of alteplase was given, followed by an IV infusion over the next half hour. The following drugs were also given: enoxaparin, metoprolol, and lisinopril.

Over the next 4 hours M.G.'s symptoms gradually subsided. M.G. now had the following vital signs: blood pressure 135/80 mm Hg, pulse 85 bpm, respirations 22/min. The next day M.G. was dismissed from the ICU with the following therapy: aspirin, clopidogrel, enoxaparin, metoprolol, lisinopril, and lovastatin. M.G.'s condition continued to improve, and a week later he was discharged from the hospital with the same drugs for postdischarge therapy.

Questions

1. M.G. complained of an unbearable chest pain. Which of the following was most likely the primary molecular mechanism that triggered his pain?

A. Activation of cardiac β_1-adrenoceptors

B. Increased activity of the Na^+/K^+ pump in the infarcted area

C. Development of metabolic alkalosis

D. Reduced adenosine triphosphate (ATP) formation in the infarcted area

E. Abnormal activity of pain transmission pathways to the brain

2. M.G.'s skin was cold and clammy. Which of the following physiological actions most likely mediated these signs?

A. Release of renin from the macula densa

B. Activation of the parasympathetic system

C. Release of endothelins from the infarcted area

D. Activation of the sympathetic system

E. Release of adenosine from the infarcted area

3. M.G.'s neck veins appeared enlarged. Which of the following actions most likely caused this sign?

A. Decreased afterload

B. Increased central venous pressure

C. Increased heart rate

D. Blockage of inferior vena cava

E. Decreased preload

4. An S3 gallop was heard on M.G.'s heart auscultation. In this patient the sound was most likely indicative of which of the following pathological conditions?

A. Impending pulmonary edema

B. Second-degree heart block

C. Left ventricular failure

D. Atrial fibrillation

E. Impending ventricular tachycardia

5. Which of the following pairs of lab exams are most indicative of M.G.'s myocardial infarction?

A. Troponin I–[K^+]

B. Troponin I–blood pH

C. Troponin I–CK-MB fraction

D. CK-MB fraction–[K^+]

E. CK-MB fraction–blood pH

F. Blood pH–[K^+]

6. After the diagnosis of myocardial infarction M.G. was immediately given a low dose of aspirin. Which of the following actions most likely mediated the therapeutic effect of the drug in the patient's disorder?

A. Coronary vasodilation

B. Increased collateral blood flow

C. Increased cardiac contractility

D. Decreased local ischemia

E. Decreased preload

7. Which of the following statements best explains why aspirin is given at a low dose to prevent platelet aggregation?

A. Higher doses would cause a longer inhibition of prostacyclin synthesis.

B. Higher doses would cause an unacceptable high risk of adverse effects.

C. Low doses also cause blockade of platelet adenosine diphosphate (ADP) receptor.

D. Low doses favor the adhesion of platelets to the vascular endothelium.

E. Higher doses favor the rupture of atherosclerotic plaques in the coronaries

8. M.G. was given nitroglycerin. Which of the following was most likely the primary action that mediated the therapeutic effect of this drug in myocardial infarction?

A. Decreased afterload

B. Increased heart contractility

C. Increased heart rate

D. Increased coronary blood flow

E. Decreased platelet aggregation

9. Which of the following endogenous compounds most likely mediated the effect of nitroglycerin in the patient's disorder?

A. Bradykinin

B. Cyclic adenosine monophosphate (cAMP)

C. Norepinephrine

D. Cyclic guanosine monophosphate (cGMP)

E. Adenosine

10. M.G.'s chest pain subsided after the IM administration of morphine. Which of the following molecular actions most likely mediated the analgesic effect of the drug?

A. Opening of Ca^{2+} channels on presynaptic nerve terminals

B. Closing of Cl^- channels on postsynaptic neurons

C. Stimulation of substance P^+ release from nociceptive nerve terminals

D. Opening of K^+ channels on postsynaptic neurons

E. Stimulation of glutamate release from nociceptive nerve terminals

11. M.G. was given an IV bolus of alteplase followed by an IV infusion of the same drug. Which of the following molecular actions most likely mediated the therapeutic effect of alteplase?

A. Inactivation of thrombin bound to fibrin in clots

B. Increased conversion of fibrinogen to fibrin

C. Increased conversion of plasminogen into plasmin

D. Inhibition of the activity of antithrombin III

E. Inhibition of plasmin binding to target fibrin

F. Increased synthesis of plasminogen

12. Because of alteplase treatment M.G. was most likely at risk of which of the following adverse effects?

A. Disseminate intravascular coagulation

B. Acute liver failure

C. Hemorrhagic stroke

D. Pulmonary embolism

E. Ulcerative colitis

13. M.G. was given IV enoxaparin. Which of the following endogenous compounds was most likely the molecular target of this drug?

A. Plasmin

B. Vitamin K

C. Antithrombin III

D. Glycoprotein IIb/IIIa

E. Fibrinogen

14. Which of the following is an advantage of enoxaparin over the standard unfractionated heparin?

A. Decreased risk of bleeding complications

B. Good oral bioavailability

C. No risk of drug-induced thrombocytopenia

D. Pronounced antiplatelet activity

E. No risk of allergic reactions

15. M.G. was given metoprolol IV. The reduced activity of which of the following enzymes most likely mediated the therapeutic effect of the drug in the patient's disease?

A. Guanylate cyclase

B. Phospholipase C

C. Phospholipase A2

D. Adenylate cyclase

E. Tyrosine kinase

16. When M.G. was dismissed from the hospital metoprolol was prescribed as chronic therapy. Which of the following actions was most likely an important determinant of the long-term therapeutic effect of the drug in the patient's disease?

A. Downregulation of β-adrenoceptors

B. Increased renin secretion

C. Decreased myocardial remodeling

D. Decreased gluconeogenesis

E. Increased preload

17. When M.G. was dismissed from the hospital, clopidogrel was prescribed in addition to aspirin. The blockade of which of the following platelet receptors most likely mediated the therapeutic effect of the drug in the patient's disease?

A. Thromboxane receptors

B. Platelet glycoprotein IIb/IIIa receptors

C. Serotonin receptors

D. Glycoprotein Ia receptors

E. ADP receptors

18. Which of the following was the most likely reason for the addition of clopidogrel to aspirin?

A. To achieve synergism between the two drugs

B. To decrease the gastric toxicity of aspirin

C. To avoid aspirin resistance

D. To increase the aspirin duration of action

E. To increase aspirin bioavailability

19. When M.G. was dismissed from the hospital, lisinopril was prescribed as chronic therapy. Which of the following molecular actions most likely mediated the therapeutic effect of the drug in the patient's disease?

A. Stimulation of metabolism of bradykinin

B. Inhibition of synthesis of angiotensin II

C. Blockade of angiotensin II receptors

D. Decreased metabolism of angiotensin I

E. Increased metabolism of angiotensin II

20. During the long-term therapy with lisinopril, M.G. was most likely at risk of which of the following adverse effects of the drug?

A. Hypokalemia

B. Hypertension

C. Dry cough

D. Metabolic acidosis

E. Agranulocytosis

Answers and Explanations

▶ *Learning objective:* Explain the main molecular mechanism that causes the pain of myocardial infarction.

1. Answer: D

The pain of myocardial infarction is a typical example of ischemic pain. The mechanisms responsible for this pain are complex and not entirely understood, but a primary mechanism is that the decreased oxygen supply to cardiac cells reduces the oxidative phosphorylation needed to generate ATP. This decreases the entrance of pyruvate into the citric acid cycle, causing a shift to lactic acid production (see the patient's low blood pH). In other words, there is a shift from aerobic to less effective anaerobic metabolism. Outcomes are the loss of the normal sodium-potassium pump and the release of chemical substances that stimulate chemosensitive and mechanoreceptive receptors innervated by unmyelinated nerve cells found within the heart muscle fibers and around the coronary vessels. The pain substances that are released include lactate, serotonin, bradykinin, histamine, reactive oxygen species, and adenosine. All can contribute to the ischemic pain of myocardial infarction, but adenosine seems to be the most likely culprit compound.

A Cardiac β$_1$-adrenoceptors are usually activated in myocardial infarction because the decreased cardiac output triggers an activation of the sympathetic nervous system, but this activation is not the primary reason for the chest pain.

B The activity of the Na⁺/K⁺ pump in cardiac cells is decreased, not increased, because of the decreased formation of ATP.

C Acidosis, not alkalosis, is the most likely sign of myocardial infarction, because of lactic acid production (see the patient's low blood pH).

E The pain of myocardial infarction is an ischemic pain due to activation of pain receptors. It is therefore a type of nociceptive pain. Abnormal activity of pain transmission pathways to the brain is a feature of neuropathic, not nociceptive, pain.

▶ *Learning objective:* Explain the reasons for cold and clammy skin of a patient suffering from the onset of a myocardial infarction.

2. Answer: D

Most myocardial infarctions reduce cardiac output. This reduction triggers immediately the activation of the sympathetic nervous system, which in turn causes the following:

▶ Skin vasoconstriction (cold skin), mediated by the activation of α_1-adrenoceptors that are predominant on skin vessels

▶ Sweating (clammy skin), mediated by the activation of M_3 cholinergic receptors (postganglionic neurons innervating the sweat glands are sympathetic cholinergic neurons)

A Release of renin from the macula densa increases the synthesis of angiotensin II, which is a vasoconstricting agent. Angiotensin II levels are increased in myocardial infarction, but this is not the primary cause of skin vasoconstriction.

B The activation of the parasympathetic nervous system should have caused skin vasodilation, not vasoconstriction.

C Endothelins are increased after myocardial infarction. They are powerful vasoconstricting agents, but they are cleared rapidly after release. Therefore a systemic vasoconstricting effect is unlikely.

E Adenosine is released from the infarcted area but would cause vasodilation, not vasoconstriction.

▶ *Learning objective:* Explain the reasons for bulging jugular veins in a patient suffering from the onset of a myocardial infarction.

3. Answer: B

The jugular veins carry blood from the head to the superior vena cava that empties into the heart. The external jugular vein is closest to the skin and can sometimes be seen as a ropelike bulge on the side of the neck. This bulge is an indirect indicator of the central venous pressure (i.e., the pressure in the thoracic vena cava), which is often a good approximation of right atrial pressure. Myocardial infarction affects predominantly the left ventricle. The decreased contractility of the ventricle causes an acute impairment of left atrial empting during systole, which in turn causes an increase in left atrial pressure, in pulmonary vein pressure, and, eventually, in right atrial pressure.

A, E A decreased afterload or preload would improve the pumping activity of the heart; therefore the central venous pressure would decrease, not increase.

C An increased heart rate would increase cardiac output and thus decrease, not increase, the central venous pressure.

D Blockage of the inferior vena cava decreases preload; therefore the central venous pressure would decrease, not increase.

▶ *Learning objective:* Explain the pathological condition that can cause an S3 gallop on heart auscultation.

4. Answer: C

The S3 gallop is caused by blood from the left atrium slamming into an already overfilled ventricle during diastolic filling. It is called a gallop because tripling of heart sounds resembles the three-beat gallop of a horse. S3 is heard in several illnesses. It can normally be heard in healthy children and adults up to age 40. S3 heard after 40 years of age usually indicates an illness. Although having only intermediate sensitivity, the S3 is a highly specific finding among older adults with heart failure. Most myocardial infarctions lead to acute heart failure due to the sudden, large decrease in heart contractility.

Among several proposed theories, the most likely explanation for S3 is that when the rush of blood into the heart ventricles during filling comes to a sudden halt (i.e., it reaches maximum filling) the kinetic energy of the blood movement is converted to vibration. These vibrations can sometimes be heard. The higher the inflow rate and the higher the filling rate, the greater the blood deceleration and the more likely an S3 will occur.

A Left ventricular failure can cause an impending pulmonary edema, but pulmonary edema is not the cause of S3.

B, D, E These arrhythmias can occur after myocardial infarction, but they are not the cause of the third heart sound.

▶ *Learning objective:* Recognize the pairs of lab exams that are most indicative of an ongoing myocardial infarction.

5. Answer: C

Troponin I and CK-MB ratio are the two cardiac markers most frequently used to assist the diagnosis of myocardial infarction. The elevation of both troponin I and CK-MB fraction in the present patient are consistent with myocardial necrosis.

▶ Troponin I is a protein unique to the heart muscle and highly concentrated in cardiomyocytes. It is released with very small areas of heart damage as early as 1 to 3 hours after injury, and levels return to normal within 5 to 14 days. The more damage there is to the heart, the greater the amount of troponin I there will be in the blood. The very high troponin I level in M.G.'s blood indicates that the infarct was quite extensive. The troponin I test has high sensitivity and specificity and is the preferred test to assist the diagnosis of myocardial infarction. Elevated troponin levels are considered diagnostic.

▶ The CK-MB fraction measures the blood level of CK-MB, the bound combination of two variants (isoenzymes CKM and CKB) of the enzyme phosphocreatine kinase. CK-MB typically begins to rise 4 to 6 hours after the onset of infarction, and elevations return to baseline within 36 to 48 hours. This means that CK-MB, unlike troponins, cannot be used for the late diagnosis of an acute myocardial infarction but can be used to suggest reinfarction if levels rise again after declining.

A, D, F Blood K^+ levels are increased, due to the necrosis of cardiac cells, but this sign occurs in many diseases that are due to, or associated with, cell necrosis.

B, E, F Acidosis (see the low plasma pH) occurs frequently in myocardial infarction, but can also occur in many other disorders.

▶ *Learning objective:* Explain the hemodynamic consequence of the early aspirin administration to a patient with a myocardial infarction.

6. Answer: D

It has been clearly shown that acute use of aspirin can decrease both mortality and recurrence of a myocardial infarction. Virtually all vascular occlusive events, including acute myocardial infarction and occlusive cerebrovascular accidents, are initiated by platelet activation and aggregation, with subsequent activation of the clotting cascade. Aspirin works by inhibiting platelet aggregation, which in turn decreases thrombus expansion and local ischemia.

A, B Aspirin causes effects opposite to those listed.

C, E Aspirin has no effects on cardiac hemodynamics.

▶ *Learning objective:* Explain why aspirin is given at low doses to prevent platelet aggregation.

7. Answer: A

Aspirin irreversibly inhibits the activity of cyclooxygenase type 1 (COX-1) in the platelets to inhibit the production of thromboxane A2 (TA2; a promoter of platelet aggregation) and at higher doses the activity of cyclooxygenase type 2 (inducible, COX-2) in the endothelial cells to inhibit the synthesis of prostacyclin (PGI2; an inhibitor of platelet aggregation). However, endothelial cells produce new cyclooxygenase in a matter of hours, whereas the anuclear platelets cannot replenish the enzyme. Therefore the low dose used is sufficient for causing an inhibition of TA2 production that lasts for the life of the platelets. Higher doses are potentially less efficacious because of a longer inhibition of prostacyclin production, which would cause an increase in platelet aggregation.

B Most adverse effects of aspirin are dose-dependent, but the decreased risk of adverse effects is not the reason why aspirin is given at low doses.

C Aspirin has no effect on platelet ADP receptor. This receptor is irreversibly blocked by P2Y12 receptor antagonists like clopidogrel.

D Adhesion of platelets to the vascular endothelium is a consequence of platelet aggregation. Aspirin inhibits, not favors, platelet aggregation.

E The rupture of an atherosclerotic plaque occurs when a thin-cap fibroatheroma is broken by the coronary pressure. Aspirin is not involved in plaque rupture.

▶ *Learning objective:* Explain the main action that mediates the therapeutic effect of nitroglycerin in myocardial infarction.

8. Answer: D

Sublingual, intravenous, and oral nitrate preparations are currently used in the management of myocardial infarction. The two main effects that mediate the therapeutic efficacy of these drugs are

- ▶ dilatation of large coronary arteries and arterioles, which may lead to increased perfusion of ischemic zones
- ▶ dilatation of large veins that decreases preload, reduces ventricular volumes, and causes a fall in pulmonary capillary wedge pressure

The main scope of giving nitroglycerin to patients with myocardial infarction is to allay chest pain. Since this ischemic pain is most likely due to the release of pain-producing substances from the infarcted area, an increased perfusion of the ischemic zones can decrease this release, thereby decreasing the pain.

An additional effect is the drug-induced decrease in preload due to the dilation of the large veins. In conclusion, nitroglycerin can allay pain by both decreasing oxygen demand and increasing oxygen supply in the infarcted area.

A Nitroglycerin can dilate arteries, thus decreasing afterload, but the effect is less pronounced than the dilation of large veins and is not the primary action that mediates the pain-reducing activity of this drug.

B, C, E All these can be actions of high doses of nitroglycerin, but they are not the primary action that mediates the pain-reducing activity of this drug.

▶ *Learning objective:* Identify the endogenous compound that mediates the pharmacological action of nitrates.

9. Answer: D

Nitrates release free nitrite ions, which in turn are converted into nitric oxide. Nitric oxide causes the activation of guanylyl-cyclase, leading to an increase in cGMP, which in turn produces dephosphorylation of myosin light chain. Myosin is no longer able to interact with actin, resulting in vascular smooth muscle relaxation.

A Bradykinin is one of the metabolites produced during myocardial ischemia and infarction that can activate cardiac spinal (sympathetic) sensory neurons to cause chest pain. It is not involved in the mechanism of action of nitroglycerin.

B Myocardial infarction can either increase the heart cAMP (through activation of the sympathetic system) or decrease it (by decreasing oxygen supply to cardiac cells), but nitroglycerin does not directly affect cAMP.

C Myocardial infarction can increase the heart norepinephrine (through activation of the sympathetic system), but nitroglycerin does not directly affect this neurotransmitter.

E Adenosine is released from the infarcted area, but nitroglycerin has no direct activity on adenosine actions.

▶ *Learning objective:* Explain the molecular mechanism that mediates the analgesic effect of morphine.

10. Answer: D

The analgesic effect of opioids like morphine is mediated by the activation of opioid receptors. These receptors are primarily inhibitory receptors, coupled with G proteins. The main transduction mechanisms of these receptors are activation of phospholipase C or inhibition of adenylyl cyclase. Two well established consequences of this transduction are

▶ at the presynaptic level, blockade of voltage-gated Ca^{2+} channels, thereby reducing the release of a large number of neurotransmitters (most often glutamate but also acetylcholine, norepinephrine, serotonin, and substance P)
▶ at the postsynaptic level, opening of ligand-gated K^+ channels, thereby evoking an inhibitory postsynaptic potential (IPSP)

A Presynaptic voltage-gated Ca^{2+} channels are blocked, not opened, by opioids.

B Closing of Cl^- channels on postsynaptic neurons would cause depolarization of the cell membranes, thereby evoking an excitatory postsynaptic potential. Opioids do not affect Cl^- channels.

C Substance P is an excitatory neurotransmitter of nociceptive nerve terminals. Its release would cause an increase in pain transmission. Opioids inhibit, not stimulate, substance P release.

E Glutamate is an excitatory neurotransmitter of nociceptive nerve terminals. Its release would cause an increase in pain transmission. Opioids inhibit, not stimulate, glutamate release from nociceptive nerve terminals.

▶ *Learning objective:* Explain the molecular mechanism of action of alteplase.

11. Answer: C

It has been shown that fibrinolytic drugs like alteplase can substantially decrease the mortality of myocardial infarction when given within 12 hours of symptom onset. However, these drugs are less effective and have more adverse effects than percutaneous coronary intervention, and are therefore used when this procedure cannot be performed, as in the present case. All fibrinolytic drugs act by catalyzing the conversion of plasminogen to plasmin. The older compounds of this class (very rarely used today) activate both plasminogen in the blood and plasminogen that is already bound to fibrin, whereas the newer compounds (alteplase, reteplase, tenecteplase), preferentially activate plasminogen bound to fibrin. This would avoid, at least in part, the induction of a systemic lytic state.

A Fibrinolytic drugs do not affect thrombin bound to fibrin. This thrombin is resistant even to inactivation by antithrombin III.

B This would be the mechanism of action of thrombin.

D This would be the mechanism of action of heparin.

E This would inhibit, not promote, fibrinolysis.

F Fibrinolytic drugs do not affect the synthesis of plasminogen.

▶ *Learning objective:* Describe a serious adverse effect that can occur after the administration of alteplase.

12. Answer: C

Bleeding (most common in cerebral and intestinal vessels) is the most frequent adverse effect of fibrinolytic drugs like alteplase. These drugs can cause what is called a systemic lytic state because the systemic formation of plasmin destroys coagulation factors. Bleeding is dose-dependent, and hemorrhagic stroke can occur in up to 2% of patients receiving the drug.

A Disseminated intravascular coagulation is a pathological process characterized by the widespread activation of the clotting cascade, which in turn causes the formation of blood clots in the small blood vessels throughout the body. Fibrinolytic drugs do not cause this disorder.

B Acute liver failure can cause bleeding, but alteplase-induced bleeding does not cause acute liver failure.

D Pulmonary embolism can be treated, not caused, by alteplase.

E Patients suffering from ulcerative colitis are at increased risk of alteplase-induced bleeding, but alteplase does not cause ulcerative colitis.

▶ *Learning objective:* Identify the endogenous compound that functions as a molecular target of enoxaparin.

13. Answer: C

Enoxaparin is a low-molecular-weight heparin (LMWH).

Antithrombin III (ATIII) is a protease inhibitor that slowly neutralizes many activated coagulation factors, especially thrombin and Xa, by forming stable complexes with them (a "suicide substrate"). Both regular heparin and LMWHs accelerate the activity of ATIII by increasing (up to 1,000-fold) the rate of ATIII-coagulation factor reaction. Once ATIII and the coagulation factor have formed a complex, heparin quickly dissociates and binds to other ATIII molecules. The combination of ATIII unfractionated heparin increases degradation of both factor Xa and thrombin, whereas LMWHs more selectively increase degradation of factor Xa.

A Plasmin is an enzyme present in blood that degrades many blood plasma proteins, including fibrin clots. The synthesis of plasmin is activated by fibrinolytic drugs.

B Vitamin K is the vitamin involved in the synthesis of II, VII, IX, and X coagulation factors as well as the endogenous anticoagulant proteins C and S.

D Glycoprotein IIb/IIIa is a protein that activates a specific receptor on platelets. This activation is the final common pathway on an enzyme involved in the final pathway for platelet aggregation.

E Fibrinogen is the coagulation factor I that is converted by the thrombin into fibrin.

▶ *Learning objective:* Describe an advantage of enoxaparin over the standard unfractionated heparin.

14. Answer: A

LMWHs, such as enoxaparin, cause a lower incidence of bleeding complications, which could be related to the fact that these agents preferentially inhibit factor Xa (thrombin inhibition requires a larger heparin molecule). The risk of bleeding complication is decreased but not abolished, because bleeding complications can occur even with LMWHs.

B The oral bioavailability of both HMW and LMW heparins is zero.

C High-molecular-weight heparin (HMWH) causes transient thrombocytopenia in up to 15% of patients and severe thrombocytopenia (which is antibody mediated) in up to 5% of patients. LMWH causes thrombocytopenia is < 1%. Therefore the risk of thrombocytopenia is reduced, but not abolished.

D LMWHs do not have antiplatelet activity.

E HMWH causes an allergic reaction in about 10% of patients. LMWHs cause allergic reactions in about 1% of patients. Therefore the risk of allergic reaction is reduced, but not abolished.

▶ *Learning objective:* Describe the molecular mechanism of action of metoprolol.

15. Answer: D

Metoprolol is a selective β-receptor blocker. Activation of all β-receptors increases the synthesis of cAMP through an increased activity of adenylate cyclase. By blocking these receptors, all β-blockers do the opposite (i.e., the activity of adenylate cyclase is decreased).

A Guanylate cyclase catalyzes the synthesis of cGMP. Its activity can be reduced, indirectly, by antimuscarinic drugs, not by β-blockers.

B Phospholipase C catalyzes the synthesis of inositol 1,4,5-triphosphate/diacylglycerol (IP3/DAG). Its activity can be reduced by antimuscarinic drugs, not by β-blockers.

C Phospholipase A2 catalyzes the synthesis of eicosanoids. Its activity can be reduced by glucocorticoids, not by β-blockers.

E Tyrosine kinase enzyme is a transmembrane receptor that mediates the action of several endogenous compounds, including insulin. Its activity is not reduced by β-blockers.

▶ *Learning objective:* Describe a long-term therapeutic effect of metoprolol in patients with myocardial infarction.

16. Answer: C

Cardiac remodeling is defined as alteration in the structure (dimensions, mass, shape) of the heart (called cardiac or ventricular remodeling) in response to hemodynamic load and/or heart injury in association with neurohormonal activation. It may occur after myocardial infarction, hypertension, myocarditis, and valvular disorders. Cardiac remodeling is generally accepted as a determinant of the clinical course of heart failure, and patients with major remodeling have an increase of ventricular mass and volume that progressively worsens cardiac function. The two neurohormonal systems that are primarily involved in the cardiac remodeling process are the renin–angiotensin–aldosterone system and the sympathetic system. This explains why angiotensin-converting enzyme inhibitors, angiotensin blockers, aldosterone antagonists, and selective β-blockers like metoprolol can reduce remodeling.

A By blocking β-adrenoceptors chronically, all β-blockers cause an upregulation, not a downregulation, of β-adrenoceptors.

B By blocking $β_1$-adrenoceptors in the macula densa, all β-blockers decrease, not increase, renin secretion.

D Nonselective β-blockers decrease gluconeogenesis by blocking $β_2$-adrenoceptors in the liver, but metoprolol is a selective β-blocker; therefore it has negligible effects on gluconeogenesis. Moreover, a decreased gluconeogenesis has nothing to do with the long-term therapeutic effect of the drug in the patient's disease.

E β-Blockers have minor effects on preload because the increased diastolic time would increase preload, but the vasodilation, caused by the decreased renin secretion, would decrease it. An increased preload would adversely affect heart failure.

17. Answer: E

Clopidogrel is an antiplatelet drug that causes an irreversible inhibition of ADP receptors, thereby inhibiting ADP-mediated platelet aggregation. Aspirin is the first-line antiplatelet drug for prevention of recurrence of myocardial infarction, but clopidogrel is frequently added to aspirin.

A, B, C, D The blockade of all these receptors can decrease platelet aggregation, but these receptors are not blocked by clopidogrel.

▶ *Learning objective:* Explain why clopidogrel is often administered with aspirin to patients with myocardial infarction.

18. Answer: A

A platelet ADP receptor inhibitor like clopidogrel is often administered in addition to aspirin to patients with STEMI. The two drugs are synergistic and enhance each other's effects. This is in accordance with the general rule of pharmacology that synergism is most likely when the same final effect of both drugs is reached through different mechanisms of action.

B Gastric toxicity of aspirin is quite rare with the antiplatelet dosage of the drug. Regardless, clopidogrel cannot decrease this toxicity.

C Aspirin resistance can occur after long-term use, but clopidogrel cannot decrease this resistance.

D, E Clopidogrel does not affect the pharmacokinetics of aspirin.

▶ *Learning objective:* Explain the molecular mechanism of action of lisinopril.

19. Answer: B

Lisinopril is an ACE inhibitor. The converting enzyme peptidyl dipeptidase hydrolyzes angiotensin I to angiotensin II and catalyzes bradykinin breakdown.

By inhibiting this enzyme, ACE inhibitors lead to

▶ inhibition of the renin–angiotensin system
▶ increased plasma levels of bradykinin

Both actions lead to relaxation of vascular smooth muscle, but the first action is the most important.

A ACE inhibitors can inhibit, not stimulate, the metabolism of bradykinin.

C Blockade of angiotensin II receptors is the mechanism of action of angiotensin blockers like losartan, not of ACE inhibitors.

D By inhibiting the synthesis of angiotensin II, more angiotensin I is available, and therefore its metabolism would be increased, not decreased.

E By inhibiting the synthesis of angiotensin II less angiotensin II is available; therefore its metabolism is indirectly decreased, not increased.

▶ *Learning objective:* Describe a common adverse effect of ACE inhibitors.

20.   Answer: C

A dry, disturbing cough is a typical adverse effect of ACE inhibitors that occurs in up to 20% of patients and is most likely due to the increased plasma levels of bradykinin, as kinins are known to cause contraction of nonvascular smooth muscle.

A By blocking aldosterone synthesis ACE inhibitors tend to cause hyperkalemia, not hypokalemia.

B ACE inhibitors are antihypertensive agents, so hypertension is unlikely.

D, E ACE inhibitors do not cause these effects.

Case 32

Parkinson's Disease

G.I., a 52-year-old man, was admitted to the neurology clinic because of a mild, intermittent resting tremor in his right hand that had worsened over the past 2 months and had recently progressed to the contralateral hand. He admitted that it took a little more effort to get movement started and that his muscles felt a little stiff. The patient also noticed a loss in the sense of smell and excessive sweating, especially during the night.

G.I.'s medical history was significant for hypercholesterolemia, partially controlled with lovastatin. The patient never smoked and denied the use of alcohol or illicit drugs. His family history was unremarkable.

Physical examination showed a well-nourished man with a notable lack of normal changes in facial expression. He spoke slowly with a monotone voice. A right-sided resting tremor of the pill-rolling type was noted, which decreased during finger-to-nose coordination testing. A cogwheel rigidity was elicited by passively bending both arms. An impairment with fine coordination was made apparent by the rapid alternating movements and finger taps. G.I.'s gait was slow but otherwise normal, with slightly bent posture, and he had no problem with his balance. A handwriting sample was progressively smaller in size, indicating micrographia.

A diagnosis of early, mild Parkinson's disease was made, and the patient was dismissed from the clinic with a prescription of rasagiline. His symptoms did not improve after 2 months of therapy, and the neurologist discontinued rasagiline and prescribed pramipexole.

Four months later, G.I. returned to the neurology clinic for a routine follow-up visit. He stated that his slowness and stiffness had improved but the tremor was minimally changed, and he still suffered occasionally from insomnia. He also noted that he sometimes had the urge to walk a great distance, with no purpose or destination, and he underwent binge eating at times. The neurologist explained that G.I.'s symptoms were most likely related to pramipexole. The daily dose of the drug was decreased, and benztropine was added to the therapy.

One year later G.I. was admitted to the neurology clinic because of worsening of his disease, in spite of the ongoing therapy with pramipexole and benztropine. G.I. reported that he no longer had trouble with compulsive behavior, but he felt an increased rigidity, stiffness, and tremor. He was slower in all activities and was tired throughout much of the day. Physical examination confirmed the patient's report and revealed a loss of balance resulting in gait abnormalities. The neurologist decided to add to the ongoing therapy a levodopa/carbidopa combination and entacapone.

After 2 years of levodopa/carbidopa therapy, G.I. started experiencing periods of substantial immobility lasting for a few minutes that occurred 2 to 4 hours after the last levodopa intake. Sometimes these periods were followed by a sudden switching to a fluidlike state of improved mobility, but often by a period of dyskinetic activity. The neurologist added amantadine to the current therapy and tried to change the dose and time of administration of levodopa, with little success. Eventually he decided to prescribe subcutaneous injections of apomorphine. He also prescribed another drug to counteract a disturbing adverse effect of apomorphine.

Questions

1. G.I. was diagnosed with Parkinson's disease. Which of the following pairs of brain structures was most likely primarily involved in the pathogenesis of the disease?

A. Locus ceruleus–raphe nuclei

B. Locus ceruleus–globus pallidus

C. Locus ceruleus–subthalamic nucleus

D. Globus pallidus–subthalamic nucleus

E. Raphe nuclei–subthalamic nucleus

F. Raphe nuclei–globus pallidus

2. Which of the following neuronal proteins is thought to play a primary role in the pathogenesis of Parkinson's disease?

A. Syntaxin

B. Synaptobrevin

C. Synuclein

D. Ankyrin

E. Spectrin

3. G.I. showed several symptoms and signs typical of Parkinson's disease. Which of the following symptoms and signs could also most likely affect this patient?

A. Dry mouth

B. Choreiform movements

C. Symmetric leg weakness

D. Aphasia

E. Insomnia

4. Rasagiline was prescribed to G.I. The inhibition of which of the following enzymes most likely mediated the therapeutic effect of the drug in the patient's disease?

A. DOPA decarboxylase

B. Monoamine oxidase B

C. Dopamine β-hydroxylase

D. Tyrosine hydroxylase

E. Catechol O-methyltransferase

5. Pramipexole was prescribed to G.I. Which of the following molecular actions most likely mediated the therapeutic effect of the drug in the patient's disease?

A. Blockade of presynaptic dopaminergic receptors

B. Increased synthesis of dopamine in the striatum

C. Decreased peripheral biotransformation of levodopa

D. Activation of postsynaptic dopaminergic receptors

E. Inhibition of central dopamine metabolism

F. Upregulation of dopaminergic receptors in the striatum

6. Which of the following adverse effects would most likely occur during the first days of pramipexole treatment?

A. Diplopia

B. Visual impairment

C. Peripheral edema

D. Nausea

E. Diarrhea

F. Muscle cramps

7. Benztropine was prescribed to G.I. Which of the following actions most likely mediated the therapeutic effect of the drug?

A. Inhibition of levodopa metabolism in the striatum

B. Inhibition of the abnormally high cholinergic tone in the striatum

C. Activation of dopaminergic receptors in the striatum

D. Blockade of nicotinic neuronal receptors in the cerebral cortex

E. Increased GABAergic activity in the subthalamic nucleus

8. Benztropine was most likely given to improve which of the following of G.I.'s signs?

A. Gait disturbances

B. Tremor

C. Bradykinesia

D. Insomnia

E. Pramipexole-related symptoms

9. G.I. started a treatment with a levodopa/carbidopa combination. Which of the following actions most likely mediated the therapeutic effect of levodopa in the patient's disease?

A. Downregulation of dopaminergic receptors in striatal neurons

B. Increased synthesis of dopamine in subthalamic neurons

C. Increased synthesis of dopamine in striatal neurons

D. Inhibition of DOPA decarboxylase in striatal neurons

E. Inhibition of catechol O-methyltransferase in nigral neurons

10. Carbidopa is almost always added to levodopa in the therapy of Parkinson's disease. Which of the following statements best explains the reason for this addition?

A. More levodopa is available to enter the brain.

B. Active transport of dopamine into the brain is increased.

C. Carbidopa activates brain dopamine receptors.

D. Carbidopa counteracts most central adverse effects of levodopa.

E. Peripheral biotransformation of dopamine is increased.

11. The risk of which of the following adverse effects of levodopa could increase by adding carbidopa to the treatment?

A. Nausea and vomiting

B. Tachycardia

C. Postural hypotension

D. Dyskinesias

E. Diarrhea

12. Entacapone was prescribed to G.I. The inhibition of which of the following enzymes most likely mediated the therapeutic effect of the drug in the patient's disease?

A. DOPA decarboxylase

B. Monoamine oxidase B

C. Dopamine β-hydroxylase

D. Tyrosine hydroxylase

E. Catechol O-methyltransferase

13. G.I. started experiencing periods of immobility that occurred 2 to 4 hours after the last levodopa intake (wearing-off reactions) or periods of akinesia alternating with normal motility (on–off reactions). Which of the following was most likely the pathological basis of these motor fluctuations?

A. Decreased activity of central glutamatergic pathways

B. Increased intestinal absorption of levodopa

C. Insufficient dopamine delivery to central receptors

D. Increased peripheral inhibition of DOPA-decarboxylase

E. Decreased activity of central catechol O-methyltransferase

14. Amantadine was prescribed to G.I. Which of the following molecular actions most likely contributed to the therapeutic effect of the drug in the patient's disease?

A. Inhibition of levodopa metabolism

B. Increased dopamine synthesis and release

C. Activation of N-methyl-D-aspartate (NMDA) receptors

D. Activation of muscarinic receptors

E. Activation of adenosine receptors

15. Apomorphine was prescribed to G.I. Activation of which of the following brain receptors most likely mediated the therapeutic effect of the drug in the patient's disease?

A. α-adrenoceptors

B. 5-hydroxytryptamine 2 (5-HT2) receptors

C. Muscarinic receptors

D. D_2 receptors

E. α-Amino-3-hydroxy-5-methyl-4-isoxazolepropionic acid (AMPA) receptors

283

16. Which of the following drugs was most likely prescribed to counteract the most disturbing adverse effect of apomorphine?

A. Trimethobenzamide

B. Ondansetron

C. Scopolamine

D. Diphenhydramine

E. Meclizine

Answers and Explanations

▶ *Learning objective:* Identify the two brain structures most likely involved in the pathogenesis of Parkinson's disease.

1. Answer: D

Parkinson's disease involves primarily the basal ganglia of the brain. These are a group of interconnected subcortical nuclei that include the striatum, substantia nigra, globus pallidus, and subthalamic nucleus. Basal ganglia function via a series of reciprocal innervations among themselves and the cortex.

The striatum receives inputs from the cerebral cortex and substantia nigra and sends output to the thalamus via the globus pallidus and subthalamic nucleus. The thalamus then feeds back information to the motor cortex.

Two pathways connect the striatum to the thalamus:

▶ A direct pathway (excitatory)
▶ An indirect pathway (inhibitory), through the globus pallidus and the subthalamic nucleus

Both pathways receive input from dopaminergic neurons of the substantia nigra, pars compacta. The cell membranes of the striatal neurons that form the direct pathway have mainly D_1 excitatory receptors, whereas the cell membranes of neurons of the indirect pathway have mainly D_2 inhibitory receptors.

In Parkinson's disease more than 50% of nigral neurons are lost. The destruction of dopaminergic neurons decreases the activity of the excitatory direct pathway and increases the activity of the inhibitory indirect pathway.

The net result is that excitatory thalamic feedback to the cortex is reduced.

Excitatory cholinergic interneurons are also present in the striatum. The destruction of dopaminergic neurons in the substantia nigra leads to excessive cholinergic activity of these neurons.

A, B, C, E, F The locus ceruleus and raphe nuclei are not basal ganglia and are not primarily involved in Parkinson's disease.

▶ *Learning objective:* Identify the brain protein that is thought to play a primary role in the pathogenesis of Parkinson's disease.

2. Answer: C

Synuclein is a presynaptic neuronal and glial cell protein, which can form insoluble fibrils in Lewy bodies. Although there are rare cases of Parkinson's disease without Lewy bodies, the pathological hallmark of Parkinson's disease remains synuclein-filled Lewy bodies in the nigrostriatal system; therefore the disease is today widely recognized as a *synucleinopathy*. Because this synucleinopathy can occur in many other parts of the nervous system, including the lower brain stem, the hypothalamus, the thalamus, and the neocortex, many experts believe that Parkinson's disease is a relatively late development of a brain synucleinopathy.

A, B Syntaxins and synaptobrevins are membrane proteins of secretory vesicles participating in exocytosis.

D, E Ankyrins and spectrins are cytoskeletal proteins that play an important role in maintenance of plasma membrane integrity and cytoskeletal structure.

▶ *Learning objective:* Identify a very common symptom of Parkinson's disease.

3. Answer: E

Insomnia is very common in Parkinson's disease, affecting over 50% of the patients. It may result from nocturia, from excessive nighttime sweating, or simply from the inability to turn in bed. Insomnia may contribute to depression, exacerbate cognitive impairment, or cause excessive daytime sleepiness.

A Sialorrhea and drooling, not dry mouth, are typical symptoms of Parkinson's disease thought to be caused by impaired or infrequent swallowing, rather than hypersecretion.

B Choreiform movements suggest Huntington's disease, not Parkinson's disease.

C Symmetric weakness is a common sign of a motor neuron disease, not of Parkinson's disease.

D Aphasia is a language impairment that results from dysfunction of the language centers in the cerebral cortex and basal ganglia or of the pathways that connect them. Aphasia can be, very rarely, associated with severe and long-lasting Parkinson's disease.

▶ *Learning objective:* Select the enzyme that can be inhibited by rasagiline.

4. Answer: B

Rasagiline and selegiline are selective irreversible inhibitors of monoamine oxidase B. Two types of monoamine oxidase have been distinguished in the nervous system. Monoamine oxidase A metabolizes norepinephrine, dopamine, and serotonin; monoamine oxidase B metabolizes dopamine selectively. By inhibiting the enzyme, these drugs increase the availability of dopamine in the striatum. Rasagiline seems preferable to selegiline because it does not have amphetamine metabolites and is preferentially used for early treatment of Parkinson's disease, as in the present case. However, the therapeutic effect of monoamine oxidase inhibitors is modest when given alone.

A DOPA decarboxylase is an enzyme that catalyzes several different decarboxylation reactions, including the conversion of L-DOPA to dopamine.

C Dopamine β-hydroxylase is the enzyme that catalyzes the conversion of L-DOPA to dopamine.

D Tyrosine hydroxylase is the enzyme that catalyzes the conversion of tyrosine to DOPA.

E Catechol O-methyltransferase is an enzyme that catalyzes the metabolism of catecholamines.

▶ *Learning objective:* Identify the molecular mechanism of action of pramipexole.

5. Answer: D

Pramipexole is a dopamine D_2 and D_3 receptor agonist. Dopaminergic agonists are used as monotherapy for mild Parkinson's disease or as adjunctive therapy in advanced-stage disease. They are especially effective in patients under 65, as in the present case. Although these drugs are not as effective as levodopa they have a number of potential advantages. Because they act directly on dopamine receptors they do not require conversion to an active product. Therefore, unlike levodopa, which needs a normal dopaminergic neuron for dopamine synthesis, they act independently of degenerating dopaminergic neurons. They have a longer half-life than levodopa formulations, reducing the need for multiple daily dosing. Moreover, the initial therapy with dopamine agonists is associated with a lower incidence of response fluctuations and dyskinesias. As a drug class, these drugs provide adequate control of symptoms in up to 80% of patients with early disease stage, and this control is sustained for 2 to 3 years or more in most cases.

A Pramipexole is a dopamine agonist, not antagonist.

B This would be the mechanism of action of levodopa.

C This would be the mechanism of action of carbidopa.

E Dopaminergic receptors in the striatum are already upregulated because of the decreased availability of dopamine. Activation of dopamine receptors would cause downregulation, not upregulation of these receptors.

▶ *Learning objective:* Identify a very common adverse effect of pramipexole.

6. Answer: D

Nausea, with or without vomiting, can occur in up to 45% of patients and can be a significant problem during therapy with dopamine agonists. The symptom is primarily due to activation of dopamine receptors in the nucleus of tractus solitarius (a purely sensory nucleus located in the medulla oblongata) and chemoreceptor trigger zone (located in the area postrema, on the floor of the fourth ventricle). Nausea is the adverse effect that most commonly causes treatment discontinuation, but with continued use, many patients develop tolerance to this effect.

A, B, C, E, F All these adverse effects can occur with pramipexole, but their incidence is < 5%.

▸ *Learning objective:* Explain the mechanism of action of benztropine in Parkinson's disease.

7. Answer: B

Benztropine is an antimuscarinic drug. In Parkinson's disease, the loss of dopaminergic neurons results in a loss of the balance that normally exists between excitatory acetylcholine-mediated and inhibitory dopamine-mediated neurotransmission. Antimuscarinic drugs, such as trihexyphenidyl and benztropine (the two antimuscarinic most frequently used in Parkinson's disease), are thought to act by blocking muscarinic receptors in the striatum, thus decreasing the abnormally high cholinergic tone resulting from lack of the inhibitory activity of dopamine.

A, C, D, E Antimuscarinic drugs do not have these effects.

▸ *Learning objective:* Identify the signs of Parkinson's disease that are primarily improved by benztropine.

8. Answer: B

Benztropine is an antimuscarinic drug. Centrally acting anticholinergic drugs have been used for many years in Parkinson's disease and continue to have a useful role for patients who are less than 70 years of age and have disturbing tremor. They also may be useful in patients with more advanced disease who have persistent tremor despite treatment with dopamine agonists, as in the present case. Anticholinergic drugs are relatively contraindicated

in the elderly, for whom adverse effects are particularly troublesome.

A, C, D, E Anticholinergic drugs do not significantly improve these symptoms.

▸ *Learning objective:* Select the action that mediates the therapeutic effect of levodopa in Parkinson's disease.

9. Answer: C

Dopamine cannot cross the blood–brain barrier and therefore has no therapeutic effects in Parkinson's disease when given via the peripheral circulation. However, levodopa, the immediate precursor of dopamine, is readily carried across the blood–brain barrier by the neutral amino acid transporter. In the brain, levodopa is biotransformed into dopamine within the presynaptic terminals of dopaminergic neurons in the striatum. These neurons are therefore able to increase the synthesis and release of dopamine, and this balances the loss of dopaminergic neurons, which constitutes the pathological basis of Parkinson's disease.

A Dopaminergic receptors are upregulated, not downregulated, due to the decreased availability of dopamine in the striatum.

B Subthalamic neurons are mainly glutamatergic, not dopaminergic.

D This action would decrease, not increase, the availability of dopamine in the basal ganglia.

E The inhibition of catechol O-methyltransferase would increase the availability of dopamine, but this is an action of catechol O-methyltransferase inhibitors, not of levodopa.

▸ *Learning objective:* Explain why carbidopa is added to levodopa in the therapy of Parkinson's disease.

10. Answer: A

All effects of levodopa, both central and peripheral, are due to its transformation to dopamine, a reaction catalyzed by the enzyme DOPA decarboxylase. Carbidopa is an inhibitor of DOPA decarboxylase that cannot cross the blood–brain barrier. When levodopa is given in combination with carbidopa, the peripheral metabolism of levodopa is reduced, resulting in higher plasma levels of levodopa; thus more levodopa is available to enter the brain. Concomitant administration of levodopa and carbidopa may reduce the daily requirement for levodopa by about 75%.

B Dopamine cannot enter the brain.

C Central dopamine agonists, such as pramipexole, ropinirole, and rotigotine, not carbidopa, activate brain dopamine receptors.

D By decreasing the peripheral conversion of levodopa to dopamine, carbidopa can decrease most peripheral adverse effects of levodopa because they are all related to dopamine. However, the increased central concentration of levodopa can increase, not decrease, the central adverse effects of levodopa.

E Because less dopamine is available peripherally, its peripheral biotransformation is decreased, not increased.

▶ *Learning objective:* Identify the adverse effect of levodopa that could increase by adding carbidopa to the treatment.

11. Answer: D

By inhibiting DOPA decarboxylase, carbidopa diminishes the peripheral metabolism of levodopa, increasing its availability to enter the central nervous system. Therefore, the needed dose of levodopa can be lowered by about fivefold, and the risk of peripheral adverse effects of levodopa are consequently reduced. On the contrary the risk of central adverse effects of levodopa, such as dyskinesias, is increased because more levodopa can enter the brain.

A Nausea and vomiting are due to activation of D2 receptors on the chemoreceptor trigger zone located in the brain stem but outside the blood–brain barrier. Nausea and vomiting occur in about 80% of patients when levodopa is given alone but are reduced to less than 20% of patients when the drug is given with carbidopa.

B, C, E These are peripheral adverse effects of levodopa. Their risk is decreased, not increased, by adding carbidopa to the treatment.

▶ *Learning objective:* Identify the enzyme that can be inhibited by entacapone.

12. Answer: E

Entacapone is a peripheral inhibitor of catechol O-methyltransferase. Substrates of the enzyme are levodopa and catecholamines. The inhibition of DOPA decarboxylase by carbidopa is associated with compensatory activation of catechol O-methyltransferase that catalyzes the transformation of levodopa into 3-O-methyldopa in the gut and the liver. Elevated levels of 3-O-methyldopa have been associated with a poor therapeutic response to levodopa, perhaps in part because the metabolite competes with levodopa for an active carrier mechanism that transports the drug across the blood–brain barrier.

By inhibiting catechol O-methyltransferase, entacapone causes the following actions:

▶ More levodopa becomes available for active transport into the central nervous system.
▶ Less 3-O-methyldopa can compete with levodopa for active transport into the central nervous system.

A DOPA decarboxylase is an enzyme that catalyzes several different decarboxylation reactions, including the conversion of L-DOPA to dopamine.

B Monoamine oxidase is an enzyme that catalyzes the metabolism of catecholamines.

C Dopamine β-hydroxylase is the enzyme that catalyzes the conversion of L-DOPA to dopamine.

D Tyrosine hydroxylase is the enzyme that catalyzes the conversion of tyrosine to DOPA.

▶ *Learning objective:* Explain the most likely reason for the wearing-off and on–off reactions in Parkinson's disease.

13. Answer: C

Wearing-off and on–off reactions are almost invariable consequences of long-term levodopa treatment in patients with Parkinson's disease. The exact pathophysiological basis of these reaction is still uncertain but is most likely related to insufficient delivery of dopamine to central receptors. Early in the course of the disease, sufficient dopaminergic neurons remain that can store dopamine derived from levodopa administration and release it in a more physiological manner. These neurons act as a buffer against fluctuating levodopa concentrations. As the disease progresses dopamine terminals are lost, and the capacity to store dopamine presynaptically is diminished. This can impair buffering of the rising and falling concentrations of levodopa. Consequently, dopamine receptors are subject to intermittent or pulsatile phasic stimulation rather than by a more physiological tonic stimulation. This explanation is in line with the clinical observation that wearing-off and on–off reactions may be diminished by the administration of dopamine agonists that act directly on dopamine receptors. However, several patients experience motor fluctuations despite a treatment regimen that includes a dopamine agonist, as in the present case.

A Overactivity, not decreased activity, of central glutamatergic pathways may be involved in wearing-off and on–off reactions.

B, D, E These actions would increase, not decrease, the delivery of dopamine to central receptors.

▶ *Learning objective:* Identify the most likely mechanism of action of amantadine in Parkinson's disease.

14. Answer: B

Amantadine is an antiviral agent that also has relatively weak antiparkinsonian properties. The exact mechanism of the antiparkinsonian action of the drug is still uncertain, but amantadine probably acts by increasing dopamine synthesis and release and by blocking dopamine reuptake. The drug can also block NMDA glutamate receptors, adenosine receptors, and muscarinic receptors, and these actions likely can contribute to the antiparkinsonian effect of the drug. Amantadine is used mainly as an adjunctive agent in managing levodopa-induced dyskinesias, as in

the present case. It has been shown that the drug can cause about 50% reduction in dyskinesia severity and duration without adversely impacting motor performance.

A Inhibition of levodopa metabolism would be the mechanism of action of carbidopa.

C NMDA receptors can be blocked, not activated, by amantadine.

D Muscarinic receptors can be blocked, not activated, by amantadine.

E Adenosine receptors can be blocked, not activated, by amantadine.

▶ *Learning objective:* Identify the action of brain receptors that most likely mediates the therapeutic effect of apomorphine in Parkinson's disease.

15. Answer: D

Apomorphine is a potent dopaminergic agonist that has good affinity for D_2, D_3, D_4, and D_5 receptors, but low affinity for D_1 receptors. The drug, injected subcutaneously, has a rapid onset of action (5–10 minutes), and a short duration (60–90 minutes). Because of these properties, apomorphine is approved as a rescue treatment (given occasionally or several times a day) for patients with severe periods of immobility who are unresponsive to other measures, as in the present case.

A Apomorphine can cause blockade, not activation, of α-adrenoceptors.

B Apomorphine can cause blockade, not activation, of 5-HT2 receptors.

C, E Apomorphine has no significant actions on these receptors.

▶ *Learning objective:* Select the drug that is commonly prescribed to counteract the most frequent adverse effect of apomorphine.

16. Answer: A

Apomorphine is a highly emetogenic drug, most likely because it activates D_2 adrenoceptors in the chemoreceptor trigger zone. The development of nausea and vomiting is almost universal when subcutaneous apomorphine is administered, and the drug was used in the past to induce vomiting in cases of poisoning. A pretreatment with an antiemetic, such as trimethobenzamide, for 3 days is recommended before apomorphine is introduced and is then continued as long as apomorphine is administered. Trimethobenzamide most likely acts by blocking D_2 receptors in the chemoreceptor trigger zone.

B Serotonin antagonists, such as ondansetron, are effective antiemetics, but their combination with apomorphine is contraindicated because it may cause severe hypotension.

C, **D**, **E** These drugs are used when nausea and vomiting are due to motion sickness. They are not effective in cases of apomorphine-induced vomiting.

Case 33

Peptic Ulcer Disease

S.T., A 72-year-old woman, presented to her family physician complaining of having had epigastric pain for more than 1 month and feeling weak for the past week. The pain occurred daily, was nonradiating, and increased at night and between meals. The pain seemed to decrease on ingesting food or antacids. The patient also stated that 3 days ago she noticed tarry stools with no blood. She denied decreased appetite, weight loss, nausea, or vomiting. S.T. smoked one pack of cigarettes daily and drank 1 to 2 cans of beer per week.

S.T. had been suffering with osteoarthritis for 2 years and had been taking acetaminophen two to three times daily to relieve her pain. One year ago, S.T. suffered from an episode of traveler's diarrhea that disappeared after an appropriate antibiotic therapy. Recently she had been diagnosed with a small atherosclerotic plaque on the right external carotid artery and had been taking lovastatin since then.

Physical examination showed a well-nourished woman in slight distress with the following vital signs: blood pressure 136/82 mm Hg, pulse 68 bpm, respirations 18/min. Abdomen examination showed normal bowel sounds and mild epigastric tenderness. Rectal examination disclosed melenic stools in the rectal vault. The rest of physical examination was unremarkable.

The physician ordered endoscopy and blood exams. Endoscopy results indicated a 3 cm clean-based gastric ulcer, and a biopsy of the ulcer site identified *Helicobacter pylori*. A 14-day triple therapy was prescribed with clarithromycin, metronidazole, and omeprazole, followed by omeprazole alone for 4 weeks.

Two weeks later S.T. underwent a urea breath test that turned out to be positive, indicating that the *H. pylori* infection was not eradicated. The physician decided to start a new therapy that contained tetracycline, bismuth subsalicylate, metronidazole, and omeprazole.

Questions

1. S.T. was found to have a 3-cm gastric ulcer. Secretion of hydrochloric acid from the stomach cells plays a primary role in the pathophysiology of peptic ulcer disease. Which of the following transport systems mediates the hydrogen secretion into the stomach lumen?

A. Lipid diffusion

B. Aqueous diffusion

C. Bulk flow transport

D. Facilitated diffusion

E. Active transport

2. S.T. complained of epigastric pain that increased at night. Which of the following mediators of hydrochloric acid secretion best explains this symptom?

A. Prostaglandins

B. Norepinephrine

C. Adenosine

D. Acetylcholine

E. Somatostatin

3. S.T.'s epigastric pain was relieved by antacids. These drugs are able to antagonize the effects of the hydrochloric acid secreted by gastric parietal cells. Which of the following pharmacological terms best defines this acid–antacid antagonism?

A. Competitive

B. Noncompetitive

C. Functional

D. Chemical

E. Pharmacokinetic

4. S.T. was found to have a 3 cm gastric ulcer. Which of the following facts of the patient's history most likely contributed to the appearance of her disorder?

A. Osteoarthritis disease

B. Acetaminophen use

C. Smoking

D. Drinking beer

E. Carotid artery plaque

F. Traveler's diarrhea

5. *Helicobacter pylori* was identified in S.T.'s ulcer site. Which of the following molecular actions most likely contributes to the bacterium-induced decrease in gastric mucosal defense?

A. Inhibition of interleukin-1 secretion

B. Activation of vasoactive intestinal peptide (VIP)

C. Blockade of muscarinic M_3 receptors

D. Inhibition of somatostatin secretion

E. Activation of prostaglandin receptors

6. S.T.'s therapy included omeprazole. Which of the following enzymes was most likely inhibited by this drug?

A. Na^+/K^+ ATPase

B. H^+/K^+ ATPase

C. Protein kinase A

D. Adenylyl cyclase

E. Ca^{2+} ATPase

7. Omeprazole has a half-life of about 1 hour, but the drug is usually given once daily. Which of the following statements best explains the long duration of action of the drug?

A. It accumulates inside the gastric cells.

B. It is biotransformed into a compound with a long half-life.

C. It remains in the gastric lumen for a long time.

D. It inactivates H^+/K^+ ATPase irreversibly.

E. It undergoes enterohepatic cycling.

8. Proton pump inhibitors inhibit both fasting and meal-stimulated hydrochloric acid secretion. Which of the following is the percent inhibition of 24-hour hydrochloric acid secretion of a standard dose of these drugs?

A. 75%

B. 80%

C. 85%

D. 90%

E. > 95%

9. After oral administration a high concentration of proton pump inhibitors occurs in the stomach lumen. Which of the following pharmacokinetic actions can account for this high concentration?

A. Negligible systemic drug absorption
B. Ion-trapping mechanism
C. Inhibition of stomach emptying
D. Fast conversion from inactive prodrug
E. Fast dissolution of the pharmaceutical form

10. Clarithromycin was prescribed to S.T. Which of the following structures of bacterial cells represents the primary site of action of the drug?

A. Cytoplasmic membrane
B. Outer membrane
C. Porin channels
D. Peptidoglycan layer
E. Ribosomes
F. DNA

11. Metronidazole was prescribed to S.T. because *H. pylori* is quite sensitive to this antibiotic. Which of the following properties of this bacterium best explains the reason for its sensitivity to metronidazole?

A. Gram-negative
B. Urease-positive
C. Microaerophilic
D. Oxidase-positive
E. Lactose-negative

12. A triple therapy with omeprazole, clarithromycin, and metronidazole was prescribed to S.T. Which of the following statements best explains why this drug regimen is a first-line therapy for *H. Pylori*–associated ulcers?

A. Omeprazole is rapidly bactericidal against *H. pylori*.
B. The regimen eliminates almost completely the risk of ulcer recurrence.
C. Clarithromycin greatly enhances the bactericidal activity of omeprazole.
D. Metronidazole greatly enhances the bactericidal activity of omeprazole.
E. The regimen can cure the ulcer in up to 70% of cases.

13. A combination of clarithromycin and metronidazole is currently used to treat *H. pylori*–associated ulcers. Which of the following statements best explains the most likely reason for this combination?

A. To reach bactericidal effect
B. To kill concomitant bacteria
C. To increase metronidazole half-life
D. To reduce drug resistance
E. To improve metronidazole absorption

14. Bismuth salt was prescribed to S.T. Which of the following actions most likely mediated the therapeutic effect of the drug in the patient's disease?

A. Increased gastric mucus secretion
B. Blockade of H_2 histamine receptors in parietal cells
C. Formation of a protective layer over the ulcer
D. Inhibition of H^+/K^+ ATPase
E. Blockade of M_3 muscarinic receptors in parietal cells

Answers and Explanations

▸ *Learning objective:* Identify the transport system that mediates the hydrogen secretion into the stomach lumen.

1.   Answer: E

Hydrochloric acid (HCL) is secreted by parietal cells that contain an extensive secretory network (deep invaginations of the plasma cell membrane called canaliculi). Chloride and hydrogen ions are secreted separately from the cytoplasm of parietal cells, which are mixed in the canaliculi. Hydrochloric acid is then secreted into the lumen of the oxyntic gland and gradually reaches the main stomach lumen. Hydrogen is formed in the parietal cells by carbonic anhydrase that splits carbonic acid into H^+ and bicarbonate. Hydrogen is then secreted by the enzyme H^+/K^+ adenosine triphosphatase (ATPase) (an antiporter named the proton pump). This pump is unique to the parietal cells and transports the H^+ against a concentration gradient of about 3 million to 1, which is the steepest ion gradient formed in the human body. A transport system that works against a concentration gradient is referred to as active transport.

A, B, C, D All these transport systems are passive (i.e., they do not require metabolic energy from the cell.

▸ *Learning objective:* Identify the mediator of hydrochloric acid secretion that most likely facilitates the nocturnal gastric pain in patients with peptic ulcer.

2.   Answer: D

The pain from gastric ulcer is related to an increased concentration of hydrochloric acid on the ulcer crater. It is well known that parasympathetic activity increases during the night, which in turn increases acetylcholine (ACh) secretion. ACh can activate the proton pump through four distinct physiological events:

▸ In the body of the stomach, the vagal postganglionic muscarinic nerves release ACh, which directly activates the proton pump.

▸ In the lamina propria of the body of the stomach, ACh triggers histamine secretion from enterochromaffin-like cells. Histamine also activates the proton pump.
▸ In the stomach antrum, ACh released from preganglionic vagal neurons activates peptidergic postganglionic neurons, which release gastrin-release peptide. This peptide in turn stimulates antral G cells to produce and release gastrin. Gastrin stimulates acid secretion directly by activation of the proton pump and indirectly by stimulation of histamine secretion by enterochromaffin-like cells.
▸ In both the antrum and the corpus, the vagus nerve inhibits D cells, thus reducing their release of somatostatin and reducing background inhibition of gastrin release.

A, B, C, F All these mediators inhibit, not stimulate, hydrochloric acid secretion.

▸ *Learning objective:* Explain the definition of chemical antagonism.

3.   Answer: D

Antacid drugs are weak bases that react chemically with gastric hydrochloric acid to form a salt and water. In this way, gastric acidity is reduced. This acid–antacid antagonism does not involve pharmacokinetic action or receptor occupancy but only a chemical combination between two molecules. It is therefore defined as chemical antagonism.

A, B, C All these antagonisms involve receptor occupancy.

E Pharmacokinetic antagonism occurs when a drug prevents the absorption or stimulates the elimination of the drug to be antagonized, reducing its concentration at the site of action.

▸ *Learning objective:* Identify a risk factor for the development of gastric ulcer.

4.   Answer: C

Cigarette smoking is a risk factor for the development of peptic ulcer and its complications. Smoking impairs ulcer healing and increases the incidence of recurrence.

Risk correlates with the number of cigarettes smoked per day. The smoking risk is thought to be primarily related to nicotine, which can have several actions decreasing the gastric mucosa defense against aggressive factors. The most important of these actions include the following:

▶ Activation of neuronal nicotinic receptors on ganglionic parasympathetic neurons, which, in turn causes an acetylcholine-mediated stimulation of the proton pump and a stimulation of pepsinogen secretion
▶ Stimulation of the synthesis of platelet-activating factor and endothelin, two potent ulcerogenic agents
▶ Stimulation of release of vasopressin, which can play an aggressive role in peptic ulcer formation through its vasoconstricting activity
▶ Inhibition of prostaglandin biosynthesis in the gastric mucosa

A, B Osteoarthritis per se is not a risk factor for peptic ulcer but is thought to be associated with the disease because of the frequent concomitant use of nonsteroidal anti-inflammatory drugs as analgesics that can cause gastric cell damage. In the present case, however, acetaminophen was used as the analgesic. The drug is a very weak prostaglandin inhibitor in peripheral tissues and does not cause gastric cell damage.

D Although alcohol is a strong promoter of hydrochloric acid secretion, the patient's alcohol consumption was quite small. No definite data link moderate amounts of alcohol to the development of peptic ulcer.

E, F These are not risk factors for peptic ulcer disease.

▶ *Learning objective:* Describe a mechanism that most likely contributes to *H. pylori*–induced decrease in gastric mucosal defense.

5. Answer: D

Helicobacter pylori is a gram-negative, microaerophilic bacterium that has adapted to thrive in acid. It can cause gastritis, peptic ulcer disease, gastric adenocarcinoma, and low-grade gastric

lymphoma. The microorganism disrupts the normal mucosal defense and repair through several mechanisms, one of which is thought be the inhibition of somatostatin secretion. Somatostatin is the most important hormone that inhibits gastrin release. It is secreted by the D cells of the stomach antrum, and its release is stimulated by a fall in the gastric pH to less than 3. In the absence of somatostatin, high gastrin levels cause increased local release of histamine, which stimulates the gastric parietal cells to secrete increased levels of acid.

A Interleukin-1 is an inflammatory cytokine. *H. pylori* causes an infection, and, therefore, inflammatory cytokines are activated, not inhibited.

B, C, E All these actions would cause a decrease of hydrochloric acid activity that is instead increased by *H. pylori*.

▶ *Learning objective:* Identify the enzyme that is inhibited by omeprazole.

6. Answer: B

Omeprazole is the prototype of proton pump inhibitors, a class of drugs that inhibit the enzyme H^+/K^+ ATPase (proton pump) in the gastric parietal cells, suppressing the secretion of hydrogen ions into the gastric lumen.

A Na^+/K^+ ATPase is a transport protein found in all mammals' cells. It is inhibited by cardiac glycosides.

C Protein kinases are enzymes that phosphorylate several substrates, modulating their action. Inhibitors of specific protein kinases (tyrosine kinase) are used in the treatment of cancer.

D Adenylyl cyclase is the enzyme that catalyzes cyclic adenosine monophosphate synthesis.

E Ca^{2+} ATPase is a transport protein in the plasma membrane of cells that serves to remove Ca^{2+} from the cell.

▶ *Learning objective:* Explain the reason for the long duration of action of omeprazole.

7. Answer: D

All proton pump inhibitors have short half-lives (1–2 hours), but they inactivate H^+/K^+ ATPase irreversibly. Therefore, their pharmacological activity lasts more than 18 hours, which is the time needed for the synthesis of new H^+/K^+ ATPase molecules. However, because not all proton pump molecules are inactivated with the first dose of the drug, 3 to 4 days of daily medication are required for full antacid activity of the drug.

A, B, C, E Omeprazole does not display these actions.

▶ *Learning objective:* Identify the percent inhibition of 24-hour hydrochloric acid secretion of a standard dose of proton pump inhibitors.

8. Answer: E

Proton pump inhibitors are the most effective inhibitors of hydrochloric acid secretion. When standard doses are administered they inhibit > 95% of daily hydrochloric acid secretion. Equivalent doses of the different agents on the market show little difference in clinical efficacy.

A, B, C, D See correct answer explanation.

▶ *Learning objective:* Explain the pharmacokinetic action that can account for the high concentration of omeprazole in the stomach lumen.

9. Answer: B

Oral proton pump inhibitors are inactive prodrugs that are formulated as acid-resistant, enteric-coated capsules or tablets. After passing through the stomach into the duodenal lumen the enteric coating dissolves, and the prodrug is absorbed. Proton pump inhibitors are weak bases, with pK_a of 4 to 5, and are mainly nonionized (i.e., lipid soluble) in the extra- and intracellular fluids, where pH is > 7. Therefore, the prodrug diffuses readily across all cell membranes and can reach the canaliculi of the parietal cell of the stomach. Since the pH of the canaliculi is the same as that of the stomach lumen (< 2) the prodrug becomes ionized and is trapped in the gastric fluid, where it can be concentrated more than 1,000-fold. The prodrug also rapidly undergoes conversion into its active form, which can bind covalently the H^+/K^+ ATPase, irreversibly inactivating the enzyme.

A Proton pump inhibitors are well absorbed from the duodenal lumen.

C Inhibition of stomach emptying can retard drug absorption, because most drugs are mainly absorbed from the duodenal lumen, but proton pump inhibitors do not retard stomach emptying.

D Proton pump inhibitors must be converted to their active metabolites, but this conversion is not the reason for the high concentration of these agents in the stomach lumen.

E The enteric-coated pharmaceutical form dissolves into the duodenal lumen and cannot account for the high concentration of the drug in the stomach lumen.

▶ *Learning objective:* Identify the site of action of erythromycin.

10. Answer: E

Clarithromycin is a macrolide antibiotic. These drugs act by binding reversibly to the 50S subunit of the bacterial ribosome, which is therefore the primary cellular site of action of macrolides.

A, B, C, D, F Macrolide antibiotics do not bind to these structures.

▶ *Learning objective:* Describe the property of *H. pylori* that makes it very sensitive to metronidazole.

11. Answer: C

Metronidazole is an antibiotic that can kill most microaerophilic and anaerobic bacteria and anaerobic protozoa. Its selectivity for microaerophilic and anaerobic bacteria is a result of the ability of these microorganisms to reduce metronidazole to its active form intracellularly. This process includes intracellular electron transport proteins, such as ferredoxin, which is found only in microaerophilic and anaerobic bacteria. *H. pylori* is a microaerophilic bacterium, which explains its sensitivity to metronidazole.

A, B, D, E All these are properties of *H. pylori*, but they cannot explain its sensitivity to metronidazole.

▶ *Learning objective:* Explain why a three-drug regimen is the first-line therapy for *H. pylori*–associated ulcers.

12. Answer: B

For the *H. pylori*–associated ulcers there are two therapeutic goals: eradicate *H. pylori* and heal the ulcer. The first goal is important because it has been shown that eradication of *H. pylori* almost completely eliminates the risk of ulcer recurrence. The most effective regimens for *H. pylori* eradication are combinations of two antibiotics and a proton pump inhibitor. After completion of triple therapy, the proton pump inhibitor should be continued for 3 to 6 weeks to ensure complete ulcer healing. This regimen heals the peptic ulcer and prevents almost completely the risk of ulcer recurrence.

A, C, D Omeprazole has no bactericidal activity against *H. pylori*. It does create a hostile environment for *H. pylori* by increasing gastric pH.

E The triple regimen can cure the ulcer in more than 90%, not in up to 70%, of cases.

▶ *Learning objective:* Explain the reason for the concomitant use of two antibiotics for the treatment of *H. pylori*–associated peptic ulcer.

13. Answer: D

Resistance strains to all antibiotics used against *H. pylori* infection have been discovered. Overwhelming evidence indicates that this resistance is essentially due to chromosomal mutations. Therefore, a concomitant treatment with two different antibiotics can significantly increase the success of the therapy. For example, if the frequency of mutation for the acquisition of resistance to one drug is 10^{-6} and that for a second drug

is 10^{-5}, the probability of two simultaneous, independent mutations in a single cell is the product of the two frequencies (i.e., 10^{-11}).

A Both clarithromycin and metronidazole exert a bactericidal effect against *H. pylori*.

B *H. pylori* infection is not a mixed infection, because other bacteria cannot survive in the acidic environment of the stomach.

C, E Metronidazole pharmacokinetics is not modified by the concomitant administration of another antibiotic.

▶ *Learning objective:* Explain the mechanism of action of bismuth salt in peptic ulcer disease.

14. Answer: C

When a first-line triple therapy fails to eradicate *H. pylori*, a second-line therapy is usually attempted, as in the present case. This therapy often includes bismuth compounds that exert several useful actions in peptic ulcer treatment. The most important is thought to be the protection of the damaged mucosa. The salts bind to the base of the ulcer, forming a protective layer that hinders the action of hydrochloric acid and pepsin.

A Increased gastric mucus secretion would be a mechanism of action of prostaglandins.

B Blockade of H_2 histamine receptors in parietal cells would be the mechanism of action of H_2 antagonists.

D Inhibition of H^+/K^+ ATPase would be the mechanism of action of proton pump inhibitors.

E Blockade of M_3 muscarinic receptors in parietal cells would be the mechanism of action of antimuscarinic drugs.

Case 34

Perimenopause and Osteoporosis

H.L., a 49-year-old woman, visited her gynecologist with the complaints of a sudden feeling of warmth on her chest and flushing of her skin, followed by sweating and chills, all of which would occur in episodes three to four times a day for the last 2 months. The symptoms would subside on their own, usually within 5 to 10 minutes. She reported that for the past 2 weeks, the symptoms had become more bothersome at night, when she would waken to find herself shivering and drenched in sweat.

H.L.'s menses had always been regular until 1 year ago. Her last menstrual period was 3 weeks ago, and she had had six menses in the last year. She was sexually active and reported that every time she did a pregnancy test after missing a period on the expected date, the results were negative. She was not using any hormonal contraceptive, only male condoms, and those only occasionally.

H.L. had no history of surgery or of thromboembolic disorders. She had no family history of breast or endometrial cancer. She had hypertension that was well controlled on hydrochlorothiazide and ramipril.

Physical examination was normal for a 49-year-old woman. Body mass index (BMI) was 25 kg/m². Vital signs were as follows:

- Blood pressure while lying: 122/78 mm Hg
- Blood pressure while standing: 120/74 mm Hg
- Pulse: 80 bpm
- Respirations: 16/min

Some laboratory tests were ordered with the following results:

Blood hematology

- Hemoglobin (Hb): 13 g/dL (normal 12–16)
- White blood cell count (WBC): 6,500/mm³ (normal 4,500–11,000)
- Calcium (Ca^{2+}): 9.5 mg/dL (normal 9–11)
- Estradiol: 30 pg/mL (normal 50–350)
- Follicle-stimulating hormone (FSH): 70 mIU/L (normal 1.6–15)
- Luteinizing hormone (LH): 42 IU/L (normal 1.30–10)
- Thyroid-stimulating hormone (TSH): 2.4 mIU/L (normal 0.5–4.5)
- Creatinine: 1 mg/dL (normal 0.6–1.2)
- Blood urea nitrogen (BUN): 10 mg/dL (normal 7–18)
- Sodium (Na^+): 136 mEq/L (normal 135–146)
- Potassium (K^+): 4 mEq/L (3.5–5.5)

Dual-energy X-ray absorptiometry (DEXA)

T-score: −2.5 (normal: −1 and above)

H.L.'s gynecologist explained to her that these symptoms, called hot flashes, occur in many women of her age and prescribed appropriate oral drugs to manage H.L.'s symptoms. She was also given a therapy for osteoporosis. During a follow-up visit after 3 months, she reported that she was no longer experiencing frequent symptoms of hot flashes and sudden sweating, but she complained about gastric acidity, which caused severe piercing pain in the upper part of her abdomen. Her doctor revised her osteoporosis treatment by substituting it with a nonoral drug that needed to be administered only once a year.

During her follow-up visit a year later, her doctor evaluated her condition and stopped the drugs that she was taking for the management of hot flashes.

One year later, she visited her physician again, complaining of vaginal itching and pain during intercourse. Examination showed that her labia minora were thin and the vaginal mucosa was pale, thin, and dry. She asked her doctor to prescribe the same drugs that she had taken for managing her hot flashes, because she had had a satisfactory sexual life while she was on that therapy. However, her doctor explained to her that the same therapy was no longer required and prescribed an appropriate drug formulation to treat her symptoms.

Questions

1. H.L. had episodic symptoms of sudden warmth on her skin, sweating, and chills. Which of the following medical conditions most likely caused these symptoms?

A. Perimenopause

B. Menopause

C. Endometrial carcinoma

D. Migraine

E. Pheochromocytoma

2. H.L.'s lab results revealed that her FSH and LH levels were above the normal range. Which of the following changes in her physiology resulted in elevation of gonadotropin levels?

A. Decreased gonadotropin-releasing hormone secretion

B. Decreased estrogen synthesis in the adipose tissue

C. Increased synthesis of adrenal sex hormones

D. Decrease in ovarian steroidogenesis

E. Increased catecholamine synthesis in the adrenal medulla

3. Which of the following changes in biochemical mediators is postulated to be the cause of vasomotor symptoms in a woman traversing the menopausal phase?

A. Increase in FSH and LH

B. Decrease in serotonin and increase in norepinephrine

C. Decrease in dopamine and increase in serotonin

D. Increase in histamine and decrease in epinephrine

E. Increase in TSH

4. The patient was prescribed an appropriate therapy to treat the symptoms of hot flashes. Which of the following agents did her physician most likely prescribe?

A. Conjugated equine estrogen

B. Medroxyprogesterone

C. Conjugated equine estrogen + medroxyprogesterone

D. Ethinyl estradiol

E. Levonorgestrel

5. The patient was also prescribed a progestin along with an estrogen. Addition of a progestin to the patient's hormonal therapy would most likely be beneficial in preventing the development of which of the following disorders?

A. Osteoporosis

B. Breast carcinoma

C. Hypertriglyceridemia

D. Endometrial cancer

E. Thromboembolism

6. H.L.'s DEXA scan suggested that she had moderate osteoporosis (T-score −2.5). Which of the following drugs would be most appropriate for long-term treatment of her osteoporosis?

A. Alendronate

B. Calcium and vitamin D

C. Teriparatide

D. Calcitonin

E. Sevelamer

7. Which of the following actions most likely mediated the therapeutic effect of bisphosphonates in osteoporosis?

A. Inhibition of binding of receptor activator of nuclear factor κ-B ligand (RANKL) to RANK

B. Inhibition of osteoclast activity by interfering with biochemical pathways inside osteoclasts

C. Increase in new bone formation by stimulating osteoblast activity

D. Increase in bone preservation by stimulating estrogen receptors

E. Inhibition of the interaction of parathyroid hormone with its receptors

301

8. The patient was tolerating the hormonal replacement therapy (HRT) well. How long is the HRT recommended to continue to manage vasomotor symptoms?

A. Lifelong

B. 1–2 years

C. 5–10 years

D. Until endometrial hyperplasia develops

E. Until age 60

9. It is recommended that the HRT be continued for the shortest period of time with the smallest effective doses of gonadal hormones to treat moderate to severe vasomotor symptoms. The risk of which of the following diseases precludes long-term use of HRT?

A. Stroke

B. Osteoporosis

C. Atrophic vaginitis

D. Melanoma

E. Type 2 diabetes mellitus

10. H.L. started experiencing vaginal dryness, itching, and painful coitus after a year of stopping HRT. Which of the following drugs/drug formulations would be most appropriate for relieving her symptoms?

A. Oral estrogen therapy

B. Vaginal estrogen cream

C. Transdermal estrogen/progestin patch

D. Vaginal dinoprostone gel

11. H.L. developed gastritis that prompted her physician to switch to an alternative treatment for her osteoporosis. Which of the following was most likely this alternative treatment?

A. Intramuscular prednisone

B. Intravenous zoledronate

C. Subcutaneous teriparatide

D. Intravenous calcium gluconate

12. For a woman who has contraindications for the use of HRT, which of the following drugs could be an appropriate choice to treat menopausal vasomotor symptoms?

A. Sumatriptan

B. Phenytoin

C. Octreotide

D. Propranolol

E. Venlafaxine

Answers and Explanations

▶ *Learning objective:* Define perimenopause and menopause.

1. Answer: A

Menopause is defined as the last spontaneous episode of physiological uterine bleeding, and it is identified only retrospectively after 12 months of amenorrhea. Therefore a woman is already postmenopausal when she is identified as having reached menopause a year ago.

Perimenopause precedes menopause, usually by 2 to 3 years. During the perimenopausal phase, an age-related accelerated degeneration of oocytes occurs, and the ovaries become increasingly resistant to gonadotropin action. Due to these changes, a woman may experience irregular menses and vasomotor symptoms (hot flashes and night sweats). At menopause all ovarian follicles have been depleted.

A hot flash, is a subjective sensation of intense warmth of the upper body, typically lasting for 4 to 5 minutes, which can be preceded by palpitations or headache and weakness. The episode ends with profuse sweating and a cold sensation that causes shivering. The flash is due to vasomotor instability in response to declining estrogen levels.

B The patient had not reached menopause, because she had had her last menstrual period 3 weeks before visiting her physician.

C The irregular vaginal bleeding can be a symptom of endometrial carcinoma. Usually it is manifested as unexpected vaginal bleeding/spotting between periods. However, the vasomotor symptoms are typical of estrogen deficiency associated with menopause transition. Nevertheless, the patient would be examined to rule out any urogenital disorder before starting the treatment of her symptoms.

D Patient neither had a history nor presented with the signs and symptoms suggestive of migraine.

E Pheochromocytoma can cause hot flashes and sweating, but these are commonly associated with high blood pressure and postural hypotension. Both signs were absent in this patient.

▶ *Learning objective:* Describe the feedback regulation of the hypothalamus–pituitary–ovarian axis during menopause.

2. Answer: D

During perimenopause, there is an age-related acceleration in oocyte degeneration, resulting in decreased ovarian estrogen/progestin synthesis as well as decreased response of the ovaries to gonadotropins (FSH and LH). The hypothalamus–pituitary–ovarian reproductive axis is regulated by feedback responses from the ovarian hormones inhibin, estrogen, and progestins. A decrease in the levels of these hormones results in upregulation of gonadotropin release. However, gonadotropins cannot exert any stimulatory effect on the degenerated ovaries. Due to this, the levels of gonadotropins start increasing during the perimenopausal period. Menopause is characterized by a > 90% decrease in estrogen levels. FSH levels are increased 10- to 20-fold, and those of LH are about threefold higher at menopause. These levels peak around 2 to 3 years after menopause and stay elevated thereafter. Gonadotropins can be extracted from the urine of postmenopausal women and purified, and they were once used for therapeutic purposes as menotropins.

A GnRH secretion is increased, not decreased, in the absence of feedback from the ovarian hormones.

B Estrogen synthesis in the adipose tissue is increased, not decreased, because after menopause fat is one of the primary tissues where androstenedione is converted to estrone by the action of aromatase.

C Adrenal hormone synthesis is not under the control of the reproductive axis.

E Catecholamines from the adrenal medulla are not involved in regulating the reproductive axis.

▶ *Learning objective:* Describe the pathophysiology of vasomotor symptoms of menopause.

3. Answer: B

Vasomotor symptoms and genitourinary atrophy are associated with declining estrogen levels. Hot flashes, one type of vasomotor symptoms, are experienced by about 50 to 80% of women transitioning through menopause. Although the prevalence of vasomotor symptoms is highest during the 2 years after menopause, the onset of symptoms can begin during the perimenopause, as in the present case. Studies have shown that the vasomotor symptoms can persist for longer than 1 year in 80% and longer than 5 years in 25% of women.

Emergence of hot flashes is associated with declining estrogen levels that occur during menopause. Serotonin and norepinephrine are involved in temperature regulation. It has been suggested that a decline in estrogen levels leads to a decrease in serotonin levels and an increase in the levels of norepinephrine. Fluctuations in the levels of serotonin and norepinephrine cause activation of the body's heat-release mechanisms, leading to cutaneous vasodilation and sweating, as seen in hot flashes.

A, C, D, E These are not the triggers that cause hot flashes.

E Thyroid dysfunction can be a cause of menstrual irregularities. It is important to rule out thyroid dysfunction while evaluating a patient for menopausal symptoms. H.R.'s thyroid function was normal, as indicated by her TSH levels.

▶ *Learning objective:* List the estrogen and progestin compounds, routes of administration, and different regimens used to treat menopausal hot flashes.

4. Answer: C

Due to ovarian follicle degeneration, the ovaries stop responding to gonadotropins, so the steroidogenesis is suppressed, resulting in a decline in estrogen and progestin levels. The hot flashes are the result of a decline in estrogen levels. In a woman with an intact uterus, who experiences vasomotor symptoms due to menopause or transition through menopause, hormonal replacement therapy is started with both the ovarian hormones, an estrogen and a progestin.

Commonly used hormone formulations are oral, transdermal patch, and vaginal ring. Progestin can also be given via an intrauterine device. Some examples of estrogen–progestin replacement formulations are oral conjugated equine estrogens (CEE) + medroxyprogesterone acetate (MPA) and oral or transdermal estradiol-17β + norethindrone acetate.

The hormone replacement can be accomplished either by using the cyclic or the continuous method. With the cyclic method, withdrawal bleeding would occur during the hormone-free period, and in the continuous method, no hormone-free period is provided, so no withdrawal bleeding would occur. One of the adverse effects of hormone therapy is regular bleeding, bleeding that occurs apart from the withdrawal bleeding related to the hormone-free period of the cyclic method. Regular bleeding is more common (80% women) in women using the continuous method, even though these women do not have a cyclic withdrawal bleeding period.

A, D, E These are either estrogen-alone or progestin-alone preparations.

▶ *Learning objective:* Identify the disorder that can be prevented by adding a progestin to the estrogen in the menopausal replacement therapy.

5. Answer: D

Although hot flashes occur mainly due to estrogen deficiency, in a woman who has an intact uterus, a progestin is also added to the estrogen therapy. Use of hormone replacement therapy with an estrogen alone increases the risk of endometrial cancer 2- to 10-fold. The higher the dose and duration of estrogen therapy, the greater the risk of developing endometrial cancer. Increased risk persists for at least 5 years after discontinuation of estrogen therapy. Estrogen has proliferating effects on the endometrial lining and can cause endometrial hyperplasia that could progress to endometrial carcinoma. Progestin counteracts estrogen's proliferating effects, so addition of a progestin attenuates or eliminates the risk of endometrial cancer. Therefore, in a woman with an intact uterus, a progestin should be added to estrogen therapy. If the uterus was removed before menopause, there is no need to add a progestin to estrogen therapy.

A, B, C, E The addition of a progestin does not decrease the risk of these disorders.

▶ *Learning objective:* Identify the most appropriate drug for long-term treatment of osteoporosis.

6. Answer: A

H.L. had osteoporosis as indicated by the T-score. The T-score is the number of standard deviations above or below the mean for healthy 20- to 29-year-olds, as determined by dual energy X-ray absorptiometry. Osteoporosis is defined as a T-score of ≤ -2.5. A T-score between -2.5 and -1 indicates low bone density. A T-score of ≥ -1 is normal.

Osteoporosis due to menopause is due to declining levels of estrogen. Hormone replacement therapy (HRT) with estrogen alone or in combination with progestin is effective in preventing bone loss associated with menopause. HRT is indicated primarily to treat vasomotor symptoms and not osteoporosis. The bone protection effects of HRT are additional benefits. As long as the hormone replacement continues for the treatment of vasomotor symptoms, bone density will be maintained. However, bone loss resumes on discontinuation of HRT. Therefore, an alternative therapy should be considered for the long-term treatment of osteoporosis so that bone protection could continue even after the HRT is discontinued. Bisphosphonates (alendronate, zoledronate, pamidronate, risedronate, ibandronate) are currently the first-line drugs to treat and prevent osteoporosis, unless there is a contraindication (such as renal impairment) to their use. This is the reason H.L.'s renal function test was ordered, which had a normal result.

B Calcium and vitamin D alone would not be able to treat osteoporosis. These are added to the osteoporosis treatment, so as to provide adequate amounts of calcium to the bones to facilitate bone remodeling.

C Teriparatide, a recombinant parathyroid hormone, is recommended for the treatment of severe osteoporosis in patients who fail to respond adequately to other osteoporosis therapies.

D Calcitonin is not an effective drug to treat osteoporosis; moreover, its effects on bone are short lasting. This is a drug that can be used to manage hypercalcemia of malignancy for a short period of time (usually a few days, until the action of other drugs kicks in).

E Sevelamer is a drug used to manage hyperphosphatemia in chronic renal failure. This drug acts by chelating phosphate in the gastrointestinal tract to prevent its absorption.

▶ *Learning objective:* Describe the mechanism of action of bisphosphonates.

7. Answer: B

Bone resorption and bone formation are coupled by an interaction between osteoblasts and osteoclasts that follows these steps:

- ▶ Parathyroid hormone, shear stress, and transforming growth factor-β (TGF-β) cause osteoblast precursors to express the osteoclast differentiation factor RANKL.
- ▶ RANKL binds to RANK, a receptor expressed on osteoclast precursors.
- ▶ The RANKL–RANK binding interaction, together with macrophage colony-stimulating factor (M-CSF), causes osteoclast precursors to differentiate into mature osteoclasts.

- ▶ As mature osteoclasts resorb (erode) bone, matrix-bound factors, such as TGF-β, insulin-like growth factor-1 (IGF-1), other growth factors, and cytokines are released.
- ▶ These liberated factors stimulate osteoblast precursors to develop into mature osteoblasts, which begin to refill the resorption pits excavated by the osteoclasts.

Bisphosphonates are currently the most widely used antiresorptive drugs for treating osteoporosis. Once these agents enter the circulation, they reach the bone and are incorporated into the bone mineral, where they remain unmetabolized and biologically active. Once the bone is resorbed (eroded) by osteoclasts, the acid secreted by osteoclasts dissociates bisphosphonates from the bone mineral, and bisphosphonates are internalized by osteoclasts. Within the osteoclasts, bisphosphonates block a step in the mevalonate pathway. Disruption of this process decreases prenylation, the covalent attachment of certain lipids (farnesyl) to multiple proteins, including intracellular regulatory enzymes, such as guanosine triphosphatases. This impairs a number of osteoclastic functions and ultimately causes osteoclast apoptosis. This is how bisphosphonates inhibit bone erosion by osteoclasts.

A This would be the mechanism of denosumab.

C This would be the mechanism of teriparatide.

D This would be the mechanism of action of estrogens.

E This action would be counterintuitive to treat osteoporosis.

▶ *Learning objective:* Explain the appropriate duration of menopausal hormone therapy.

8. Answer: B

The primary indication for using HRT in a woman with menopause is to treat vasomotor symptoms (hot flashes and night sweats). About 40% of women in menopause experience vasomotor symptoms. In most of them, these symptoms subside with time without any treatment. In the rest, hormone therapy will most likely provide relief. In contrast to earlier beliefs and understanding about the management of the menopausal period with replacement therapy with estrogen and progestins for a prolonged period, several studies have provided a greater deal of insight into the effects of HRT on women in menopause, including the many adverse effects that can occur with long-term HRT. The results of these studies have suggested that HRT should be used with minimal effective doses of hormones for the shortest period of time, only to manage vasomotor symptoms. In most of the patients who experience vasomotor symptoms, the symptoms subside in 1 or 2 years, and then cessation of therapy can be tried by tapering the doses gradually.

A Lifelong hormone replacement therapy is not recommended as explained.

C Duration of 5 to 10 years is too long and is not recommended.

D One of the adverse effects of the estrogen component of HRT is endometrial hyperplasia that can progress to cause endometrial carcinoma. Waiting until the endometrial hyperplasia develops is incorrect.

E The median age of menopause in the developed world is 45 to 55 years. Continuing the HRT until age 60 is too long a period.

▶ *Learning objective:* Describe the adverse effects of menopausal HRT.

9. Answer: A

The results of the Women's Health Initiative study have suggested that long-term use of HRT in a postmenopausal woman can increase the risk of cardiovascular events, stroke, and certain cancers, such as breast and endometrial cancer. The longer the exposure to HRT, the greater the risk. The elevated risk of breast and endometrial cancer persists for at least 5 years after discontinuation of HRT. Studies have also suggested that the risk of breast cancer is greater in patients taking progestin-containing HRT compared to estrogen replacement alone. Estrogen replacement also doubles the risk of venous thromboembolic disease (deep vein thrombosis and pulmonary thrombosis).

B, C Estrogen replacement provides protection against osteoporosis and atrophic vaginitis.

D The association between development of melanoma and HRT has not been reported.

E HRT use has not been found to cause diabetes mellitus.

▶ *Leaning objective:* Describe an appropriate drug preparation for managing vaginal atrophy associated with menopause.

10. Answer: B

Deficiency of estrogen causes vaginal atrophy, and, unlike the vasomotor symptoms, vaginal atrophy does not reverse on its own with time. The vaginal mucosa appears pale, thin, and dry, causing the symptoms of pruritus and painful coitus. The mucosa of the urethra is also affected, resulting in increased incidence of urinary tract infections. About 10 to 40% of postmenopausal women experience these symptoms, and only 25% of those affected seek medical attention. Estrogen has growth-promoting effects on the urogenital mucosa and can reverse the atrophic changes.

A, C A systemic (oral or transdermal) HRT with estrogen alone or in combination with a progestin, depending upon if the patient has an intact uterus, is attempted only to treat vasomotor symptoms. When a woman does not have vasomotor symptoms and has only local urogenital symptoms, local therapy with estrogen alone is recommended. Local therapy would avoid unnecessary systemic exposure to gonadal hormones and their adverse effects.

D Dinoprostone is a prostaglandin analogue used to promote labor through ripening of the cervix.

▶ *Learning objective:* Describe the adverse effects of oral bisphosphonate therapy and alternative treatment options.

11. Answer: B

One of the adverse effects of bisphosphonate therapy with oral agents is gastritis and erosive esophagitis. To avoid this, especially the erosive esophagitis, a patient is advised to take the drug on an empty stomach in the morning with plenty of water and to maintain an upright posture for about 30 minutes after taking the drug.

If severe gastritis develops, as in the present case, the intravenous route can be used for administering the bisphosphonate drug. Two agents, zoledronate and pamidronate, are available for intravenous use. Zoledronate is administered by intravenous infusion over 30 minutes once a year.

A Prednisone is a glucocorticoid agent. Osteoporosis is one of the adverse effects of glucocorticoid therapy.

C Teriparatide is a recombinant parathyroid hormone. It is usually recommended in severe cases of osteoporosis when other drugs fail to achieve the desired therapeutic effects.

D Intravenous calcium gluconate is used to reverse hypocalcemic emergencies.

▶ *Learning objective:* Describe the alternatives to HRT to treat vasomotor symptoms of menopause.

12. Answer: E

Many selective serotonin reuptake inhibitors (SSRIs) and serotonin and norepinephrine reuptake inhibitors (SNRIs) have found to be effective in controlling vasomotor symptoms. Their efficacy is thought to be due to their effect on serotonin and norepinephrine levels. Two agents, venlafaxine and paroxetine, have been most studied for this indication and are considered the drugs of choice from this class of drugs. Venlafaxine is an SNRI and paroxetine is an SSRI. These drugs have therapeutic effects only in controlling vasomotor symptoms; they do not have any protective effect on bone mineral density or urogenital mucosa. The doses of these agents used for controlling the vasomotor symptoms of menopause are much lower than what is used for their antidepressant effects. Some of the common adverse effects of venlafaxine are dry mouth, decreased appetite, nausea, constipation, and increased blood pressure.

A, B, C, D All these drugs have no therapeutic role in controlling vasomotor symptoms of menopause.

Case 35   Pheochromocytoma

E.F., a 36-year-old black woman, was admitted to the hospital because of paroxysmal epi-sodes of increased heart rate, profuse sweating, throbbing headache, dyspnea, and squeezing chest pain, all of which began together abruptly. Each episode lasted about 30 minutes and subsided gradually. These episodes started 1 month ago and occurred weekly. The patient noticed that they were often precipitated by bending or by other movements that com-pressed the abdomen. Occasionally the episodes were accompanied by nausea, anxiety, and a sense of impending doom. E.F. also noticed that her first episode occurred a few hours after she took a tablet of an over-the-counter preparation for nasal decongestion.

Two weeks ago, E.F. was diagnosed with hypertension. Her blood pressure was staying near 180/120 mm Hg. She was prescribed a low-sodium diet, hydrochlorothiazide, and nife-dipine. After 2 weeks of therapy, her blood pressure was somewhat reduced (165/105 mm Hg), but she was still hypertensive.

E.F.'s father died at age 68 from a myocardial infarction. E.F.'s mother died at the age of 42 from Sipple's syndrome (medullary thyroid carcinoma, pheochromocytoma, and hyperpara-thyroidism). E.F. had only one brother, aged 45, who had been suffering from chronic obstruc-tive pulmonary disease (COPD) and recently recovered from a non-Hodgkin's lymphoma.

E.F. married 25 years ago to a white man, now aged 50. Her husband was healthy and both enjoyed a daily walk of about 1 hour. They had four children, all living and well.

The patient did not smoke, denied the use of illicit drugs, and drank alcohol occasionally.

Physical examination showed a well-developed and nourished black female who looked her age and was in no acute distress. She was 162 cm and weighed 68 kg.

Vital signs were as follows:

▶ Blood pressure while lying: 182/112 mm Hg (left arm), 178/110 mm Hg (right arm)
▶ Blood pressure while standing: 160/92 mm Hg (left arm), 154/96 mm Hg (right arm)
▶ Heart rate: 88 bpm and regular
▶ Respirations: 16/min and regular

The remainder of the physical examination was unremarkable.

Pertinent laboratory results on admission were as follows:

Blood hematology

▶ Red blood cell count (RBC): 4.8 x 10^6/μL (normal 4-6)
▶ Hemoglobin (Hb): 13 g/dL (normal 12–16)
▶ Hematocrit (HCT): 54% (normal 36–48)
▶ Mean corpuscular volume (MCV): 90 fL (normal 80–100)
▶ White blood cell count (WBC): 8 × 10^3/μL (normal 4–10)

Blood chemistry

▶ Fasting glucose: 152 mg/dL (normal 70–110)

- Creatinine: 1.1 mg/dL (normal 0.5–1.4)
- Blood urea nitrogen (BUN): 30 mg/dL (normal 5–25)
- Uric acid: 8 mg/dL (normal 4–8.5)
- Sodium (Na$^+$): 152 meq/L (normal 135–146)
- Potassium (K$^+$): 3.2 meq/L (normal 3.5–5.5)

Electrocardiography

Sinus tachycardia with some ventricular premature contractions

From the patient's report and examination, a preliminary diagnosis of pheochromocytoma was made and several tests were performed to confirm the diagnosis. The results were the following:

24 hours urinary catecholamine excretion

- Epinephrine: 90 µg/dL (normal 1.7–22.4)
- Norepinephrine: 855 µg/dL (normal 12.1–85.5)
- Total metanephrines: 18.8 mg/dL (normal < 1.3)

Clonidine test

- Plasma norepinephrine before clonidine: 1,500 pg/mL
- Plasma norepinephrine after clonidine: 1,300 pg/mL
- *(Normal response: norepinephrine falls to < 400 pg/mL)*

Positron emission tomography

A 4-cm left adrenal mass was detected.

The antihypertensive therapy was discontinued, and E.F. was prescribed phenoxybenzamine (10 mg twice daily initially, then increased by 10 mg increments every other day to a maintenance dosage of 30 mg twice daily). Two days later, propranolol was added. After 2 weeks of therapy E.F. was feeling well. She was free of headaches and was no longer having palpitations or episodes of sweating. She was scheduled for surgery to remove the left adrenal mass, and 5 days before the operation she was given metyrosine.

During surgery E.F.'s blood pressure fluctuated widely. Initially, with manipulation of the adrenal mass, her blood pressure rose to 200/100 mm Hg and her heart rate was 92 bpm. Intravenous (IV) labetalol was administered, and a few minutes later E.F.'s blood pressure went back to 140/88 mm Hg, and her heart rate was 64 bpm.

Postoperatively E.F.'s blood pressure remained normal, she felt well, and 4 days later she was discharged from the hospital. A follow-up appointment to monitor her blood pressure was planned and her children were being carefully evaluated to detect possible asymptomatic pheochromocytoma or multiple endocrine neoplasm (MEN) syndromes.

Questions

1. E.F. was diagnosed with pheochromocytoma. This tumor originates from which of the following cell types?

A. Smooth muscle cells

B. Endothelial cells

C. Lymphocytes

D. Chromaffin cells

E. Plasma cells

F. Glandular cells

2. Which of the following triad of symptoms, when occurring during paroxysmal attacks, strongly suggests the diagnosis of pheochromocytoma?

A. Headache–diarrhea–drowsiness

B. Urinary incontinence–drowsiness–dry mouth

C. Headache–profuse sweating–tachycardia

D. Drowsiness–joint pain–tachycardia

E. Joint pain–blurred vision–tachycardia

F. Drowsiness–diarrhea–blurred vision

3. E.F. stated that her first paroxysmal episode occurred a few hours after she took a tablet of an over-the-counter drug for nasal congestion. The physician thought that the intake of this medication most likely triggered the paroxysmal episode. Which of the following was most likely the drug taken by the patient?

A. Propranolol

B. Atropine

C. Pseudoephedrine

D. Loratadine

E. Prazosin

F. Caffeine

4. The antihypertensive treatment prescribed for E.F. was only partially effective. Which of the following statements best explains the reason for this modest effect?

A. The nifedipine dosage was very low.

B. Nifedipine acts as a functional antagonist of catecholamines.

C. Epinephrine increases nifedipine metabolism.

D. In pheochromocytoma L-type calcium channels are desensitized.

E. In pheochromocytoma most arterioles underwent sclerosis.

5. Which of the following data from E.F.'s family history would suggest an inherited cause of her pheochromocytoma?

A. The father's disease

B. The mother's disease

C. The brother's COPD

D. The brother's lymphoma

6. Which of the following phrases best explains the most likely cause of E.F.'s chest pain felt during the paroxysmal episodes?

A. Catecholamine-induced coronary vasoconstriction

B. Heart oxygen demand higher than oxygen supply

C. Dyspnea-induced intercostal muscle spasm

D. Sharp increase in pulmonary artery pressure

7. Which of the following cardiovascular effects was most likely induced by E.F.'s disease?

A. Decreased pulse pressure

B. Postural hypotension

C. Coronary vasoconstriction

D. Increased cardiac output

311

8. Activation of which of the following adrenoceptors most likely contributed to the increase in E.F.'s fasting plasma glucose level?

A. α_2

B. α_1

C. β_1

D. D_1

E. D_2

9. E.F. was given the clonidine test. Which of the following actions on brain autonomic receptors most likely mediates the diagnostic activity of this drug?

A. Activation of α_2-adrenoceptors

B. Blockade of imidazoline receptors

C. Activation of β_2-adrenoceptors

D. Blockade of muscarinic receptors

E. Activation of GABA receptors

10. Clonidine was barely able to modify E.F.'s plasma norepinephrine levels. Which of the following phrases best explains the reason for his result?

A. Pheochromocytoma strongly increases central sympathetic outflow.

B. Secretion of tumor catecholamines is autonomous.

C. Tumor catecholamines are very slowly metabolized.

D. Pheochromocytoma secretes mainly epinephrine.

11. E.F. was given phenoxybenzamine. Which of the following pairs of adrenoceptors represent the molecular targets of this drug?

A. α_1–β_1

B. α_1–β_2

C. α_1–α_2

D. α_2–β_1

E. α_2–β_2

F. β_1–β_2

12. Which of the following of E.F.'s symptoms and signs was most likely best antagonized by the phenoxybenzamine treatment?

A. Sweating

B. Palpitations

C. Bronchodilation

D. Hyperglycemia

E. Increased gluconeogenesis

13. Five days before surgery E.F. was given metyrosine. Which of the following molecular actions most likely mediated the therapeutic effect of this drug?

A. Blockade of β_1-adrenoceptors

B. Inhibition of catecholamine biosynthesis

C. Blockade of α_1-adrenoceptors

D. Stimulation of catecholamine biotransformation

E. Blockade of α_2-adrenoceptors

14. Two days after initiating therapy with phenoxybenzamine, propranolol was added to E.F.'s treatment. The primary reason for this addition was to counteract which of the following pheochromocytoma-induced effects?

A. Peripheral vasoconstriction

B. Increase in heart rate

C. Hyperglycemia

D. Sweating

E. Throbbing headache

15. E.F. was given labetalol during surgery. Which of the following sets of action depicted in the attached table most likely occurred shortly after the administration of this drug?

Set	Total peripheral resistance	Renin secretion	Heart rate
A.	↑	↑	↓
B.	↔	↓	↓
C.	↓	↔	↑
D.	↓	↓	↓
E.	↔	↔	↑

↑ = increased; ↓ = decreased; ↔ = negligible effect

Answers and Explanations

▶ *Learning objective:* Identify the cell type that can originate pheochromocytoma.

1. Answer: D

Pheochromocytoma is a tumor of chromaffin cells that secrete catecholamines. In 90% of cases pheochromocytomas are found in the adrenal medulla, but they may also be found in other tissues derived from neural crest cells (paraganglia of the sympathetic chain, carotid body, genitourinary system, brain). Chromaffin cells appear malignant upon microscopic examination, but the tumor is considered benign in 90% of cases (no metastases) and is curable if correctly diagnosed and properly treated. If misdiagnosed or improperly treated, it is usually fatal.

A Smooth muscle cells can originate leiomyomas or leiomyosarcomas.

B Endothelial cells can originate endotheliomas.

C Lymphocytes can originate lymphoblastic and lymphocytic leukemias.

E Plasma cells can originate plasmacytoma and multiple myeloma.

F Glandular cells can originate adenocarcinomas.

▶ *Learning objective:* Describer the triad of symptoms that strongly suggest the diagnosis of pheochromocytoma.

2. Answer: C

Paroxysmal attacks of headache, sweating, and tachycardia are so common that the lack of all three would virtually exclude the diagnosis of pheochromocytoma. Hypertension, the most prominent feature, may be paroxysmal (45%) or persistent (50%) and is rarely (5%) absent.

Other common symptoms include tachypnea, angina, nausea and vomiting, epigastric pain, paresthesias, constipation, and a sense of impending doom.

Epinephrine, norepinephrine, and dopamine are secreted by the adrenal medulla, and most of the symptoms of pheochromocytoma are due to the exces-

sive amount of catecholamines released during the paroxysmal attack. By activating β_1 (and to a lesser extent β_2) receptors in the heart catecholamines increase myocardial contractility, conduction, excitability, frequency, and oxygen consumption. Tachycardia is most often sinus tachycardia or supraventricular tachycardia. Catecholamines produce a prompt increase in the metabolic rate (likely due to cutaneous vasoconstriction and increased muscular activity) and then a delayed increase probably due to oxidation of lactate in the liver. This calorigenic action stimulates sweating. The sudden release of catecholamines causes a sharp increase of blood pressure, which is the most likely cause of the severe headache in these patients.

A, B, D, E, F All these items contain at least one symptom that is absent in pheochromocytoma patients.

▶ *Learning objective:* Identify the drug that can trigger paroxysmal symptoms in a patient with from pheochromocytoma.

3. Answer: C

Pseudoephedrine is an indirect-acting sympathomimetic drug. It is a component of some over-the-counter preparations used as nasal decongestants. The drug acts, at least in part, by releasing catecholamines from postganglionic sympathetic terminals. In pheochromocytoma, catecholamine stores within sympathetic nerve endings are increased because the catecholamines produced by the tumor are, in part, taken up by the sympathetic terminals. Therefore the intake of a medication containing pseudoephedrine can trigger a paroxysmal episode in a patient with pheochromocytoma.

A Propranolol is a β-adrenoceptor antagonist. The drug could counteract, not trigger, some symptoms of pheochromocytoma (tachycardia).

B Atropine is an antimuscarinic drug. Atropine could trigger some symptoms of pheochromocytoma (tachycardia), but could counteract other symptoms (sweating).

D Loratadine is an antihistamine drug. The drug cannot trigger a pheochromocytoma attack.

E Prazosin is an α_1-adrenoceptor antagonist. The drug could counteract, not trigger, some symptoms of pheochromocytoma (hypertension).

F Caffeine is a central nervous system stimulant. The drug could trigger some symptoms of pheochromocytoma (tachycardia) but could counteract other symptoms (headache).

▶ *Learning objective:* Explain why a calcium channel blocker is usually not fully effective in decreasing the hypertension of a patient suffering from pheochromocytoma.

4. Answer: B

E.F.'s physician overlooked the possibility of pheochromocytoma. Even if only 1 out of 1,000 hypertensive patients turn out to be affected by this disease, pheochromocytoma should always be suspected in patients with hypertension, and this diagnosis should be excluded only after appropriate investigation. Nifedipine is a calcium channel blocker that, at therapeutic doses, blocks only L-type calcium channels on the smooth muscle membrane. By reducing calcium entry the drug provokes a vasodilation, mainly on the arterioles. Therefore it antagonizes the vasoconstricting action of catecholamines by acting on receptors different from those activated by catecholamines. In conclusion, it can be defined as a functional antagonist of norepinephrine and epinephrine. A general rule in pharmacology is that a functional antagonist is less effective than a pharmacological antagonist, in most cases.

A The nifedipine dose was the standard antihypertensive dose.

C Epinephrine has no effect on nifedipine metabolism.

D, E Pheochromocytoma does not cause these effects.

▶ *Learning objective:* Describe the parents' disease that can suggest an inherited cause of pheochromocytoma.

5. Answer: B

Up to 25% of pheochromocytomas are considered to be inherited and associated with other endocrine tumors. E.F. has a posi-

tive family history for multiple endocrine neoplasia (MEN 2A, also called Sipple's syndrome), which suggests that the tumor could be inherited as an autosomal dominant disorder.

A A positive family history for myocardial infarction is known to be a major risk factor for cardiovascular disease but not for pheochromocytoma.

C A positive family history for COPD can barely increase the risk of the disease but not the risk of pheochromocytoma.

D A positive family history for lymphoma can be a risk factor for blood cancers but not for pheochromocytoma.

▶ *Learning objective:* Explain the reason for chest pain in a patient with pheochromocytoma.

6. Answer: B

Catecholamine-induced tachycardia requires an increased amount of oxygen, but, in spite of coronary vasodilation, oxygen demand is higher than oxygen supply, causing a relative heart ischemia. The ischemic muscle releases pain-producing substances. This is why cardiac efficiency (i.e., the proportion of work done by the heart to the oxygen used to perform that work) is always decreased by sympathomimetic drugs.

A Catecholamines cause coronary vasodilation, not vasoconstriction, because the heart relies primarily on metabolic mechanisms to adapt the caliber of its coronary vessels to the need of oxygen. Because tachycardia increases this need, vasodilation occurs.

C Dyspnea is the result, not the cause, of intercostal muscle spasm.

D Only extremely high tachycardia can increase pulmonary artery pressure, due to the increased left diastolic volume. Moreover, pulmonary hypertension rarely causes squeezing chest pain.

▶ *Learning objective:* Describe a common cardiovascular effect in a patient with pheochromocytoma.

7. Answer: B

An excessive fall in blood pressure that occurs on assuming the upright position is called postural (or orthostatic) hypotension. It occurs primarily for two reasons:

- The baroreceptor reflex cannot function properly, because there is an impairment of the afferent, central, or efferent portion of the autonomic reflex arc.
- There is volume depletion by any cause.

Under normal conditions, the gravitational stress of sudden standing normally causes pooling of blood in the venous capacitance vessels of the legs and trunk. The subsequent transient decrease in venous return and cardiac output results in reduced blood pressure, which, in turn, decreases the stretching of baroreceptors located in the carotid sinus and in the aortic arch. This leads to the removal of the inhibitory influences on vasomotor centers in the brain, resulting in a compensatory reflex increase in sympathetic drive. Therefore heart rate, myocardial contractility, and total peripheral resistance increase, thereby restoring the blood pressure to normal.

Postural hypotension affects about 70% of patients with pheochromocytoma. Even if the ultimate cause is uncertain, it is likely that the two main causes of postural hypotension are operative. Pheochromocytoma can cause volume depletion because of chronic vasoconstriction and profuse sweating. Pheochromocytoma can impair the baroreceptor function because of chronic activation of sympathetic receptors.

The fact that E.F. has an elevated hematocrit and that her BUN is elevated in the presence of a normal serum creatinine level (see laboratory results) suggests that she has some degree of intravascular volume depletion.

A The patient's pulse pressure was increased, not decreased.

C Coronary vasodilation, not vasoconstriction, occurs in pheochromocytoma because the increased heart work needs an increased oxygen supply.

D Pheochromocytoma usually causes a decrease, not an increase, in cardiac output due to volume depletion.

▶ *Learning objective:* Identify the adrenoceptor that most likely contributed to the hyperglycemia in a patient with pheochromocytoma.

8. Answer: A

Catecholamines have several different actions that can increase blood glucose. These include the following:

- Inhibition of insulin secretion (the activation of α_2-receptors in pancreatic cells, which inhibits the secretion, predominates over the activation of β_2-receptors, which stimulates the secretion).
- Stimulation of glycogenolysis in the liver (through activation of β_2-adrenoceptors). Glycogenolysis is stimulated also in muscle, but the glucose is used by the muscle cells to provide energy.
- Stimulation of gluconeogenesis in the liver (though activation of β_2-adrenoceptors).
- Stimulation of glucagon secretion (through activation of β_2-adrenoceptors), which in turn stimulates liver glycogenolysis.

B Activation of α_1-adrenoceptors causes vasoconstriction all over the body. By decreasing oxygen supply to the liver the glucose output should be decreased, not increased.

C Activation of β_2-, not β_1-adrenoceptors in the liver can increase glucose output.

D, E Activation of dopamine D_1- and D_2-adrenoceptors does not affect blood glucose.

▶ *Learning objective:* Explain the molecular mechanism of action of clonidine.

9. Answer: A

Clonidine is an α_2-adrenoceptor agonist that acts mainly on presynaptic receptors in the rostral ventrolateral medulla (the vasomotor center). This action reduces the efferent sympathetic discharge, thereby decreasing the catecholamine release from the adrenal medulla in a normal person. This is the basis for the clonidine test.

315

B Clonidine can cause activation, not blockade, of imidazoline receptors located in the rostral ventrolateral medulla (the vasomotor center). This action also contributes to the reduction of the efferent sympathetic discharge.

C, D, E Clonidine does not bind these receptors.

▶ *Learning objective:* Explain why clonidine cannot significantly decrease catecholamine secretion in a patient with pheochromocytoma.

10. Answer: B

Unlike normal chromaffin cells, pheochromocytoma cells are not innervated and therefore not susceptible to manipulation by drugs that decrease central sympathetic outflow.

In a patient without pheochromocytoma, plasma norepinephrine should fall to < 400 pg/mL after clonidine. The modest decrease in the present case supports the diagnosis of pheochromocytoma.

A Pheochromocytoma has no direct action on central sympathetic outflow. Since it causes a sympathetically mediated vasoconstriction, the central sympathetic outflow should be decreased, not increased.

C There is no difference between normal and tumor catecholamine metabolism.

D Unlike the normal adrenal medulla, which secretes ~ 85% epinephrine, most pheochromocytomas secrete predominantly norepinephrine.

▶ *Learning objective:* Explain the molecular mechanism of action of phenoxybenzamine.

11. Answer: C

Phenoxybenzamine is a noncompetitive nonselective α-adrenoceptor antagonist. Noncompetitive antagonists bind to the agonist receptor site in an irreversible (or quasi-irreversible) fashion (often the bond is covalent), or they bind to a secondary site, within the receptor, altering the binding property of the agonist site (allosteric interaction). In both cases the final result is that no change in the antagonist occupancy takes place when the agonist is applied (that is the antagonism is nonsurmountable). By blocking α_1-adrenoceptors the drug lowers the blood pressure and is the first-line agent for the preoperative management of pheochromocytoma.

A, B, D, E, F Phenoxybenzamine does not block β-adrenoceptors.

▶ *Learning objective:* Identify the pheochromocytoma/symptom that is best antagonized by phenoxybenzamine.

12. Answer: D

Both epinephrine and norepinephrine activate α_2-adrenoceptors in the pancreas. This activation decreases insulin secretion, leading to hyperglycemia, a well-known effect of pheochromocytoma. By blocking α_2-adrenoceptors, phenoxybenzamine counteracts the epinephrine-induced decrease of insulin secretion. Therefore more insulin can be secreted, and hyperglycemia is reduced.

A Sweating is a sympathomimetic effect, but the receptors involved are mainly cholinergic; therefore sweating cannot be blocked by an α-antagonist. Moreover, in patients with pheochromocytoma the effect is most likely indirect, related to the hypermetabolism induced by catecholamine excess.

B, C, E All these actions are due to activation of β-adrenoceptors and therefore are not blocked by phenoxybenzamine.

▶ *Learning objective:* Explain the molecular mechanism of action of metyrosine.

13. Answer: B

Metyrosine is the α-methyl analogue of tyrosine (α-methyltyrosine). It is a competitive inhibitor of tyrosine hydroxylase, the rate-limiting enzyme in catecholamine biosynthesis. The drug is given sometimes for 5 to 10 days preoperatively in order to decrease catecholamine production, as in the present case. A dose of 1 g daily can provide up to 70% inhibition of catecholamine biosynthesis.

A, C, D, E See correct answer explanation.

▶ *Learning objective:* Explain why a β-blocker is usually given after phenoxybenzamine to a patient with pheochromocytoma.

▶ *Learning objective:* Describe the effect of labetalol on total peripheral resistance, renin secretion, and heart rate in a patient with pheochromocytoma.

14. Answer: B

Propranolol is a nonselective β-adrenoceptor blocker. It is given to pheochromocytoma patients in order to control the heart rate. It must be given only after α-adrenergic blockade has been introduced. If given in the absence of α-adrenergic blockade, propranolol would cause serious (and sometimes life-threatening) adverse effects because of the following:

▶ The decrease in heart contractility that is essential for maintaining a normal blood flow in the face of the α_1-mediated increase in systemic vascular resistance. An acute cardiac failure could ensue.

▶ The blockade of β_2-mediated coronary vasodilation that could unmask the unopposed α_1-mediated vasoconstriction. An acute myocardial infarction could ensue.

A Propranolol can block β_2-adrenoceptor-mediated vasodilation, but this would increase, not counteract, peripheral vasoconstriction.

C, D, E Propranolol can counteract these catecholamine-mediated effects, but this is not the primary reason for the use of this drug in pheochromocytoma.

15. Answer: D

Labetalol is an $\alpha\beta$-adrenoceptor antagonist. By blocking β_1-adrenoceptors in juxtaglomerular cells the drug inhibits renin secretion.

The increased blood pressure during surgery was likely due to massive release of preformed epinephrine that most likely caused vasoconstriction and tachycardia (epinephrine can activate both α_1-adrenoceptors, causing vasoconstriction, and β_2-adrenoceptors, causing vasodilation, but at very high doses vasoconstriction predominates). By blocking α_1-adrenoceptors labetalol counteracts the epinephrine-induced vasoconstriction. The α_1-blocking actions of the drug are weak compared with its β_1-blocking actions but are nevertheless sufficient to counteract the epinephrine-induced vasoconstriction (remember the difference between blocking vasoconstriction and causing vasodilation), leading to a decreased total peripheral resistance, as in the present case (see decreased diastolic pressure). By blocking β_1-adrenoceptors labetalol counteracts the epinephrine-induced tachycardia, leading to normal heart rate, as in the present case. By blocking β_1-adrenoceptors in juxtaglomerular cells the drug inhibits renin secretion.

A These effects would be caused by an IV injection of norepinephrine to a normal person.

B These effects would be caused by an IV injection of a selective β_1-adrenoceptor blocker to a normal person.

C These effects would be caused by an IV injection of a selective α_1-adrenoceptor blocker to a normal person.

E These effects would be caused by an IV injection of a muscarinic M_2 antagonist to a normal person.

Case 36

Pneumonia

D.W., a 67-year-old man, was admitted to the hospital with a 3-day history of fever, worsening shortness of breath, chills, productive cough, and complaints of a knifelike chest pain that was made worse by coughing and breathing. The patient stated that his shortness of breath started about 10 days ago after a walk in extremely cold weather.

Pertinent medical history included a 5-year history of chronic bronchitis that produced one cup of sputum per day. One year earlier the patient underwent an episode of bronchitis exacerbation that was treated successfully with levofloxacin. He had been taking the same drug prophylactically during the winter months since then.

D.W. did not smoke and denied use of alcohol or illicit drugs. He was retired from work as a bank clerk and lived at home with his wife.

Physical examination showed an elderly man in moderate distress, with the following vital signs: blood pressure 143/78 mm Hg, heart rate 102 bpm, respirations 32/min, temperature 100.9°F (38.3°C). Chest auscultation revealed fine crackling rales in the lower base of the right lung. Examination of the left lung was normal.

Pertinent laboratory exam results on admission were as follows:

Blood hematology

- ► Red blood cell count (RBC): $3.9 \times 10^6/\mu L$ (normal, men 4.0–6.0)
- ► White blood cell count (WBC): $16 \times 10^3/\mu L$ (normal 4–10)
- ► Neutrophils: 85% (normal 45–75)
- ► Lymphocytes: 8% (normal 16–47)
- ► Platelets: $250 \times 10^3/\mu L$ (normal 130–400)
- ► Hemoglobin (Hb): 11 g/dL (normal 12–16)
- ► Hematocrit (Hct): 34% (normal 36–48)

Blood chemistry

- ► pH: 7.38 (normal 7.35–7.45)
- ► Creatinine: 1.3 mg/dL (normal 0.6–1.2)
- ► Blood urea nitrogen (BUN): 30 mg/dL (normal 8–25)
- ► Sodium (Na^+): 138 mEq/L (normal 135–146)
- ► Potassium (K^+): 4.2 mEq/L (normal 3.6–5.3)
- ► Glucose: 102 mg/dL (normal 60–110)

Arterial blood gases

- ► PO_2: 75 mm Hg (normal 80–100)
- ► PCO_2: 42 mm Hg (normal 38–45)
- ► SaO_2: 92% (normal > 95)

Sputum Gram's stain

▶ Epithelial cells: < 10/high-power field
▶ Polymorphonuclear leukocytes: > 25/high-power field
▶ Gram-negative rods: many

Chest radiography

A right lung lobar infiltrate with lobar consolidation

A diagnosis of community-acquired pneumonia was made, and the patient started treatment with ceftriaxone and azithromycin, pending sputum culture. Over the next 48 hours the patient's clinical status did not improve substantially, and the sputum culture revealed *Haemophilus influenzae* as the main offending pathogen. The rod was found to be resistant to ceftriaxone, azithromycin, and levofloxacin but susceptible to tobramycin. The current therapy was changed, tobramycin was given, and the patient steadily improved with decreasing fever, tachypnea, cough, and chest pain. One week later D.W. had recovered and was discharged from the hospital.

Questions

1. D.W. was diagnosed with community-acquired pneumonia. Which of the following pairs of bacteria are among the most commonly identified pathogens in this disease?

A. *Klebsiella pneumoniae–Pseudomonas aeruginosa*

B. *Pseudomonas aeruginosa–Mycoplasma pneumoniae*

C. *Streptococcus pneumoniae–Mycoplasma pneumoniae*

D. *Streptococcus pneumoniae–Klebsiella pneumoniae*

E. *Pseudomonas aeruginosa–Streptococcus pneumoniae*

F. *Mycoplasma pneumoniae–Klebsiella pneumoniae*

2. Community-acquired pneumonia is differentiated from hospital-acquired pneumonia mainly because of the most common bacteria causing the disease. Which of the following bacteria is the most common cause of pneumonia acquired in intensive care settings and in immunocompromised patients?

A. *Mycoplasma pneumoniae*

B. *Chlamydophila pneumoniae*

C. *Moraxella catarrhalis*

D. *Legionella pneumophila*

E. *Pseudomonas aeruginosa*

F. *Bacteroides fragilis*

3. D.W.'s chest radiograph showed a lobar infiltrate. Which of the following statements best defines the cause of infiltration of lungs?

A. Bronchioles are abnormally dilated.

B. Alveoli are filled with pus, proteins, or blood.

C. Bronchial arterioles are filled with microthrombi.

D. Alveoli break to form much bigger sacs.

E. Alveoli are abnormally inflated.

4. D.W. was treated with levofloxacin during his bronchitis exacerbation. The inhibition of which of the following bacterial enzymes most likely mediated the therapeutic effect of the drug in the patient's disease?

A. Peptidyl transferase

B. Transglycosylase

C. Dihydrofolate reductase

D. DNA-dependent RNA polymerase

E. Dihydropteroate synthetase

F. Topoisomerase II

5. Fluoroquinolones are antibiotics with a very broad activity spectrum. Which of the following sets of activity spectrum is correct for this class of drugs?

Set	*Klebsiella pneumoniae*	*Mycoplasma pneumoniae*	*Legionella pneumophila*	*Enterococcus faecalis*	*Treponema pallidum*
A.	Resistant	Sensitive	Sensitive	Resistant	Sensitive
B.	Sensitive	Sensitive	Sensitive	Sensitive	Resistant
C.	Sensitive	Resistant	Resistant	Resistant	Sensitive
D.	Sensitive	Resistant	Resistant	Sensitive	Sensitive

321

6. D.W. started a treatment that included ceftazidime, a third-generation cephalosporin with a broad activity spectrum. Which of the following sets of activity spectrum is correct for this drug subclass?

Set	Klebsiella pneumoniae	Mycoplasma pneumoniae	Legionella pneumophila	Enterococcus faecalis	Streptococcus pneumoniae
A.	Resistant	Sensitive	Sensitive	Resistant	Sensitive
B.	Sensitive	Resistant	Resistant	Sensitive	Sensitive
C.	Sensitive	Sensitive	Sensitive	Sensitive	Resistant
D.	Sensitive	Resistant	Resistant	Resistant	Sensitive

7. Which of the following bacterial structures most likely represents the primary binding site for cephalosporins?

A. Ribosomes

B. Peptidoglycan layer

C. Inner plasma membrane

D. Cytoplasm

E. Plasmid

F. DNA

8. D.W. started a treatment that included azithromycin. Which of the following molecular actions on bacterial cells most likely mediated the therapeutic effect of the drug in the patient's disease?

A. Inhibition of DNA-dependent RNA polymerase

B. Inhibition of DNA gyrase

C. Production of aberrant bacterial proteins

D. Blockade of translocation reaction

E. Blockade of transfer RNA (tRNA) binding to the ribosome

9. *Haemophilus influenzae* was found to be the cause of D.W.'s pneumonia, and the rod was resistant to ceftazidime, azithromycin, and levofloxacin. Which of the following mechanisms most likely accounts for the resistance to all of these antibiotics?

A. Alteration of ribosomal binding site that prevents drug binding

B. Production of bacterial β-lactamases

C. Decreased production of autolytic enzymes

D. Increased activity of a bacterial efflux pump

E. Increased bacterial cell membrane permeability

10. D.W. started a treatment with tobramycin. Which of the following molecular actions most likely contributed to the therapeutic effect of the drug in the patient's disease?

A. Inhibition of topoisomerases

B. Inhibition of transpeptidases

C. Blockade of initiation complex formation

D. Blockade of peptidoglycan chain elongation

E. Blockade of peptidoglycan chain elongation

F. Inhibition of DNA-dependent RNA polymerase

Answers and Explanations

▸ *Learning objective:* Select the two most common identified pathogens in community-acquired pneumonia.

1. Answer: C

Community-acquired pneumonia develops in people with limited or no contact with medical institutions. The most common identified typical organisms are *Streptococcus pneumoniae* and *Haemophilus influenzae*, while the most common identified atypical organisms are *Mycoplasma pneumoniae* and *Chlamydophila pneumoniae.*

A, B, E *Pseudomonas aeruginosa* usually causes hospital-acquired pneumonia.

A, D, F *Klebsiella pneumoniae* causes a rare and severe pneumonia, usually among diabetic patients and alcoholics.

▸ *Learning objective:* Identify the bacterium common in pneumonia acquired in intensive care settings and in immunocompromised patients.

2. Answer: E

Pseudomonas aeruginosa is found chiefly in soil and water, but it is also found on the skin in moist areas, and some people carry it in the normal colon flora. It is primarily an opportunistic pathogen that causes infection in hospitalized patients, mainly in those who are immunosuppressed or have chronic respiratory disease (e.g., cystic fibrosis). In many hospitals it is the most common cause of nosocomial pneumonia.

A, B, C, D All these bacteria usually cause community-acquired pneumonias.

F Pneumonia caused by *Bacteroides fragilis* is exceedingly rare.

▸ *Learning objective:* Explain the most likely cause of infiltration of lungs.

3. Answer: B

A lung infiltrate is due to alveoli filled with fluid consisting of white blood cells, pus, protein, or blood. Airspace filling causes the areas of increased density on X-ray (i.e., the infiltrates). Lung infiltrates can occur in several lung disorders, including actinomycosis, cystic fibrosis, and fungal infection, and are common in pneumonia, as in the present case.

A, C, D, E None of these events causes lung infiltrates.

▸ *Learning objective:* Identify the enzyme specifically inhibited by levofloxacin.

4. Answer: F

Levofloxacin is a fluoroquinolone antibiotic. These agents inhibit bacterial DNA function in gram-negative bacteria by blocking topoisomerase II (also called DNA gyrase). The blockade prevents the relaxation of supercoiled DNA, which is required for normal transcription.

A Peptidyl transferase is inhibited by chloramphenicol.

B Transglycosylase is inhibited by vancomycin.

C Dihydrofolate reductase is inhibited by trimethoprim.

D DNA-dependent RNA polymerase is inhibited by rifamycins.

E Dihydropteroate synthase is inhibited by sulfonamides.

▸ *Learning objective:* Identify the correct activity spectrum of fluoroquinolones.

5. Answer: B

Fluoroquinolones are effective against the following:

▸ Many gram-positive bacteria (including *Enterococcus faecalis*)
▸ Most gram-negative rods (including *Klebsiella pneumoniae* and *Legionella pneumophila*)
▸ Most atypical bacteria (including *Mycoplasma pneumoniae*)

Fluoroquinolones are not effective against spirochetes (*Treponema pallidum*).

A This would be a correct antibacterial spectrum for macrolides.

C This would be a correct antibacterial spectrum for third- and fourth-generation cephalosporins.

D This would be a correct antibacterial spectrum for carbapenems.

Learning objective: Identify the correct activity spectrum of third-generation cephalosporins.

6. Answer: D

Third-generation cephalosporins are effective against the following:

- Many gram-positive bacteria (including *Streptococcus pneumoniae*)
- Many gram-negative rods (including *Klebsiella pneumoniae*)

Cephalosporins are not effective against enterococci (*Enterococcus faecalis*), mycoplasmas (*Mycoplasma pneumoniae*), and legionellae (*Legionella pneumophila*).

A This would be a correct antibacterial spectrum for macrolides.

B This would be a correct antibacterial spectrum for carbapenems.

C This would be a correct antibacterial spectrum for fluoroquinolones.

Learning objective: Identify the primary site of action of ceftriaxone.

7. Answer: C

Ceftazidime is a β-lactam antibiotic. All β-lactam drugs bind to proteins called penicillin-binding proteins *located on the inner plasma membrane* of certain bacteria. These proteins are enzymes endowed with various catalytic functions, which are inhibited by the binding with the antibiotic. The most important enzymes inhibited are transpeptidases, which catalyze the final cross-link step in the synthesis of murein (also called peptidoglycan). Since peptidoglycan layers are constituents of bacteria cell wall, the synthesis of this wall is blocked.

A, B, D, E, F β-Lactam antibiotics do not bind to these bacterial structures.

Learning objective: Explain the mechanism of action of azithromycin.

8. Answer: D

Azithromycin is a macrolide antibiotic. These drugs inhibit bacterial protein synthesis, mainly by blocking the translocation of the newly synthesized peptidyl-tRNA from the acceptor site to the donor site of the ribosome. They are mainly bacteriostatic, but they may be bactericidal at higher doses.

A This would be the mechanism of action of rifampin.

B This would be the mechanism of action of quinolones.

C This would be the mechanism of action of aminoglycosides.

E This would be the mechanism of action of tetracyclines.

Learning objective: Identify the common mechanism for bacterial resistance to cephalosporins, macrolides, and fluoroquinolones.

9. Answer: D

Efflux pumps are transport proteins involved in the extrusion of toxic substrates from within cells into the external environment. These proteins are found in both gram-positive and gram-negative bacteria as well as in eukaryotic organisms. Microorganisms can overexpress efflux pumps and then expel antibiotics to which the microbes would otherwise be susceptible. Efflux pumps are prominent mechanisms of resistance to virtually all classes of clinically relevant antibiotics.

A This would be a mechanism of resistance to macrolides like azithromycin but not to ceftriaxone or levofloxacin.

B This would be a mechanism of resistance to β-lactam drugs like ceftriaxone but not to azithromycin or levofloxacin.

C, E This mechanism would decrease, not increase, the resistance of the offending pathogen to the listed antibiotics.

Learning objective: explain the molecular mechanism of action of aminoglycosides.

10. Answer: C

Tobramycin is an aminoglycoside antibiotic. These drugs inhibit bacterial protein synthesis, but their mechanism includes at least the following three different actions:

- Blockade of the formation of the initiation complex
- Misreading of the code of the messenger RNA (mRNA) template, leading to an incorrect amino acid

incorporation into the bacterial polypeptide chain

▶ Blockade of translocation of peptidyl-tRNA

The misreading of the mRNA template could explain, at least in part, the bactericidal effect of these drugs.

A This would be the mechanism of action of fluoroquinolones.

B, D These events belong to the mechanism of action of β-lactam antibiotics.

E Inhibition of DNA-dependent RNA polymerase would be the mechanism of action of rifamycins.

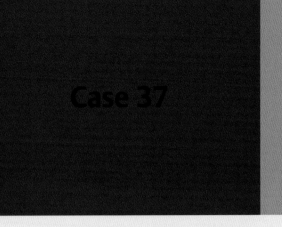

P.C., a 22-year-old woman, presented to her gynecologist because of excessive hair growth on her face, legs, and abdomen. Her menstrual periods had always been irregular. Her first menstrual period occurred at the age of 13. The longest interval between her periods had been 3 to 4 months and the shortest 20 days. She reported that whenever she had periods, they were quite heavy, and the bleeding would last for more than 7 days. She was sexually active and used male condoms.

Her mother had type 2 diabetes mellitus (DM2), and her father had DM2 and hypertension. She was a nonsmoker and an occasional alcohol drinker.

Physical examination revealed a white American woman with a body mass index of 32 kg/m². Her vital signs were pulse 80 bpm, blood pressure 120/78 mm Hg, respiration 20/min.

Some pertinent lab tests were ordered with the following results:

Blood hematology

- Hemoglobin (Hb): 13 g/dL (normal 12–16)
- Fasting blood glucose: 107 mg/dL (normal 70–110)
- 24-hour postprandial glucose: 130 mg/dL
- Free testosterone: 6.0 pg/mL (normal 0.7–3.6)
- Luteinizing hormone (LH): 24 mIu/L (normal 5–20)
- Follicle-stimulating hormone (FSH): 8 mIu/L (normal 5–20)
- LH/FSH: 3 (normal near 1 in the early half of the menstrual cycle)
- Thyroid-stimulating hormone (TSH): 2.8 mIu/L (normal 0.4-4.0)
- Prolactin: 8 ng/mL (normal 2–29)

Transvaginal ultrasonography

Several immature ovarian cysts were seen in her ovaries.

A diagnosis of polycystic ovarian syndrome (PCOS) was made. Her physician advised her to join training sessions to lose weight and prescribed an oral combination hormonal contraceptive (CHC).

She did not like changes in her mood that occurred after she started taking her CHC. Her doctor informed her that in the majority of patients these adverse effects subside within a short time span and suggested she to continue the medicine for a few months.

She did well on the oral CHC. Her menstruation became regular, and her unwanted body hair growth reduced dramatically within 1 year of treatment.

During a follow-up visit a year later, P.C. presented with tiredness and increased frequency of urination. She reported that she had noticed increased growth of unwanted body hair again. Her lab reports revealed fasting glucose levels 120 mg/dL and HbA$_{1c}$ of 8%. The doctor added an appropriate drug to her therapy. Six months later, her blood glucose levels were under control and she was feeling better.

P.C. got married and decided to discontinue CHC because the couple desired to have children. However, P.C. failed to conceive, even after 2 years of not using any contraceptive method. Meanwhile, P.C. had gained weight and was not practicing her weight loss program strictly. Her doctor conducted some tests on her and her husband. Her husband had a normal sperm count with normal morphology, but she was found to have anovulatory cycles. Her physician prescribed a drug to induce ovulation. P.C. needed to visit her physician for regular examinations while on this therapy. After 4 cycles of unsuccessful treatment with the drug, the physician decided to attempt therapy with another drug. However, within 3 months of starting therapy with the new drug, P.C. started experiencing sudden episodes of a warm sensation over her face, neck, and chest, accompanied with sweating and chills, so the drug was discontinued. After a year of unsuccessful therapy, she was scheduled for therapy with gonadotropins. Follicle-stimulating hormone (FSH) and human chorionic gonadotropin (HCG) were used for the treatment. The gonadotropin therapy was successful, and P.C. was overjoyed at being pregnant.

Questions

1. P.C. presented with unwanted hair growth on her face, abdomen, and legs. An increase in which of the following processes is most likely the direct cause of these symptoms?

A. Aromatization of adrenal androgens

B. Ovarian androgen synthesis

C. Ovarian estrogen synthesis

D. Cortisol synthesis

E. Secretion of FSH

2. P.C. complained of irregular menstrual periods. Which of the following pathophysiological changes is most likely the cause of this symptom?

A. Impaired ovarian follicle maturation

B. Apoptosis of theca cells

C. Hyperplasia of granulosa cells

D. Ectopic endometrial tissue around the ovaries

E. Pancreatic beta cell failure

3. P.C. revealed that when she had menstrual periods, her menstrual flow was heavy and prolonged. Which of the following changes in her reproductive tract was related to this symptom?

A. Ovarian atresia

B. Endometrial atrophy

C. Endometrial carcinoma

D. Ovarian swelling

E. Endometrial thickening

4. P.C. was prescribed an oral CHC for treating hirsutism. Which of the following hormonal agents were the components in the most likely CHC preparation that was prescribed for her?

A. Ethinyl estradiol and norethindrone

B. Ethinyl estradiol and mifepristone

C. Ethinyl estradiol and anastrozole

D. Ethinyl estradiol and norgestimate

E. Ethinyl estradiol and spironolactone

5. Which of the following effects best explains the mechanism of oral CHCs in treating hirsutism in patients with PCOS?

A. Increased secretion of ovarian estrogens

B. Increased secretion of adrenal androgens

C. Decreased secretion of ovarian androgens

D. Decreased secretion of SHBG

E. Increased secretion of gonadotropins

6. P.C. was prescribed an oral CHC for treatment of hirsutism. Had she not responded to oral CHC well, which of the following drugs could be added to her therapy?

A. Leuprolide

B. Luteinizing hormone

C. Spironolactone

D. Anastrozole

E. Ketoconazole

7. P.C. was found to have increased fasting glucose levels. Her androgenic symptoms also started worsening after an initially good response to her CHC. Which of the following drugs could be added to her therapy at this stage?

A. Insulin

B. Metformin

C. Glimepiride

D. Sitagliptin

E. Drospirenone

8. P.C. wanted to become pregnant but could not conceive after trying for 2 years. Which of the followings drugs was most likely prescribed for inducing ovulation?

A. Clomiphene

B. Spironolactone

C. Ulipristal

D. Tamoxifen

E. Fulvestrant

9. P.C. did not respond to clomiphene after four cycles of its use. Which of the following drugs can also be used for induction of ovulation?

A. Spironolactone

B. Finasteride

C. Flutamide

D. Cabergoline

E. Letrozole

10. P.C. experienced hot flashes after she started taking letrozole. Which of the following molecular actions most likely mediated the adverse effect of this drug?

A. Inhibition of estrogen synthesis

B. Increased gonadotropin secretion

C. Antagonism of estrogen receptors

D. Decreased uptake of norepinephrine

E. Increased release of serotonin

11. P.C. underwent successful therapy with gonadotropins. She was administered FSH for stimulating development of ovarian follicles and then was injected with HCG to induce ovulation on the appropriate day. Which of the following receptors does HCG act upon to bring about its ovulation-inducing effect?

A. FSH receptors

B. LH receptors

C. Gn-RH receptors

D. Estrogen receptors

E. Progesterone receptors

Answers and Explanations

▶ *Learning objective:* Describe the pathophysiology of PCOS.

1. Answer: B

PCOS is characterized by ovarian dysfunction, hyperandrogenism, hyperinsulinemia, and polycystic ovaries. Ovarian dysfunction is manifested by oligo-ovulation or anovulation. Patients present with irregular menstrual cycles. Hyperandrogenism is manifested by clinical signs of acne and hirsutism and is caused by hyperandrogenemia (elevated total and free testosterone plasma levels). More than half the patients have an increased LH/FSH ratio and are obese.

Three mechanisms appear to be involved in the pathophysiology of PCOS:

▶ **Inappropriate gonadotropin secretion:** There is an increased LH secretion, whereas the FSH secretion remains normal, causing an increased LH/FSH ratio. P.C.'s LH/FSH was 3. Usually the levels of these two hormones are near equal in the first half of the menstrual cycle. This relative change in the levels of these two hormones is enough to disrupt the normal ovarian function. Increased LH secretion relative to FSH, too early in the menstrual cycle, results in failure of development of a dominant follicle, which would result in anovulation. Due to anovulation, the woman does not enter the luteal phase and has very low progesterone. This results in unopposed estrogen that causes endometrial hyperplasia, leading to increased risk of endometrial carcinoma. In the short term, failure to enter into the luteal phase would result in failure of withdrawal bleeding, resulting in amenorrhea. Even when menstrual bleeding occurs, it usually marks the end of an anovulatory cycle.

▶ **Excess androgen production:** In PCOS, increased LH and insulin levels cause increased androgen production in the ovaries. Normally, LH acts on the theca cells to stimulate synthesis of androstenedione. Androstenedione is converted to testosterone, then these androgens enter the granulosa cells where aromatase converts them to estrone and estradiol, respectively. In PCOS ovaries, steroidogenesis is directed more toward testosterone synthesis, resulting in elevated testosterone levels in the circulation and hyperandrogenism (acne and hirsutism). Also, because testosterone levels are high, subsequently, due to its aromatization, there is elevation of estradiol levels too, which again contributes toward endometrial hyperplasia.

▶ ***Hyperinsulinemia:*** Insulin resistance is found in patients with PCOS, which seems to be tissue-selective. Resistance is increased in the skeletal muscle and fat, which results in compensatory hyperinsulinemia to facilitate uptake and utilization of glucose. However, ovarian theca cells show increased sensitivity to insulin, which results in increased testosterone synthesis. Insulin also decreases the synthesis of sex hormone–binding globulin (SHBG), a protein to which a large fraction of testosterone is bound in the circulation, resulting in elevated levels of free testosterone and hyperandrogenism.

A Increased aromatization of androgens results in increased estrogen synthesis. Increased levels of estrogens are not the cause of androgenic symptoms. Moreover, there is no increase in aromatization of adrenal androgens.

C Increased estrogen synthesis can occur as a result of increased synthesis of testosterone in the ovaries, but it is not the cause of hyperandrogenism.

D Increased cortisol synthesis is not associated with pathophysiology of PCOS.

E LH secretion increases in PCOS. FSH secretion remains near normal.

▶ *Learning objective:* Describe the cause of irregular menstrual periods in polycystic ovarian syndrome.

2. Answer: A

The LH/FSH ratio is found to be increased in 20 to 60% of PCOS patients. In normal menstrual cycles, in the first half, FSH increases to stimulate graafian follicle maturation, and from midcycle, LH increases to induce ovulation and the start of the luteal phase. If fertilization does not occur, the endometrium sheds off as menstrual bleeding. In PCOS, increased LH secretion that starts in the first half of the menstrual cycle results in failed development of a dominant fol-

licle, which would result in anovulation. Due to anovulation, the woman does not enter the luteal phase and would have very low progesterone. This results in unopposed estrogen, which causes endometrial hyperplasia. As this continues, there is no real menstrual cycle until endometrial thickening progresses so much that it has to shed off, which might not occur until after a few months. Also, it is possible that ovulation occasionally occurs between the anovulatory cycles and the bleeding actually follows the luteal phase. Due to the uncertain occurrence of ovulatory cycles in PCOS, caused by the mechanisms already described, menstruation becomes irregular, and many times a patient will not menstruate for many months, followed suddenly by a heavy period. CHCs are useful for regulating menstrual cycles in these patients. With the use of a cyclic CHC for a 28-day menstrual cycle, a patient could choose a preparation that provides 21 days with active hormone followed by 7 hormone-free days to experience withdrawal bleeding. However, CHCs will not necessarily convert anovulatory to ovulatory cycles.

B, C Atrophy of theca cells or hyperplasia of granulosa cells does not occur in PCOS.

D Ectopic endometrial tissue is found in endometriosis, not in PCOS.

E Pancreatic beta cell failure is seen in DM; moreover, it is not the cause of irregular menstruation in PCOS.

▶ *Learning objective:* Describe the cause of heavy menstruation in PCOS.

3. Answer: E

Due to anovulatory cycles in PCOS, a woman does not enter the luteal phase and so would have low progesterone levels. This results in unopposed estrogen, which causes endometrial hyperplasia. As this continues, there is no real menstrual cycle until endometrial thickening progresses so much that it has to shed off as uterine bleeding. Because of continuous thickening of the endometrial lining resulting from the absence of normal regular monthly withdrawal bleeding, whenever menstrual bleeding occurs, it is heavy.

Treatment with CHCs would regulate the menstrual cycles of a woman with PCOS, so menstrual periods would occur at regular intervals. Regular menstrual cycles would avoid endometrial thickening and thus would alleviate heavy periods.

A Ovarian atresia is seen at menopause, not in PCOS.

B Endometrial hyperplasia, not atrophy, occurs in women with PCOS.

C Endometrial carcinoma can be a consequence of long-term endometrial hyperplasia. Patients with PCOS can be at risk of developing endometrial carcinoma. Usually a patient presents with vaginal bleeding occurring during the cycle. The clinical picture of P.C. was not consistent with endometrial carcinoma.

D Ovarian hyperstimulation can occur in response to therapy with drugs to stimulate development of ova and induce ovulation. The condition is characterized by swelling in the ovaries, and the patient may present with lower abdominal pain, nausea, vomiting, diarrhea, and sudden weight gain. Severe symptoms include difficulty in breathing, pleural effusion, darker urine, and marked abdominal bloating and distension. These symptoms were absent in the present patient.

▶ *Learning objective:* Describe the appropriate preparations of combined hormonal contraceptives for the treatment of hirsutism in PCOS.

4. Answer: D

A CHC is a preparation that contains both an estrogen and a progestin. CHCs are indicated in PCOS to treat hormonal dysregulation. They are effective in regulating menstrual cycles and treating menorrhagia (heavy periods) and hyperandrogenism.

There are different oral CHCs (also called combined oral contraceptives) available. In most of them the estrogen component is ethinyl estradiol. Different progestin agents can be used; for example, there are oral CHC preparations containing norethindrone, levonorgestrel, norgestimate, or drospirenone.

Synthetic progestins are derived either from C-21 or 19-nortestosterone substrates.

Traditional oral CHCs contain original 19-nor derivatives, such as norethindrone. These progestins have some androgenic actions that manifest as androgenic adverse effects (acne, hirsutism). Newer 19-nor derivatives, called gonanes, including norgestimate and levonorgestrel, have less androgenic activity. Most of the newer CHC preparations contain progestins from the gonane class so as to decrease the chances of androgenic adverse effects. P.C. was prescribed an oral CHC preparation that contained norgestimate to avoid aggravation of her hirsutism.

A This oral CHC would not be appropriate for a woman suffering from hirsutism.

B, C, E These do not represent combined oral contraceptives; mifepristone is a progestin antagonist; anastrozole is an aromatase inhibitor; spironolactone is an antagonist of mineralocorticoid and androgen receptors.

▶ *Learning objective:* Explain how CHCs act to decrease free androgen levels.

5. Answer: C

Combined hormonal contraceptives act to decrease free testosterone levels by the following two mechanisms:

▶ **Increasing synthesis of SHBG by the liver:** A free form of androgens in the bloodstream is the form that can enter the cells and interact with intracellular receptors to exert its androgenic effects. The plasma protein (SHBG)-bound form is largely nonbioavailable for biological effects. Increased synthesis of SHBG in the liver, in response to the estrogen component of oral CHCs, results in increased binding of plasma androgens to SHBG and a decrease in bioavailable free plasma androgen levels.

▶ **Decreasing androgen synthesis in the ovaries:** Through feedback regulation, the estrogen component of CHCs decreases FHS release from the anterior pituitary, which, in addition to suppressing the development of a dominant graafian follicle, also suppresses the ovarian steroidogenesis. Suppression of steroidogenesis results in decreased synthesis of both ovarian androgens and estrogens, thus resulting in a decrease in plasma androgen levels.

A A CHC preparation would decrease the synthesis of both ovarian androgens and estrogens, but it is the decreased secretion of androgens, not of estrogens, that mediates its therapeutic effects for treating hirsutism associated with PCOS.

B Adrenal sex hormone production is not under the control of the hypothalamic–pituitary axis.

D A CHC increases, not decreases, the secretion of SHGB.

E A CHC decreases, not increases, the secretion of gonadotropins.

▶ *Learning objective:* Describe the drugs that can be used to treat androgenic symptoms related to PCOS.

6. Answer: C

Spironolactone acts as an aldosterone receptor antagonist, a weak androgen receptor antagonist, a weak inhibitor of testosterone synthesis, and a weak inhibitor of 5α-reductase. Due to its ability to block aldosterone receptors, it is used as a potassium-sparing diuretic, and due to its ability to suppress androgen action and biosynthesis, it can be used to manage signs and symptoms of hyperandrogenism.

When the symptoms of hyperandrogenism in a patient with PCOS do not respond adequately to CHCs, spironolactone can be added to the treatment, or used alone. Spironolactone can cause birth defects when taken during pregnancy, so when used alone, it is important to provide adequate contraception to prevent pregnancy. One of the adverse effects of spironolactone is to cause hyperkalemia. Drospirenone is one of the progestins that has antiandrogenic activity and so is used as a progestin component in CHCs for patients with hyperandrogenism; however, the drug can cause hyperkalemia as its adverse effect. Because of the danger of add-on risk of hyperkalemia, use of spironolactone with drospirenone-containing CHCs is contraindicated.

A Leuprolide is a gonadotropin-releasing hormone (Gn-RH) agonist that exerts differential effects depending on whether it is administered in a pulsatile manner via a pump or as a depot injection for continuous delivery. By pulsatile delivery it causes stimulation of gonadotropin secretion and eventually an increase in gonadal steroidogenesis. By continuous delivery, it shuts down the reproductive axis. Either result is not desirable in treating hirsutism in a woman with PCOS. Leuprolide is useful in endometriosis by shutting down the reproductive axis and in the treatment of infertility by stimulating gonadotropin secretion.

B LH is used in the treatment of infertility to provide an LH surge for ovulation.

D Anastrozole is an aromatase inhibitor that is indicated in the treatment of endometriosis and breast cancer and for induction of ovulation.

E Ketoconazole is an antifungal agent. It also inhibits human steroidogenesis in a nonselective manner. It can be used for the pharmacological management of Cushing's syndrome, where it reduces cortisol synthesis and the synthesis of other steroidal hormones.

▶ *Learning objective:* Describe the role of metformin in the management of PCOS and DM2.

7. Answer: B

Insulin resistance is found in patients with PCOS, which seems to be tissue-selective. Resistance is increased in the skeletal muscle and fat, resulting in compensatory hyperinsulinemia to facilitate uptake and utilization of glucose. However, ovarian theca cells show increased sensitivity to insulin, which results in increased testosterone synthesis. Insulin also decreases the synthesis of SHBG, a protein to which a large fraction of testosterone is bound in the circulation, resulting in elevated levels of free testosterone and hyperandrogenism (acne and hirsutism).

Insulin resistance in the periphery can progress to cause overt hyperglycemia to cause DM2 in PCOS patients. It becomes more difficult to manage PCOS when risk factors such as DM and dyslipidemia are present.

P.C. also had a strong family history of diabetes. She developed DM2 while her periods became regular and her hirsutism responded well on CHC therapy. Metformin is a first-line agent for treating DM2 unless a patient has contraindications to its use. It reduces both glucose output from the liver and insulin resistance in the periphery. In PCOS, metformin has been shown to correct hormonal dysfunction by reducing relative hyperinsulinemia. Metformin is also effective for weight loss (2–3 kg), which would be beneficial for P.C. Therefore, metformin was an appropriate choice.

A A patient with PCOS already has relative hyperinsulinemia, so exogenous insulin will further increase the insulin levels and thus increase androgen secretion from the theca cells. Also, insulin therapy can increase weight gain, which would not have been desirable for P.C., who was already overweight.

C Glimepiride increases insulin secretion from the pancreatic beta cells; although it can control blood glucose levels, it will cause weight gain. This would not be a desirable outcome for P.C.

D Sitagliptin acts by inhibiting degradation of incretin hormones; thus it increases insulin secretion. It can be useful in controlling hyperglycemia but has not been studied for therapeutic effects in PCOS.

E Drospirenone is a progestin compound that has antialdosterone and antiandrogenic activity. CHCs containing drospirenone are one of the preferred preparations for treating hyperandrogenism and regulating menstrual cycles in a woman with PCOS. However, it has no therapeutic effects in controlling hyperglycemia.

▸ *Learning objective:* Describe the pharmacology of clomiphene for inducing ovulation.

P.C. was having anovulatory cycles, which was why she was not able to conceive.

PCOS is the most common cause of anovulatory infertility. Lifestyle changes (hypocaloric diet, weight reduction) alone are considered the first-line treatment for the management of infertile anovulatory women with PCOS who are overweight or obese. P.C. was instructed to follow a weight loss program but failed to stick to the program.

Clomiphene, an ovulation inducer, is the first-line drug to treat infertility in women with PCOS. It is a partial agonist at estrogen receptors and blocks estrogen receptors in the hypothalamus and anterior pituitary, leading to inhibition of estradiol's negative feedback on gonadotropin secretion. This results in increased secretion of FSH and LH from the anterior pituitary, which stimulate the development of ovarian follicles and, eventually, result in induction of ovulation.

Clomiphene is administered daily for 5 days, started on day 5 after a spontaneous or progestin-induced menstruation. Graafian follicle maturation and ovulation are monitored by ultrasonography. Most of the women with PCOS would ovulate within three or four cycles of clomiphene therapy, but if not, further treatment is not recommended because of the concern of ovarian cancer. Adverse effects of clomiphene or other ovulation-inducing agents include ovarian hyperstimulation.

B Spironolactone is an aldosterone and androgen antagonist. It does not act as an ovulation inducer.

C Ulipristal is a selective progestin receptor modulator used for emergency contraception.

D Tamoxifen is a selective estrogen receptor modulator used in the adjunctive therapy of breast carcinoma.

E Fulvestrant is a pure estrogen receptor antagonist used in the treatment of breast carcinoma in postmenopausal women with hormone receptor–positive metastatic breast cancer that has progressed on tamoxifen.

▸ *Learning objective:* Describe drugs that can be used to induce ovulation in PCOS.

Most of the women with PCOS would ovulate within three or four cycles of clomiphene therapy, but if not, further treatment with this drug is not recommended because of the concern of ovarian cancer. Metformin acts as a second-line treatment at this stage, but the patient was already taking this drug for controlling hyperglycemia. In this situation, other ovulation inducers can be used. Letrozole can be used before trying gonadotropins.

Letrozole is an aromatase inhibitor. Aromatase enzyme catalyzes the conversion of androgens to estrogens. The enzyme converts androstenedione to estrone and testosterone to estradiol. By inhibiting the enzyme, letrozole reduces the levels of estrogens and results in increased gonadotropin secretion via feedback regulation. Increased levels of gonadotropins stimulate follicular development in the ovaries, which would culminate in ovulation.

A Spironolactone is an aldosterone and androgen antagonist. It does not act as an ovulation inducer.

B Finasteride inhibits the conversion of testosterone to dihydrotestosterone by inhibiting the activity of 5α-reductase. It is useful in benign prostate hyperplasia and in male pattern baldness.

C Flutamide is an androgen receptor antagonist and can be used to treat hyperandrogenism.

D Cabergoline is a long-acting dopamine D_2-receptor agonist. It can be used in the treatment of hyperprolactinemia associated with a prolactinoma.

▶ *Learning objective:* Describe the adverse effects of letrozole.

10. Answer: A

Letrozole inhibits estrogen synthesis by inhibiting the activity of aromatase. It has been suggested that decline in estrogen levels leads to a decrease in serotonin levels and an increase in the levels of norepinephrine. Serotonin and norepinephrine are involved in temperature regulation. Fluctuations in the levels of serotonin and norepinephrine cause activation of the body's heat-release mechanisms, leading to cutaneous vasodilation and sweating as seen in hot flashes.

B By inhibiting estrogen synthesis letrozole, via a feedback mechanism, increases the release of gonadotropins from the anterior pituitary. However, increased gonadotropin is not the cause of estrogen deficiency and hot flashes.

C Letrozole does not inhibit estrogen receptors. Fulvestrant is an estrogen receptor antagonist.

D, E Letrozole does not directly decrease the uptake of norepinephrine nor does it increase the release of serotonin. Emergence of hot flashes is associated with declining estrogen levels that occur during natural menopause. Serotonin and norepinephrine are involved in temperature regulation. It has been suggested that a decline in plasma estrogens leads to decreased, not increased, serotonin levels and increased, not decreased, norepinephrine levels.

▶ *Learning objective:* Describe the role of HCG in gonadotropin therapy for induction of ovulation.

11. Answer: B

FSH, LH, and HCG are glycoproteins. Because HCG and LH are structurally similar, and HCG can bind to LH receptors to bring about LH effects, HCG can be used for providing an LH surge to induce ovulation. These hormones bind to cell membrane–bound G-protein coupled receptors on the theca and granulosa cells, and stimulate adenylyl cyclase activity (increased intracellular cyclic adenosine monophosphate) to promote ovarian steroidogenesis.

Initially FSH is injected every day, with doses mimicking the levels in the normal menstrual cycle, until the ovarian follicles attain an adequate size (as monitored by transvaginal ultrasonography). When adequate size is attained, HCG is injected to provide an LH surge to induce ovulation. Ovulation occurs in the next 24 to 48 hours after HCG is injected. Multiple ova mature and are released in response to the gonadotropin therapy, so when natural insemination is allowed around the expected time of ovulation, multiple births can occur.

A FSH, not LH, binds to FSH receptors.

C Gn-RH is released in a pulsatile manner from the hypothalamus and reaches the anterior pituitary through the portal circulation. In the anterior pituitary, it binds to membrane-bound Gn-RH receptors on the surface of gonadotrope cells to stimulate gonadotropin (FSH and LH) secretion into the circulation.

D, E HCG does not bind to estrogen or progestin receptors.

P.A., a 43-year-old woman, was admitted to the hospital because of severe fatigue, loss of appetite, nausea, vomiting, and diarrhea over the last 3 weeks. She revealed that she had been feeling progressively tired for the last 2 months. She had lost weight and felt muscle weakness, irritability, and depression. She said these symptoms had worsened gradually over time. She also reported that her hand creases and skin over the knees, elbows, knuckles, and malleoli looked darker in complexion than before. Her history was significant for decreased libido for the past few months, which was unusual compared to her earlier levels of libido. She was a nonalcoholic and a nonsmoker.

She had no history of exposure to tuberculosis. Her sister had a history of Graves' disease, and her father died of a stroke 2 years ago.

Physical examination revealed a white woman in distress, lethargic and dehydrated. Her vitals were blood pressure 98/65 mm Hg, pulse 110 bpm, respirations 30/min.

Pertinent lab results on admission were as follows:

Blood hematology

- Red blood cell count (RBC): $2.9 \times 10^6/\mu L$ (normal 4.0–6.0)
- Hemoglobin (Hb): 11 g/dL (normal 12–16)
- White blood cell count (WBC): $10 \times 10^3 /\mu L$ (normal 4–10)
- Neutrophils: 50% (normal 40–70)
- Lymphocytes 38% (20–40)
- Eosinophils 1% (normal 1–3)
- Basophils 0% (normal 0–1)
- Monocytes 4% (normal 3–7)

Blood chemistry

- Fasting blood glucose: 60 mg/dL (normal 70–110)
- Sodium (Na^+): 129 mEq/L (normal 136–145)
- Potassium (K^+): 5.8 mEq/L (normal 3.5–5.2)
- Blood urea nitrogen (BUN): 30 mg/dL (normal 7–18)
- Creatinine: 1.5 mg/dL (normal 0.6–1.2)
- Cortisol: 3 µg/dL (normal > 18, at 6–8 a.m.)
- Adrenocorticotropic hormone (ACTH): 1,000 pg/dL (normal 400–2,000)
- Thyroid-stimulating hormone (TSH): 2.5 mIU/L (normal 0.5–3.5)

Cosyntropin-stimulation test

Abnormal response (failed to raise serum cortisol levels)

Antiadrenal antibodies

Positive

Interferon-gamma release assay (IGRA)

Negative

A diagnosis of primary chronic adrenal insufficiency (Addison's disease) was established, and an appropriate treatment was initiated. Her pharmacotherapy included a drug that was to be administered twice a day, the first dose in the morning (~ 70% of the total daily dose) and a second, smaller dose (~ 30% of the total daily dose) in the evening. The patient responded well and rapidly to the therapy. Thereafter, she visited the clinic for follow-up every 3 months.

A year later, P.A. was brought to the emergency department in an unconscious state. Her son told the attending physician that she was having flu and had been feeling exhausted before her condition worsened to the unconscious stage. Her vital signs on admission were blood pressure 86/58 mm Hg, cardiac rate 130 bpm, respiration 26/min.

Given her history of Addison's disease, she was promptly administered intravenous (IV) hydrocortisone and fluids. With this therapy, the patient recovered well. After 3 days the patient was discharged on her old prescription of oral replacement therapy with adrenocortical hormones.

Questions

1. P.A.'s blood pressure was low when she first presented with the constellation of symptoms of Addison's disease. Which of the following molecular actions most likely mediated low blood pressure in this patient?

A. Increased sodium loss in the urine

B. Increased potassium loss in the urine

C. Decreased renin secretion

D. Decreased antidiuretic hormone (ADH) secretion

E. Decreased epinephrine secretion by adrenal medulla

2. P.A.'s lab exams indicated a very low level of cortisol. Which of the following is the most likely cause of cortisol decrease in this patient?

A. Decreased release of ACTH

B. Autoantibody-induced loss of adrenocortical cells

C. Decreased perfusion of the adrenal gland

D. Tuberculosis of adrenal glands

E. Diversion of precursors toward adrenal androgen synthesis

3. P.A. complained about increased pigmentation of the skin, especially over the knees, elbows, knuckles, and malleoli. What is the cause of increased pigmentation in this patient?

A. Autoantibody-induced skin damage

B. Enhanced activity of ACTH on the adrenal cortex

C. Decreased activity of enzymes involved in cortisol synthesis

D. Decreased activity of enzymes involved in aldosterone synthesis

E. Enhanced action of melanocyte-stimulating hormone on the skin

4. P.A.'s lab results revealed elevated levels of blood urea nitrogen and creatinine. Which of the following is the most likely cause of these results?

A. Dehydration

B. Glomerulonephritis

C. Urolithiasis

D. Increased renal blood flow

E. Posterior pituitary dysfunction

5. In a patient with Addison's disease, which of the following organs, other than the adrenal glands, has the possibility of being affected by autoimmunity?

A. Pancreas

B. Anterior pituitary

C. Thyroid

D. Stomach

E. Bone joints

6. Which of the following pathological findings would likely be noticed in P.A.'s adrenal gland?

A. Adrenal hypertrophy

B. Shrunken adrenal cortex

C. Cortex dominated by zone reticularis cells

D. Shrunken adrenal medulla

E. Hemorrhage in the cortex

7. P.A. was diagnosed with primary chronic adrenocortical insufficiency. What drug/drugs would she most likely need for the lifelong management of her condition?

A. Only hydrocortisone

B. Hydrocortisone and fludrocortisone

C. Only fludrocortisone

D. Hydrocortisone, fludrocortisone, and dehydroepiandrosterone

8. Which of the following is the reason for adding fludrocortisone to P.A.'s replacement therapy rather than achieving optimal mineralocorticoid effects by administering higher doses of hydrocortisone?

A. High hydrocortisone dose increases the risk of osteoporosis.

B. Hydrocortisone cannot bind to mineralocorticoid receptors.

C. Hydrocortisone is inactivated rapidly by the cells of renal tubules.

D. Hydrocortisone cannot enter inside the renal tubular cells.

9. P.A. experienced myriad symptoms related to cortisol deficiency. Which of the following is one of the critical body functions that requires normal levels of cortisol?

A. Cardiac contractility

B. Electrolyte balance

C. Gluconeogenesis

D. Respiration

E. Skeletal growth

10. Which of the following molecular actions most likely mediates the physiological effects of cortisol?

A. Cortisol is converted to cortisone, which activates cortisol receptors.

B. The cortisol-receptor complex binds to specific nucleotide sequences of DNA.

C. The cortisol-receptor complex binds to surface receptors of most cell membranes.

D. Cortisol stimulates tyrosine kinase activity of the surface-bound receptors.

11. Fludrocortisone was added to P.A.'s adrenocortical replacement therapy. Which of the following processes is stimulated by fludrocortisone to achieve replacement of deficient mineralocorticoid effects in the patient?

A. Transcription of epithelial sodium channel gene

B. Angiotensin II synthesis

C. Gluconeogenesis

D. Vasopressin synthesis

E. Expression of adrenoceptors on the renal vasculature

12. A year later, P.A. was brought to the emergency room in an unconscious state. Which of the following disorders most likely caused the patient's unconsciousness?

A. Myxedema coma

B. Lactic acidosis

C. Acute renal failure

D. Adrenal crisis

E. Diabetic ketoacidosis

13. Which of the following disorders could develop if P.A. continued taking double the recommended dose of hydrocortisone on a chronic basis even after the resolution of her acute illness?

A. Osteoporosis

B. Retinal damage

C. Hypoparathyroidism

D. Hypoglycemia

E. Hyperthyroidism

Answers and Explanations

▶ *Learning objective:* Explain the pathophysiology of low blood pressure associated with Addison's disease.

1.   Answer: A

In general, clinical manifestations of primary adrenocortical insufficiency do not appear until at least 90% of the cortex is compromised. Initially, the patient starts experiencing gradual progression of symptoms of fatigue and weakness. The development of low blood pressure is due mainly to the following two reasons:

▶ **Lack of aldosterone (by far the primary mechanism):** The decreased aldosterone levels cause sodium loss in the urine, which in turn leads to hyponatremia and extracellular volume depletion. This is the ultimate cause of decreased blood pressure.

▶ **Lack of cortisol:** Cortisol acts as a permissive agent for catecholamine activity. Cortisol deficiency diminishes the catecholamine activation of α_1-adrenoceptors, contributing to the decrease in blood pressure.

B Aldosterone causes an increased renal excretion of potassium. In Addison's disease the opposite effect occurs.

C Renin secretion might increase, not decrease, in the absence of aldosterone (by a feedback mechanism) in an attempt to counteract aldosterone deficiency, but without much beneficial outcome because the end organ (adrenal glands) has lost its function.

D ADH secretion is primarily regulated by plasma osmolality and stimulates free water reabsorption from the renal tubules in cases of increased plasma osmolality. Its release is not decreased in Addison's disease.

E Addison's disease does not involve adrenal medulla, and secretion of epinephrine is not affected.

▶ *Learning objective:* Describe the pathophysiology of primary adrenocortical insufficiency.

2. Answer: B

There are three main causes of adrenal cortical damage: autoimmunity, infections, and hemorrhage. In cases of hemorrhage, adrenal damage is acute, and the appearance of symptoms is sudden. But in the present case, the patient experienced gradual progression of symptoms, which happens due to insidious damage to the adrenocortical cells, resulting in primary chronic adrenocortical insufficiency.

In developed countries, autoimmune adrenalitis accounts for most cases (~ 70%) of primary chronic adrenocortical insufficiency. This involves insidious autoimmune destruction of adrenal cortical hormone–secreting cells, leading to damage of the entire adrenal cortex. Autoantibodies against several steroidogenic enzymes (e.g., 21-hydroxylase, 17-hydroxylase) can be detected in these patients, as in the present case.

Infectious causes could involve, especially in the developing nations, tuberculosis and meningococcemia. Tuberculous adrenalitis usually follows an insidious course. In contrast, adrenal hemorrhage due to septicemia caused by *Neisseria meningitidis* results in a rather fast onset of symptoms of acute adrenocortical insufficiency.

A Decreased levels of ACTH are seen in secondary adrenocortical insufficiency. In primary adrenocortical insufficiency, ACTH levels are elevated.

C Decreased perfusion could eventually develop due to decreased cortical mass, but this is not the cause of decreased adrenocortical hormone synthesis in the present case.

D Tuberculous adrenalitis may cause primary chronic adrenocortical insufficiency. However, the tuberculin test (IGRA) was negative for the present patient.

E Congenital adrenal hyperplasia is a group of disorders in which deficiency or decreased activity of enzymes of the glucocorticoid and mineralocorticoid pathways results in the diversion of hormone precursors toward the synthesis of adrenal androgens. This is a congenital disorder; signs and symptoms appear quite early in life and vary according to the degree of deficiency of activity of these enzymes. In this disorder, the levels of ACTH are high, not normal, resulting in adrenal hypertrophy.

▶ *Learning objectives:* Explain the cause of increased pigmentation in patients with primary adrenocortical insufficiency.

3. Answer: E

Corticotropin-releasing hormone (CRH) from the hypothalamus reaches the anterior pituitary and binds to G protein–coupled receptors on the surface of corticotroph cells to stimulate synthesis of pro-opiomelanocortin (POMC). POMC is a precursor peptide that is cleaved into multiple peptide hormones, including ACTH, melanocyte-stimulating hormone (MSH), lipotropin, and β-endorphin.

In primary adrenocortical insufficiency, the decreasing levels of cortisol increase the release of CRH by a feedback mechanism. Increased levels of CRH result in increased synthesis of POMC, which in turn increases levels of ACTH and MSH. MSH binds to its receptors on skin melanocytes and stimulates melanin synthesis, which causes increased pigmentation. Also, because of similarities between ACTH and MSH peptide sequences, high levels of ACTH can bind to MSH receptors to stimulate melanogenesis.

A, B, C, D These actions are not the causes of increased pigmentation associated with primary adrenocortical insufficiency.

▶ *Learning objective:* Explain the cause of elevated BUN and creatinine levels in Addison's disease.

4. Answer: A

In Addison's disease the decreased aldosterone levels cause sodium loss, resulting in hyponatremia. Loss of sodium is associated with loss of water in urine, resulting in decreased intravascular volume and dehydration. Because of dehydration, the glomerular filtration rate diminishes and the same amounts of BUN and creatinine are now present in smaller amounts of intravascular fluid. This is the reason for elevated BUN and creatinine levels in patients with Addison's disease.

B, C This patient has no signs of glomerulonephritis or nephrolithiasis.

D Increased renal blood flow would increase the glomerular filtration rate; therefore BUN levels would not be elevated.

E In Addison's disease posterior pituitary function is not impaired.

▶ *Learning objective:* Identify the concomitant organ that is more likely affected by autoimmunity in a patient with Addison's disease.

5. Answer: C

In about 50% of patients with primary adrenal insufficiency due to autoimmune dysfunction, it is likely to find other concomitant autoimmune disorders. Autoimmune thyroid disorders (Hashimoto's thyroiditis or Graves' disease) are the most common in such cases. Therefore, it is important to test for dysfunction of other endocrine organs in patients presenting with symptoms indicating primary adrenal insufficiency. This is the reason for testing thyroid function in this patient, which was normal.

A An autoimmune disorder affecting the pancreas would be type 1 diabetes mellitus.

B An autoimmune disorder affecting the anterior pituitary would be autoimmune hypophysitis, an inflammation of the pituitary gland due to autoimmunity.

D An autoimmune disorder affecting the stomach would be pernicious anemia.

E An autoimmune disorder affecting the bone joints would be rheumatoid arthritis.

▶ *Learning objective:* Describe the pathological changes in adrenal glands of a patient with Addison's disease.

6. Answer: B

Primary autoimmune adrenalitis is characterized by irregularly shrunken glands. The glandular tissue mass decreases so much that it may be difficult to identify it within the suprarenal adipose tissue. Histologically, the cortex contains only scattered residual cortical cells in a collapsed network of connective tissue.

A The adrenal cortex is damaged by autoantibodies in Addison's disease. Shrinkage, not hypertrophy, of the adrenal cortex is the result of this damage.

C The entire cortex is damaged, including the zona reticularis cells.

D A variable lymphoid infiltrate is present in the cortex and may extend into the subjacent medulla. The adrenal medulla is otherwise preserved.

E Hemorrhage would cause fast onset of symptoms of adrenocortical insufficiency and is usually caused by trauma or meningococcal septicemia.

▶ *Learning objective:* Identify the drugs to be used for hormone replacement therapy in a female patient with Addison's disease.

---

7. Answer: D

In a patient who is experiencing signs and symptoms of primary adrenocortical insufficiency, it is critical to replace cortisol immediately. The principle that is followed is that the therapy is initiated with the lowest effective dose of hydrocortisone while mimicking the normal diurnal adrenal rhythm of cortisol release (this is the reason for administering hydrocortisone in two divided doses—a 70% dose in the morning and a 30% dose in the evening). Because mineralocorticoid activity of 50 mg hydrocortisone is approximately equal to 0.1 mg fludrocortisone (a synthetic mineralocorticoid), the effect of hydrocortisone on the patient's plasma sodium and potassium levels is monitored too. If the hyperkalemia persists despite administering optimal doses of hydrocortisone, fludrocortisone can be added to achieve optimal mineralocorticoid effects. Most patients with primary adrenal insufficiency eventually require mineralocorticoid replacement to prevent sodium loss, intravascular volume depletion, and hyperkalemia.

In women, the inner layer of the adrenal cortex (i.e., the zona reticularis) is the primary source of androgens. Dehydroepiandrosterone (DHEA) from the adrenal cortex is converted to androgens and estrogens in the periphery. A decrease in adrenal androgen synthesis is associated with a loss of libido in these patients. Clinical trial data suggest that replacement with 50 mg of DHEA daily may be beneficial for outcomes such as improved mood, psychological well-being, and sexual life of female patients with primary adrenocortical insufficiency.

In view of this information, a female patient with Addison's disease would need hydrocortisone, fludrocortisone, and DHEA for lifelong replacement therapy. Male patients with Addison's disease would not need DHEA, because the testes are the primary organ for androgen supply.

A, C Both glucocorticoid and mineralocorticoid replacements are needed in Addison's disease.

B This would be an appropriate therapy for male patients with Addison's disease.

▶ *Learning objective:* Describe the rationale for adding fludrocortisone to the adrenal replacement therapy for achieving optimal mineralocorticoid effects.

---

8. Answer: A

Aldosterone is the principal mineralocorticoid that controls sodium and potassium exchange in the distal nephron. Aldosterone interacts with mineralocorticoid receptors in the kidney, whereby sodium is retained and potassium is secreted in the renal tubules. The sensitivities of both the glucocorticoid receptor and the mineralocorticoid receptor for cortisol, in vitro, are similar. Therefore cortisol (hydrocortisone) can interact with aldosterone receptors in the kidneys. Then why is fludrocortisone needed for producing mineralocorticoid effects?

Cortisol circulates in much higher concentrations than aldosterone, and yet normally, it does not interact with mineralocorticoid receptors in the kidney to produce physiologically required mineralocorticoid effects. However, small changes in aldosterone quite rapidly affect sodium and potassium exchange in the kidney. The intracellular enzyme 11β-hydroxysteroid dehydrogenase type 2 (HSD2) inside the distal nephron cells metabolizes cortisol to the inactive cortisone and protects the mineralocorticoid receptor from cortisol binding. However, when the levels of cortisol are much higher than the physiological levels (as would occur with high doses of hydrocortisone, and in Cushing's syndrome), this enzymatic inactivation of cortisol is overwhelmed, and cortisol becomes capable of interacting with the mineralocorticoid receptors, resulting in sodium retention, volume expansion, hypertension, and hypokalemia (mineralocorticoid effects).

Therefore higher doses of hydrocortisone could achieve mineralocorticoid effects, but it will be at the cost of producing a number of adverse effects related to high levels of cortisol. All the signs and symptoms that are exhibited by a patient with Cushing's disease (due to high cortisol levels), such as moon facies, osteoporosis, hyperglycemia, cataract, mental disturbances, redistribution of fat, increased risk of opportunistic infections, among others, could occur by administering very high doses of hydrocortisone. Thus it is prudent to add fludrocortisone to the ongoing therapy with minimally optimal replacement doses of hydrocortisone, in order to achieve optimal mineralocorticoid effects, rather than trying to achieve these effects by increasing the hydrocortisone dose.

B Hydrocortisone shows equal affinity for both glucocorticoid and mineralocorticoid receptors in vitro. For further explanation, see above.

C Hydrocortisone, when present in normal levels, is inactivated by renal HSD2, but this is not the reason for not administering higher does to achieve mineralocorticoid effects.

D Hydrocortisone is a lipid-soluble molecule and can cross all cell membranes easily.

▶ *Learning objective:* Describe the role of cortisol in maintaining normal homeostasis.

9.   Answer: C

Cortisol has widespread effects on body function. It has profound effects on messenger RNA expression. About 10% of all human genes are estimated to have glucocorticoid response elements (GREs). Activation of GREs affecting expression of such a large number of genes explains the critical role cortisol plays in most tissues.

Cortisol plays a critical role in maintaining normal energy homeostasis. This is done primarily by the action of the hormone on glucose metabolism. Cortisol antagonizes insulin action and promotes gluconeogenesis to increase blood glucose levels. Along with other mediators, it stimulates enzymes of the gluconeogenesis pathway to increase glucose output from the liver. This is a critical function to maintain normal plasma glucose levels during the fasting state, for example, to supply glucose to vital organs, such as the brain, during nighttime sleep (when the body is fasting). In conditions of cortisol deficiency, gluconeogenesis is impaired, and hypoglycemia can occur, which can rapidly compromise vital organ functions.

Normal levels of cortisol are so critical for the normal function of the body that in a patient with primary chronic adrenal insufficiency, acute deficiency of cortisol (acute adrenal crisis) would cause intractable vomiting, abdominal pain, hypotension, coma, and vascular collapse. If replacement with hydrocortisone is not started promptly, death can occur rapidly.

A, B, D, E These body functions can be influenced by cortisol, but its role is not as critical as the one of maintaining glucose homeostasis.

▶ *Learning objective:* Describe the molecular mechanism of action of cortisol.

10.   Answer B

Cortisol is a lipid-soluble hormone. Its free form in plasma can rapidly cross cell plasma membranes by lipid diffusion. Inside the cells, cortisol binds to cortisol receptors. The cortisol-receptor complex translocates into the nucleus to interact with specific nucleotide sequences of DNA (i.e., GREs) to modulate gene expression.

At physiological plasma levels of cortisol, cortisol undergoes inactivation and reactivation through the cortisol-cortisone shunt. In the distal tubular cells of the kidneys, cortisol is inactivated to cortisone by HSD2, thus preventing cortisol's interaction with the mineralocorticoid receptors. Cortisone then enters the circulation and is reactivated in the liver to cortisol by HSD1.

A Cortisone is the inactive form of cortisol and does not interact with glucocorticoid or mineralocorticoid receptors.

C Cortisol receptors are not located on cell membranes.

D Cortisol does not interact with cell surface receptors to stimulate tyrosine kinase activity. An example of a molecule that does this is insulin.

▶ *Learning objective:* Describe the mechanism of action of fludrocortisone.

11. Answer: A

Stimulation of mineralocorticoid receptors by fludrocortisone in the distal renal tubular cells results in stimulation of transcription of genes responsible for gene products required for translation of epithelial sodium channels, a protein that is required for sodium reabsorption.

B Angiotensin II synthesis is stimulated by the action of renin on angiotensinogen to convert it to angiotensin I, and then by the action of angiotensin-converting enzyme in the pulmonary vasculature to convert angiotensin I to angiotensin II. Angiotensin II acts on the adrenal zona glomerulosa to stimulate the release of aldosterone, which binds to mineralocorticoid receptors in the distal renal tubules to stimulate reabsorption of sodium in exchange with potassium.

C Gluconeogenesis is stimulated by cortisol and by epinephrine (via β_2-adrenoceptor activation in the liver).

D Vasopressin synthesis and release from the posterior pituitary gland are mainly regulated by plasma osmolality.

E Cortisol is involved in modulating expression of adrenoceptors on the vasculature; aldosterone or its analogues (fludrocortisone) do not have this action.

▶ *Learning objective:* Identify the disorder that can most likely cause unconsciousness in a patient with primary chronic adrenocortical insufficiency.

12. Answer: D

P.A. developed acute adrenal crisis. She had flu that had increased her stress level; therefore her body required more than the usual amount of hydrocortisone. The normal adrenal glands of a normal person increase cortisol production during stressful conditions. However, dysfunctional adrenal glands of a patient with primary adrenocortical insufficiency cannot compensate for the increased need during conditions of increased physiological stress

imposed, for example, by an acute illness. During an acute illness, such patients usually require double the dose of hydrocortisone to maintain homeostasis. Such stress-related dose adjustment must be continued until the condition resolves, in order to prevent the development of adrenal crisis.

Because the patient's hydrocortisone dose was not modified to deal with the increased physical stress of the acute illness, and because she might have missed some doses of her medicine due to nausea and vomiting, she developed acute adrenal crisis.

A Myxedema coma is a consequence of untreated hypothyroidism.

B Lactic acidosis can occur as an adverse effect of drugs like metformin.

C The patient's history and signs and symptoms did not support the diagnosis of acute renal failure.

E Diabetic ketoacidosis develops in poorly controlled hyperglycemia in type 1 diabetes mellitus.

▶ *Learning objective:* Describe the adverse effects of supraphysiological doses of hydrocortisone.

13. Answer: A

A patient with manifestations of primary chronic adrenocortical insufficiency requires lifelong replacement therapy with adrenal cortical hormones. The first hormone that needs to be replaced quickly is cortisol (known as hydrocortisone when used as a medication). Because the goal is to replace deficient hormones in order to restore and maintain normal physiological functions, minimal optimal doses of hydrocortisone are used. During acute stresses, the dosage of hydrocortisone needs to be increased to deal with increased physical stress. When the acute illness resolves, drug dosage needs to be decreased to the original minimal dose required for maintaining homeostasis.

Glucocorticoids have two broad indications. One is for replacement therapy (as in the present case), and the second is for achieving anti-inflammatory or immunosuppressive effects. For achieving the latter effects, doses of glucocorticoid agents are much higher than those used for replacement therapy. There are greater chances for the development of numerous adverse effects (similar to signs and symptoms of Cushing's syndrome), most of which can be viewed as exaggerated physiological effects.

Glucocorticoids are the most common cause of drug-induced osteoporosis when given at a dosage higher than that required for replacement therapy. The mechanism of this effect includes the following actions:

► Increased urinary excretion of calcium and decreased intestinal calcium absorption, by inhibition of renal calcitriol production. The resulting negative calcium balance leads to increased parathyroid hormone release. Increased parathyroid hormone acts on bones to mobilize calcium.

► Decline in bone formation mediated by direct inhibition of osteoblast proliferation and differentiation and by an increase in the apoptosis rates of mature osteoblasts and osteocytes.

► Enhancement of bone resorption by stimulating osteoclast proliferation.

B, C, D, E These disorders are not caused by supraphysiological dosage of hydrocortisone.

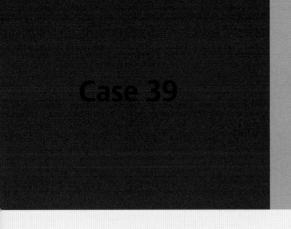

K.L., a 73-year-old African American man, visited his physician complaining of urinary problems that had started 2 months ago but worsened over time. His complaints included increased urinary frequency, nocturia five to six times per night, bedwetting (nocturnal enuresis), a need to strain to void, difficulty in starting voiding (hesitancy), diminished and interrupted stream, and postvoid dribbling. Occasionally his urine appeared cloudy and red. The patient also complained of fatigue and bone pain that started 2 weeks ago and was increasing over the last few days.

K.L.'s medical history was significant for hypertension, presently treated with hydro-chlorothiazide and long-acting nifedipine. Ten years earlier, he underwent surgery to remove colon cancer. The patient's prostate-specific antigen (PSA), done 2 years earlier, was normal.

The patient's father died from prostate cancer at age 65, and his mother from liver cancer at age 82. K.L. never smoked and denied alcohol or illicit drug use.

K.L. was admitted to the hospital for further evaluation. Physical examination showed a man in moderate discomfort with the following vital signs: blood pressure 142/82 mm Hg, pulse 80 bpm, respirations 16/min.

Substantial pain was elicited by touching his spine or his left femur or moving his left leg. On rectal examination his prostate was markedly enlarged and asymmetric to the left with no nodules.

Pertinent lab exam results on admission were as follows:

Urinalysis

- Red blood cell count (RBC): 200/high-power field (normal < 3)
- Rare bacteria, no albumin, no ketones

Blood chemistry

- Acid phosphatase: 12 ng/mL (normal < 2.5)
- Creatinine: 2.1 mg/dL (normal 0.6–1.2)
- Calcium (Ca^{2+}): 16 mg/dL (normal 8.8–10.4)
- Blood urea nitrogen (BUN): 30 mg/dL (normal 8–25)
- Total PSA: 12 ng/mL (normal < 4 ng/mL)

A prostate biopsy revealed that 90% of the tissue had no glandular differentiation, but a pattern of cords and sheets of cells with prominent hyperchromatic nuclei and scant cytoplasm.

A bone scan showed areas of increased uptake (hot spots) in the lumbar spine, left femur, and left pelvis.

A diagnosis of metastatic prostate cancer was made. The tumor was diagnosed inoperable, and the patient was dismissed from the hospital with a postdischarge therapy that included leuprolide (administered as a depot preparation), flutamide, and pamidronate.

Questions

1. K.L. was diagnosed with prostate cancer. Which of the following was most likely the pathological type of his cancer?

A. Chondrosarcoma

B. Squamous cell carcinoma

C. Osteosarcoma

D. Adenocarcinoma

E. Plasmacytoma

F. Ductal carcinoma

2. K.L.'s prostate cancer most likely arose in which of the following regions of the prostate?

A. Anterior fibromuscular stroma

B. Central zone

C. Peripheral zone

D. Periurethral zone

E. Transition zone

3. Prostate cancer is usually staged to define the extent of the tumor and its aggressiveness. Gleason's grading system, based on the glandular pattern and degree of differentiation, is commonly used. Which of the following grades most likely represent the best classification for K.L.'s cancer?

A. 2

B. 4

C. 6

D. 7

E. 10

4. Which of the following triads of K.L.'s lab exams most likely indicated that his cancer has already metastasized?

A. PSA–calcium–acid phosphatase

B. PSA–bone scan–calcium

C. BUN–calcium–bone scan

D. BUN–calcium–acid phosphatase

E. Acid phosphatase–bone scan–calcium

F. BUN–PSA–calcium

5. Most prostate cancers are found by screening with PSA. Which of the following disorders can cause PSA elevation in up to 50% of patients without prostate cancer (i.e., a false-positive result)?

A. Urinary tract infection

B. Benign prostatic hyperplasia

C. Urinary bladder cancer

D. Renal cancer

E. Prostate infarct

6. K.L. complained of urinary problems. Which of the following was most likely the primary reason for the patient's urinary symptoms?

A. Associated urinary infection

B. Spreading of cancer to the bladder

C. Stromal hyperplasia of prostate periurethral glands

D. Urethral obstruction due to cancer-induced compression

E. Reactive inflammation of periurethral tissue

7. Leuprolide was prescribed to K.L. Which of the following was most likely the primary reason for this therapy?

A. Induction of cancer cell apoptosis

B. Increase in serum estradiol levels

C. Reduction of serum testosterone levels

D. Reduction of serum dihydrotestosterone levels

E. Reduction of angiogenesis in the prostate gland

8. Which of the following is the primary site of action of leuprolide?

A. Gonadotroph cells of the pituitary

B. Hypothalamic neurons

C. Leydig's cells of the testes

D. Gland cells of the prostate

E. Cells of the zona reticularis in the adrenals

9. Which of the following molecular actions most likely mediated the therapeutic effect of leuprolide in K.L.'s disease?

A. Downregulation of androgen receptors

B. Desensitization and downregulation of Gn-RH receptors

C. Blockade of androgen receptors in the testes

D. Inhibition of tyrosine kinase of cancer cells

E. Activation of Gn-RH synthesis in the hypothalamus

10. Flutamide was prescribed for K.L. Which of the following molecular actions most likely mediated the therapeutic effect of the drug in the patient's disease?

A. Inhibition of aromatase enzyme

B. Inhibition of 5α-reductase enzyme

C. Irreversible blockade of LH receptors

D. Competitive blockade of androgen receptors

E. Inhibition of P-450 enzymes

11. Which of the following is a rare but life-threatening adverse effect of flutamide that is also mentioned as a "black box warning" on the drug's label?

A. Pemphigus

B. Peptic ulcer

C. Chronic kidney disease

D. Hepatic necrosis

E. Agranulocytosis

F. Stroke

12. Which of the following adverse effects could most likely occur during the leuprolide/flutamide therapy, considering the mechanisms of action of both drugs?

A. Hypotension

B. Gynecomastia

C. Thrombosis

D. Peptic ulcer

E. Thrombocytopenia

F. Angioneurotic edema

13. Pamidronate was prescribed to K.L. Which of the following was most likely a reason for this prescription?

A. Treatment of urinary incontinence

B. Treatment of kidney insufficiency

C. Prevention of bone fractures

D. Prevention of lung metastases

E. Improvement of overall survival

14. Which of the following actions most likely mediated the therapeutic effect of pamidronate in the patient's disease?

A. Stimulation of osteoblast activity

B. Stimulation of intestinal calcium absorption

C. Inhibition of renal calcium excretion

D. Inhibition of osteoclast activity

E. Stimulation of renal synthesis of calcitriol

15. Which of the following is a rare but significant adverse effect that may occur with high-dose pamidronate treatment?

A. Osteomalacia

B. Osteoporosis

C. Acute tendinitis

D. Jaw osteonecrosis

E. Acute gingivitis

Answers and Explanations

▶ *Learning objective:* Identify the pathological type of prostate cancer.

1. Answer: D

More than 90% of prostate cancers are adenocarcinomas that usually arise in the peripheral zone of the gland. In contrast to benign glands, prostate cancer glands are smaller, more crowded, and lined in a single, uniform layer, as found in K.L.'s biopsy.

B, F These cancer types can rarely affect the prostate.

A, C, E These cancer types do not involve the prostate.

> ▶ *Learning objective:* Identify the region of the prostate where prostate cancer most likely begins.

2. Answer: C

Most prostatic adenocarcinomas arise in the peripheral zone of the prostate, which accounts for approximately 70% of the total prostate volume. Because of this location, many prostatic adenocarcinomas can be palpated by digital rectal examination.

A The peripheral zone is deficient anteriorly. This area is filled by the anterior fibromuscular stroma.

B The central zone takes up 25% of the prostate volume and contains the ejaculatory ducts.

D The periurethral zone is a narrow area of the prostate consisting of the short ducts adjacent to the prostatic urethra.

E The transition zone is the middle area of the prostate, between the peripheral and central zones. It surrounds the urethra as it passes through the prostate.

> ▶ *Learning objective:* Explain the microscopic Gleason grading system of prostate cancer.

3. Answer: E

Gleason's grading system refers to the microscopic appearance of the cancer. It starts with the best-differentiated tumors (grade 2) and ends with tumors that are totally undifferentiated (grade 10).

K.L.'s cancer has no glandular differentiation and therefore belongs to the highest level of Gleason's scale.

A, B, C, D See correct answer explanation.

> ▶ *Learning objective:* Identify three lab exams that most likely indicate a metastasized prostate cancer.

4. Answer: E

K.L. had a high acid phosphatase level and a positive bone scan.

Acid phosphatases are enzymes widely distributed in tissues. However, acid phosphatase activity is 100 time higher in the prostate gland than in other tissues. Elevated levels of acid phosphatase usually indicate metastatic prostate cancer, because once the carcinoma has spread, the prostate starts releasing the enzyme.

Bone scan hot spots in a patient with suspected bone metastasis are highly indicative of bone metastases.

Metastatic cancer in the skeleton can cause calcium to leak into the bloodstream. This can weaken the bone, increasing the risk of fractures. Hypercalcemia in turn can cause a variety of problems, including weakness, constipation, and dehydration.

A, B, C, F PSA cannot confirm that the cancer has metastasized, even if PSA scores tend to correlate with the risk of spread. However, K.L.'s PSA scores were not very high.

C, D, F BUN cannot suggest bone metastases.

> ▶ *Learning objective:* Describe the disease that can cause a false-positive result in patients with high PSA levels.

5. Answer: B

Although PSA is elevated in 25 to 90% of patients with prostate cancer, it can also be moderately elevated in up to 50% of patients with benign prostatic hyperplasia. However, the likelihood of cancer increases with increasing PSA levels. The test, together with clinical examination, can reliably suggest the diagnosis.

A, E These diseases can sometimes cause positive PSA, but the frequency of false-positives is much lower than that for benign prostatic hyperplasia.

C, D These diseases do not cause PSA elevations.

> ▶ *Learning objective:* Explain the cause of urinary problems in a patient with prostate cancer.

6. Answer: D

K.L.'s urinary symptoms were most likely due primarily to anatomical outlet obstruction. A growing tumor of the prostate starts squeezing the urethra. Also, the prostate gland is surrounded by a fibromuscular capsule that is not readily distensible. Obstruction leads to a chronically distended bladder that loses its ability to contract. This causes overflow incontinence (i.e., urinary leakage) resulting from an overfilled and distended bladder that is unable to empty. Overflow incontinence is the result of urethral overactivity, bladder underactivity, or a variable combination of both, as in the present case. In fact, the initial urethral hyperactivity due to urethral narrowing caused, over time, bladder underactivity.

A Urinary symptoms are common in urinary infections, but K.L.'s urinalysis was not indicative of an infection (bacteria were rare).

B An advanced prostate cancer can spread to the bladder, but this is not the primary reason for urinary problems in this disease.

C Stromal hyperplasia of the prostate periurethral glands is one of the earliest findings in patients with benign prostatic hyperplasia. Even if a benign prostate enlargement and cancer often coexist, K.L.'s biopsy did not mention a concomitant benign prostatic hyperplasia.

E Reactive inflammation of periurethral tissue can occur in prostate cancer but is not the primary reason for urinary problems in this disease.

▶ *Learning objective:* Explain the reason for leuprolide therapy in prostate cancer.

7. Answer: C

Leuprolide is a gonadotropin-releasing hormone (Gn-RH) agonist. Other members in this drug group include goserelin, buserelin, and triptorelin. Continuous administration of these drugs can decrease the release of luteinizing hormone (LH) and follicle-stimulating hormone (FSH). Prostate cancer is, at least initially, a hormone-dependent adenocarcinoma. In the past castration was found effective in reducing the cancer progression. Today it has been shown that reduction in serum testosterone levels with Gn-RH agonists causes a reduction of serum testosterone levels equal to that achieved with bilateral orchiectomy.

A Leuprolide has no direct action on cancer cell apoptosis.

B Estradiol levels are reduced, not increased, by leuprolide.

D It was once believed that dihydrotestosterone played a role in the development and exacerbation of benign prostatic hyperplasia as well as prostate cancer, but this has largely been disproved.

E Reduction of angiogenesis in the prostate gland can have an anticancer effect, but leuprolide does not reduce angiogenesis.

▶ *Learning objective:* Identify the site of action of leuprolide.

8. Answer: A

Leuprolide is an analogue of Gn-RH and acts on the gonadotroph cells of the pituitary to affect the release of LH and FSH.

B Leuprolide can cause a feedback inhibition of secretion of Gn-RH from hypothalamic neurons, but these neurons are not the primary site of action of leuprolide.

C Leydig's cells of the testes produce testosterone in the presence of LH. Therefore, they are involved in the leuprolide action but are not the primary target of leuprolide.

D Gland cells of the prostate secrete a slightly alkaline fluid that constitutes roughly 30% of the volume of the semen. This secretion is not affected by Gn-RH or its analogues.

E Cells of the zona reticularis in the adrenals synthesize testosterone, but they are under the control of adrenocorticotropic hormone, not of Gn-RH or its analogues, such as leuprolide.

▶ *Learning objective:* Explain the molecular mechanism of action of leuprolide.

9. Answer: B

The Gn-RH is released in a pulsatile way, which is crucial for the proper synthesis and release of gonadotropins by the pituitary gonadotroph cells. The continuous administration of Gn-RH (due to administration of a depot preparation that continuously releases the drug) leads to desensitization and downregulation of Gn-RH receptors in the pituitary gonadotroph cells. This produces a decline in the release of FSH and LH. Ultimately the levels of these hormones and consequently of testosterone become profoundly suppressed.

351

A Because testosterone synthesis is impaired, androgen receptors are upregulated, not downregulated.

C Leuprolide has no direct action on androgen receptors.

D Inhibition of tyrosine kinase of cancer cells may have an anticancer effect, but this inhibition is the mechanism of action of several monoclonal antibodies (imatinib, erlotinib, sorafenib), not of leuprolide.

E Leuprolide can cause a feedback inhibition, not activation, of Gn-RH synthesis in the hypothalamus.

▶ *Learning objective:* Explain the molecular mechanism of action of flutamide.

---

10. Answer: D

Flutamide, bicalutamide, and nilutamide are competitive androgen receptor antagonists that are approved for hormonal therapy of prostate cancer. The drugs are most effective when used simultaneously with Gn-RH agonists, such as leuprolide acetate, as in the present case.

A This would be the mechanism of action of aromatase inhibitors. Because aromatase is the enzyme that converts testosterone into estradiol, this inhibition would be irrational in prostate cancer.

B 5α-reductase is the enzyme that catalyzes the transformation of testosterone into dihydrotestosterone. Flutamide does not inhibit the enzyme. Moreover, it has been shown that the inhibition of this enzyme increases the incidence of prostate cancer.

C, E Flutamide cannot cause these effects.

▶ *Learning objective:* Identify a rare but life-threatening adverse effect of flutamide.

---

11. Answer: D

Hepatotoxicity is a rare (< 0.5%) but serious adverse effect of flutamide, because the disease can progress to hepatic encephalopathy and death related to acute liver failure. Flutamide hepatotoxicity appears to be due primarily to hepatic necrosis, even if reversible hepatitis has been reported. Approximately half the reported cases occurred in the first 3 months of flutamide treatment. Hepatotoxicity is reversible in some cases if flutamide is discontinued promptly. Patients should undergo periodic monitoring of liver function tests. Liver function tests should also be obtained at the onset of symptoms such as nausea, vomiting, abdominal pain, fatigue, anorexia, flulike symptoms, hyperbilirubinuria, jaundice, or right upper quadrant tenderness. Flutamide should be immediately discontinued in patients with jaundice or with liver transaminases above two to three times the upper limit of normal.

A, B, C, E, F The risk of these adverse effects in patients taking flutamide is < 0.01%.

▶ *Learning objective:* Identify an adverse effect common to both leuprolide and flutamide.

---

12. Answer: B

Gynecomastia is a condition in which the glandular tissue in the breasts becomes enlarged in boys or men, sometimes causing discomfort or nipple tenderness. About 10 to 20% of gynecomastia cases are due to drugs that can decrease the activity of testosterone, favoring an increased activity of estrogens. Leuprolide and flutamide have different mechanisms of action, but the final effect of both is a decreased activity of testosterone. Gynecomastia occurs in about 7% of leuprolide-treated patients and in about 9% of flutamide-treated patients. Because K.L. received both drugs the risk of gynecomastia was most likely substantial.

A, C, D, E, F These adverse effects can occur with leuprolide or flutamide, but their incidence is < 3%.

▶ *Learning objective:* Explain a reason for the use of pamidronate in metastasized prostate cancer.

---

13. Answer: C

Pamidronate is a bisphosphonate drug. These agents are used for the treatment of hypercalcemia and prevention of bone fractures in prostate and breast cancers. They can also reduce the pain caused by bone metastases. It is worth noting that, although quite uncommon, long-term use of bisphosphonates has been associated with atypical fractures.

A, **B**, **D** Pamidronate cannot treat or prevent these diseases.

E Pamidronate cannot improve overall survival in patients with cancer.

▶ *Learning objective:* Explain the action mediating the therapeutic effect of pamidronate.

---

14.   Answer: D

Bisphosphonate drugs like pamidronate are called osteoclast inhibitors because they are incorporated into the bone matrix and inhibit the activity of osteoclasts in a dose-dependent manner. This inhibitory effect apparently involves two primary mechanisms:

▶ The drugs are incorporated into adenosine triphosphate analogues that accumulate within the osteoclast, thereby promoting osteoclast apoptosis.
▶ The drugs interfere with the anchoring of cell surface proteins to the osteoclast membrane, thereby preventing osteoclast attachment to bone.

A Stimulation of osteoblast activity would be an indirect action of both parathyroid hormone and calcitriol.

B Stimulation of intestinal calcium absorption would be an action of calcitriol.

C Inhibition of renal calcium excretion would be an action of both parathyroid hormone and calcitriol.

E Inhibition of renal synthesis of calcitriol would be an action of parathyroid hormone.

▶ *Learning objective:* Identify a rare but serious adverse effect of pamidronate treatment.

---

15.   Answer: D

Osteonecrosis, primarily of the jaw, has been described in patients receiving bisphosphonates. Typical signs and symptoms of osteonecrosis of the jaw include pain, swelling, infection, loosening of the teeth, a feeling of heaviness in the jaw, and drainage of exposed bone. Dental surgery may exacerbate the condition. Most reported cases have occurred in cancer patients after invasive dental procedures, such as tooth extraction.

A Osteomalacia is defined as a decreased bone mass with decreased ratio of mineral to matrix. The disorder is treated with calcium and vitamin D or calcitriol.

B Osteoporosis is defined as a decreased bone mass with a normal ratio of mineral to matrix. Bisphosphonate drugs are able to treat, not cause, osteoporosis.

C, **E** These disorders do not occur after bisphosphonate drug treatment.

Psoriasis

H.J., a 36-year-old woman, presented to the dermatology clinic because of worsening of her psoriasis.

H.J.'s medical history indicated that she was diagnosed with plaque psoriasis when she was 20. The psoriasis initially responded to topical combination therapy with betamethasone and calcipotriene. Salicylic acid and coal tar compounds were also used topically from time to time. Subsequently the patient underwent photochemotherapy using oral methoxsalen (a psoralen agent) and psoralen plus ultraviolet A (PUVA) phototherapy with good results. Some years later, however, the therapy was no longer effective, and flare-ups were managed first with oral acitretin with limited success. At that time a change in therapy was implemented, and over the years the patient received various drugs, including methotrexate, cyclosporine, and ustekinumab.

H.J. suffered from an episode of acute bronchiolitis when she was 5 but had no other diseases besides psoriasis.

The family history indicated that H.J.'s father was diagnosed with psoriasis at the age of 65 and died 6 years later from heart failure. Her mother was alive and well. H.J. was married and had one 14-year-old son. In the past the patient had smoked two to four cigarettes daily, but she had quit smoking when she was 22. She denied the use of illicit drugs but admitted drinking a glass of scotch almost every evening.

Upon skin examination, confluent plaque psoriasis was noted. Erythematous plaque-like lesions were present on the scalp, abdomen, trunk, arms, and legs. Lesions were red to violet in color and were loosely covered with silvery-white scales. There were no pustules or vesicles. The patient admitted that the lesions were quite disturbing and that she often scratched them. The rest of the physical examination was noncontributory.

Questions

1. H.J. had psoriasis. Which of the following is the approximate percentage of the population affected by this disease worldwide?

A. < 0.1%

B. 0.1–0.5%

C. 1–5%

D. 9–10%

E. 11–12%

2. H.J. was diagnosed with plaque psoriasis. With appropriate treatments, which of the following is most likely the mean duration of this disease?

A. 5 years

B. 10 years

C. 15 years

D. 20 years

E. Lifelong

3. Which of the following was most likely a significant risk factor for H.J.'s psoriasis?

A. Smoking

B. Drugs

C. Infections

D. Genetic factors

E. Gender

4. Psoriasis is a well-known chronic dermatosis. A biopsy of H.J.'s skin would most likely show which of the following pairs of skin lesions?

A. Smaller papillary vessels–neutrophil microabscesses

B. Parakeratosis–thicker stratum granulosum

C. Parakeratosis–smaller papillary vessels

D. Thicker stratum granulosum–neutrophil microabscesses

E. Thicker stratum granulosum–smaller papillary vessels

F. Parakeratosis–neutrophil microabscesses

5. Current pathophysiological studies indicate that psoriasis belongs most likely to which of the following disease types?

A. Infective

B. Autoimmune

C. Allergic

D. Preneoplastic

E. Degenerative

6. An initial topical treatment of H.J.'s psoriasis included an ointment containing betamethasone and calcipotriene. Activation of which of the following receptors on epidermal cells most likely mediated the therapeutic effect of calcipotriene in the patient's disease?

A. Tumor necrosis factor receptors

B. Interferon receptors

C. IL-10 receptors

D. Vitamin D receptors

E. IL-6 receptors

7. Betamethasone was given topically to H.J. Which of the following adverse effects could likely occur with the topical long-term use of this drug?

A. Cataract

B. Weight loss

C. Skin hyperpigmentation

D. Hypotension

E. Skin atrophy

8. Salicylic acid was given topically to H.J. Which of the following actions most likely mediated the therapeutic effect of the drug in the patient's disease?

A. Antipruritic

B. Anti-inflammatory

C. Keratolytic

D. Counterirritant

E. Antiseptic

F. Astringent

9. H.J. underwent PUVA photochemo-therapy. Which of the following statement best explains why psoralens are associated with ultraviolet therapy?

A. Psoralens protect the skin from ultraviolet-induced burning.

B. Psoralens need photoactivation to produce a therapeutic effect.

C. Ultraviolet A counteracts most adverse effects of psoralens.

D. Ultraviolet A strongly increases the duration of psoralen action.

10. Acitretin was given orally to H.J. Which of the following epidermal cell structures most likely represents the primary site of action of this drug?

A. Plasma membrane

B. Mitochondria

C. Smooth endoplasmic reticulum

D. Rough endoplasmic reticulum

E. Nucleus

F. Ribosomes

11. Which of the following laboratory tests would be crucial to monitor monthly, after starting acitretin therapy in this patient and for 2 to 3 years after discontinuation of the therapy?

A. Liver function tests

B. Pregnancy test

C. Complete blood count

D. Cholesterol levels

E. Urinalysis

12. Methotrexate was given to H.J. Because of the long-term therapy with this drug and the patient's history, which of the following toxic effects should be especially taken into account during H.J.'s treatment?

A. Liver fibrosis

B. Stroke

C. Heart failure

D. Ulcerative colitis

E. Osteoarthritis

13. Cyclosporine was given to H.J. Which of the following actions most likely mediated the therapeutic effect of the drug in the patient's disease?

A. Stimulation of synthesis of tumor necrosis factor

B. Stimulation of B cell differentiation into memory B cells

C. Inhibition of the apoptosis pathway in target cells

D. Stimulation of gene expression for IL-2 production

E. Inhibition of calcineurin

14. During cyclosporine therapy, H.J. was most likely at risk of which of the following drug-induced adverse effects?

A. Nephrotoxicity

B. Hypotension

C. Weight loss

D. Pulmonary fibrosis

E. Toxic megacolon

15. If cyclosporine had to be discontinued because of adverse effects, which of the following drugs could be an appropriate therapy for H.J.'s psoriasis at that time?

A. Hydroxychloroquine

B. Trastuzumab

C. Infliximab

D. Abciximab

E. Ketorolac

F. Ibuprofen

Answers and Explanations

▶ *Learning objective:* Identify the approximate percentage of the population affected by psoriasis worldwide.

1. Answer: C

Psoriasis is a skin inflammatory disease that affects about 1 to 5% of the population worldwide. Light-skinned people are at greater risk. Peak onset is roughly bimodal, most often at ages 20 to 39 and at ages 55 to 70, but the disorder can occur at any age.

A, B, D, E See correct answer explanation.

▶ *Learning objective:* Estimate the mean duration of psoriasis when treated appropriately.

2. Answer: E

There are five types of psoriasis: plaque, guttate, inverse, pustular, and erythrodermic. Plaque psoriasis, also known as psoriasis vulgaris, makes up about 90% of cases. Plaque psoriasis is an incurable disease. Even the most appropriate treatments can control symptoms for a while, but the disease waxes and wanes repeatedly and is lifelong.

A, B, C, D See correct answer explanation.

▶ *Learning objective:* Identify a significant risk factor for psoriasis.

3. Answer: D

Psoriasis has long been known to occur in families. Approximately 40% of patients with psoriasis have a family history of this disorder in first-degree relatives, as in the present case. Moreover, genome-wide association studies have identified multiple susceptibility loci for psoriasis, many of which contain genes involved in regulation of the immune system.

A Smoking may be a risk factor for psoriasis, but the amount was too low to be significant in the present case.

B Multiple drugs are associated with psoriasis or psoriasis-like drug eruptions. The most common offenders are β-blockers, lithium, and antimalarial drugs, nonsteroidal anti-inflammatory drugs, and tetracycline. There was no mention of these drugs in H.J.'s medical history.

C Infections have been linked to psoriasis but H.J.'s only infectious disease occurred several years before the appearance of psoriasis.

E There is no clear gender predilection for psoriasis.

▶ *Learning objective:* Describe the pathological lesions most likely found in a biopsy of psoriatic skin.

4. Answer: F

Psoriasis is characterized by an abnormally excessive and rapid growth of the epidermal layer of the skin. Skin cells are replaced every 3 to 5 days in psoriasis rather than the usual 28 to 30 days. This results in epidermal hyperplasia and parakeratosis (retention of nuclei in the stratum corneum) with concomitant inflammation. Neutrophils are prominent in lesions of psoriasis and are found in collections throughout the epidermis, forming microabscesses (named Munro's microabscesses). The neutrophil chemoattractant interleukin-8 (IL-8) is highly elevated in psoriatic skin.

A, C, E Dermal papillary vessels are dilated, not smaller.

B, D, E The stratum granulosum is thinner or even absent, not thicker.

▶ *Learning objective:* Identify the type of pathological disease that most likely includes psoriasis.

5. Answer: B

Although early concepts of the pathogenesis of psoriasis focused primarily on keratinocyte hyperplasia, dysregulation of the immune system is now recognized as the critical event, and psoriasis is considered an autoimmune disorder today.

The following is a basic sequence of the immunologic events that are theorized to occur in psoriasis:

▶ Antigenic stimuli contribute to the activation of dendritic cells and other innate immune cells in the skin.
▶ These immune cells move from the dermis to the epidermis and secrete inflammatory cytokines, such as tumor necrosis factor-α, IL-1, and IL-6, that stimulate the activation of myeloid dendritic cells in the skin.
▶ Myeloid dendritic cells produce cytokines that stimulate the attraction, activation, and differentiation of T cells.

▶ Recruited T cells produce cytokines that stimulate keratinocytes to proliferate and produce proinflammatory cytokines.
▶ These cytokines perpetuate the inflammatory process via participation in positive feedback loops.

A Patients with psoriasis can have an increased risk of skin infections, especially if they are treated with immunosuppressive agents, but psoriasis is not an infective disorder.
C Although psoriasis and allergies both involve the immune system, psoriasis is an autoimmune, not an allergic disease.
D Preneoplastic (also called precancerous) disease refers to a lesion or process that has a high risk of becoming malignant with time. Psoriasis does not become malignant with time.
E A degenerative disease results from a continuous process based on degenerative cell changes, affecting tissues or organs, which will increasingly deteriorate over time. Psoriasis is an inflammatory, not a degenerative, disorder.

▶ *Learning objective:* Identify the receptors activated by calcipotriene.

6. Answer: D
Calcipotriene is a synthetic vitamin D_3 derivative that is effective in the treatment of plaque psoriasis of moderate severity. The exact mechanism of action of the drug is unknown, but it binds to vitamin D receptors on epidermal cells, inducing inhibition of keratinocyte proliferation and induction of keratinocyte differentiation. The drug is often given together with betamethasone, because the combination has been shown more effective than its individual ingredients. Calcitriol, the active form of vitamin D_3, can also be given topically in psoriasis and is similar in efficacy to calcipotriene.
A, B, C, E All these receptors are cytokine receptors that are ubiquitously present throughout several cells and tissues. Calcipotriene does not activate these receptors.

▶ *Learning objective:* Describe the adverse effect that can occur after long-term use of topical betamethasone.

7. Answer: E
Glucocorticoids remain the mainstay of topical psoriasis treatment despite the development of newer agents. These drugs are only partially absorbed through the normal skin, but absorption is increased severalfold when the skin is inflamed. Topical glucocorticoids are safer than systemic glucocorticoids. Nevertheless, cutaneous and systemic side effects can occur, particularly with potent agents, or with extensive use. Local effects of topical glucocorticoids are many, including skin atrophy, acne, rosacea, purpura, hypopigmentation, delayed wound healing, perioral dermatitis, and hypertrichosis. Skin atrophy presents as shiny, often wrinkled-appearing skin with prominent telangiectases. The pathogenesis of this adverse effect is likely multifactorial, involving an inhibitory effect on keratinocyte proliferation, inhibition of dermal collagen synthesis, and inhibition of hyaluronic acid synthesis.
A Cataract is an adverse effect of systemic glucocorticoids. This adverse effect can occur rarely with chronic periorbital application of topical glucocorticoids.
B, C, D Glucocorticoids tend to cause adverse effects opposite to those listed.

▶ *Learning objective:* Describe the action that most likely mediated the therapeutic effect of salicylic acid in psoriasis.

8. Answer: C
Salicylic acid has been extensively used topically in dermatologic therapy as a keratolytic agent. The mechanism of this action is still uncertain, but it seems that the drug solubilizes cell surface proteins that function as intercellular cement. This reduces keratinocyte adhesion, resulting in desquamation of keratitic debris.
A, B, D, E, F Salicylic acid exhibits most of these actions, but they are not involved in the therapeutic effect of the drug in psoriasis.

▸ *Learning objective:* Explain why oral psoralens are associated with ultraviolet therapy in the treatment of psoriasis.

9. Answer: B

Psoralens, such as methoxsalen, can be considered prodrugs because they must be photoactivated by long-wavelength light to produce their beneficial effects. A number of possible mechanisms have been postulated to explain antiproliferative PUVA's effects. Most likely psoralens intercalate with DNA and, after UV irradiation, they cause interstrand cross-links that inhibit DNA function. About 90% of psoriatic patients have clearing of skin disease after 30 PUVA treatment with methoxsalen, and remission can last for more than 6 months.

A Psoralens are not sunscreening agents.

C, D Ultraviolet A does not affect the action of psoralens. The light simply activates the prodrugs, causing both their therapeutic and their adverse effects.

▸ *Learning objective:* Describe the cell structure that represents the primary site of action of retinoids

10. Answer: E

Acitretin is a retinoid used orally for patients with severe psoriasis. Retinoids are analogues of vitamin A with important functions in the body, including regulation of cell proliferation and differentiation. They are used both topically and systemically, mainly to treat acne or disorders of keratinization, as in the present case. Retinoids exert their effects on gene expression by activating receptors that are members of the superfamily of nuclear receptors, which includes steroids, vitamin D, and thyroid hormone receptors. Retinoid receptors have different isoforms and a given retinoid binds to a specific receptor isoform. The retinoid–receptor complex is transported to the nucleus, where it binds specific DNA sequences, activating transcription of genes, whose products produce the desired pharmacological effects of these drugs, as well as their unwanted adverse effects.

A, B, C, D, F Retinoids do not act on these structures.

▸ *Learning objective:* Identify the lab test that must be monitored in a young woman taking retinoid therapy.

11. Answer: B

Acitretin is a second-generation retinoid. All retinoids are strong teratogenic drugs (pregnancy Food and Drug Administration category X) and must not be used by females who are pregnant or who intend to become pregnant. Therefore a woman of child-bearing age should have at least monthly pregnancy testing, even if the patient is using a form of effective contraception regularly. Women must avoid pregnancy for at least 2 to 3 years following discontinuation of therapy, due to the long-term teratogenic potential of these drugs.

A, C, D, E Retinoids can cause liver toxicity, and increased liver enzymes can occur in > 30% of patients receiving the drug. Therefore all the listed exams must be done frequently during therapy but can be discontinued when therapy is terminated.

▸ *Learning objective:* Recognize the adverse effect that can occur after long-term therapy with methotrexate in a patient that drinks alcohol regularly.

12. Answer: A

The folic acid antagonist methotrexate has been used successfully in the treatment of psoriasis for more than 20 years. In the past it was thought that the mechanism of action was related to the antiproliferative effects of methotrexate on DNA synthesis in epidermal cells. Further studies, however, support the concept that it is the immunosuppressive effects of methotrexate on activated T cells that controls psoriasis. Methotrexate is relatively safe and well tolerated, but the two most significant adverse effects of the drug are myelosuppression and cumulative liver toxicity (fibrosis and cirrhosis), which is potentially fatal. Liver toxicity is even more likely in the present case, because the patient drank alcohol regularly. Alcohol and methotrexate constitute a particularly potent hepatotoxic combination.

B, C, D, E The risk of all these toxic effects is very low or absent during methotrexate therapy.

▶ *Learning objective:* Describe the mechanism of action of cyclosporine.

13. Answer: E

Cyclosporine is an immunosuppressant drug, and several studies support its status as a highly and rapidly effective treatment. Improvement is generally observed within 4 weeks. The activity of cyclosporine is mediated through reversible inhibition of T cell function, particularly T-helper cells. The drug binds to a T-helper cell cytoplasmic cyclophilin, and then the complex binds to calcineurin (a phosphatase) and inhibits its action. This inhibition is thought to prevent activation of nuclear factors involved in the gene transcription of IL-2 and other cytokines. Because IL-2 is needed for T cell activation and proliferation, these T cell functions are suppressed.

A, B, C, D All these actions would activate, not inhibit, immunity processes.

▶ *Learning objective:* Identify a very common adverse effect of cyclosporine.

14. Answer: A

The patient was most likely at risk of cyclosporine-induced nephrotoxicity, which is the most common adverse effect of the drug, occurring in up to 80% of treated patients. The pathophysiology of this adverse effect is still uncertain, but is likely related to a glomerular hypoperfusion secondary to vasoconstriction of the afferent arteriole.

B Cyclosporine usually causes hypertension, not hypotension.

C Weight gain, not loss, is more likely with cyclosporine because the drug may cause appetite stimulation.

D, E Cyclosporine does not cause these effects.

▶ *Learning objective:* Identify a drug that can be used to treat psoriasis.

15. Answer: C

Infliximab is a tumor necrosis factor-α (TNF-α) inhibitor. The drug is a monoclonal antibody that binds to both the soluble and the membrane-bound TNF-α, blocking the binding of TNF-α to its receptors.

Some TNF-α inhibitors, including infliximab, etanercept, and adalimumab, are used to treat moderate to severe chronic plaque psoriasis. Some meta-analyses support the designation of infliximab as the most effective of these biologic agents.

A Hydroxychloroquine is a disease-modifying antirheumatic drug used in rheumatoid arthritis.

B Trastuzumab is a monoclonal antibody to human epidermal growth factor receptor 2 used in breast cancer.

D Abciximab is an antiplatelet monoclonal antibody used in acute coronary syndromes.

E, F Ketorolac and ibuprofen are nonsteroidal anti-inflammatory drugs.

Case 41

Pulmonary Embolism

Q.R., a 64-year-old man, underwent total right knee replacement for severe degenerative joint disease. Three days after surgery, he presented with acute onset of shortness of breath, right side chest pain worsened by breathing, cough, and red-stained sputum. The patient's medical history was significant for an episode of deep venous thrombosis on the left leg that occurred 3 years ago and was successfully treated with heparin and warfarin. Before surgery Q.R. received cefazolin for antimicrobial prophylaxis. Postsurgical treatment included anticoagulant therapy with heparin and ketorolac for postsurgical pain.

Physical examination showed a patient in moderate respiratory distress with the following vital signs: blood pressure 110/70 mm Hg, pulse 125 bpm, respirations 30/min. Lung auscultation gave some inspiratory crackles. Cardiac examination revealed tachycardia but was otherwise unremarkable. The right lower extremity was postsurgical and was healing well, with + 2 pitting edema, calf tenderness, and erythema.

Pertinent lab exam results were:

Arterial blood gases

- PO2: 72 mm Hg (normal 80–100)
- PCO2: 44 mm Hg (normal 38–45)
- SaO2: 90% (normal > 95)

Ventilation/perfusion (V/Q) scanning

Substantial increase of the whole lung V/Q ratio.

Computer tomography scan

Complete occlusion of an inferior branch of the right pulmonary artery.

A diagnosis of pulmonary thromboembolism was made, and emergency therapy was started with oxygen, intravenous (IV) unfractionated heparin, and oral dabigatran.

Questions

1. Q.R. was diagnosed with pulmonary thromboembolism. Which of the following is the most common clinical presentation of thromboembolism in the general population?

A. No symptoms

B. Tachycardia

C. Dyspnea

D. Hemoptysis

E. Lung crackles

2. An acute pulmonary thromboembolism can cause sudden death. Which of the following mechanisms most likely mediates this death?

A. Massive lung atelectasis

B. Lung hemorrhage

C. Acute right heart failure

D. Myocardial infarction

E. Glottis edema

3. Q.R.'s pulmonary thromboembolus most likely originated in which of the following cardiovascular structures?

A. Right superior pulmonary artery

B. Left femoral artery

C. Right popliteal vein

D. Right heart atrium

E. Left dorsal metatarsal vein

F. Left superior pulmonary vein

4. A thromboembolic disease starts with thrombus formation that is triggered by the activation of the extrinsic coagulation cascade. The activation of which of the following coagulation factors was most likely the primary event leading to the thrombus formation?

A. Factor IX

B. Factor X

C. Factor II

D. Factor XII

E. Factor VII

F. Factor IV

5. Q.R. suffered from chest pain worsened by breathing. Which of the following organs was most likely the source of his pain?

A. Heart

B. Intercostal muscles

C. Aorta

D. Pleura

E. Diaphragm

F. Bronchi

6. Q.R. underwent measurement of the V/Q ratio. Which of the following is most likely the alveolar ventilation in a normal adult person at rest (in L/min)?

A. 2.5

B. 4.2

C. 5.5

D. 6.0

E. 6.5

7. Q.R.'s lab exams showed a substantial increase of the whole lung V/Q ratio. Which of the following statements best explains the reason for this result?

A. Increased ventilation, increased perfusion

B. Normal ventilation, increased perfusion

C. Normal ventilation, decreased perfusion

D. Decreased ventilation, normal perfusion

E. Decreased ventilation, increased perfusion

8. Q.R.'s vital signs included tachycardia. Which of the following was most likely the cause of his increased heart rate?

A. Generalized bronchoconstriction

B. Increased firing from aortic baroreceptors

C. Decreased pulmonary vascular resistance

D. Increased right ventricle afterload

E. Decreased peripheral vasoconstriction

9. Cefazolin was given to Q.R. as antimicrobial prophylaxis before surgery. Which of the following bacterial species most likely represented the main target of the drug in this patient?

A. Klebsiellae

B. Enterococci

C. Bacteroides

D. Chlamidiae

E. Staphylococci

F. Mycobacteria

10. Q.R. was treated with unfractionated heparin IV. The drug acts by inhibiting the activation of many coagulation factors. Which of the following factors is most sensitive to this inhibition?

A. VIIa

B. I

C. XII

D. IIa

E. V

F. IX

11. Protamine is commonly given in cases of heparin overdose. Which of the following statements best explains the mechanism of action of protamine?

A. Speed up the metabolism of heparin by the liver

B. Blocks the synthesis of heparin in mast cells and basophils

C. Binds to antithrombin III, preventing binding to heparin

D. Combines with heparin in the blood, deactivating it

E. Activates the coagulation cascade, overriding the action of heparin

12. Which of the following lab exams should be performed frequently during the heparin treatment to predict a serious adverse effect of the drug?

A. Prothrombin time

B. Bleeding time

C. Fibrinolysis time

D. Red blood cell count

E. Platelet count

F. White blood cell count

13. Which of the following lab tests is most commonly used to monitor the anticoagulant activity of unfractionated heparin?

A. Prothrombin time

B. Bleeding time

C. Fibrinolysis time

D. Activated partial thromboplastin time

E. Plasminogen activity

F. Protein C antigen

14. Q.R. was treated with oral dabigatran. Which of the following coagulation factors is the primary molecular target of this drug?

A. Factor IX

B. Factor X

C. Factor IIa

D. Factor VII

E. Factor XIIa

F. Factor IV

15. Which of the following drugs could be used in a case of severe dabigatran overdose?

A. Vitamin K

B. Protamine sulfate

C. Desmopressin

D. Abciximab

E. Idarucizumab

Answers and Explanations

▶ *Learning objective:* Describe the most common clinical outcome of pulmonary thromboembolism in the general population.

1. Answer: A

Pulmonary emboli are quite common, but most patients with pulmonary embolism have no obvious symptoms at presentation. Rather, pulmonary embolism can cause symptoms only when sufficiently large, and the diagnosis is made ante mortem in only 10 to 20% of cases. When present, symptoms may vary from sudden catastrophic hemodynamic collapse to gradually progressive dyspnea. The diagnosis of pulmonary embolism should be suspected in patients with respiratory symptoms unexplained by an alternative diagnosis.

B, C, D, E All these are Q.R.'s symptoms, which indicate that his thromboembolus was medium to large.

▶ *Learning objective:* Identify the most common cause of sudden death in acute pulmonary thromboembolism.

2. Answer: C

A pulmonary embolus that occludes the main pulmonary artery, or one of its primary branches, can cause a sudden increase in pulmonary pressure. In normal individuals, the pulmonary circulation is a low resistance, high capacitance system capable of accommodating a three- to four-fold increase in right ventricular stroke volume without significantly raising pulmonary pressures. However, the thin right ventricular wall makes the right chamber poorly tolerant of acute pulmonary hypertension. In normal individuals, the right ventricle is unable to acutely generate a mean pressure > 40 mm Hg, and stroke volume decreases linearly as right ventricular afterload increases. Rapid elevations in afterload can cause acute right ventricle dilation, damaging the contractile sarcomere apparatus with resultant right ventricular failure.

A Because the airways are not obstructed, the lung does not collapse and there is no atelectasis.

B Lung hemorrhage can occur in pulmonary embolism, but this is not the cause of sudden death.

D Myocardial infarction can occur in the very rare cases of chronic massive pulmonary embolism, but this is not the cause of sudden death in acute pulmonary thromboembolism.

E Edema is not a feature of acute pulmonary thromboembolism.

▶ *Learning objective:* Identify the site of origin of the patient's pulmonary thromboembolus.

3. Answer: C

Thromboemboli almost never originate in the pulmonary circulation; they arrive there by a venous route. More than 95% of pulmonary thromboemboli arise from thrombi in the deep veins of the lower extremities—the popliteal, femoral, and iliac veins. Risk factors for these thrombi include immobilization, especially following orthopaedic surgery and local vascular damage, as in the present case. Since the patient was operated in the right leg, the thromboembolus most likely originated in the right popliteal vein.

A, B Thromboemboli originate in the veins, not in the arteries.

D Thromboemboli can originate in the pelvic, renal, or upper extremity veins, or in the right heart chambers, but this is a very rare event.

E Since the patient was operated in the right leg, his thromboembolus most likely originated in the right, not in the left, leg.

F Thromboemboli almost never originate in the pulmonary circulation.

▶ *Learning objective:* Identify the coagulation factor whose activation is the primary event leading to the thrombus formation.

4. Answer: E

The coagulation cascade is a sequence of enzymatic events. Coagulation factors circulate as inactive proenzymes. These proenzymes are activated by the activated factor that precedes them in the cascade. Because the activation reaction is catalytic, amplification occurs (e.g., one unit of factor Xa can generate 40 units of thrombin). This robust amplification process generates a large amount of fibrin.

The coagulation cascade has traditionally been divided traditionally as follows:

▶ **Extrinsic coagulation pathway (ECP):** It begins with enzymes located outside the blood.
▶ **Intrinsic coagulation pathway (ICP):** It begins with enzymes located in the blood.
▶ **Final common pathway**

The ICP is activated in vitro by factor XII (Hageman's factor).

The ECP is activated in vivo by tissue factors at the site of vascular injury, which in turn activates factor VII (stable factor or proconvertin).

Because factor VII can in turn activate factor X (a key factor in the coagulation cascade), the ECP is regarded as the primary pathway for coagulation in vivo.

A Factor IX (Christmas factor) activates factor X.

B Factor X (Stuart–Prower's factor) activates factor II.

C Factor II (prothrombin) activates factor I (fibrinogen).

D Factor XII (Hageman factor) activates factor XI.

F Factor IV (calcium) is a cofactor that facilitates several steps of the coagulation cascade.

▶ *Learning objective:* Describe the most likely source of chest pain in a patient with pulmonary thromboembolism.

5. Answer: D

A chest pain worsened by breathing is defined pleuritic chest pain. This pain occurs in about 50% of patients with pulmonary embolism and is mainly due to pleural effusion. The pleural effusion associated with pulmonary emboli is almost always an exudate. In other words, pleural effusion is most likely related to pleural inflammation. The primary mechanism by which pulmonary emboli produce pleural inflammation is by increasing the perme-

ability of the capillaries in the lung. This results in increased pulmonary interstitial fluid. The main factor responsible for the increased permeability of pulmonary capillaries is probably the release of inflammatory mediators from the platelet-rich thrombus. It is likely that vascular endothelial growth factor (VEGF) plays a role in this increased permeability. Platelets contain large quantities of VEGF, which is one of the most potent factors known for increasing capillary permeability. The pleural cavity normally contains a small amount of lubricating fluid that allows the two layers to slide over each other during breathing. When the pleura becomes inflamed, the layers rub together, causing chest pain.

A, B, C, E, F All these organs can be a source of chest pain, but this pain is not of respiratory origin and usually is not worsened by breathing.

▶ *Learning objective:* Identify the alveolar ventilation (in L/min) in a normal adult person at rest.

6. Answer: B

In pulmonary physiology *ventilation* refers to the air that reaches the alveoli in a minute. It can be calculated as follows: tidal volume (TV) − dead space (DS) × respiratory rate (RR). In a normal adult person at rest, this ventilation is

$$[VT (0.5 L) - DS (0.15 L)] \times RR (12/min)$$
$$= 4.2 \ L/min.$$

A, C, D, E See correct answer explanation.

▶ *Learning objective:* Explain the reason for an increased V/Q ratio in a patient with pulmonary thromboembolism.

7. Answer: C

Pulmonary thromboembolism most often results from an embolus in a branch of the pulmonary artery. This causes a large perfusion defect in the area supplied by that branch, whereas the ventilation in the same area remains normal. Therefore the whole lung V/Q ratio is increased. This "mismatched" defect is highly specific (97%) for pulmonary embolism.

A This event would not change the V/Q ratio.

B, D, E All these events would decrease, not increase, the V/Q ratio.

▶ *Learning objective:* Identify the main cause of tachycardia in a patient with pulmonary thromboembolism.

8. Answer: D

Tachycardia is a common symptom of acute pulmonary thromboembolism. The reason is that the thromboembolus causes a sudden increase in right ventricular afterload, which in turn elicits a decrease in cardiac output. When cardiac output is decreased activation of the sympathetic nervous system occurs within 30 to 60 seconds, leading to compensatory tachycardia.

A Mild to moderate hypoxemia is a common finding in pulmonary thromboembolism. Hypoxemia causes bronchodilation, not bronchoconstriction.

B When cardiac output is decreased blood pressure decreases, causing a decreased, not an increased, firing from baroreceptors.

C Pulmonary vascular resistance is increased, not decreased, because of the occlusion or subocclusion in the pulmonary artery bed.

E Activation of the sympathetic system causes an increase, not a decrease, in peripheral vasoconstriction.

▶ *Learning objective:* Identify the bacterial species that is the most likely target of cefazolin in prophylaxis for orthopaedic surgery.

9. Answer: E

Antibiotic prophylaxis is given to prevent infections and should be used when efficacy has been demonstrated and benefits outweigh the risks. Surgical wound infections are a major category of nosocomial infections, and risk factors for those infections include orthopaedic surgery. Optimal antimicrobial agents for prophylaxis should be bactericidal, nontoxic, and active against the typical pathogens that can cause postoperative surgical infection. In most hospitals, cefazolin is the antibiotic of choice for preoperative prophylaxis in patients undergoing total joint replacement procedures. The reason for this is that cefazolin (a first-generation cephalosporin) has excellent activity against staphylococci that constitute the normal flora of the skin (mainly *Staphylococcus epidermidis*) and are common pathogens in orthopaedic surgery with hardware insertion.

A All cephalosporins, including cefazolin, are very active against klebsiellae, but these bacteria are not common pathogens in orthopaedic surgery.

B, C, D, F These bacteria do not belong to the normal skin flora and are not sensitive to cefazolin.

▶ *Learning objective:* Identify the coagulation factor that is most sensitive to heparin-induced inhibition.

10. Answer: D

Antithrombin III (ATIII) is a protease inhibitor that slowly neutralizes many activated coagulation factors by forming stable complexes with them (a "suicide substrate"). Heparin accelerates the activity of ATIII by increasing the rate of reaction to ATIII-coagulation factor. Thrombin (factor IIa) is the most sensitive to inhibition (in this case the rate is increased at least 1,000-fold). Once ATIII and thrombin have formed a complex, heparin quickly dissociates and binds to other ATIII molecules.

A Heparin has very little activity against factor VIIa.

B, C, E, F All these are proenzymes, not activated enzymes. Heparin acts only on activated coagulation factors.

▶ *Learning objective:* Explain the mechanism of action of protamine in cases of heparin overdose.

11. Answer: D

Protamine sulfate is a highly basic peptide that combines with heparin (which is a highly acidic compound) as an ion pair to form a stable complex devoid of anticoagulant activity. The drug has a rapid onset of action with an effect lasting about 2 hours.

A, B, C, E Protamine does not display these actions.

▶ *Learning objective:* Identify the lab exam that should be done frequently during heparin therapy.

12. Answer: E

Unfractionated heparin can cause transient thrombocytopenia (called type I) in up to 15% of patients and severe thrombocytopenia (called type II) in up to 5% of patients. Type II thrombocytopenia is due to antibody-mediated platelet aggregation and has a mortality rate up to 30% (it can cause paradoxical thromboembolism, leading to stroke, myocardial infarction, etc.). Therefore a platelet count should be performed frequently during heparin treatment. Any thrombocytopenia appearing during treatment should be considered suspicious for heparin-induced thrombocytopenia, and the drug should be substituted with another anticoagulant.

A Prothrombin time is a test used to monitor the anticoagulant activity, not to predict a serious adverse effect of heparin. Moreover it is not a sensitive test for heparin.

B Bleeding time is normal in the presence of coagulation disorders other than thrombocytopenia or von Willebrand's disease. It can be increased in cases of heparin-induced thrombocytopenia, but the platelet count is a much more reliable test.

C This test evaluates fibrinolytic activity. Heparin does not alter fibrinolysis.

D, F These exams are not needed during heparin treatment.

▶ *Learning objective:* Identify the lab exam most commonly used to monitor the anticoagulant activity of unfractionated heparin.

13. Answer: D

The activated partial thromboplastin time is used to detect deficiency in the intrinsic coagulation pathway. Because unfractionated heparin inhibits the activation of several factors of the intrinsic pathway the test is most sensitive to heparin action.

A Heparin can increase prothrombin time, but this test is less sensitive than activated partial thromboplastin time and is not the standard test used to monitor the anticoagulant activity of unfractionated heparin.

B Bleeding time is normal in the presence of coagulation disorders other than thrombocytopenia or von Willebrand's disease.

C, E, F These tests are used to detect specific inherited or acquired bleeding disorders.

▶ *Learning objective:* Identify the coagulation factor that represents the molecular target of dabigatran.

14. Answer: C

Dabigatran belongs to the subclass of direct thrombin inhibitors. These drugs bind to the active site of both free and fibrin-bound thrombin (factor IIa), preventing its coagulant activity. In patients with acute thromboembolism pulmonary anticoagulation is recommended, with the objective of preventing both early death and recurrent symptomatic or fatal thromboembolism. The standard duration of anticoagulation should cover at least 3 months. Within this period, acute-phase treatment consists of administering parenteral anticoagulation (unfractionated heparin or low-molecular-weight heparin) over the first 5 to 10 days. This parenteral anticoagulation should overlap with the initiation of warfarin or of one of the new oral anticoagulants, such as dabigatran, as in the present case.

A, B, D The synthesis of these factors is inhibited by warfarin. Dabigatran has no action on the synthesis of these proenzymes.

E Dabigatran has no action on factor XIIa.

F Factor IV is calcium, which acts as a cofactor at several steps of the coagulation cascade. It is not involved in the action of dabigatran.

▶ *Learning objective:* Identify the drug to be used in cases of serious dabigatran overdose.

15. Answer: E

New oral anticoagulants like dabigatran have lower bleeding rates compared to warfarin, but bleeding can occur with all anticoagulant overdose. Idarucizumab is a monoclonal antibody designed to antagonize the anticoagulant effects of an excessive dose of dabigatran. A large study found that idarucizumab effectively reversed anticoagulation by dabigatran within minutes. Because all monoclonal antibodies can have serious adverse effects idaru-cizumab should be used only in cases of severe dabigatran overdose.

A Vitamin K is the antidote for an overdose of warfarin.

B Protamine sulfate is the antidote for an overdose of heparin.

C Desmopressin has a procoagulant, not an anticoagulant, effect by increasing factor VIII activity. It is used to treat hemophilia and von Willebrand's disease.

D Abciximab is an antiplatelet drug used in unstable angina.

Case 42

Rheumatoid Arthritis

K.L., a previously healthy 48-year-old woman, was admitted to the hospital because of generalized muscle and joint pain. For the past 6 months, she had been suffering from morning stiffness and joint pain that would last for several hours after she got up, and from afternoon fatigue and malaise. She reported that her joints of both hands were swollen and painful and that she had been taking a large amount of analgesics (including ibuprofen, ketorolac, piroxicam, and acetaminophen) to control her pain. However, in spite of the therapy, her symptoms had worsened during the past month, and she had been forced to limit her physical activities to some degree. She also noted that her eyes seemed unusually red and dry and that she had dry mouth and a dry cough most of the day.

K.L.'s vital signs were blood pressure 128/82 mm Hg, pulse 72 bpm, respirations 15/min. Physical examination revealed bilateral symmetrical swelling, tenderness, and warmth of the radiocarpal, metacarpophalangeal (MCP), and proximal interphalangeal joints of both hands and the metatarsophalangeal joints of the feet.

Pertinent laboratory results on admission were as follows:

Blood hematology

- ▶ Erythrocyte sedimentation rate (ESR): 58 mm/h (normal < 20)
- ▶ Hemoglobin (Hb): 10.1 gm/dL (normal 12–16)
- ▶ Hematocrit (Hct): 33% (normal 36–48)
- ▶ Iron: 45 mg/dL (normal 60–180)
- ▶ Rheumatoid factor (RF): 69 U/mL 0 to 20

Urinalysis

Normal results

X-ray

The patient's hands and feet showed juxta-articular osteopenia, narrowing of joint spaces, and marginal erosion of the articular surfaces.

A diagnosis of rheumatoid arthritis was made, and K.L. was given a prescription for a nonsteroidal anti-inflammatory drug (NSAID) and hydroxychloroquine. The prescribed therapy was initially effective in reducing pain, tenderness, and swelling of the joints, but 6 months later the pain and inflammation progressively worsened, and K.L. returned to the hospital for further evaluation.

It was found that there were significant deficits in range of motion in both hands and feet, and joint deformities in both hands. Two subcutaneous nodules were evident on the extension surface of both forearms. The rheumatologist decided to remove the NSAID and to add methotrexate.

After 2 months of therapy K.L.'s condition was not much improved, and the rheumatologist decided to remove hydroxychloroquine and add leflunomide to the treatment.

The methotrexate–leflunomide therapy worked quite well, slowing the progression of the disease, but 8 months later K.L. was again admitted to the hospital because of reactivation of her disease at a higher level of severity. This time the rheumatologist decided to add a biologic disease-modifying antirheumatic drug (DMARD) to her current therapy and prescribed etanercept.

Questions

1. K.L. was diagnosed with rheumatoid arthritis (RA). This disease affects what percentage of the population worldwide?

A. 1%

B. 3%

C. 6%

D. 10%

E. 15%

2. RA can occur at any age. However, which of the following is the age range (in years) with the most frequent onset of RA?

A. 10–15

B. 20–30

C. 35–50

D. 55–65

E. 70–75

3. Because no single laboratory or clinical finding is specific for RA, the diagnosis of this disease is primarily based on multiple clinical and laboratory criteria. According to the American College of Rheumatology, four out of seven different clinical and laboratory data must be present to classify a patient as having RA. The seven criteria most likely include which of the following?

A. Increased erythrocyte sedimentation rate

B. Involvement of distal interphalangeal joints

C. Symmetric arthritis for ≥ 6 weeks

D. Articular osteosclerosis

E. Crystals on synovial fluid examination

4. K.L.'s X-ray showed changes typical for RA. Which of the following is usually the earliest plain radiological finding in RA?

A. Joint space expansion

B. Articular osteosclerosis

C. Juxta-articular osteoporosis

D. Osteophytosis

E. Subchondral necrosis

5. RA primarily affects joints. Which of the following pairs of joints are most frequently involved in the establishment of RA?

A. Metatarsophalangeal–distal interphalangeal

B. Metatarsophalangeal–acromioclavicular

C. Radiocarpal–metacarpophalangeal

D. Metacarpophalangeal–distal interphalangeal

E. Radiocarpal–acromioclavicular

6. RA is an autoimmune chronic joint disorder. Which of the following sets of cytokines shown in the attached table is thought to play the most central role in the pathogenesis of RA?

Set			
A.	TNF	IL-10	IL-4
B.	TNF	IL-6	IL-1
C.	IL-1	IL-4	IL 11
D.	IL-6	IL-10	IL 4
E.	IL-10	IL-4	IL-1

Abbreviations: TNF, tumor necrosis factor; IL, interleukin.

7. RA is a systemic disease that can involve extra-articular manifestations, often occurring as a syndrome. Taking into account K.L.'s symptoms, which of the following syndromes was most likely associated with her disease?

A. Horner's syndrome

B. Barret's syndrome

C. Sjögren's syndrome

D. Cushing's syndrome

E. Nephrotic syndrome

F. Carcinoid syndrome

373

8. K.L. was found to have two subcutaneous nodules, 6 months after the beginning of the RA therapy. A histological examination of these nodules would most likely match which of the following descriptions?

A. A compact collection of macrophages and epithelioid cells

B. A central area of fibrinoid necrosis surrounded by palisading macrophages and lymphocytes

C. A compact mass of mature adipocytes surrounded by a fibrous capsule

D. A central area of liquefactive necrosis surrounded by a fibrous capsule

9. K.L. was found to have a low plasma iron level, which was most likely secondary to chronic NSAID ingestion. Which of the following statements best explains a reason why these drugs can cause gastrointestinal (GI) damage and bleeding?

A. Increased histamine secretion by gastric enterochromaffin-like cells

B. Activation of muscarinic M_3 receptors on gastrointestinal cells

C. Activation of gastrin receptors on gastrointestinal cells

D. Reduced secretion of mucus and bicarbonate by gastrointestinal cells

E. Inhibition of platelet aggregation

10. NSAIDs were initially effective in reducing pain and swelling of K.L.'s joints. Which of the following actions best explains why NSAIDs can reduce swelling of the joints?

A. Decreased synthesis of IL-1 and IL-2

B. Inhibition of platelet aggregation

C. Increased renal blood flow

D. Decreased blood flow in the inflamed area

E. Increased margination of neutrophils

11. An NSAID was prescribed to K.L. together with hydroxychloroquine. Which of the following NSAIDs would be an appropriate choice for this patient?

A. Piroxicam

B. Ibuprofen

C. Diclofenac

D. Indomethacin

E. Celecoxib

F. Ketorolac

12. Hydroxychloroquine was prescribed to K.L. Which of the following statements best explains the main advantage of this drug over NSAIDs in the therapy of RA?

A. It provides a complete cure of the disease.

B. It is a more effective analgesic drug.

C. It can retard cartilage destruction.

D. Its onset of action is fast, usually < 1 week.

E. It inhibits the rate-limiting step of eicosanoid biosynthesis.

13. It is known that prolonged treatment with hydroxychloroquine can cause a specific adverse effect. Which of the following tests/exams should be performed periodically during therapy to monitor this potential adverse effect?

A. Electrocardiography

B. Liver function tests

C. Ophthalmoscopic exam

D. Kidney function tests

E. Electroencephalography

14. Methotrexate was prescribed to K.L. Which of the following mechanisms of action most likely contributes to the therapeutic efficacy of low doses of methotrexate in RA?

A. Inhibition of apoptosis of T-helper cells

B. Stimulation of IL-6 synthesis

C. Activation of IL-1 receptors

D. Enhanced extracellular concentrations of adenosine

E. Stimulation of calcineurin enzyme synthesis

15. Which of the following adverse effects was K.L. most likely to experience from methotrexate after 1 to 2 weeks of treatment?

A. Erythema multiforme

B. Portal fibrosis

C. Osteonecrosis

D. Pulmonary fibrosis

E. Oral ulcers

F. Skin necrosis

16. Leflunomide was prescribed for K.L. Which of the following is most likely the mechanism of the immunosuppressive action of this drug?

A. Inhibition of IL-10 receptors

B. Activation of TNF-α receptors

C. Inhibition of T cell proliferation

D. Inhibition of COX-2

E. Stimulation of antibody production by B cells

17. It is known that leflunomide can rarely cause a life-threatening adverse effect. Which of the following lab exams should be performed before, and then monthly after, starting the therapy to monitor this potential toxicity in the patient?

A. Activated partial thromboplastin time

B. Blood urea nitrogen

C. Creatinine clearance

D. Glucose-6-phosphate dehydrogenase

E. Alanine aminotransferase

18. Because nonbiologic DMARDs were no longer effective in K.L.'s disease, the rheumatologist decided to add a biologic DMARD to the therapy. Which of the following statements best explains a primary advantage of biologic over nonbiologic DMARDs?

A. They have a lower risk of adverse effects.

B. Their therapeutic effect occurs after 2 to 3 days of therapy.

C. They can improve RA resistance to nonbiologic DMARDs.

D. They can be easily administered by oral route.

E. They can reverse the existing joint damage.

19. Etanercept was prescribed for K.L. Which of the following molecular actions would most likely mediate the therapeutic effectiveness of this drug in the patient's RA?

A. Decreased gene expression of TNF-α

B. Blockade of TNF-α receptors

C. Binding to TNF-α in the extracellular fluids

D. Stimulation of TNF-α metabolism

E. Increased renal excretion of TNF-α

20. With etanercept therapy K.L. was most likely at increased risk of which of the following diseases?

A. Psoriasis

B. Heart failure

C. Opportunistic infection

D. Lupus-like syndrome

E. Secondary malignancy

Answers and Explanations

▶ *Learning objective:* Identify the percentage of people affected by RA worldwide.

1. Answer: A

RA affects about 1% of the population worldwide but varies greatly between geographic regions. In the United States approximately 1.5 million individuals have RA. Women are affected two to three times more often than men.

B, C, D, E See correct answer explanation.

▶ *Learning objective:* Identify the age range during which onset of RA is most frequent.

2. Answer: C

The onset of RA is most often between 35 and 50 years of age, but it can arise during childhood (juvenile idiopathic arthritis) or old age. Since RA is a long-lasting disease, its prevalence increases with advancing age up to the seventh decade.

A, B, D, E See correct answer explanation.

▶ *Learning objective:* Identify a clinical sign that is included in the seven clinical and laboratory data criteria typical for RA.

3. Answer: C

According to the American College of Rheumatology, any four of the following criteria must be present to classify patients as having RA:

▶ Arthritis of ≥ 3 joints (for ≥ 6 weeks)
▶ Arthritis of hand ≥ 3 joints (for ≥ 6 weeks)
▶ Symmetric arthritis (for ≥ 6 weeks)
▶ Morning stiffness ≥ 1 hour (for ≥ 6 weeks)
▶ Rheumatoid nodules
▶ Higher than normal levels of serum rheumatoid factor
▶ Imaging changes (hand X-ray changes typical for RA)

A Increased ESR is often present in RA but is by no means a specific sign.

B The joints involved in RA include primarily proximal, not distal, interphalangeal joints

D Articular osteosclerosis is a sign of osteoarthritis, not of RA.

E Crystals on synovial fluid examination are a sign of gouty arthritis, not of RA.

▶ *Learning objective:* Identify the earliest radiological finding usually present in RA.

4. Answer: C

The radiographic hallmarks of RA are as follows:

▶ Osteoporosis: initially juxta-articular, and later generalized
▶ Soft tissue swelling (fusiform and periarticular)
▶ Symmetrical joint space narrowing
▶ Marginal erosions

The juxta-articular osteoporosis is usually the earliest radiographic finding, even if soft tissue swelling may be the early/only radiographic finding.

A Joint spaces are narrowed, not expanded, in RA.

B, D These findings are typical of osteoarthritis, not of RA.

E Subchondral necrosis can sometimes be associated with RA (mainly in patients under corticosteroid therapy), but this is not an early radiological finding.

▶ *Learning objective:* Describe the pair of joints most frequently involved in the establishment of RA.

5. Answer: C

The joints affected most frequently by RA are small joints of the wrists (radiocarpal), hands (metacarpophalangeal and proximal interphalangeal), and feet (metatarsophalangeal). In addition, elbows, shoulders, hips, knees, and ankles may be involved.

A, D The distal interphalangeal joints are rarely involved in RA. When this occurs, it is more often due to a coexisting osteoarthritis.

B, E The acromioclavicular is the joint between the end of the clavicle and the lateral end of the spine of the scapula. It is rarely affected by RA.

▶ *Learning objective:* Identify the set of cytokines that is thought to play a central role in the pathogenesis of RA.

6. Answer: B

RA begins with inflammation of the synovial lining that surrounds the joint space. As in any other kind of inflammatory disorder, proinflammatory cytokines are secreted by leukocytes, macrophages, and other cells in the inflammatory area.

Tumor necrosis factor-α (TNF-α), interleukin (IL)-6, and IL-1 are proinflammatory cytokines thought to play the most central role in the pathogenesis of RA. In RA these cytokines stimulate cartilage destruction, osteoclast-mediated bone resorption, synovial inflammation, and prostaglandins (which potentiate inflammation). In healthy individuals the inflammatory process is regulated by balancing the ratios of proinflammatory cytokines with anti-inflammatory cytokines. In the synovium of patients with RA, however, this balance is heavily weighted toward the proinflammatory cytokines, which results in chronic inflammation and tissue destruction.

A, C, D, E All these sets have two anti-inflammatory cytokines, such as IL-4, IL-10, and IL-11.

▶ *Learning objective:* Identify the syndrome that was most likely associated with the patient's RA.

7. Answer: C

Sjögren's syndrome is a chronic, autoimmune, systemic inflammatory disorder characterized by dryness of the mouth, eyes, and other mucous membranes due to lymphocytic infiltration of the exocrine glands. It is classified as primary when there is no other associated disease, but in about 30% of cases it is secondary (i.e., associated with other autoimmune disorders). The syndrome affects about 10% of patients with RA. The K.L.'s symptoms of dry eyes, dry mouth, and dry cough indicate that she was most likely suffering from secondary Sjögren's syndrome.

A Horner's syndrome is a combination of symptoms and signs that arises when a group of nerves of the sympathetic trunk is damaged. It is characterized by miosis, partial ptosis, and apparent anhidrosis. K.L. did not show these symptoms.

B Barret's syndrome occurs when the inner lining of the esophagus changes (metaplasia) to resemble the intestinal lining. It is caused by long-standing gastrointestinal reflux. K.L. did not show symptoms of gastrointestinal reflux.

D Cushing's syndrome is a collection of signs and symptoms due to prolonged exposure (for whatever reason) to a glucocorticoid. The main signs include hypertension, weight gain, skin changes, hirsutism, hyperglycemia, and hypercholesterolemia. K.L. did not show these symptoms.

E Nephrotic syndrome refers to urinary excretion of > 2 g of protein/day due to glomerular disease. K.L. did not show proteinuria.

F Carcinoid syndrome is a paraneoplastic syndrome secondary to carcinoid tumors. It is usually caused by endogenous secretion of mainly serotonin. The syndrome includes flushing and diarrhea. K.L. did not show these symptoms.

▶ *Learning objective:* Describe the microscopic appearance of rheumatoid nodules.

8. Answer: B

Rheumatoid nodules are usually subcutaneous necrotizing granulomas. Histology usually shows a central area of fibrinoid necrosis surrounded by palisading macrophages and lymphocytes. Rheumatoid nodules in the subcutaneous tissues have been reported at initial presentation in 7% of patients with RA and are found at some time during the disease course in 20 to 40% of patients. These nodules are seen most commonly on the extensor surface of the elbows, forearm, and hands but may also be seen on the feet and in some internal organs (e.g., the lungs and heart). The vast majority of patients with rheumatoid nodules have positive tests for rheumatoid factor, as in the present case. In general, patients with rheumatoid nodules tend to have a severe RA phenotype, with more rapid progression of joint destruction.

A A compact collection of macrophages and epithelioid cells would be the histology of nonnecrotizing granulomas.

C A compact mass of mature adipocytes surrounded by a fibrous capsule would be the histology of lipomas.

D A central area of liquefactive necrosis surrounded by a fibrous capsule would be the histology of abscesses.

▶ *Learning objective:* Explain the mechanism of NSAID-induced gastric damage.

9. Answer: D

NSAIDs appear to produce gastric damage by two mechanisms: a systemic action and a local action.

The systemic action is related to the cytoprotection provided by prostaglandin action on the GI mucosa, brought about by maintaining blood flow and stimulating bicarbonate and mucus production. By blocking prostaglandin biosynthesis, NSAIDs impair the ability of the GI mucosa to defend itself against aggressive factors.

The local action occurs via an ion-trapping mechanism. Most NSAIDs are weak acids with a pK_a < 5. Therefore, they are mainly nonionized (i.e., lipid-soluble) in the stomach lumen and can cross the cell membrane by lipid diffusion. In the alkaline environment of the cytoplasm, they become ionized (i.e., water-soluble) and are trapped inside the cell, causing cell damage.

A, B, C All these actions could cause gastric bleeding, but NSAIDs do not cause these actions.

E NSAIDs can inhibit platelet aggregation, but this is not the cause of gastrointestinal damage and bleeding, although it can be a factor for increased bleeding.

▶ *Learning objective:* Explain the NSAID-induced reduction of joint swelling in RA.

10.   Answer: D

Prostaglandins generally promote acute inflammation, and both prostaglandin E_2 and prostaglandin I_2 markedly enhance edema formation by promoting blood flow in the inflamed region. By blocking prostaglandin biosynthesis NSAIDs decrease blood flow in the inflamed area, reducing swelling of the joints.

A NSAIDs have negligible effects on IL synthesis, which is instead inhibited by glucocorticoids.

B NSAIDs can inhibit platelet aggregation, but this is not the cause of the decreased swelling.

C, E These actions can be prostaglandin mediated; therefore they would be decreased, not increased, by NSAIDs.

▶ *Learning objective:* Identify the appropriate NSAID to be used in a patient suffering from NSAID-induced gastric damage.

11.   Answer: E

The patient already suffered from NSAID-induced gastric damage. Therefore, a selective cyclooxygenase-2 (COX-2) inhibitor like celecoxib would be a rational choice. The anti-inflammatory effect of NSAIDs is mediated by the inhibition of cyclooxygenase, the enzyme that catalyzes the synthesis of prostaglandins, which are known inflammatory mediators.

Two different isoforms of cyclooxygenase have been found, cyclooxygenase-1 (COX-1) and cyclooxygenase-2 (COX-2). COX-1 is expressed in most tissues of the body, and

its inhibition is thought to mediate the analgesic and antipyretic effect of NSAIDs as well as most of their adverse effects. Inflammatory mediators such as cytokines upregulate COX-2 expression, leading to high levels of COX-2 in inflamed tissues. Most NSAIDs are nonselective COX inhibitors; namely, they inhibit both isoforms of the enzyme. Selective COX inhibitors like celecoxib inhibit only COX-2, and have anti-inflammatory, analgesic, and antipyretic activity but lower incidence of certain adverse effects like gastrointestinal toxicity.

A, B, C, D, F All these drugs are nonselective COX inhibitors and are therefore more prone to cause gastrointestinal toxicity.

▶ *Learning objective:* Explain the main advantage of hydroxychloroquine over NSAIDs in the therapy of RA.

12.   Answer: C

Hydroxychloroquine is an antimalarial drug that was proven effective in RA. It belongs to a group of drugs called disease-modifying antirheumatic drugs (DMARDs). Unlike NSAIDs, which offer mainly symptomatic relief in RA, DMARDs can slow the progression of the disease by retarding cartilage destruction.

DMARDs can be subdivided into nonbiologic drugs (usually small molecules) and biologic drugs (namely, drugs manufactured in a living system, which are usually big molecules).

Hydroxychloroquine is currently used for patients with low RA disease activity, no features of poor prognosis, and disease duration less than 24 months, as in the present case.

A There is no cure for RA. DMARDs can improve the function during the first 3 to 10 years, but considerable decline usually occurs thereafter.

B Hydroxychloroquine has negligible analgesic properties.

D The onset of action of nonbiologic DMARDs is slow. The therapeutic effect may take months to become clinically evident.

E Antimalarials like hydroxychloroquine do not affect the rate-limiting step of eicosanoid biosynthesis, which is instead inhibited by glucocorticoids.

▶ *Learning objective:* Identify the test/exam that should be performed periodically during therapy with hydroxychloroquine.

13.   Answer: C

Hydroxychloroquine is usually well tolerated, but it can cause ocular toxicity, mainly at dosages > 250 mg/d. Because the daily dose for RA is 400 to 600 mg, this toxicity must be taken into account. Ocular toxicity includes the following:

▶ Corneal deposits that may appear as early as 3 weeks after hydroxychloroquine initiation. They can cause blurred vision, halos around lights, and photophobia.

▶ Retinal damage that usually occurs in patients who have received long-term or high-dosage therapy. It can cause visual field defects, such as scotomas, with decreased visual acuity or abnormal color vision. Retinopathy is dose-related and has occurred within several months to several years of daily therapy. In a number of patients, early retinopathy diminished or regressed completely after therapy was discontinued, but retinopathy can continue to progress even after the drug is discontinued, and irreversible retinal damage has been observed in some cases.

A, **B**, **D**, **E** Brain, heart, liver, and kidney are not significant targets for hydroxychloroquine toxicity.

▶ *Learning objective:* Explain a mechanism that can contribute to the therapeutic efficacy of low doses of methotrexate in RA.

14.   Answer: D

Methotrexate was originally used as a chemotherapy treatment for cancer. When used in much lower doses for RA and other rheumatic diseases, methotrexate works to reduce inflammation and to decrease joint damage. It is today a first-line agent for treating RA. The drug is a structural analogue of folic acid that can competitively inhibit the binding of folic acid and dihydrofolic acid (DHF) to dihydrofolate reductase, the enzyme responsible for reducing DHF to tetrahydrofolic acid (THF), the active intracellular metabolite. Thus methotrexate decreases the amount of intracellular THF available and affects the metabolic pathways that are THF dependent. These pathways include purine and pyrimidine metabolism, as well as amino acid and polyamine synthesis.

Methotrexate is a prodrug that becomes active only when polyglutamated within cells. The process of polyglutamation is slow and takes several weeks to reach steady state. This delay explains the time to achieve the plateau effect of clinical response.

The mechanism by which the low doses of methotrexate used in RA can improve the symptoms and signs of the disease is still uncertain. One of the most likely hypotheses is related to the drug-induced dephosphorylation of adenosine monophosphate, which in turn enhances the extracellular concentrations of adenosine, a potent inhibitor of inflammation.

Other mechanisms could also be operative. The drug can induce apoptosis in most rapidly proliferating cells, including activated peripheral T-helper cells. These cells are the major effector cells in several autoimmune diseases; therefore inducing apoptosis in these cells represents an important goal in any immunosuppressive treatment.

A, **B**, **C**, **E** All these actions would be proinflammatory, not anti-inflammatory.

▶ *Learning objective:* Identify an early adverse effect that can occur during methotrexate therapy.

15.   Answer: E

Approximately 10% of RA patients treated with methotrexate experience oral ulcers. They are likely related to folic acid deficiency, because folinic acid supplementation is found to minimize this adverse effect.

A, **B**, **C**, **D**, **F** All these adverse effects can occur during methotrexate therapy, but they occur in < 1% of cases and usually after long-term treatments.

► *Learning objective:* Explain the mechanism of the immunosuppressive action of leflunomide.

16. Answer: C

Leflunomide is a nonbiologic DMARD that is often used either alone or in combination with methotrexate for patients who have not responded adequately to methotrexate alone, as in the present case. The agent is a prodrug that is converted, both in the intestine and in plasma, to its active metabolite. This metabolite inhibits dihydroorotate dehydrogenase, an enzyme located in cell mitochondria, which catalyzes a key step in de novo pyrimidine synthesis. This inhibition leads to a decrease in ribonucleotide synthesis and the arrest of cell growth in the G1 phase. Consequently, leflunomide inhibits T-cell proliferation, causing an immunosuppressive effect.

A IL-10 is an anti-inflammatory cytokine. Inhibition of IL-10 receptors would cause an inflammatory reaction.

B TNF-α is a mediator of inflammatory reactions. Activation of TNF-α receptors would cause an inflammatory reaction.

D Inhibition of COX-2 would cause an anti-inflammatory reaction, but leflunomide does not inhibit this enzyme.

E Stimulation of antibody production can be a part of an anti-inflammatory reaction, but leflunomide does not cause this effect.

► *Learning objective:* Identify the lab exam that should be performed frequently during leflunomide treatment to prevent a potential life-threatening effect of this drug.

17. Answer: E

Potential liver toxicity is the greatest concern with leflunomide. The drug can cause transient serum alanine aminotransferase elevations above three times the upper limit of normal (ULN) in 1 to 4% of patients. In addition, leflunomide is associated with rare instances of clinically apparent liver injury that can be severe. The liver injury usually arises after 1 to 6 months of therapy (often associated with diarrhea) and begins to resolve within a week of stopping therapy, although some cases of acute liver failure and some fatal cases have been reported. When alanine aminotransferase (ALT) levels rise above three times ULN, repeat testing is recommended, as well as discontinuation if levels remain above this cut off. The risk of liver injury is increased if a patient is already taking drugs, such as methotrexate, that have the potential to cause hepatotoxicity, as in the present case. The hepatic injury due to leflunomide is thought to occur by the production of a toxic intermediate. Because both leflunomide and the active metabolite have very long half-lives as a result of extensive enterohepatic cycling, cholestyramine can be given to speed up their elimination.

A Activated partial thromboplastin time is used to monitor bleeding disorder. Leflunomide can cause, albeit rarely, hematuria, but this adverse effect is not life-threatening.

B, C Blood urea nitrogen and creatinine clearance monitor kidney toxicity. The risk of kidney toxicity due to leflunomide is negligible.

D Patients with glucose-6-phosphate dehydrogenase deficiency are at risk of hemolytic anemia. The risk of hemolytic anemia due to leflunomide is negligible.

► *Learning objective:* Identify the advantage of biologic over nonbiologic DMARDs in the treatment of RA.

18. Answer: C

It has been consistently shown that biologic DMARDs (i.e., drugs manufactured by recombinant technology) can improve RA that has become resistant to a previous therapy. Because of this, they have changed the therapeutic approach to the disease. Today the disease is treated earlier and more aggressively with much higher expectations for patient outcomes. Rheumatologists now recognize that the first year is a critical time to treat RA. Often much of the bone and joint damage occurs early, within a few weeks of onset. Biologic DMARDs do not reverse existing damage, but they can protect the joints against continued damage and have been shown to slow the progression of the disease substantially, even in cases of resistance to previous therapy.

A Biologic DMARDs carry a risk of adverse effects that is equal to, or even higher than, that of nonbiologic DMARDs.

B Biologic DMARDs tend to work a little more quickly than conventional DMARDs, but it still takes several weeks or months before the patient receives their full benefit.

D All biologic DMARDs are proteins and therefore not active by the oral route.

E No therapy can reverse the existing joint damage of RA.

▶ *Learning objective:* Identify the molecular action that mediates the therapeutic efficacy of etanercept in RA.

19. Answer: C

Etanercept is a TNF-α inhibitor. Although a wide range of cytokines are expressed in the joints of RA patients, TNF-α appears to be particularly important in the inflammatory process through the activation of specific membrane-bound TNF receptors. Five biologic DMARDs that inhibit TNF-α have been approved for the therapy of RA and other rheumatic diseases. These agents are etanercept, adalimumab, certolizumab, golimumab, and infliximab. Etanercept binds to TNF-α in the extracellular fluids, thereby neutralizing it. The drug has a higher affinity for TNF-α than the natural soluble and cellular TNF-α receptors.

A Decreased gene expression of TNF-α would be a mechanism of action of glucocorticoids.

B Etanercept binds to TNF-α, not to TNF-α receptors.

D, **E** The pharmacokinetics (metabolism, excretion) of TNF-α is not affected by etanercept.

▶ *Learning objective:* Identify the risk of disease that can occur in patients under treatment with etanercept.

20. Answer: C

The greatest concern with all biologic DMARDs, including etanercept, is the risk of serious infections because these drugs interfere with the immune system. In clinical trials, 27 to 81% of patients receiving the drug had an infection, such as a bacterial, viral, or fungal infection. TNF-α has a central role in mycobacterial infections and several cases of active tuberculosis have been reported worldwide with the use of therapeutic agents that inhibit TNF-α.

A, **B**, **D**, **E** All these adverse effects can be associated with etanercept therapy but are reported in < 0.1% of patients receiving the drug.

Case 43

Schizophrenia

B.E., a 23-year-old man, was brought to the emergency department of the local psychiatric hospital by the police after he created a disturbance at a local fast-food restaurant. As he entered the department he repeatedly screamed, "I cannot stay here; I got to go home."

B.E. was extremely agitated, moved about constantly, frequently shouted at the nurses and doctors, and threatened the interviewer when asked questions regarding his illness. He said repeatedly he had bought some food at the restaurant, and when he sat down to eat it somebody accused him of stealing the food and called the police.

B.E. stated that he came to this town with his parents 3 years ago, but he had lost touch with his family and had been living in a Christian guest house for the past 2 years. He had no close friends and did not trust most people. He heard voices of "dead people" who wanted to kill him. He said that "people in the street are reading my mind and telling everyone my personal secrets." These problems had been disturbing him for the past 6 months. B.E. had no history of a previous psychiatric illness and had never been hospitalized. He denied alcohol or illicit drug use and admitted he had never held steady employment and relied on Social Security income and money from strangers to survive.

The hospital records revealed that B.E.'s mother was hospitalized twice for unspecified psychotic episodes. A monozygotic twin of the patient committed suicide at the age of 18. Another brother with autism was living at home with his family. An uncle of the patient had been an alcoholic and had hanged himself 5 years ago.

Physical examination showed a thin, disheveled-looking man with very poor hygiene, who appeared much older than his stated age, with the following vital signs: blood pressure 125/72 mm Hg, pulse 92 bpm, respirations 25/min, body temperature 97.7°F (36.5°C).

A complete neurological examination was noncontributory.

Mental examination disclosed a patient extremely suspicious of the interviewer and his surroundings, who continually asked, "Whom do you work for? What do you want?"

B.E.'s thought process exhibited loose associations, such as "What are you doing to me? Don't you like my dressing?" He seemed to be responding to internal stimuli, mumbling to himself and answering his own questions. He was extremely anxious and nervous, concerned that the "dead people" were going to track him down and "bury me alive." His affect was blunted, with a minimal range of reactivity to his emotions. His memory (immediate, recent, and remote) seemed to be intact. The patient was oriented to person, place, time, and situation, but his insight and judgment were poor, as evidenced by denial of his illness and the need for treatment.

All laboratory tests on admission, including complete blood count with differential, a comprehensive metabolic panel, and thyroid and liver function tests, were within normal limits. The urinalysis and urine drug screen were negative.

A diagnosis of schizophrenia was made. B.E. was admitted to the psychiatric hospital, received three intramuscular injections of haloperidol during the next 24 hours, and his agitation resolved. The therapy was continued orally for the next 2 days. On the third day B.E. presented with a stiff neck, protruding tongue, and spasm of the jaw and an oculogyric crisis (eyes rolling back into head). The patient was very upset and wanted to leave the hospital. An intravenous (IV) injection of benztropine was started, and a few minutes later the motor symptoms had improved substantially. The same drug was also prescribed orally for a week. Because of the adverse effects of haloperidol, the psychiatrist decided to change the antipsychotic therapy, and the patient started an oral treatment with risperidone. During the following 4 weeks of treatment, the daily dose was increased gradually, and B.E. became more sociable, his hallucinations and suspiciousness disappeared, and his thought disorder improved. B.E. was dismissed from the hospital with the same postdischarge therapy, and he agreed to follow a rehabilitation program.

Six months later most of B.E.'s psychotic symptoms had substantially improved, but he was readmitted to the psychiatric hospital because of a motor syndrome that involved the face (blinking, grimacing), the tongue (chewing, writhing), the lips (smacking, puckering), the neck (torticollis), and the limbs (toe tapping, pill rolling). The patient also noted an unusual increased size of his breasts. Risperidone was discontinued and the syndrome gradually subsided. A few days later B.E. was dismissed from the hospital with a postdischarge therapy that included aripiprazole.

One year later B.E. was readmitted to the psychiatric hospital because of a failed attempt to commit suicide. In spite of his strict adherence to the prescribed treatment, hallucinations, delusions, and thought disorders had returned and were most likely the reason for his suicide attempt. A diagnosis of resistant schizophrenia was made, aripiprazole was discontinued, and another atypical antipsychotic was prescribed.

Questions

1. B.E. was diagnosed with schizophrenia. Which of the following pairs of the patient's symptoms are most likely characteristic of this disease?

A. Hearing voices of "dead people"–orientation to person, place, and time

B. Orientation to person, place, and time–extreme anxiety

C. Hearing voices of "dead people"–worrying about being buried alive

D. Orientation to person, place, and time–worrying about being buried alive

E. Extreme anxiety–worrying about being buried alive

F. Hearing voices of "dead people"–extreme anxiety

2. Schizophrenia symptoms are usually subdivided into positive and negative. Which of the following of B.E.'s symptoms can most likely be classified as negative?

A. Suspiciousness

B. Disorganized speech

C. Nervousness

D. Blunted affect

E. Auditory hallucinations

3. The cause of schizophrenia is unknown, but evidence for a genetic component is strong. Which of the following events in B.E.'s family history best explains this genetic component?

A. The mother's psychotic episodes

B. The twin brother's suicide

C. The uncle's suicide

D. The brother's autism

4. Some hypotheses imply the involvement of different neurotransmitters in the pathogenesis of schizophrenia. Which of the following sets of neurotransmitters is most likely related to the biochemical hypotheses of schizophrenia?

A. Norepinephrine–serotonin–acetylcholine

B. Dopamine–glutamate–acetylcholine

C. Serotonin–γ-aminobutyric acid (GABA)–glutamate

D. Norepinephrine–GABA–dopamine

E. Dopamine–serotonin–glutamate

F. Norepinephrine–GABA–acetylcholine

5. Schizophrenia is thought to be associated with disorders of brain neural pathways. Which of the following pairs of neuronal pathways were most likely involved in the pathogenesis of this disease?

A. Mesolimbic–tuberoinfundibular

B. Corticospinal–tuberoinfundibular

C. Corticospinal–mesocortical

D. Tuberoinfundibular–mesocortical

E. Mesolimbic–corticospinal

F. Mesolimbic–mesocortical

6. B.E. was treated with haloperidol, a typical antipsychotic drug. It is known that antipsychotic drugs can block central and peripheral receptors with different affinity. This can explain several adverse effects of these drugs. Which of the following sets of adverse effects (from A to D) is most likely to be correct for haloperidol?

Set	EPS	SE	Hypo	A-ch
A.	++	+++	+++	+++
B.	0	+++	+++	+++
C.	+	++	0	0
D.	+++	+	0	0

Abbreviations: EPS, extrapyramidal symptoms; SE, sedation; Hypo, hypotension; A-ch, anticholinergic effects.

7. B.E. underwent some motor adverse effects after a few days of haloperidol treatment. Which of the following brain structures was most likely involved in the pathogenesis of those effects?

A. Locus ceruleus

B. Striatum

C. Nucleus accumbens

D. Amygdala

E. Hippocampus

8. After 6 months of treatment with risperidone, B.E. presented with abnormal involuntary movements in different organs. Which of the following is the correct name for this drug-induced syndrome?

A. Akathisia

B. Acute dystonia

C. Parkinsonism

D. Tardive dyskinesia

E. Tourette's syndrome

F. Huntington's chorea

9. After risperidone treatment B.E. noted an unusual increase in the size of his breasts. A blockade of receptors located in which of the following organs/tissues most likely mediated this drug-induced increase?

A. Testes

B. Anterior pituitary

C. Adrenal glands

D. Mammary glands

E. Frontal cortex

F. Basal ganglia

10. B.E. was treated with aripiprazole. This drug decreases dopamine actions in CNS areas where high levels of dopamine occur and increases dopamine actions in CNS areas where levels of dopamine are low. Which of the following agonist/antagonist terms best describes this drug?

A. Full agonist

B. Partial agonist

C. Competitive antagonist

D. Irreversible antagonist

E. Inverse agonist

11. Aripiprazole can act on D_2 receptors, but its antipsychotic effects is most likely also mediated by a pronounced activity on which of the following brain receptors?

A. $5-HT_{2A}$ receptors

B. α_2-adrenoceptors

C. H_1 receptors

D. Muscarinic receptors

E. NMDA receptors

F. μ-receptors

12. B.E. was diagnosed with resistant schizophrenia. Which of the following antipsychotic drugs was most likely prescribed to manage the patient's disorder?

A. Chlorpromazine

B. Thioridazine

C. Fluphenazine

D. Clozapine

E. Haloperidol

F. Olanzapine

13. Which of the following blood tests should be performed weekly during the first 6 months of treatment with the drug chosen for the therapy of resistant schizophrenia?

A. Creatinine

B. Blood urea nitrogen

C. Transaminases

D. Neutrophil count

E. Hemoglobin

F. Red blood cell count

Answers and Explanations

▶ *Learning objective:* Identify two target symptoms of schizophrenia.

1. Answer: C

According to the *Diagnostic and Statistical Manual of Mental Disorders* (Fifth Edition), (*DSM-V*), in order to meet the criteria for the diagnosis of schizophrenia, two (or more) of the following symptoms must be present for a significant portion of time during a 1-month period:

- ▶ Delusions (fixed false beliefs)
- ▶ Hallucinations (false perceptions)
- ▶ Disorganized speech (e.g., frequent derailment or incoherence)
- ▶ Grossly disorganized or catatonic behavior
- ▶ Negative symptoms (diminished emotional expression or avolition)

The patient exhibits delusions (thinking to be buried alive) and hallucinations (hearing voices of "dead people"). Even if no clinical sign or symptom is pathognomonic for schizophrenia, delusion and hallucinations are typical symptoms of this disease.

A, B, D Orientation to person, place and time is a normal mental symptom.

B, E, F Extreme anxiety can be a symptom of schizophrenia but can be present in a vast array of other mental disorders.

- ▶ *Learning objective:* Identify a negative symptom of schizophrenia.

2. Answer: D

Schizophrenia symptoms are usually subdivided into positive and negative, and they are the basis for assessing the change in the clinical status and the response to medications.

Positive symptoms include delusions, hallucinations, thought disorders, and movement disorders.

Negative symptoms include blunted affect, anhedonia, difficulty beginning and sustaining activities, poverty of speech, and asociality.

A, B, C, E All these are positive, not negative, symptoms of schizophrenia.

- ▶ *Learning objective:* Identify the event of the patient's family history that best indicates a genetic component in the pathogenesis of his schizophrenia.

3. Answer: B

The current belief is that there are a number of genes that contribute to susceptibility to or pathology of schizophrenia. The estimated number of genetic variations linked to schizophrenia is approximately 10. These genetic variations are common in every population, but it is likely that if a person has a number of these genetic variations the risk of developing schizophrenia begins to rise. The stronger genetic risk of developing schizophrenia is an identical twin with the disease. In this case the risk is > 50%. B.E. had a twin brother who committed suicide at the age of 18. Suicide is the single leading cause of premature death in patients with schizophrenia. Suicide attempts are made by 20 to 50% of schizophrenic patients, and eventually 10 to 15% commit suicide, usually in the initial stage of their illness. Most schizophrenic suicide victims are young, unmarried men, as was the twin brother of the patient. It is therefore quite likely that the suicide of the twin brother was related to undetected schizophrenia.

A, D These family events can increase the risk of schizophrenia, but this increase is much lower than that of a twin brother with the disease.

C The suicide of the patient's uncle was most likely due to alcoholism. Suicide is 120 times more prevalent among adult alcoholics than in the general population.

- ▶ *Learning objective:* Identify the set of neurotransmitters that is most likely related to the biochemical hypotheses of schizophrenia.

4. Answer: E

The main biochemical hypotheses of schizophrenia are as follows:

- ▶ ***The dopamine hypothesis:*** The hypothesis proposes that schizophrenia results from an abnormality in dopamine neurotransmission in certain neuronal pathways of the brain. The hypothesis is supported by the following observations:
  - – Typical antipsychotic drugs strongly block D2 receptors in the central nervous system (CNS), and there is a very strong correlation between clinical potency of these drugs and their in vitro affinity for these receptors. These drugs can improve positive symptoms of schizophrenia, but they do not improve, or may even worsen, negative symptoms.

– Drugs that increase dopaminergic activity in the limbic system (cocaine, amphetamines, levodopa, apomorphine, etc.) can induce schizophrenic-like behavior and exacerbate the symptoms of schizophrenia.

– An increased density of dopamine receptors has been found postmortem in brains of untreated schizophrenic patients.

– Imaging studies have shown increased striatal dopamine synthesis and release in schizophrenic patients.

▶ **The serotonin hypothesis:**
The hypothesis proposes that schizophrenia results from an abnormality in serotonin neurotransmission.

The hypothesis is supported by the following observations:

– 5-HT$_{2A}$-receptor stimulation is the basis for the hallucinatory effects of hallucinogenic drugs.

– Most atypical antipsychotic drugs are weak D$_2$ receptor antagonists but strong 5-HT$_{2A}$ receptor antagonists.

– Serotonin modulates dopamine neurotransmission (activation of 5-HT$_{2A}$ receptors inhibits dopamine release in nigrostriatal and tuberoinfundibular pathways; these actions may explain low extrapyramidal and hyperprolactinemic symptoms with atypical antipsychotics)

– Serotonin modulates glutamate neurotransmission (activation of 5-HT$_{2A}$ receptors leads to depolarization of glutamate neurons)

▶ **The glutamate hypothesis:**
The hypothesis proposes that schizophrenia results from an abnormality in glutamate neurotransmission.

The hypothesis is supported by the following observations:

– Phencyclidine and ketamine are noncompetitive inhibitors of the N-methyl-D-aspartate (NMDA) receptors that exacerbate the symptoms of schizophrenia.

– Phencyclidine and related drugs cause a variety of cognitive impairments in primates. Atypical antipsychotic drugs are much more potent than dopaminergic antagonists in blocking these effects.

– Activation of NMDA receptors located on GABAergic neurons increases GABA release. Hypofunction of NMDA receptors can induce disinhibition of downstream excitatory activity, which can lead to hyperstimulation of cortical neurons.

A, B, F Acetylcholine is the neurotransmitter thought to be involved in Alzheimer's disease.

C, D, F GABA is the neurotransmitter thought to be involved in anxiety disorders.

A, D, F Norepinephrine is the neurotransmitter thought to be involved in depressive disorders.

▶ *Learning objective:* Identify the two neuronal pathways most likely involved in the pathogenesis of schizophrenia.

5. Answer: F

According to the dopamine hypothesis schizophrenia is related to an abnormality in dopamine neurotransmission. The main neuronal pathways of the brain dopaminergic system are the following:

▶ **Mesocortical:** from midbrain ventral tegmentum to prefrontal cortex and frontal cortex
▶ **Mesolimbic:** from midbrain ventral tegmentum to amygdala, olfactory tubercle, nucleus accumbens
▶ **Nigrostriatal:** from substantia nigra to striatum
▶ **Tuberoinfundibular:** from hypothalamic and periventricular neurons to posterior pituitary

The mesocortical pathway is thought to mediate cognition, communication, social functions, and response to stress, whereas the mesolimbic pathway is thought to mediate stimulus processing, motivation for rewarding stimuli, the perception of pleasure, and learning of motor function related to reward.

An abnormality of dopamine neurotransmission in mesocortical pathway could explain symptoms such as cognitive deficits, delusions, disorganized speech, and social dysfunction. An abnormality of dopamine neurotransmission in the mesolimbic pathway could explain symptoms such as hallucinations, restricted range of emotions, and anhedonia.

B, C, E The corticospinal pathway is a white matter motor pathway starting at the cortex that terminates on motor neurons in the spinal cord, controlling movements of the limbs and trunk. The neurotransmitter of this pathway is glutamate, not dopamine.

A, B, D The tuberoinfundibular pathway is a dopaminergic pathway that regulates dopamine release. It is minimally involved in the pathogenesis of schizophrenia but can mediate some adverse effects of antipsychotic drugs.

▶ *Learning objective:* Identify the right set of adverse effects for haloperidol.

6. Answer: D

Haloperidol has a high receptor affinity for D_2 receptors that can explain the high risk of extrapyramidal effects, and low or no affinity for histaminergic or autonomic receptors that can explain the low risk of sedative or autonomic effects.

A This set would be right for chlorpromazine.

B This set would be right for clozapine.

C This set would be right for aripiprazole.

▶ *Learning objective:* Identify a brain structure that is most likely involved in some motor adverse effects of haloperidol.

7. Answer: B

The motor adverse effects exhibited by B.E. (stiff neck, protruding tongue, etc.) after a few days of haloperidol treatment were most likely an acute dystonic reaction that can occur in > 10% of patients receiving the drug. Dystonic reactions are classic extrapyramidal effects of typical antipsychotic drugs and are thought to be due to blockade of D_2 receptors in the nigrostriatal pathway. Extrapyramidal effects are less pronounced with atypical antipsychotic agents, and this is one of the main reasons for the current preference of these drugs in the treatment of schizophrenia.

A The locus ceruleus is a nucleus located in the pons and involved with physiological responses to stress and panic. It is the principal site for brain synthesis of norepinephrine.

C The nucleus accumbens is a basal ganglia nucleus located just in front of the hypothalamic preoptic area involved in responses to pleasurable stimuli.

D The amygdala is a region of the brain located deep within the temporal lobes, responsible for detecting fear and preparing for emergency events.

E The hippocampus is a region of the brain located within the brain's medial temporal lobes, primarily responsible for regulating memory, in particular longterm memory.

▶ *Learning objective:* Describe the antipsychotic-induced tardive dyskinesia.

8. Answer: D

The patient was most likely suffering from tardive dyskinesia, a syndrome characterized by involuntary choreoathetoid movements (most commonly perioral movements) that occurs in patients taking long-term antipsychotics. The minimum treatment period for the appearance of the syndrome is 3 months, but the disorder can occur even after several years of treatment. Typical antipsychotics are more frequently involved, but some atypical antipsychotics can also cause the syndrome. Specifically the incidence of tardive dyskinesia with risperidone is up to 5%. Risk factors for the syndrome include higher daily doses and the history of an extrapyramidal syndrome early in the treatment, as in the present case. For most patients a mild syndrome can be reversed with the prompt discontinuation of the antipsychotic agent. However, when the syndrome is severe it is irreversible in most cases. The causes of tardive dyskinesia are still unknown, but a supersensitivity of postsynaptic dopamine receptors is the most likely hypothesis. Once the syndrome is diagnosed the best management is to discontinue the offending drug. When continuing treatment is clearly indicated, the favored strategy is to switch antipsychotic therapy to a drug with negligible risk of tardive dyskinesia.

A Akathisia is a neuropsychiatric syndrome characterized by subjective and objective psychomotor restlessness. It is a recognized adverse effect of antipsychotic drugs, but symptoms are different from those of tardive dyskinesia.

B Dystonia is a state of abnormal muscle tone resulting in muscular spasm and abnormal posture. It is a recognized adverse effect of antipsychotic drugs. Dystonia and tardive dyskinesia share several similar features, because both involve movements of the head, arms, legs, hand, feet, lips, and tongue. However, dystonia is usually acute, starting after a few days of treatment, whereas the minimum treatment period for the appearance of tardive dyskinesia is 3 months.

C Parkinsonism is a neurologic syndrome characterized by rhythmic muscular tremors, rigidity of movement, festination, droopy posture, and masklike facies. It is a recognized adverse effect of antipsychotic drugs, but symptoms are different from those of tardive dyskinesia.

F Huntington's chorea is an inherited disorder that results in death of brain cells. The earliest symptoms are often subtle problems with mood or mental abilities. A general lack of coordination and an unsteady gait often follow. It is not caused by antipsychotic drugs, which are in fact sometimes used to treat some symptoms of the syndrome.

▶ *Learning objective:* Identify the cause of antipsychotic-induced gynecomastia.

9. Answer: B

The drug-induced effect was gynecomastia. Most antipsychotic drugs can cause hyperprolactinemia by blocking dopamine receptors on the mammotroph cells of the anterior pituitary. Hyperprolactinemia can cause several effects, including amenorrhea/galactorrhea in women and gynecomastia in men. Chronic hyperprolactinemia may result in weight gain and loss of bone density in both males and females. Atypical antipsychotics have fewer hyperprolactinemic effects than typical antipsychotics, but they can also cause these effects. Risperidone has the highest and aripiprazole the lowest risk for prolactin elevation.

A, C Gynecomastia can be caused by drugs that block testosterone receptors in the testes and adrenal glands, but antipsychotics do not act on these receptors.

D Prolactin causes enlargement of the mammary glands by activating prolactin receptors on mammary tissue, but antipsychotic drugs do not block these receptors.

E, F Antipsychotic drugs block dopamine receptors at these sites, but activation of these receptors does not cause hyperprolactinemia.

▶ *Learning objective:* Identify the receptor properties of aripiprazole.

10. Answer: B

Aripiprazole is an atypical antipsychotic drug that acts as a partial agonist at CNS D_2 receptors. Partial agonists are drugs that are able to activate the receptor but cannot evoke a maximal response. In other words, the intrinsic activity of a partial agonist is higher than zero but lower than 100%. Because of this property, when both a partial agonist and a full agonist are present at the receptor site, the partial agonist acts as an agonist when the concentration of the full agonist is low, but it acts as a competitive antagonist when the concentration of the full agonist is high.

Aripiprazole has a negligible risk of tardive dyskinesia, and this was most likely a reason for the choice of this drug to substitute risperidone in the treatment of the patient's schizophrenia.

A A full agonist is a drug that can bind a receptor, activate it, and produce a maximal response.

C A competitive antagonist is a drug that can bind a receptor but fails completely to produce any activation of that receptor. Its action can be overcome by increasing the concentration of the agonist.

D An irreversible antagonist is a drug that can bind a receptor but fails completely to produce any activation of that receptor. Its action cannot be overcome by increasing the concentration of the agonist.

E An inverse agonist is a drug that can bind a receptor and decrease the constitutive activity of a receptor.

▶ *Learning objective:* Identify the CNS receptor affected by aripiprazole.

11. Answer: A

Aripiprazole is an atypical antipsychotic drug. Although all effective antipsychotic drugs block D_2 receptors, atypical antipsychotics share the ability to alter the activity of 5-HT_{2A} receptors. Specifically aripiprazole acts as a partial agonist at D_2 receptors and as a competitive antagonist at 5-HT_{2A} receptors. Most atypical antipsychotics have an affinity for 5-HT_{2A} receptors greater than that of typical antipsychotics.

B, C, D, E, F The affinity of aripiprazole for these receptors is negligible or none.

▶ *Learning objective:* Identify the antipsychotic drug to be used for the management of resistant schizophrenia.

12. Answer: D

The prescribed drug was most likely clozapine, an atypical antipsychotic drug. Clozapine is the only agent that has shown superiority over other antipsychotic drugs for the management of resistant schizophrenia. Symptomatic improvement with clozapine in the treatment of resistant patients often occurs slowly, and as many as 60% of patients may improve if clozapine is used for up to 6 months. Clozapine is also the only antipsy-

chotic indicated to reduce the risk of suicide, which was most likely a further reason for the choice of the drug in the present case.

A, B, C Chlorpromazine, thioridazine, and fluphenazine are typical antipsychotic drugs from the phenothiazine class.

E Haloperidol is a typical antipsychotic drug from the butyrophenone class.

F Olanzapine is an atypical antipsychotic drug. In spite of the chemical similarity with clozapine, the drug has negligible effects for the management of resistant schizophrenia.

▶ *Learning objective:* Identify the blood test to be performed frequently in a patient treated with the first-line drug for resistant schizophrenia.

13. Answer: D

The first-line drug to treat patients with resistant schizophrenia is clozapine. The drug can cause agranulocytosis, a potentially lethal adverse effect that occurs in about 1% of patients receiving the drug. Because of this the U.S. Food and Drug Administration requires regular monitoring and registry reporting of neutrophil counts. This should be done weekly during the first 6 months of clozapine administration, every other week for the second 6 months, and every 4 weeks after 1 year, for the duration of treatment.

A, B Clozapine does not increase the risk of kidney disease (indicated by increased creatinine and blood urea nitrogen).

C Clozapine does not increase the risk of liver diseases (indicated by increased transaminases).

E, F Clozapine does not increase the risk of anemias (indicated by decreased hemoglobin and red blood cell count).

Case 44

Solid Organ Transplantation

M.P., a 58-year-old African American woman with stage D heart failure, was in the coronary intensive care unit, where she had been receiving continuous inotropic therapy for 3 weeks.

Three years earlier M.P. had had an acute myocardial infarction, followed 1 year later by a coronary artery bypass graft. Over the past year the patient underwent several admissions for exacerbation of heart failure and an episode of sudden cardiac death 2 months ago. M.P. had been suffering from hypertension and hypercholesterolemia for 8 years. Her most recent lab exams showed a left ventricular ejection fraction of 15, severe mitral regurgitation, and moderate pulmonary hypertension.

M.P. was being treated with milrinone, losartan, dabigatran, furosemide, spironolactone, and lovastatin. Her vital signs were blood pressure 130/78 mm Hg; heart rate 72 bpm; respirations 26/min; temperature, 98.3°F (36.8°C).

Recent blood exam results were as follows:

- ► Sodium (Na⁺): 138 mEq/L (normal 135–145)
- ► Potassium (K⁺): 4.1 mEq/L (normal 3.4–4.6)
- ► Total calcium 9.2 mg/dL (normal 8.5–10.5)
- ► Chloride (Cl⁻): 92 mEq/L (normal 95–105)
- ► Carbon dioxide (CO₂): 33 mEq/L (normal 24–30)
- ► Blood urea nitrogen (BUN): 22 mg/dL (normal 8–25)
- ► Creatinine: 1.2 mg/dL (normal 0.6–1.2)
- ► Total bilirubin: 1.8 mg/dL (normal 0.1–1.0)
- ► Aspartate aminotransferase (AST): 40 U/L (normal, women 10–35)
- ► Alanine aminotransferase (ALT): 16 U/L (normal, women 7–35)
- ► Lactate dehydrogenase (LDH): 180 U/L (normal 50–150)
- ► Alkaline phosphatase: 100 U/L (normal 30–120);
- ► Cholesterol: 225 mg/dL (normal < 200)
- ► Triglycerides: 92 mg/dL (normal < 150)

M.P. was placed on the waiting list for heart transplantation and 10 days later underwent heart transplant surgery. Before the operation the patient received mycophenolate mofetil, methylprednisolone, omeprazole, vancomycin, cefoperazone, and trimethoprim–sulfamethoxazole. After surgery intravenous (IV) infusions of dopamine (low doses), milrinone, nitroglycerin, isoproterenol, and methylprednisolone were started. Later, M.P. was transferred to the cardiac surgery intensive care unit for posttransplantation care. The following medications were given: vancomycin, cefoperazone, trimethoprim–sulfamethoxazole, methylprednisolone, omeprazole, mycophenolate mofetil, and tacrolimus. The patient was also maintained on continuous IV infusions of dopamine, nitroglycerin, milrinone, and isoproterenol.

Two days later the patient was extubated. She was hemodynamically stable, and the cardiovascular drugs were discontinued, whereas the immunosuppressive therapy was continued.

The patient was discharged after 20 days in the hospital with the following postdischarge therapy: methylprednisolone, tacrolimus, mycophenolate mofetil, omeprazole, and lovastatin.

Two weeks later M.P. was readmitted to the hospital following an episode of tonic-clonic seizure that the physicians believed to be drug induced. Biopsy results indicated a moderate-grade rejection of her transplanted heart. M.P.'s immunosuppressive therapy was updated, and she was now receiving the following immunosuppressive drugs: methylprednisolone (higher dose), mycophenolate mofetil, and sirolimus.

Questions

1. Before and after her heart transplant, M.P. had been receiving inotropic support that included parenteral administration of milrinone. Which of the following molecular actions most likely mediated the therapeutic effect of this drug?

A. Cyclic adenosine monophosphate (cAMP)-mediated increase in cardiac intracellular Ca^{2+} levels

B. Cyclic guanosine monophosphate (cGMP)-mediated dephosphorylation of myosin light chain

C. Opening of K^+ channels in cardiac cell membrane

D. Increased binding of Ca^{2+} to calmodulin

E. Activation of 1 Ca^{2+}/3 Na^+ antiporter

2. Omeprazole was given to M.P. before and after surgery. The administration was done most likely to counteract a potential adverse effect of which of the following drugs?

A. Mycophenolate mofetil

B. Milrinone

C. Vancomycin

D. Cefepime

E. Methylprednisolone

3. Before and after surgery, M.P. received antibiotic prophylaxis that included vancomycin, cefoperazone, and trimethoprim–sulfamethoxazole. Vancomycin was most likely added because it is effective against which of the following pairs of bacterial genera that are resistant to cefoperazone?

A. *Pseudomonas–Klebsiella*

B. *Salmonella–Serratia*

C. *Enterococcus*–methicillin-resistant (MR) *Staphylococcus*

D. *Enterobacter–Haemophilus*

E. *Mycoplasma–Chlamydia*

4. The antibiotic prophylaxis given to M.P. included trimethoprim–sulfamethoxazole. This antibiotic combination was most likely given primarily to prevent infection caused by which of the following pairs of microbial agents?

A. *Mycoplasma pneumoniae–Clostridium difficile*

B. *Bacteroides fragilis–Aspergillus fumigatus*

C. *Pneumocystis jiroveci–Toxoplasma gondii*

D. *Enterococcus faecalis–Mycobacterium tuberculosis*

E. *Pseudomonas aeruginosa–Cryptococcus neoformans*

5. Soon after surgery, M.P. was treated with several drugs that included low doses of dopamine. Which of the following was most likely the main reason for dopamine administration to this patient?

A. To increase atrial contractility

B. To improve diuresis

C. To increase total peripheral resistance

D. To decrease preload

E. To increase coronary blood flow

6. Isoproterenol was given to M.P. after transplantation. Activation of which of the following pairs of autonomic receptors most likely mediated the therapeutic effect of the drug in the patient's disease?

A. $\alpha_1 - \beta_2$

B. $\alpha_1 - M_2$

C. $\beta_2 - M_2$

D. $\alpha_1 - \beta_1$

E. $\beta_1 - \beta_2$

F. $\beta_1 - M_2$

7. Nitroglycerin was given to M.P. after transplantation. Which of the following actions most likely contributed to the therapeutic effect of the drug in the patient's disease?

A. Decreased preload

B. Decreased atrioventricular conduction

C. Decreased heart rate

D. Increased diuresis

E. Decreased risk of arrhythmia

8. After transplantation M.P. received a triple immunosuppressive therapy that included tacrolimus. The drug most likely acts by binding to which of the following molecular targets?

A. Cyclophilin

B. Tumor necrosis factor (TNF)

C. Interleukin-6

D. FK-binding protein

E. Dihydroorotate dehydrogenase

9. After transplantation, M.P. received a triple immunosuppressive therapy that included mycophenolate mofetil. This drug selectively inhibits the proliferation of which of the following pairs of cells of the innate immune system?

A. T-helper cells–neutrophils

B. Natural killer cells–neutrophils

C. B lymphocytes–macrophages

D. Neutrophils–macrophages

E. T-helper cells–natural killer cells

F. Natural killer cells–macrophages

10. M.P.'s postdischarge therapy included lovastatin. Which of the following liver cell structures was most likely the primary site of action of that drug?

A. Plasma membrane

B. Nucleus

C. Endoplasmic reticulum

D. Mitochondria

E. Lysosomes

F. Golgi body

11. Which of the following actions most likely mediated the therapeutic effect of lovastatin in M.P.'s disease?

A. Decreased synthesis of high-density lipoprotein (HDL)

B. Decreased synthesis of hepatic transaminase

C. Increased hepatic endocytosis of low-density lipoprotein (LDL)

D. Increased synthesis of lipoprotein lipase

E. Increased synthesis of mevalonic acid

12. M.P. was readmitted to the hospital following an episode of tonic-clonic seizure that physicians believed to be drug-induced. Which of the following drugs taken by the patient most likely caused her seizure?

A. Prednisolone

B. Mycophenolate mofetil

C. Omeprazole

D. Lovastatin

E. Tacrolimus

13. After the diagnosis of moderate-degree rejection, M.P.'s immunosuppressive therapy was updated by including sirolimus. The inhibition of which of the following enzymes most likely mediated the therapeutic effect of the drug in the patient's disease?

A. Dihydroorotate dehydrogenase

B. Dihydrofolate reductase

C. Mammalian kinase

D. Calcineurin

E. Inosine monophosphate dehydrogenase

Answers and Explanations

▶ *Learning objective:* Identify the molecular action mediating the positive inotropic effect of milrinone.

1. Answer: A

Milrinone is a phosphodiesterase inhibitor. These drugs inhibit the cAMP phosphodiesterase 3 isozyme (localized mainly in the heart and vascular smooth muscle) with a resulting increase in cAMP levels. The cAMP increase causes the following effects:

▶ In the myocardium: the phosphorylation of a protein kinase, which ultimately increases the availability of free intracellular Ca^{2+}, leading to an increased contractility

▶ In the smooth muscle: the inactivation of myosin light chain kinase, which causes vascular smooth muscle relaxation, leading to a decreased afterload

Both effects are useful in heart failure. Phosphodiesterase inhibitors are very effective, but they can cause an increase in mortality if used chronically. Therefore they are approved by the U.S. Food and Drug Administration for the acute or short-term treatment of heart failure, as in the present case.

B Phosphodiesterase inhibitors do not inhibit the cGMP phosphodiesterase isozyme. Moreover, the dephosphorylation of myosin light chain would lead to relaxation, not contraction, of cardiac myocytes.

C The increased cAMP level does not trigger the opening of K^+ channels. Additionally, this opening would cause hyperpolarization of the cell membrane, which would adversely affect cardiac contractility.

D The increased availability of intracellular Ca^{2+} would increase the binding of Ca^{2+} to troponin C, not to calmodulin, in cardiac myocytes.

E This would be the mechanism of action of digoxin.

▶ *Learning objective:* Identify the drug that can cause adverse effects that are counteracted by omeprazole.

2. Answer: E

Omeprazole was most likely given to M.P. in order to prevent methylprednisolone-induced gastric damage. It is well recognized that glucocorticoids can be ulcerogenic agents, even if this occurs mainly when they are given at high doses for long periods. Glucocorticoids can inhibit prostaglandin biosynthesis, thereby decreasing gastric bicarbonate and mucus secretion,

and they impair both angiogenesis and epithelial repair mechanisms. Omeprazole is a proton pump inhibitor. These drugs inhibit irreversibly the enzyme H^+/K^+-adenosine triphosphatase (H^+/K^+-ATPase, the so-called proton pump), which is activated during the final step of acid secretion by the parietal cells of the stomach. In this way they can exert a strong beneficial effect on both ulcer prevention and healing.

A, B, C, D The gastric damage induced by all these drugs is low or negligible.

▶ *Learning objective:* Identify the pairs of bacterial genera sensitive to vancomycin.

3. Answer: C

Solid organ transplant recipients are considered to be at "high risk" for developing infection. Therefore antibiotic prophylaxis is usually given. A broad-spectrum cephalosporin was chosen in the present case. Additionally, because infections of ventricular-assist devices and chest tubes are often due to gram-positive organisms (staphylococci, enterococci) vancomycin was added to the prophylactic treatment. Actually no β-lactam antibiotics (with the only exception of ceftaroline) are effective against MR staphylococci, and no cephalosporins are effective against enterococci. Vancomycin is quite effective against MR staphylococci, *Enterococcus faecalis*, and several strains of *Enterococcus faecium*. This explains the addition of this drug to the treatment.

A, B, D These bacterial genera are sensitive to cefoperazone but resistant to vancomycin.

E These bacterial genera are resistant to both vancomycin and cefoperazone.

▶ *Learning objective:* Identify the pairs of bacteria sensitive to trimethoprim-sulfamethoxazole.

4. Answer: C

Trimethoprim–sulfamethoxazole combination is today given universally to all transplant recipients who do not have sulfa allergies. This antibiotic combination is effective for the prevention of *Pneumocystis jiroveci* pneumonia, which occurs in many transplantation centers at an overall rate of 10 to 14%. It also provides effective prophylaxis against *Toxoplasma gondii.* Both microorganisms are resistant to most broad-spectrum antibiotics, including cefoperazone, and to vancomycin.

A, B, D, E Trimethoprim–sulfamethoxazole combination is minimally effective against all these microorganisms.

▶ *Learning objective:* Explain the primary reason for dopamine administration soon after heart transplantation.

5. Answer: B

Dopamine is a first-line agent for a decreased diuresis due to a pronounced reduction of renal blood flow. The drug is a mixed-acting adrenergic agent that, at low doses, activates D_1-adrenoceptors located primarily in renal arteriolar vessels and in the proximal tubules. Activation of these receptors causes vasodilation and inhibition of Na^+ reabsorption. Both actions contribute to increased diuresis.

A Intermediate doses of dopamine activate β_1-adrenoceptors and release of norepinephrine from nerve terminals. Both actions can increase cardiac contractility, but this is unlikely in the present case because low doses were given. Moreover, atrial contractility contributes very little to cardiac output.

C High doses of dopamine can activate α_1-adrenoceptors, increasing total peripheral resistance, but this is unlikely in the present case because low doses were given. Additionally an increase in total peripheral resistance would be detrimental for a recently transplanted heart that still has an impaired inotropic function.

D Dopamine causes arteriolar vasodilation, mainly in renal, mesenteric, and coronary beds. Therefore it can decrease afterload rather than preload.

E Activation of D_1-adrenoceptors can increase coronary blood flow, but this is not at all the main reason for giving dopamine soon after a heart transplantation.

▶ *Learning objective:* Identify the autonomic receptors activated by isoproterenol.

6. Answer: E

Isoproterenol is a nonselective β-adrenoceptor agonist (i.e., it activates all β-adrenoceptors). The drug is often used in the operating room after heart transplant because contractility and sinus node function of the new heart are temporarily impaired to varying degrees, based on the condition of the donor heart, quality of preservation, and other factors. Moreover, β-adrenoceptors of the new heart are usually upregulated, enhancing the pharmacological activity of the drug. Heart effects of the drug are due both to activation of β_1-adrenoceptors (60–80%) and to activation of β_2-adrenoceptors (20–40%).

A, B, C, D, F All these answers have at least one receptor that is not activated by isoproterenol.

▶ *Learning objective:* Identify the action of nitroglycerin that can be most useful after heart transplantation.

7. Answer: A

A transplanted heart is prone to heart failure, because normal heart contractility cannot be completely resumed in many patients. Right heart failure during the first 30 days after transplantation occurs in about 25% of cases. Nitrates are vasodilator agents that can affect mainly large veins, thereby decreasing preload. This in turn decreases the workload of the right ventricle, protecting the heart from right heart failure. Nitrates can also cause arteriolar vasodilation, thereby decreasing afterload (not listed), which can be similarly useful in heart transplantation. This explains the frequent use of nitroglycerin just after transplant.

B, C By decreasing preload nitrates could cause a reflex activation of the sympathetic system. This activation would increase, not decrease, atrioventricular conduction and heart rate.

D, E Nitrates do not have these effects.

▸ *Learning objective:* Identify the specific molecular target for tacrolimus.

8. Answer: D

Tacrolimus is an antibiotic endowed with immunosuppressive properties. It belongs to the so-called immunophilin inhibitors, which include cyclosporine, tacrolimus, and sirolimus. Tacrolimus interferes with T cell function by binding to FK-binding protein, a small protein located in the cytoplasm of T-helper cells. The tacrolimus–protein complex in turn binds to calcineurin, a cytoplasmic phosphatase, thus inhibiting calcineurin-mediated expression for production of several cytokines. In this way the drug suppresses the early cellular response to antigenic stimuli.

A Cyclophilin is the protein that binds cyclosporine.

B, C These are inflammatory cytokines. Tacrolimus does not bind to cytokines.

E This is an enzyme involved in the de novo pyrimidine biosynthesis. This enzyme is inhibited by leflunomide, not by tacrolimus.

▸ *Learning objective:* Identify the cells of the innate immune system whose proliferation was primarily inhibited by mycophenolate mofetil.

9. Answer: E

Mycophenolate mofetil is an immunosuppressive drug that inhibits inosine monophosphate dehydrogenase, an enzyme involved in the *de novo pathway* of purine biosynthesis. However, unlike other cytotoxic agents, it does not inhibit enzymes involved in the *salvage pathway* of purine biosynthesis. Thus it selectively inhibits the proliferation of all lymphocyte species (including T-helper cells and natural killer cells), because these cells lack the enzymes of the alternative salvage pathway.

A, B, C, D, F The proliferation of other cells, such as neutrophils and macrophages, is much less affected by mycophenolate mofetil, because these cells can use the salvage pathway when the de novo pathway is inhibited.

▸ *Learning objective:* Identify the site of action of lovastatin.

10. Answer: C

Lovastatin belongs to the class of 3-hydroxy-3-methylglutaryl–coenzyme A (HMG-CoA) reductase inhibitors (also called statins). These agents act by inhibiting the enzyme that is located on the liver cell endoplasmic reticulum and represents the rate-limiting step in cholesterol biosynthesis. Hyperlipidemia occurs in 60 to 83% of heart transplant recipients treated with modern, conventional immunosuppressive therapy. Many heart transplant recipients had atherosclerotic heart disease as the etiology for heart failure and were often hyperlipidemic prior to transplantation. However, some patients have a normal lipid profile prior to transplantation. New-onset hyperlipidemia in these patients most often begins at 2 weeks and stabilizes 3 months after transplant. It has been consistently shown that statin therapy improves survival rate and decreases the frequency of cardiac rejection in heart transplant recipients.

A, B, D, E, F Statins do not act on these cell structures.

▸ *Learning objective:* Describe the mechanism of action of lovastatin.

11. Answer: C

Statins inhibit HMG-CoA reductase, the enzyme that catalyzes the synthesis of mevalonic acid from HMG-CoA. The formation of mevalonic acid is the rate-limiting step in cholesterol biosynthesis. The inhibition of cholesterol synthesis in liver results in an upregulation of hepatic high-affinity LDL receptors, which in turn causes an increased removal of LDL from the blood by receptor-mediated endocytosis. Thus plasma cholesterol is reduced by both decreased cholesterol synthesis and increased LDL catabolism.

A Statins actually cause a small increase in HDL.

B Statins can increase, not decrease, the synthesis of hepatic transaminase.

D Statins do not affect directly lipoprotein lipase.

E Statins decrease, not increase, the synthesis of mevalonic acid.

▶ *Learning objective:* Describe the adverse effects of tacrolimus.

12. Answer: E

Neurotoxicity and nephrotoxicity are the two major adverse effects of tacrolimus, occurring in more than 50% of patients receiving this drug. Neurotoxicity includes headache (> 64%), insomnia, tremor, paresthesias, and seizures.

A, B The occurrence of seizures due to these drugs is very rare.

C, D These drugs do not cause seizures.

▶ *Learning objective:* Identify the enzyme that is specifically inhibited by sirolimus.

13. Answer: C

Because tacrolimus most likely caused M.P.'s neurotoxicity, the physician decided to substitute tacrolimus with sirolimus (formerly called rapamycin), an immunosuppressive drug that has negligible neurotoxic activity. Sirolimus resembles tacrolimus in that both bind to an intracellular FK-binding protein. However, whereas the tacrolimus–FK protein complex inhibits the enzyme calcineurin, the sirolimus–FK complex inhibits a *mammalian kinase* (named mammalian target of rapamycin [mTOR]), a key enzyme in cell-cycle progression that regulates cell growth, cell proliferation, cell motility, and cell survival. The blockade of mTOR causes blockade of interleukin-2-dependent lymphocyte proliferation. As a result, the drug inhibits clonal expansion of B and T lymphocytes substantially.

A Inhibition of dihydroorotate dehydrogenase would be the mechanism of action of leflunomide.

B Inhibition of dihydrofolate reductase would be the mechanism of action of methotrexate.

D Calcineurin is a protein phosphatase that is inhibited by cyclosporine and tacrolimus.

E Inhibition of inosine monophosphate dehydrogenase would be the mechanism of action of mycophenolate mofetil.

Case 45 — Stroke

Z.A., a 66-year-old woman, was admitted to the emergency department (ED) after losing consciousness at home. She regained consciousness by the time she arrived in the ED, 1 hour after the initial event.

The patient's medical history was notable for a long-standing allergic asthma presently treated with inhaled albuterol as needed. Six months earlier she suffered from a transient episode of forgetfulness and confusion lasting about half an hour. One month ago she underwent an episode of numbness and tingling of her right lower extremity lasting about 2 hours. She did not seek medical attention for these episodes.

Physical examination showed an alert and distressed woman with the following vital signs: blood pressure 188/115 mm Hg, pulse 110 bpm, respiration 22/min. The patient was unable to speak but capable of understanding what was said to her. She was able to write down her thoughts more easily than to speak them. Neurologic examination revealed paralysis of her right face and arm and loss of sensation to touch on the skin of the right face and arm. Blood exams and electrocardiography on admission were all within normal limits.

Computed tomography (CT) of the brain was performed, which failed to reveal any evidence of cerebral hemorrhage. Magnetic resonance imaging of the brain demonstrated left-sided occlusion of a cerebral artery.

A diagnosis of ischemic stroke was made, and an emergency therapy was performed. Intravenous (IV) labetalol was given, and 15 minutes later the patient's blood pressure dropped to 165/90 mm Hg. At this point an IV infusion of alteplase was started. Blood pressure was monitored and controlled by labetalol after alteplase administration.

The following day the CT scan was repeated, with no evidence of cerebral hemorrhage, and clopidogrel was included in her emergency therapy. On the following days Z.A.'s neurologic status improved, but spasticity supervened on her left arm and was relieved after the local administration of botulinum toxin.

One week later Z.A. was transferred to a stroke rehabilitation center with a postdischarge therapy that included the following drugs: clopidogrel, captopril, hydrochlorothiazide, and lovastatin.

Questions

1. Z.A. was diagnosed with stroke. Which of the following is the best definition of this disorder?

A. Sudden, focal loss of brain function due to neuron apoptosis

B. Progressive, diffuse loss of brain function due to a decrease of cerebral blood flow

C. Sudden, focal loss of brain function due to local interruption of cerebral blood flow

D. Progressive, diffuse loss of brain function due to senile plaques

E. Sudden, focal loss of brain function due to an unregulated brain electrical discharge

2. Z.A. was diagnosed with ischemic stroke. Stroke can be classified into two major subtypes based on pathogenesis: ischemic stroke and hemorrhagic stroke. Which is the approximate percent of ischemic strokes compared to all?

A. 20%

B. 40%

C. 50%

D. 70%

E. > 80%

3. Based on Z.A.'s symptoms and signs, which cerebral artery was most likely blocked?

A. Right anterior cerebral artery

B. Left middle cerebral artery

C. Right internal carotid artery

D. Left vertebral artery

E. Right posterior cerebral artery

F. Left anterior choroidal artery

4. Ischemic stroke is caused by a cerebral infarct leading to cell necrosis. Which of the following types of necrosis was most likely related to cerebral infarct?

A. Coagulative

B. Liquefactive

C. Hemorrhagic

D. Caseating

E. Fatty

5. Which of the following neurotransmitters is most likely involved in the death of neurons following a stroke?

A. γ-Aminobutyric acid (GABA)

B. Norepinephrine

C. Acetylcholine

D. Serotonin

E. Glutamate

6. A labetalol infusion was given to Z.A. to lower her blood pressure. Which of the following actions most likely contributed to the acute antihypertensive effect of the drug in this patient?

A. Decreased total peripheral resistance

B. Decreased extracellular fluid volume

C. Reflex increase in heart rate

D. Increased stroke volume

E. Increased cardiac output

7. Alteplase was given to Z.A. Binding to which of the following endogenous compounds most likely mediated the therapeutic effect of the drug in the patient's disease?

A. Thrombin

B. Antithrombin III

C. Plasminogen

D. Plasmin

E. Fibrinogen

F. Fibrin

8. The efficacy of fibrinolytic drugs in ischemic stroke is strictly related to the time of intervention. These drugs produce the best results when given within which of the following times (in hours) of onset of symptoms?

A. 3
B. 5
C. 6
D. 8
E. 10

9. Which of the following disorders would represent a contraindication to the use of alteplase in ischemic stroke?

A. Atrial fibrillation
B. Rheumatic heart disease
C. Deep venous thrombosis
D. Epilepsy
E. Major surgery within previous 14 days
F. Urinary tract infection

10. Clopidogrel was administered to Z.A. to inhibit platelet aggregation. Which of the following was the most likely reason to prefer clopidogrel to aspirin in this patient?

A. The patient suffered from a transient ischemic attack.
B. The patient's blood pressure was dangerously high.
C. The patient received an IV infusion of alteplase.
D. The patient had been suffering from allergic asthma.
E. The patient received labetalol IV.

11. Botulinum toxin was given to A.Z. Which of the following structures was most likely the primary site of the therapeutic action of this drug in the patient's disorder?

A. Nicotinic muscular receptors
B. Somatic nerve terminals
C. Muscarinic receptors
D. Autonomic nerve terminals
E. Nicotinic neural receptors

12. Z.A.'s postdischarge therapy included captopril. Which of the following actions most likely contributed to the therapeutic effect of the drug in the patient's disease?

A. Decreased bradykinin activity
B. Increased renin synthesis
C. Decreased renal prostaglandin synthesis
D. Increased Na^+ and water secretion
E. Decreased renal nitric oxide activity

13. Captopril inhibits ACE. Which of the following phrases best explains the mechanism of this inhibition?

A. Decreased ACE affinity for its substrate
B. Suicide inhibition of ACE
C. Decreased ACE biosynthesis
D. Increased ACE biotransformation
E. Concentration lower than that of the substrate

14. Z.A.'s postdischarge therapy included lovastatin. Which of the following is the primary site of action of this drug?

A. Liver cell membrane
B. Liver capillary endothelium
C. Atherosclerotic plaque
D. Liver endoplasmic reticulum
E. Brush border of intestinal cells
F. Adipocytes

15. Which of the following actions most likely mediated the therapeutic effect of lovastatin in the patient's disorder?

A. Decreased synthesis of high-density lipoprotein (HDL)
B. Decreased synthesis of hepatic transaminase
C. Increased hepatic endocytosis of low-density lipoprotein (LDL)
D. Increased synthesis of lipoprotein lipase
E. Increased synthesis of mevalonic acid

16. Chronic lovastatin therapy can increase the risk of which of the following rare but life-threatening disorders?

A. Rheumatoid arthritis
B. Rhabdomyolysis
C. Hyperthyroidism
D. Alzheimer's disease
E. Chronic kidney disease

17. In order to prevent the most serious adverse effect of statins, the serum concentration of which of the following enzymes should be measured frequently, especially during the first weeks of therapy?

A. HMG-CoA reductase
B. Aminotransferase
C. Alkaline phosphatase
D. Galactokinase
E. Creatine kinase
F. Lactate dehydrogenase

Answers and Explanations

▶ *Learning objective:* Identify the appropriate definition of stroke.

1. Answer: C

Stroke is a clinical syndrome characterized primarily by two factors:

- ▶ There is a sudden and focal loss of brain function.
- ▶ The loss is due to an abrupt interruption of cerebral blood flow.

Stroke can be further defined as a "regular stroke" when neurologic deficits last more than 1 hour and as a "transient ischemic attack" (also referred to as a ministroke) when neurologic deficits last less than 1 hour.

A Cell apoptosis is a slow process. It cannot cause a sudden loss of brain function.

B Progressive, diffuse loss of brain function due to decreased cerebral blood may define vascular dementia, not stroke.

D Progressive, diffuse loss of brain function due to senile plaques may define Alzheimer's disease, not stroke.

E Sudden, focal loss of brain function due to an unregulated brain electrical discharge may define epilepsy, not stroke.

▶ *Learning objective:* Identify the correct percentage of strokes that are classified as ischemic.

2. Answer: E

Ischemic stroke is a focal brain infarction that results from thrombotic or embolic occlusion of cerebral vessels. It accounts for > 80% of all strokes. The disorder is a leading cause of death and of serious long-term disability in the developed world. Ischemia results from thrombi or emboli. Atheromas, particularly if ulcerated, predispose to thrombi, may affect any major cerebral artery and are more common at areas of turbulent flow. Atherothrombotic occlusion usually causes neurologic symptoms that evolve over a period of time, usually hours. Emboli may lodge anywhere in the cerebral arterial tree and come more commonly from the heart (atrial fibrillation, myocardial infarction, mitral stenosis, prosthetic heart valves, etc.). Embolic occlusion usually causes neurologic symptoms that appear abruptly.

A, B, C, D See correct answer explanation.

▶ *Learning objective:* From a stroke patient's symptoms and signs, describe which cerebral artery was most likely blocked.

3. Answer: B

The loss of all sensation on the right face and arm, coupled with the paralysis of muscles in these regions, suggests that Z.A. was suffering damage of the left somatosensory and primary motor cortex. This damage causes right-sided symptoms because the motor and sensory tracts cross the midline as they travel between the cerebrum and the spinal cord. Z.A.'s language disorder is called Broca's (expressive) aphasia, and it may result from damage to the dominant Broca's motor speech area, a control center that sits just anterior to the face portion of the primary motor cortex in the left frontal lobe. The artery that supplies blood to these regions is the left middle cerebral artery. Blockage of this artery by a thrombus or embolism can cause all of this patient's signs and symptoms.

A, C, E The patient's symptoms on the right side of her body indicate that the damage was on the left, not the right, cerebral arteries.

D Both right and left vertebral arteries merge into the basilar artery. Symptoms related to vertebrobasilar occlusion include vertigo, visual disturbances, nausea and vomiting, and ataxia. These symptoms did not occur in the present case.

F Symptoms related to occlusion of the left anterior choroidal artery include right visual disturbances that did not occur in the present case.

▶ *Learning objective:* Identify the necrosis type that occurs after a cerebral infarct.

---

4. Answer: B

The necrosis of cerebral infarct is liquefactive, because the brain contains little connective tissue but high amounts of digestive enzymes and lipids. Therefore, brain cells can be readily digested by their own enzymes. Its microscopic appearance includes cyst formation with necrotic debris in the center, areas of gliosis, and numerous macrophages phagocytizing cellular debris.

A Coagulative necrosis can occur in all parts of ischemic organs other than the brain.

C Hemorrhagic necrosis occurs after profuse bleeding from ruptured blood vessels.

D Caseating necrosis is typically caused by mycobacteria, fungi, and some foreign substances.

E Fatty necrosis is a specialized necrosis of fat tissue.

▶ *Learning objective:* Identify the neurotransmitter that is most likely involved in the death of neurons following a stroke.

---

5. Answer: E

Today there is unequivocal evidence that glutamate-mediated excitotoxicity is a primary contributor to ischemic neuronal death. Excitotoxicity is the pathological process by which nerve cells are damaged or killed by excessive stimulation caused by excitatory neurotransmitters, such as glutamate. When a region of the brain becomes ischemic, neurons deep within the ischemic focus die from lack of oxygen (i.e., energy deprivation). However, at the edge of ischemic focus neurons appear to die because of a rapid elevation of extracellular glutamate levels. Glutamate activates its own ionotropic receptors, N-methyl-D-aspartate (NMDA) and amino-hydroxy-methylisoxazole-propionic acid (AMPA) located on ion channels, primarily Ca^{2+} channels. The increased Ca^{2+} influx into cells activates a number of enzymes, including phospholipases, endonucleases, and proteases, that go on to damage cell structure.

A, B, C, D All these neurotransmitters are not involved in the death of neurons that follows ischemic stroke.

▶ *Learning objective:* Describe the action that most likely mediates the acute antihypertensive effect of labetalol.

---

6. Answer: A

Labetalol is currently used to cause a prompt reduction in blood pressure. The drug decreases total peripheral resistance due to both α_1-adrenoceptor blockade in the vascular smooth muscle and to β_1-adrenoceptor blockade in the juxtaglomerular cells of the macula densa, which in turn inhibits renin secretion. A blood pressure higher than 185/110 mm Hg is a contraindication to the use of fibrinolytic drugs, which explains why Z.A. blood pressure had to be reduced before administering alteplase.

B By blocking β_1-adrenoceptor-mediated renin secretion labetalol can decrease aldosterone activity, reducing the extracellular fluid volume, but this action is mild and cannot occur at once. Therefore, it cannot explain the acute antihypertensive effect of labetalol in hypertensive crisis.

C Labetalol blocks β_1-adrenoceptors (which would decrease heart rate) and also blocks α_1-adrenoceptors (which would cause a reflex increase in heart rate). However, the drug is a stronger β-blocker than it is an α-blocker, with a ratio of 7:1 when given IV. Therefore bradycardia, not tachycardia, is the final effect. In any case, a reflex tachycardia would increase, not decrease, the blood pressure.

D, E Cardiac output is equal to stroke volume by heart rate. Blockade of β_1-adrenoceptors is more pronounced than blockade of α_1-adrenoceptors, and stroke volume and cardiac rate are usually decreased. Hence cardiac output is usually decreased, not increased.

▶ *Learning objective:* Identify the endogenous compound that represents the substrate of alteplase enzyme.

7. Answer: C

Alteplase is a fibrinolytic drug. Most drugs of this class are recombinant tissue plasminogen activators that catalyze the formation of plasmin from its precursor plasminogen. The active site of these enzymes binds plasminogen, the substrate of the enzymes. The resulting plasmin acts directly on fibrin, breaking the protein into a fibrin-split product, followed by the lysis of the clot. Tissue plasminogen activators can create a generalized lytic state when administered IV because both protective hemostatic thrombi and target thromboemboli are broken down. The newer compounds of this class (alteplase, reteplase, tenecteplase) preferentially activate plasminogen bound to plasmin, avoiding (but only partially) the creation of the systemic lytic state.

A, B, D, E, F Alteplase does not bind to these compounds.

▶ *Learning objective:* Identify the time from onset of symptoms when the administration of alteplase gives the best results.

8. Answer: A

It has been shown that fibrinolytic drugs can significantly decrease mortality from ischemic stroke when administered within 3 hours of symptom onset. Recent studies indicate that benefits can be achieved extending the window for thrombolytic therapy beyond the guideline of 3 hours, but longer times from ischemic stroke onset to initiation of treatment are associated with less absolute clinical benefit.

B, C, D, E See correct answer explanation.

▶ *Learning objective:* Identify a disorder that contraindicates the use of fibrinolytic drugs.

9. Answer: E

Fibrinolytic drugs are contraindicated in any situation in which the risk of bleeding is greater than the potential benefit. These contraindications include the following:

▶ Myocardial infarction in previous 3 months
▶ Blood glucose < 50 mg/dL
▶ Head trauma or intracranial or intraspinal surgery in the previous 3 months
▶ Prior stroke in the previous 3 months
▶ History of previous intracranial hemorrhage
▶ Acute bleeding disorders (platelet count < 100,000 mm^3, current use of anticoagulants, etc.)
▶ Major surgery within the previous 14 days
▶ Gastrointestinal or urinary tract hemorrhage within the previous 21 days
▶ Elevated blood pressure (systolic > 185 or diastolic > 110 mm Hg)
▶ Age > 80
▶ Witnessed seizure at stroke onset

Therefore, major surgery within the previous 14 days is the contraindication for the use of fibrinolytic drugs.

A, B, C These diseases can increase the risk of stroke but do not contraindicate the use of fibrinolytic drugs.

D, F These disorders do significantly affect the risk of stroke and do not contraindicate the use of fibrinolytic drugs.

▶ *Learning objective:* Explain why clopidogrel is usually preferred to aspirin in a specific patient.

10. Answer: C

Antiplatelet therapy is the mainstay for stroke treatment and secondary prevention. All patients who had an ischemic stroke or a transient ischemic attack should receive an antithrombotic agent at once.

The same agent should be taken for life to prevent stroke recurrence. The treatment usually includes aspirin, but clopidogrel can be used when the patient is at risk of aspirin hypersensitivity, as the asthmatic patient of the present case. Clopidogrel is an antiplatelet drug that causes an irreversible inhibition of adenosine diphosphate (ADP) receptors, thereby inhibiting ADP-mediated platelet aggregation. Alteplase is usually given with an antiplatelet drug.

A A previous transient ischemic attack is an indication, not a contraindication, to the use of aspirin.

B A high blood pressure is not a contraindication to aspirin.

E Labetalol IV is not a contraindication to the concomitant use of aspirin.

▶ *Learning objective:* Describe the primary site of the pharmacological action of botulinum toxin.

11. Answer: B

Botulinum toxin enters the cholinergic nerve terminals by endocytosis, where it prevents the exocytotic release of acetylcholine, causing paralysis of the skeletal muscles surrounding the site of injection. All randomized, controlled trials evaluating botulinum toxin for the treatment of upper limb spasticity after stroke have consistently demonstrated reduced muscle tone and improved patient performance. Botulinum toxin action is extremely long, and a single local injection can decrease spasticity for several weeks to several months.

A, C, E Botulinum toxin does not bind to cholinergic receptors.

D Botulinum toxin also prevents acetylcholine release from autonomic cholinergic nerve terminals, but this is not the site of the therapeutic action of the drug.

▶ *Learning objective:* Identify the action that can contribute to the therapeutic effect of captopril.

12. Answer: D

Captopril is an angiotensin-converting enzyme (ACE) inhibitor. These drugs cause a reversible inhibition of the enzyme that converts angiotensin I (inactive) into angiotensin II and can therefore inhibit most known actions of angiotensin II, including aldosterone-mediated Na^+ and water reabsorption in the distal nephron.

The association of an ACE inhibitor and a thiazide diuretic was found to cause a 42% reduction of stroke relapse. Moreover, similar results were achieved, even in patients without hypertension. Therefore, a therapy with ACE inhibitors or angiotensin antagonists plus a thiazide diuretic should be prescribed to all patient with previous ischemic stroke.

A ACE is also called kininase II because it inactivates bradykinin. By inhibiting this enzyme, the activity of bradykinin is increased, not decreased.

B By inhibiting angiotensin II synthesis, captopril increases renin synthesis (a short-loop positive feedback), but this cannot affect blood pressure because angiotensin II synthesis is inhibited. In any case, an increased renin synthesis would increase, not decrease, blood pressure.

C Renal prostaglandin synthesis is bradykinin-mediated. By increasing bradykinin activity prostaglandin synthesis would be increased, not decreased.

E Angiotensin II stimulates the production of superoxide, which can react with nitric oxide and impair its function. By inhibiting angiotensin II synthesis captopril would increase, not impair, nitric oxide activity.

▶ *Learning objective:* Explain the biochemical reason for the inhibition of ACE by captopril.

13. Answer: A

ACE inhibitors are reversible competitive inhibitors of ACE. Mathematically, the effect of a competitive inhibitor on an enzyme is to decrease the affinity of the enzyme for its substrate. Competitive ACE inhibitors decrease the affinity of ACE for angiotensin I (the natural substrate); therefore, they preferentially bind ACE, blocking its activity.

B A suicide inhibitor is an irreversible inhibitor of the enzyme. ACE inhibitors are reversible, not irreversible inhibitors.

C, D ACE inhibitors do not affect biosynthesis or biotransformation of ACE.

E Concentration of a drug depends on the given doses. Concentration alone cannot explain the action of an enzyme inhibitor.

14. Answer: D

Lovastatin is the prototype drug of 3-hydroxy-3-methylglutaryl–coenzyme A (HMG-CoA) reductase inhibitors. These agents act by inhibiting the enzyme that is located on the liver endoplasmic reticulum. It has been shown that HMG-CoA reductase inhibitors decrease the recurrence of ischemic stroke, even in patients without hyperlipidemia. Therefore, a therapy with an HMG-CoA reductase inhibitor should be prescribed to all patients with previous ischemic stroke.

A, B, C, E, F HMG-CoA reductase is minimally located on these sites.

▸ *Learning objective:* Identify the action that most likely mediated the therapeutic effect of lovastatin.

15. Answer: C

Lovastatin is the prototype drug of HMG-CoA reductase inhibitors (also named statins). These drugs inhibit the enzyme that catalyzes the synthesis of mevalonic acid from HMG-CoA. The formation of mevalonic acid is the rate-limiting step in cholesterol biosynthesis. The inhibition of cholesterol biosynthesis in liver results in an upregulation of hepatic high-affinity LDL receptors, which in turn causes an increased removal of LDL from the blood by receptor-mediated endocytosis.

A Statins actually cause a small increase in HDL.

B Statins can increase, not decrease, the synthesis of hepatic transaminase.

D This would be the mechanism of action of fibric acid derivatives.

E Statins decrease, not increase, the synthesis of mevalonic acid.

▸ *Learning objective:* Identify the organ/tissue that can be the site of a rare but serious adverse effect of lovastatin.

16. Answer: B

Myopathy is a rare but serious adverse effect of statins. The illness occurs in < 0.1%

of patients when statins are given alone, but it can occur more often when they are given concomitantly with other drugs, such as niacin or fibrates (up to 5%, when given with gemfibrozil). The spectrum of statin-related myopathy ranges from common but clinically benign myalgia (up to 10% of cases) to rare but life-threatening rhabdomyolysis. Myopathy is characterized by vacuolization of myofibers, degeneration, swelling, and eventually apoptosis. The mechanism of this adverse effect of statins is still uncertain.

A Statins have been rarely associated with rheumatoid arthritis, but the disease is not life-threatening.

C There are no reports of hyperthyroidism associated with statin treatment, and the disease is not life threatening

D Hyperlipidemia, not statin therapy, is an established risk factor for the incidence and progression of Alzheimer's disease and dementia. Some studies found that statin treatment can very rarely cause small decrements in cognition. However, the effect is not life-threatening.

E There is indirect evidence of beneficial effects, not worsening, of statins on vessel stiffening and endothelial function in patients with chronic kidney disease.

▸ *Learning objective:* Identify the enzyme whose serum concentration should be measured frequently to prevent a serious adverse effect of statins.

17. Answer: E

Creatine kinase is an enzyme found in high concentration in heart and skeletal muscle. Because this enzyme exists in relatively few organs, its serum concentration is used as a specific index of injury of myocardium or skeletal muscle. In fact, creatine kinase levels can also prove helpful in recognizing muscular dystrophy before clinical signs appear.

A HMG-CoA reductase mediates the first step in cholesterol biosynthesis.

B Aminotransferases levels are measured primarily to diagnose liver disease.

C Alkaline phosphatase is an enzyme originating mainly in the bone and liver, with some activity in the kidney and intestine. The enzyme is measured primarily as an index of bone or liver disease.

D Decreased values of this enzyme are associated with galactosemia, a rare genetic disorder.

F Lactate dehydrogenase is an enzyme widely distributed in the body tissues, and its levels are measured to provide primarily an index of pulmonary infarction.

Systemic Lupus Erythematosus

L.P., a 35-year-old Caucasian woman, was admitted to the emergency department because of a 2-day history of fever, progressive dyspnea, generalized edema, and left lower chest pain with nonproductive cough.

The patient's medical history indicated that 3 months ago she had started suffering from pain involving initially her hands and wrists and progressing, at some time later, to the knees and elbows, bilaterally. L.P. also noted a recent weight loss of 8 kg, down to 55 kg, and a severe sunburn on her face, upper neck, and back that occurred after 15 minutes of sun exposure, which was unusual for her. Two weeks before admission, L.P.'s joint pain increased and was associated with unexplained anorexia and fatigue that lasted most of the day.

Vital signs on admission were: blood pressure 145/92 mm Hg, pulse 144 bpm, respirations 32/min, body temperature 102.7°F (39.2°C). Physical examination showed a patient feeling very ill and presenting an intermittent obtunded state of consciousness. Inspection disclosed a diffuse moderate edema, an erythematous rash over the cheeks and nasal bridge, and two 3-mm aphthous ulcerations on the oral mucosa. On auscultation, heart sounds were found to be diminished, and diffuse coarse crackles were noted on both lungs, with depressed vocal transmission in the left basal thorax. Abdominal examination revealed moderate hepatomegaly.

Several laboratory exams were ordered, with the following results:

Blood hematology

- ► Erythrocyte sedimentation rate (ESR) 80 mm/h (normal 0–20)
- ► Red blood cell count (RBC): $3.1 \times 10^6/mm^3$ (normal 4.0–6.0)
- ► Hemoglobin (Hgb): 9.1 g/dL (normal 12–16)
- ► Hematocrit (Hct): 22% (normal 36–48)
- ► Mean corpuscular volume (MCV): 90 fL (normal 80–100)
- ► White blood cell count (WBC): $2.3 \times 10^3/mm^3$ (normal 4–10)
- ► Platelets: $110 \times 10^3/mm^3$ (normal 130–400)

Blood chemistry

- ► Creatinine: 2.8 mg/dL (normal 0.6–1.2)
- ► Blood urea nitrogen (BUN): 42 mg/dL (normal 8–25)
- ► Sodium (Na$^+$): 130 mEq/L (normal 135–146)
- ► Potassium (K$^+$): 5.9 mEq/L (normal 3.6–5.3)
- ► Aspartate aminotransferase: 405 U/L (normal, women 10–35)
- ► Alanine aminotransferase: 85 U/L (normal, women 7–35)
- ► Alkaline phosphatase: 135 U/L (normal 30–120)
- ► Ammonia: 38 µmol/L (normal 9–33)
- ► C-reactive protein: 110 mg/L (normal < 8)
- ► Rheumatoid factor (RF) antibody: 32 U/mL (normal < 20)
- ► Antibodies to double-stranded DNA (anti-dsDNA): 175 UI/mL (normal < 25)

Urinalysis

More than 50 leucocytes and erythrocytes per high-power field
    Proteins 700 mg/d

- ▸ Microbiological results: cultures of the blood, pleural fluid, and urine negative
- ▸ Electrocardiogram (ECG): atrial fibrillation and low voltage QRS complexes
- ▸ Chest X-ray: evident cardiomegaly and right pleural effusion
- ▸ Computed tomographic (CT) scan: large pleuropericardial effusion

A diagnosis of severe flare of systemic lupus erythematosus (SLE) was made. A renal biopsy was ordered, and an emergency therapy was implemented. The patient received intravenous (IV) fluid replacement, and an IV bolus of a high dose of a drug was given daily.

Three days later, L.P. was feeling much better. There was a remarkable edema regression, and the body temperature went back to normal. The patient was discharged from the hospital on day 10 with an appropriate postdischarge therapy that included glucocorticoids and cyclophosphamide.

One month later, L.P. was admitted to the hospital for a control visit. Lab investigation showed that her lupus nephritis was not improved, and the physician decided to substitute cyclophosphamide with another drug.

Questions

1. L.P. was diagnosed with SLE. Which of the following pairs of human features are known to increase the risk of this disease?

A. Female sex–African American race

B. Female sex–old age

C. Female sex–Caucasian race

D. Male sex–African American race

E. Male sex–old age

F. Male sex–Caucasian race

2. L.P. was diagnosed with SLE. Which of the following inflammatory cells is considered the most likely initiator of this disease?

A. Memory B cells

B. T-helper (Th) cells

C. Macrophages

D. Natural killer cells

E. Neutrophils

F. Plasma cells

3. L.P. was diagnosed with SLE. The result of which of the following laboratory tests is most likely characteristic of the patient's disease?

A. Erythrocyte sedimentation rate

B. C-reactive protein

C. Microhematuria

D. Massive proteinuria

E. RF antibody

F. Anti-dsDNA antibodies

4. In SLE, small autoimmune complexes can insert themselves into small blood vessels, joints, and glomeruli, causing symptoms. Which of the following types of hypersensitivities do these pathological findings indicate?

A. Type I

B. Type II

C. Type III

D. Type IV

5. L.P. complained of pain in her hands and wrists. An X-ray of the patient's hands would most likely show which of the following findings?

A. Normal joints

B. Erosion in the proximal joints

C. Carpal fusion

D. Bone fragmentation

E. Subchondral cysts

6. L.P. underwent a renal biopsy. The biopsy results most likely indicated which of the following kidney disorders?

A. Nephrotic syndrome

B. Kidney amyloidosis

C. Acute tubular necrosis

D. Diffuse proliferative nephritis

E. Urate nephropathy

7. The American College of Rheumatology listed 11 symptoms, signs, and lab results that are more often associated with SLE. A patient is said to have SLE if 4 or more of the 11 diagnostic criteria are present. Which one of the following sets of four symptoms, signs, and lab results indicates that L.P. was most likely suffering from SLE?

A. Serositis–atrial fibrillation–anemia–alkaline phosphatase

B. Anti-dsDNA antibody–liver disease–photosensitivity–atrial fibrillation

C. Serositis–liver disease–anemia–atrial fibrillation

D. Liver disease–photosensitivity–anti-dsDNA antibody–alkaline phosphatase

E. Serositis–Anti-dsDNA antibody–photosensitivity–anemia

8. L.P. received an emergency therapy that included a high dose of a drug administered IV. The therapeutic effect of the drug was most likely mediated by the drug binding to which of the following molecular targets?

A. Final sequence on peptidyl RNA
B. Specific nucleotide sequences on DNA
C. Final sequence on ribosomal RNA
D. Phospholipase A2
E. Interleukin-6
F. Cyclooxygenase II

9. L.P.'s postdischarge therapy included cyclophosphamide. The immunosuppressive effect of this drug is most likely mediated by which of the following actions?

A. Stimulation of synthesis of tumor necrosis factor
B. Stimulation of B cell differentiation into memory B cells
C. Inhibition of the apoptosis pathway of B cells
D. Stimulation of gene expression for interleukin-2 production
E. Cytotoxic activity against T-helper cells

10. Cyclophosphamide is an alkylating drug. Which of the following is most likely the molecular action common to this drug class?

A. Formation of covalent bonds with DNA bases
B. Enhancement of tubulin polymerization
C. Inhibition of thymidylate synthetase
D. Inhibition of DNA resealing
E. Inhibition of microtubule assembly

11. Because of cyclophosphamide therapy L.P. was most likely at increased risk of which of the following drug-induced adverse effects?

A. Liver cirrhosis
B. Hemorrhagic cystitis
C. Hemolytic anemia
D. Hypertension
E. Pulmonary fibrosis

12. Which of the following sets of drugs was most likely also included in L.P.'s post-discharge therapy?

A. Hydralazine–cobalamin–losartan
B. Hydroxychloroquine–cobalamin–hydralazine
C. Losartan–atenolol–hydroxychloroquine
D. Cobalamin–hydroxychloroquine–atenolol
E. Losartan–hydralazine–atenolol

13. Given the lack of improvement of L.P.'s lupus nephritis cyclophosphamide was substituted with another drug. Which of the following drugs was most likely given?

A. Cisplatin
B. Trastuzumab
C. Imatinib
D. Mycophenolate mofetil
E. Doxorubicin
F. Bevacizumab

14. The specific inhibition of which of the following enzymes most likely mediated the immunosuppressive effect of the drug used as a substitute for cyclophosphamide in the treatment of L.P.'s lupus nephritis?

A. Dihydrofolate reductase
B. Inosine monophosphate dehydrogenase
C. Topoisomerase II
D. Thymidylate synthetase
E. Adenosine deaminase

Answers and Explanations

▶ *Learning objective:* Identify the two factors that are known to increase the risk of SLE.

1.   Answer: A

Of all cases of SLE, 70 to 90% occur in women. Moreover, African American women are three to four times more likely than Caucasian women to get the disease.

SLE can occur at any age but occurs most frequently in women of child-bearing age, as in the present case.

B, C, D, E, F See correct answer explanation.

▶ *Learning objective:* Identify the cell type that is most likely the initiator of SLE.

2. Answer: B

SLE is an autoimmune disorder characterized by the generation of autoantibodies that leads to multisystem inflammation. T-helper cells have long been thought to play a central role in SLE pathogenesis. T-helper cells from patients with lupus show defects in both signaling and effector function, and SLE is currently believed to be a T cell–driven disease. However, the method by which each of these defects contributes to the exact clinical syndrome seen in an individual patient is still unknown.

A, C, D, E, F All these cells are involved in inflammatory processes, but they are not thought to be the initiators of SLE.

▶ *Learning objective:* Identify the laboratory test that is most characteristic of SLE.

3. Answer: F

SLE autoantibodies are primarily against fragments of nucleic acids and chromosomal proteins. Therefore, the double-stranded DNA antibody test is nearly always positive for patients with SLE. This test is more specific for SLE than for other autoimmune diseases, although this test alone is not sufficient to make the diagnosis of SLE. Autoantibodies may be present for many years before the onset of the first symptoms of SLE.

A, B These tests are positive in several chronic inflammatory disorders.

C, D These tests are positive in several kidney diseases.

E This test is positive in several diseases, including rheumatoid arthritis, SLE, tuberculosis, sarcoidosis, cancer, and viral infections.

▶ *Learning objective:* Identify the type of hypersensitivity that can occur in SLE.

4. Answer: C

In SLE endogenous antigens are continually produced, which can elicit antibody formation, forming soluble, small autoimmune complexes. Large complexes can be cleared by macrophages, but macrophages have difficulty in the disposal of small immune complexes. These immune complexes insert themselves into small blood vessels, joints, and glomeruli, causing vasculitis, arthritis, and glomerulonephritis, respectively. All these disorders can occur in SLE. Small immune complexes bound to sites of deposition (e.g., blood vessel walls) are far more capable of interacting with complement and are viewed as being highly pathogenic.

A Type I hypersensitivity occurs when immunoglobulin E (IgE) binding to immunoglobulin receptors present on mast cells and basophils causes the release of inflammatory mediators.

B Type II hypersensitivity occurs when IgG or IgM binding to receptors present on cell surfaces causes the destruction of those cells, often through complement activation.

D Type IV hypersensitivity does not involve antibody. It occurs when Th1 cells are activated by an antigen-presenting cell. When the antigen is presented again in the future, the memory Th1 cells will activate macrophages and cause an inflammatory response.

▶ *Learning objective:* Describe the X-ray finding of the hands of a patient suffering from SLE.

5. Answer: A

The arthritis of SLE is classically described as nondeforming. Unlike in rheumatoid arthritis, the joints can be realigned by manually moving them into the correct position, but the tendons lack the integrity to hold the bones in alignment.

B Erosion in the proximal joints is a classic sign of rheumatoid arthritis.

C Carpal fusion is the abnormal fusion of two or more carpal bones. It occurs primarily in osteoarthritis.

D Bone fragmentation is a radiographic feature of degenerative arthritis.

E Subchondral cysts can be seen in neuropathic arthropathy.

▶ *Learning objective:* Describe the most common type of lupus nephritis.

6. Answer: D

Nephritis can develop at any time and may be the only manifestation of SLE. It may be benign and asymptomatic or progressive and fatal. The disease is the leading cause of death in the first decade following the diagnosis. The patient's signs (edema, pleuropericardial effusion) and lab results indicate that she was suffering from lupus nephritis. Diffuse proliferative nephritis is both the most severe and the most common subtype (up to 70%). More than 50% of glomeruli are involved. Lesions can be segmental or global, with endocapillary or extracapillary proliferative lesions. Under electron microscopy, subendothelial deposits are noted, and some mesangial changes may be present. Clinically, hematuria and proteinuria are present, frequently with hypertension, as in the present case.

A Nephrotic syndrome is a glomerular disease that causes > 3 g of protein daily It can occur as part of lupus nephritis but is unlikely in the present case, since proteinuria was not so great.

B, C, E These disorders are not inflammatory. Lupus nephritis is an inflammatory renal disease.

▶ *Learning objective:* Identify the set of four symptoms and signs that can allow the diagnosis of SLE.

7. Answer: E

The 11 symptoms, signs, and lab results listed by the American College of Rheumatology are the following: malar rash, discoid rash, photosensitivity, oral ulcers, arthritis, serositis, renal disorder, neurologic disorder, hematologic disorder, antinuclear antibodies, anti-dsDNA antibody.

L.P. was suffering from serositis (see the pleuropericardial effusion), photosensitivity (see the unusual sunburn), and anemia (see the lab test results). Moreover, the patient had a high anti-dsDNA antibody titer. These are necessary and sufficient symptoms and signs (> 97% sensitivity and specificity) for the diagnosis of SLE. Other symptoms of the patient (see malar rash, oral ulcers, arthritis) can confirm the diagnosis of SLE.

A, B, C, D Atrial fibrillation, liver disease, and alkaline phosphatase are not signs that can suggest the diagnosis of SLE.

▶ *Learning objective:* Explain the molecular mechanism of action of the drug given IV to a patient with a severe flare of SLE.

8. Answer: B

Patients with severe or life-threatening manifestations of SLE secondary to major organ involvement generally require an initial period of intensive immunosuppressive therapy (induction therapy) to control the disease and halt tissue injury. Patients are usually treated for a short period of time with high doses of systemic glucocorticoids used alone or in combination with other immunosuppressive agents. Glucocorticoids cross the membrane of the target cells by passive diffusion. In the cytoplasm the drug binds to a glucocorticoid receptor bound to a heat-shock protein in the cytoplasm. After binding, the heat-shock protein is released, and the hormone–receptor complex is transported into the nucleus, where it binds to specific nucleotide sequences along the DNA, called glucocorticoid response elements. The binding to this target triggers a decreased or increased transcription of genes coding for specific proteins. Changes in the rate of synthesis of specific proteins carry out most biological actions of the hormones.

A, C Glucocorticoids bind to a specific sequence of DNA, not of RNA.

D, E, F Glucocorticoids can inhibit the activity of these enzymes, but this is due to an inhibition of their synthesis, not to a binding-induced blockade of the enzyme itself.

▸ *Learning objective:* Identify the action that most likely mediates the immunosuppressive effect of cyclophosphamide

9. Answer: E

For initial therapy in patients with diffuse or focal proliferative lupus nephritis, most experts recommend immunosuppressive therapy with either cyclophosphamide or mycophenolate mofetil, in addition to glucocorticoids. A number of clinical trials have demonstrated a benefit of cyclophosphamide plus glucocorticoids compared with glucocorticoids alone on renal survival among patients with proliferative lupus nephritis, and this explains the choice of the drug in the present case.

Cyclophosphamide is an alkylating drug. These agents exert a cytotoxic activity primarily against all rapidly dividing cells. Their immunosuppressive action seems to be primarily mediated by a cytotoxic activity against T-helper cells. In SLE, T-helper cells show abnormality in certain signaling pathways that may mediate the autoimmune disease. By damaging the DNA of these cells, alkylating drugs send them into apoptosis, thereby exerting an immunosuppressive action.

A, B, C, D All these actions would activate, not inhibit, immunity processes.

▸ *Learning objective:* Explain the molecular mechanism of action of alkylating drugs.

10. Answer: A

Alkylating drugs act by intermolecular cyclization, to form either an ethyleneimonium or a carbonium ion, which are strongly electrophilic (i.e., electron attracting). These intermediates can alkylate; that is, they can transfer alkyl groups to various cellular constituents by formation of covalent bonds with nucleophilic (i.e., electron donor) groups of these constituents. Alkylation can affect a single strand of the DNA molecule or both strands of the DNA molecule (cross-linking DNA). In both cases DNA is damaged, replication is blocked, and cell death occurs. Alkylating drugs are used mainly in cancer chemotherapy. Some of them are also used for the therapy of autoimmune diseases, and cyclophosphamide

is probably the most powerful immunosuppressive compound of this drug class.

B Enhancement of tubulin polymerization would be the mechanism of action of taxanes.

C Inhibition of thymidylate synthetase would be the mechanism of action of fluorouracil.

D Inhibition of DNA resealing would be the mechanism of action of camptothecins like topotecan.

E Inhibition of microtubule assembly would be the mechanism of action of vinca alkaloids.

▸ *Learning objective:* Identify a specific adverse effect of cyclophosphamide.

11. Answer: B

Cyclophosphamide can cause hemorrhagic cystitis with bladder mucosa edema, ulcerations, and minor to severe hemorrhage. This toxicity is thought to be due to metabolites of cyclophosphamide, including chloroethylaziridine and acrolein, which are formed by hepatic microsomes and excreted in the urine. They can concentrate in the bladder and cause mucosa damage. The incidence of hemorrhagic cystitis from cyclophosphamide administered at conventional doses is unknown, but in patients receiving high-dose regimens, it is about 10%. Prevention consists of providing adequate IV hydration and administration of 2-mercaptoethane sulfonate (mesna). This agent contains a free thiol group that can neutralize acrolein in the bladder. Mesna can prevent bladder toxicity, and its routine concurrent administration has been recommended in the treatment of all patients receiving cyclophosphamide chemotherapy.

A Cyclophosphamide can cause rarely cholestatic hepatitis, but liver cirrhosis is not reported.

C Cyclophosphamide can cause anemia due to impaired production of erythrocytes, not to hemolysis.

D Hypertension has been reported with cyclophosphamide use, but it is exceedingly rare.

E Pulmonary fibrosis has been reported with cyclophosphamide use, but it is exceedingly rare.

▶ *Learning objective:* Identify a set of drugs that can be used in SLE.

12. Answer: C

Because SLE can affect almost every organ of the body, associated disorders are common.

Antihypertensive therapy should be recommended at blood pressure levels of 140/90 mm Hg in newly diagnosed lupus patients without overt target organ involvement. In the case of lupus nephritis patients, therapy should be implemented at lower levels, such as 130/80 mm Hg. Angiotensin-converting enzyme inhibitors and angiotensin-receptor blockers (e.g., losartan) seem to be a safe and efficacious first-choice antihypertensive treatment in lupus patients, as in the present case.

SLE can be associated with various cardiac arrhythmias and β-blockers like atenolol are first-line agents in atrial fibrillation.

All patients with SLE should receive the antimalarial drug hydroxychloroquine, unless otherwise contraindicated, which is effective for the amelioration of joint symptoms as well as for the prevention of disease flares.

A, B, D Cobalamin is useless in this patient, because her anemia is not megaloblastic (see normal MCV).

A, B, E Hydralazine is an antihypertensive drug that would be contraindicated in this patient, because it can cause a drug-induced lupus.

▶ *Learning objective:* Identify the drug that can be used in cases of lupus nephritis resistant to cyclophosphamide.

13. Answer: D

The drug used to substitute for cyclophosphamide was most likely mycophenolate mofetil. When lupus nephritis is resistant to the initial immunosuppressive therapy with cyclophosphamide, a common strategy is to substitute cyclophosphamide with mycophenolate mofetil, because some studies suggest that the drug may be effective in cyclophosphamide-resistant patients.

A Cisplatin is an anticancer drug used mainly in solid tumor.

B Trastuzumab is an anticancer monoclonal antibody used mainly in breast cancer.

C Imatinib is a tyrosine kinase inhibitor used mainly in chronic myelogenous leukemia and acute lymphocytic leukemia.

E Doxorubicin is an anthracycline anticancer antibiotic used in leukemias, lymphomas, and solid tumors.

F Bevacizumab is an anticancer monoclonal antibody used in metastatic colorectal cancer.

▶ *Learning objective:* Identify the enzyme that is specifically inhibited by mycophenolate mofetil.

14. Answer: B

The immunosuppressive drug used as a substitute for cyclophosphamide in lupus nephritis was most likely mycophenolate mofetil, a prodrug that is biotransformed into mycophenolic acid. This active metabolite inhibits inosine monophosphate dehydrogenase, an enzyme involved in the *de novo pathway* of purine biosynthesis. However, unlike other cytotoxic agents, it does not inhibit enzymes involved in the *salvage pathway* of purine biosynthesis. Thus it selectively inhibits the proliferation of lymphocytes (including B and T lymphocytes), because these cells lack the enzymes of the alternative salvage pathway. Because of this, mycophenolate mofetil is cytotoxic only for lymphocytes, whereas other immunosuppressive agents, like cyclophosphamide, are cytotoxic for all rapidly growing cells.

A This enzyme catalyzes the formation of tetrahydrofolic acid.

C This enzyme breaks and reseals double-stranded DNA.

D This enzyme catalyzes the conversion of deoxyuridine monophosphate to deoxythymidine monophosphate.

E This enzyme catalyzes the conversion of adenosine to inosine.

Case 47

Torsade de Pointes

C.D., a 62-year-old woman, passed out while preparing lunch at home. She regained consciousness in a few minutes and was taken by ambulance to the emergency department. The patient's medical history was significant for an episode of cardiac arrhythmia that occurred 6 months ago and was treated with amiodarone. However, the drug was discontinued because of adverse effects and substituted with sotalol since then. Other drugs the patient had been taking included ciprofloxacin for chronic urinary tract infection, ranitidine for gastrointestinal reflux disease, pravastatin for hypercholesterolemia, and loratadine for allergic rhinitis.

C.D.'s vital signs on admission were blood pressure 135/85 mm Hg, pulse 58 bpm with some ectopic beats, respirations 15/min.

While being evaluated in the emergency department C.D. had another syncopal episode. The electrocardiogram (ECG) taken during syncope showed a heart rate of 135 bpm with disparate QRS morphologies and preceded by marked prolongation of QT intervals (600 µs: normal < 400).

A diagnosis of torsade de pointes (TDP) was made, and electrical cardioversion was performed without success. A drug was administered intravenously (IV), and the patient regained consciousness.

On recovery, C.D. complained of nausea, dizziness, and shortness of breath. Physical examination showed a patient awake on a bed and in moderate distress. Blood pressure was 140/86 mm Hg, and a pulse of 85 bpm with frequent ectopic beats. The rest of the physical examination was unremarkable.

The ECG still showed prolongation of QT intervals and several ectopic beats.

Pertinent blood test results on admission were as follows:

- ▶ Fasting glucose 140 mg/dL (normal 65–110)
- ▶ Creatinine: 1.3 mg/dL (normal 0.6–1.2)
- ▶ Blood urea nitrogen (BUN): 27 mg/dL (normal 5–25)
- ▶ Sodium (Na$^+$): 134 mEq/L (normal 135–146)
- ▶ Potassium (K$^+$): 3.1 mEq/L (normal 3.5–5.5)
- ▶ Magnesium (Mg^{2+}): 1.4 mEq/L (normal 1.8–2.6)
- ▶ Total cholesterol: 290 mg/dL (normal < 200)
- ▶ Triglycerides: 190 mg/dL (normal < 150)

During the following 8 hours, the patient's condition remained stable. Her hypokalemia and hypomagnesemia were corrected, and her admission therapy was revised. The patient recovered fully and was dismissed from the hospital. She was given instruction to avoid drugs that are prone to cause an increase in QT intervals.

Questions

1. C.D. was diagnosed with TDP. This arrhythmia belongs to which of the following arrhythmia types?

A. Sinus tachycardia

B. Monomorphic ventricular tachycardia

C. Atrioventricular reentrant tachycardia

D. Multifocal atrial tachycardia

E. Polymorphic ventricular tachycardia

F. Ectopic atrial tachycardia

2. C.D.'s ECG showed marked prolongation of the QT intervals. This interval represents which of the following phases of the heart action potential?

A. Atrial depolarization only

B. Atrial repolarization only

C. Both atrial depolarization and repolarization

D. Ventricle depolarization only

E. Ventricle repolarization only

F. Both ventricle depolarization and repolarization

3. Which of the following changes of the phases of heart action potential was most likely the primary cause of prolongation of the patient's QT intervals?

A. Increased slope of phase 0

B. Decreased slope of phase 3

C. Decreased duration of phase 2

D. Decreased duration of phase 4

E. Increased duration of phase 4

4. Which of the following changes in ionic currents on heart cell membranes most likely mediated the delayed repolarization phase in C.D.'s heart action potential?

A. Decreased inward Na^+ current

B. Decreased inward Ca^{2+} current

C. Increased inward Cl^- current

D. Decreased outward K^+ current

E. Increased outward Na^+ current

F. Increased outward Ca^{2+} current

5. The ventricular action potential in TDP is characterized by a delayed repolarization phase. Which of the following changes in the heart action potential can most likely occur as a consequence of this decrease?

A. Decreased AV conduction

B. Increased SA depolarization

C. Early afterdepolarization

D. Longer ventricular resting potential

E. Decreased action potential duration

6. C.D. had several factors that most likely increased her risk for TDP. Which of the following pairs of C.D.'s lab results most likely represent a substantial risk factor for her disorder?

A. Decreased K^+–increased glucose

B. Increased glucose–increased total cholesterol

C. Decreased K^+–decreased Mg^{2+}

D. Increased total cholesterol–decreased Mg^{2+}

E. Increased glucose–decreased Mg^2

F. Decreased K^+–increased total cholesterol

7. Which of the following sets of actions on heart ionic currents depicted in the attached table most likely mediated the therapeutic effect of amiodarone?

Set	Na^+ current	K^+ current	Ca^{2+} current
A.	↓	↓	↔
B.	↓	↔	↔
C.	↓	↓	↓
D.	↔	↑	↔
E.	↔	↔	↓

↑ = increased; ↓ = decreased; ↔ = negligible effect

8. Amiodarone has to be discontinued because of adverse effects. Which of the following adverse effects did the patient most likely suffer from?

A. Atrial fibrillation

B. Hypertension

C. Disseminate intravascular coagulation

D. Hypothyroidism

E. Hypertrophic cardiomyopathy

F. Ulcerative colitis

9. C.D. was treated chronically with sotalol to prevent recurrence of her cardiac arrhythmia. The blockade of which of the following pairs of cell structures most likely mediated the therapeutic effect of the drug?

A. Na$^+$ channels–α-adrenoceptors

B. Na$^+$ channels–β-adrenoceptors

C. K$^+$ channels–β-adrenoceptors

D. K$^+$ channels–α-adrenoceptors

E. Na$^+$ channels–K$^+$ channels

F. α-adrenoceptors–β-adrenoceptors

10. Which of the following pairs of drugs taken by C.D. most likely increased her risk of TDP?

A. Ranitidine–sotalol

B. Ranitidine–pravastatin

C. Pravastatin–ciprofloxacin

D. Ranitidine–ciprofloxacin

E. Sotalol–ciprofloxacin

F. Pravastatin–sotalol

11. C.D.'s TDP was treated aggressively most likely to prevent which of the following complications?

A. Cardiogenic shock

B. Wolff–Parkinson–White's syndrome

C. Complete AV block

D. Chronic heart failure

E. Ventricular fibrillation

12. Which of the following was most likely the antiarrhythmic drug that was able to stop C.D.'s TDP?

A. Ibutilide

B. Quinidine

C. Procainamide

D. Magnesium sulfate

E. Flecainide

13. Another strategy used to stop TDP is aimed at shortening the QT interval by increasing the underlying heart rate. Which of the following drugs is sometimes used for this purpose?

A. Albuterol

B. Atropine

C. Isoproterenol

D. Epinephrine

E. Theophylline

14. C.D. was instructed to avoid drugs that can cause TDP in patients at risk. Which of the following is the drug with the highest risk of this adverse effect?

A. Captopril

B. Quinidine

C. Adenosine

D. Simvastatin

E. Minoxidil

F. Spironolactone

Answers and Explanations

▶ *Learning objective:* Identify which type of arrhythmia TDP belongs to.

1. Answer: E

Ventricular tachycardia is defined as a series of three or more consecutive ventricular premature beats at a rate of ≥ 120 bpm. It can be subdivided as follows, according to QRS morphology:

▶ *Monomorphic:* when every QRS is the same and the rate is regular

▶ *Polymorphic:* when QRS complexes continually change in shape and the rate is irregular

The cause of polymorphic ventricular tachycardia is usually a continuously changing reentry circuit. Ventricular tachycardia can also be subdivided as follows:

▶ *Nonsustained:* when it lasts ≤ 30 seconds

▶ *Sustained:* when it lasts > 30 seconds

421

▶ TDP can be defined as a specific form of polymorphic ventricular tachycardia that is preceded by marked prolongation of QT intervals, as in the present case.

A Sinus tachycardia is due to a sinoatrial (SA) node discharge of 100 to 180 bpm.

B See correct answer explanation.

C Atrioventricular (AV) reentrant tachycardia is due to two potential pathways for conduction through the AV node. When these two pathways conduct at different velocities, reentry can occur.

D Multifocal atrial tachycardia is due to several pacemakers within the atria.

F Ectopic atrial tachycardia is due to an abnormal pacemaker within the atria.

▶ *Learning objective:* Describe the phase of the action potential represented by the QT interval of the ECG.

2. Answer: F

The various phases of the heart action potential of the atria and ventricles are represented by the ECG.

The P wave represents atrial depolarization, the QRS complex represents ventricular depolarization, and the T wave represents ventricular repolarization. Therefore the QT interval represents the entire period of depolarization and repolarization of the ventricles and reflects the duration of the ventricular action potential.

A, B, C Both atrial depolarization and repolarization are represented by the P wave.

D Ventricle depolarization is represented by the QRS complex.

E Ventricle repolarization is represented by the T wave.

▶ *Learning objective:* Describe the phase of the heart action potential that primarily mediates the prolongation of the ECG QT intervals.

3. Answer: B

The increased QT interval on ECG is due to an increased duration of ventricular action potential. The effect, in theory, can be attributed to either an increase of inward Ca^{2+} current or a decrease of outward K^+ current. Different mutations of Ca^{2+} and K^+ ion channel genes have been detected in patients with congenital QT syndrome, but K^+ channels are the most affected. Therefore it can be concluded that the most common cause of long QT intervals is a decreased repolarizing current, which in turn causes a decreased slope of phase 3, the repolarization phase of the heart action potential. This delay in repolarization can cause early afterdepolarization, the triggering event of TDP.

A The increased slope of phase 0 is due to a decreased inward Na^+ depolarizing current.

C The decreased duration of phase 2 is due to a decreased inward Ca^{2+} depolarizing current.

D, E The duration of phase 4 is related to the equilibrium potential of nonpacemaker cells of the heart. Its duration can affect the interval between two consecutive ECG complexes, not the duration of the QT interval.

▶ *Learning objective:* Describe the change in the ionic current that most likely mediates the delayed repolarization phase in the heart action potential.

4. Answer: D

The repolarization phase of heart action potential is due to a transient outward K^+ current that hyperpolarizes the membrane back toward the K^+ equilibrium potential. By decreasing this current, the repolarization phase is delayed.

A Inward Na^+ current causes depolarization. A decreased inward current would speed up, not delay, the repolarization phase.

B Inward Ca^{2+} current maintains the depolarization of phase 2. A decreased inward current would speed up, not delay, the repolarization phase.

C Inward Cl^- current caused repolarization. An increased inward current would speed up, not delay, the repolarization phase,

E There is no outward Na^+ current. Because Na^+ is more concentrated outside the cell, when Na^+ channels open, Na^+ current is inward.

F There is no outward Ca^{2+} current. Because Ca^{2+} is more concentrated outside the cell, when Ca^{2+} channels open, Ca^{2+} current is inward.

▶ *Learning objective:* Identify the change in the heart action potential that can occur because of the delayed repolarization phase.

5. Answer: C

Afterdepolarizations are abnormal depolarizations of cardiac myocytes that interrupt phase 2, phase 3, or phase 4 of the cardiac action potential in the electrical conduction system of the heart. Early afterdepolarizations occur with abnormal depolarization during phase 2 or phase 3 and are caused by an increase in the frequency of abortive action potentials before normal repolarization is completed. These afterdepolarizations are the triggering event of TDP.

A, B TDP is a type of ventricular tachycardia; therefore atrial involvement is unlikely.

D A delayed repolarization would cause a shorter, not a longer, resting potential.

E A delayed repolarization would cause an increase, not a decrease, in action potential duration.

▶ *Learning objective:* Identify the pairs of lab results that can represent a substantial risk for TDP.

6. Answer: C

The hallmark of TDP is a long QT interval. Prolongation of the QT interval indicates prolongation of action potential duration, which is related to a decreased outward K^+ current during phase 3 of the action potential. A long QT interval is present prior to the onset of tachycardia and is due to hereditary or acquired K^+ channel defects. Hypokalemia and hypomagnesemia have been reported to precipitate TDP. Hypokalemia prolongs QT, likely because it reduces, for unknown reason, K+ permeability, thus increasing the action potential duration. Hypomagnesemia can result in disturbances of nearly every organ system and can cause potentially fatal complications. Hypomagnesemia is a well-recognized cause of cardiac arrhythmias, as intracel-

lular magnesium deficiency impairs Na^+/K^+–adenosine triphosphatase. The resulting decrease in intracellular potassium disturbs the resting membrane potential and repolarization phase of myocardial cells.

A, B, E Hyperglycemia is not a risk factor for TDP.

B, D, F Hypercholesterolemia is not a risk factor for TDP.

▶ *Learning objective:* Describe the change of heart ionic currents due to amiodarone action.

7. Answer: C

Amiodarone is a class III antiarrhythmic drug with the broadest spectrum of antiarrhythmic action. This feature is most likely related to the fact that the drug is able to block not only K^+ channels but also Na^+ channels (when inactivated) and (weakly) Ca^{2+} channels. The consequence of this blockade is of course a decrease of the ionic currents related to these cations.

A This would be the action of class Ia and Ic antiarrhythmics.

B This would be the action of class Ib antiarrhythmics.

D This would be the action of class III antiarrhythmics.

E This would be the action of class IV antiarrhythmics.

▶ *Learning objective:* Describe the common adverse effects of amiodarone.

8. Answer: D

Amiodarone can cause either hyperthyroidism or hypothyroidism, although hypothyroidism is more common. Actually subclinical hypothyroidism can be detected in up to 25% of patients under amiodarone, and overt hypothyroidism occurs in about 10%. These complications are a consequence of the high iodine content of the drug. When amiodarone is metabolized in the liver, iodine molecules are released and can exert pharmacological effects. Therefore it is common to check the T4 and T3 levels periodically in patients under amiodarone therapy.

A, B, C, E, F The risks of these adverse effects in patients under amiodarone therapy are negligible or absent.

► *Learning objective:* Identify the pair of cell structures most likely blocked by amiodarone.

9. Answer: C

Sotalol is a class III antiarrhythmic drug. The primary mechanism of action of this drug class is the blockade of potassium channels, which in turn retards the repolarization phase. In addition sotalol is a nonselective β-adrenoceptor blocker. Most likely both actions contribute to the final antiarrhythmic effect of the drug.

A, B, D, E, F Na^+ channels and α-adrenoceptors are not blocked by sotalol.

► *Learning objective:* Identify two drugs that most likely contributed to the appearance of the patient's TDP.

10. Answer: E

TDP is an arrhythmia triggered by diseases or drugs that prolong the QT interval. Diseases include genetic defects, hypothyroidism, subarachnoid hemorrhage, myocarditis, hypokalemia, and hypomagnesemia. Drugs include class Ia, Ic, and III antiarrhythmic drugs, tricyclic antidepressants, neuroleptics, serotonin antagonists, macrolide antibiotics, fluoroquinolones, azole antifungals, antimalarials, some antihistamines, and some opioids. All of these drugs are able to increase action potential duration by blocking or modifying potassium channels. High doses of these drugs can trigger TDP in patients at risk. Sotalol is the only β-blocker that can block potassium channels (a property not related to β-receptor blockade), and it can cause TDP. Ciprofloxacin is a fluoroquinolone antibiotic. The concomitant use of two drugs that can both increase the risk of TDP further amplifies this risk.

A, B, C, D, F Ranitidine and pravastatin do not increase the risk of TDP.

► *Learning objective:* Identify the most serious complication of TDP.

11. Answer: E

TDP is a life-threatening disorder. It can cease spontaneously but can also degenerate into ventricular fibrillation, leading to sudden death. Therefore an aggressive therapy is mandatory.

A, B, C, D TDP does not trigger these disorders.

► *Learning objective:* Identify the most effective drug that is able to stop TDP.

12. Answer: D

Because of its efficacy, rapidity of action, and relative safety, magnesium sulfate has become the first-line agent in the acute treatment of TDP. Magnesium appears to be effective even when there is no evidence of magnesium depletion. The mechanism of action of the drug is still uncertain, but magnesium likely has a suppressive effect on the development of early afterdepolarizations responsible for TDP. Second-line agents for the acute treatment of TDP are class 1b drugs (lidocaine, mexiletine).

A, B, C, E All these drugs are contraindicated, because they can trigger TDP in patients at risk.

► *Learning objective:* Identify the drug sometimes used to shorten the QT interval in cases of TDP.

13. Answer: C

Isoproterenol is the drug sometimes used to stop TDP, even if it is less effective than magnesium sulfate. The drug is a nonselective β-adrenoceptor agonist that causes a dose-dependent increase in heart rate.

A, B, D, E All these drugs can increase heart rate, but they are useless, or even contraindicated, in TDP.

► *Learning objective:* Identify the drug with the highest risk of causing TDP.

14. Answer: B

A vast array of drugs can cause TDP, especially when given at high doses. An exception is quinidine, which can cause the disorder even at therapeutic plasma concentrations. The reason for this is still uncertain, but it is likely related to the increased action potential duration caused by this drug.

A, C, D, E, F The risk of TDP with these drugs is very low or absent.

Case 48

Type 1 Diabetes Mellitus

D.A., a 12-year-old boy, was brought to the emergency department by his parents because he had vomited three or four times in the last 2 hours, and now he was not responding clearly when his parents asked how he was feeling. His parents reported that they noticed a fruity smell from their child and also his breathing was unusual. They reported that D.A. was urinating more frequently in the past week, even getting up multiple times in the night for urination, and had noticed him being unusually lethargic.

History did not reveal any illicit drug use. There was no history of accident, head trauma, surgery, or hospitalization due to any other medical condition. He had a history of contracting flu every year. About 3 weeks ago, he had a fever, most likely due to a viral infection that lasted for 3 days.

Physical examination revealed a lethargic patient with poor skin turgor, dry mucous membranes, and sunken eyeballs.

Vital signs were blood pressure 102/60 mm Hg, heart rate 120 bpm, and respirations 22/min, irregular, and with a fruity odor.

A quick blood strip test identified high blood sugar levels (+++). Blood samples were collected for other lab tests. An intravenous (IV) line was established, and appropriate IV fluids were started promptly. An IV infusion of regular insulin was started simultaneously, after administering the initial bolus dose.

Pertinent lab results were as follows:

Blood hematology

▶ Hemoglobin A_{1c} (HbA$_{1c}$): 10% (normal < 6)
▶ Blood glucose: 550 mg/dL (normal < 140)
▶ Ketones: 5.5 mmol/L (normal < 0.6)
▶ Sodium (Na$^+$): 150 mEq/L (normal 136–145)
▶ Potassium (K$^+$): 6.0 mEq/L (normal 3.5-5.0)
▶ pH: 6.8 (normal 7.35–7.45)
▶ HCO$_3$ 10 mEq/L (normal 21–28)
▶ PCO$_2$: 20 mm Hg (normal 35–45)
▶ PO$_2$: 120 mm Hg (normal 80–100)
▶ Serum creatinine: 1.0 mg/dL (normal 0.6–1.2)

Urinalysis

▶ Glucose +++
▶ Ketones +++

After 2 days of therapy, D.A. was feeling better, normal hydration resumed, and he was responding well to verbal commands. He was still on no oral nutrients; his blood sugar was near 130 mg/dL. D.A. and his parents were scheduled for an insulin counseling session with the diabetes counselor before he could be discharged on appropriate medication. He was educated on different insulin preparations and injections and an insulin pump. He preferred the pump over the injections.

A month later, D.A. was out playing with his school friends. While playing, he passed out and was brought to the emergency department in a state of altered sensorium. He was evaluated, and an IV infusion of dextrose was started immediately. After 30 minutes, D.A.'s condition was stable.

Questions

1. Which of the following conditions did D.A. most likely suffer from when he was brought to the emergency department the first time by his parents?

A. Diabetes insipidus

B. Heat stroke

C. Bulimia

D. Diabetic ketoacidosis (DKA)

E. Syndrome of inappropriate antidiuretic hormone (ADH) secretion

2. D.A. was administered appropriate IV fluids after he was diagnosed with DKA. Which of the following was the most likely rationale for administering IV fluids to him?

A. To correct depletion of body fluids

B. To quench thirst

C. To correct insulin deficiency

D. To increase glucose entry into the brain

E. To correct the vasopressin excess in the blood

3. D.A. had a fruity breath odor when he was brought into the emergency department. Which of the following was most likely the primary cause of his fruity odor?

A. Decreased kidney function

B. Excessive protein intake

C. Excessive catabolism of muscle proteins

D. Decreased glucagon secretion

E. Increased metabolism of fatty acids

4. The levels of which of the following molecules would most likely be undetectable in D.A.'s blood?

A. Acetoacetate

B. Glucagon

C. C-protein

D. Cortisol

E. Growth hormone

5. D.A. was infused with regular insulin to treat his DKA. Which of the following actions most likely mediated the therapeutic effect of insulin in the patient's disease?

A. Inhibition of the activity of dipeptidyl peptidase-4

B. Incorporation of glucose transporters in the cell membrane

C. Activation of enzymes of the gluconeogenesis pathway

D. Inhibition of the tyrosine kinase activity of the insulin receptor

6. D.A. was administered regular insulin along with IV fluids for the treatment of DKA. Which of the following effects would be achieved by administering regular insulin to this patient?

A. Suppression of fat catabolism

B. Stimulation of glucose entry into the brain

C. Increase of renal glucose excretion

D. Inhibition of glucose filtration from the glomerulus

E. Increased catabolism of skeletal muscle proteins

7. D.A.'s lab results revealed hyperkalemia. Which of the following was the primary cause of this finding?

A. Increased activity of the Na^+/K^+ pump

B. Decreased availability of insulin

C. Decreased excretion of potassium in the urine

D. Increased reabsorption of potassium by the renal tubules

E. Increased absorption of potassium from the intestinal tract

8. On discharge, an insulin pump was set up for administering insulin replacement therapy to D.A. Which of the following types of insulins was most likely used in his insulin pump?

A. Aspart

B. Glargine

C. Detemir

D. Isophane

E. Regular

9. If D.A. had chosen to administer insulin by using a syringe or an insulin pen. Which of the following two types of insulins would he need to adequately regulate his basal as well his postprandial plasma glucose levels?

A. Glargine–detemir

B. Glargine–isophane

C. Aspart–lispro

D. Lispro–regular

E. Lispro–glargine

10. D.A. was discharged after his DKA resolved. Which of the following suggestions was most likely given to him before he was sent home on insulin therapy?

A. Do not delay intake of food more than the usual times

B. Increase daily exercise, especially in the evening

C. Increase daily food intake

D. Remove the insulin pump when flying internationally

E. Switch to oral antidiabetic medications on weekends

11. D.A.'s blood sugar levels were monitored regularly to estimate his insulin requirements. He was found to have pre-breakfast hyperglycemia, but his 3 a.m. blood glucose levels were normal. Which of the following causes is most likely responsible for prebreakfast hyperglycemia in D.A.?

A. Somogyi's effect

B. Dawn phenomenon

C. Raynaud's phenomenon

D. Lazarus's syndrome

E. Sheehan's syndrome

12. D.A. passed out while playing and was brought to the emergency department. Which of the following conditions did he develop that caused him to pass out?

A. Hyperosmolar hyperglycemic state

B. DKA

C. Hyperkalemia-induced atrioventricular block

D. Hypoglycemia

E. Diabetic nephropathy

Answers and Explanations

▶ *Learning objective:* Describe the diagnostic signs and symptoms of DKA.

1. Answer: D

D.A. had developed DKA, an acute complication of type 1 diabetes mellitus (DM1). DM1 is an autoimmune disorder in which destruction of pancreatic beta cells occurs over a variable period of time. The autoimmune pathways are triggered in genetically susceptible individuals by a variety of environmental factors, including viral infections, such as flu. Possibly the viral fever, which the patient had a history of, might be involved in causing D.A.'s disease. Absolute deficiency of insulin in DKA results in the failure of body cells (mainly skeletal muscle and adipose tissue) to utilize glucose, resulting in hyperglycemia, with blood glucose levels reaching 500 mg/dL or more. In an attempt to provide alternative fuel, catabolism of triglycerides to fatty acids, and then fatty acid metabolism in the liver to ketone bodies results in ketonemia and ketonuria. Furthermore, increased glucagon levels enhance gluconeogenesis and impair peripheral ketone utilization. Eventually, ketoacidosis ensues. As acidosis progresses to pH 7.1 or less, deep breathing with a rapid ventilation rate occurs, which can cause decreased PCO_2 and increased PO_2. Patients with previously undiagnosed DM1 can often present with DKA.

A, E Diabetes insipidus and syndrome of inappropriate ADH secretion are both disorders of abnormal ADH secretion. Hyperglycemia and an increase in ketone bodies are not seen in these conditions.

B Heat stroke can cause altered sensorium and unconsciousness, but it does not cause chronic symptoms. Also hyperglycemia and ketonemia are not seen in this condition.

C D.A. did not have any sign or history that would suggest bulimia, and the disorder is not associated with hyperglycemia and ketonemia.

▶ *Learning objective:* Describe the need for urgent administration of appropriate IV fluids in a patient with DKA.

2. Answer: A

Usually, in a previously undiagnosed DM1 patient, severe and acute insulin deficiency causes DKA, which is characterized by hyperglycemia, ketoacidosis, severe dehydration, and high plasma osmolality. In DKA, severe hyperglycemia causes osmotic diuresis, resulting in the loss of large amounts of water in urine along with glucose and electrolytes. Ketoacidosis induces nausea and vomiting, which further exacerbate dehydration by interfering with oral fluid replacement. Increased fluid loss from the body and depletion in intravascular fluid, and accumulation of solutes (glucose, ketone bodies, electrolytes), increase plasma osmolality. Plasma osmolality above 330 mOsm/kg (normal 285–295) causes impaired consciousness.

D.A. was severely dehydrated, as was evident from his poor skin turgor and dry mucous membranes. It was urgent to replenish his body's fluids in order to permit renal excretion of glucose and ketone bodies and dilute the extracellular electrolyte concentration. All these actions, along with insulin therapy, would decrease hyperglycemia, ketonemia, and osmolality.

B High levels of ketone bodies cause nausea, vomiting, and impairment of thirst sensation. Because thirst sensation is impaired, there is no sense of needing to quenching it. IV fluids are administered to replenish body fluids in DKA.

C See correct answer explanation.

D Hyperosmolality affects the level of consciousness, and rehydration with IV fluids would help in normalizing plasma osmolality. However, rehydration would not increase glucose entry into the brain. Also, the brain does not require insulin for utilizing glucose.

E Vasopressin action is not impaired. In the presence of overwhelming osmotic diuresis due to severe hyperglycemia in DKA, vasopressin action is not able to prevent water loss in the urine.

▶ *Learning objective:* Describe the reason for a fruity breath odor in patients with DKA.

3. Answer: E

In D.A., severe and acutely developed insulin deficiency resulted in failure of body cells (major organs, such as skeletal muscle and adipose tissue) require insulin to utilize glucose. This results in rapid mobilization of energy from skeletal muscle and adipose tissue. An increased flux of amino acids from the muscles to the liver results in increased gluconeogenesis and glucose output from the liver. Triglycerides in the adipose tissue release free fatty acids, which are converted to ketone bodies (acetoacetate, β-hydroxybutyrate, acetone) in the liver. Generation of excessive amounts of ketone bodies results in ketonemia, ketonuria, and ketoacidosis. The peculiar fruity odor in the breath of DKA patients is due to increased levels of acetone.

A Decreased kidney function can occur in DKA due to decreased renal blood supply resulting from depletion of intravascular volume, but it is not the cause of excessive production of ketone bodies.

B Excessive protein intake can increase amino acids and uric acid levels. This is not the cause of the fruity breath odor with DKA.

C Excessive catabolism of muscle proteins results in increased amino acid flux to the liver, where they are converted to glucose, not to ketone bodies.

D In DKA, glucagon secretion is increased, not decreased.

▶ *Learning objective:* Describe the clinical relevance of measuring plasma levels of C-peptide in the diagnosis of DM1.

4. Answer: C

Preproinsulin is a precursor molecule that is translated from the preproinsulin messenger RNA in the rough endoplasmic reticulum of beta cells of the endocrine pancreas. Preproinsulin is cleaved to form proinsulin immediately after its synthesis. Proinsulin is transported to the Golgi apparatus, where it is packaged into secretory granules. Inside the granules, proteolytic cleavage of the proinsulin peptide chain takes place, and it is converted into insulin and a smaller connecting peptide, called C-peptide. Normal mature secretory granules contain insulin and C-peptide in equimolar amounts, and in response to a secretory stimulus, both are released from the beta pancreatic cells in equimolar amounts into the circulation. C-peptide does not have any known biological function. A decrease in insulin synthesis will be accompanied with a decrease in C-peptide levels in the circulation. In DKA, there is an acute absolute deficiency of insulin because of beta cell failure, so the levels of C-peptide will also be undetectable in the circulation.

A There is increased production of ketone bodies in DKA. Acetoacetate is a ketone body.

B, D, E In response to acute deficiency of insulin, the plasma levels of counter-regulatory hormones, glucagon, corticosteroids, catecholamines, and growth hormone, are increased, not decreased.

▶ *Learning objective:* Describe the mechanism of action of insulin.

5.   Answer: B

Insulin exerts its physiological effects by binding to insulin receptors present on the surface of target cells. An insulin receptor is a large transmembrane glycoprotein composed of two α subunits linked to two β subunits by disulfide bonds to form a βααβ- heterotetramer. The larger α subunits are entirely extracellular and contain the insulin binding domain. The smaller β subunits cross the cell membrane and its cytoplasmic domain possesses a tyrosine kinase activity. Binding of insulin to the α subunit activates tyrosine kinase activity of the β subunit, resulting in phosphorylation of a network of cellular substrates, including insulin receptor substrate 1 (IRS-1) and insulin receptor substrate 2 (IRS-2). This leads to activation of additional kinases, phosphatases, and other signaling molecules involved in mediating growth effects of insulin (mitogenic pathway) and regulation of nutrient metabolism (metabolic pathway). Fat and skeletal muscle, the two major insulin target tissues involved

in the regulation of glucose metabolism, require insertion of glucose transporter 4 (GLUT4) in the cell membrane for glucose entry inside their cells. Activation of insulin receptors stimulates translocation of GLUT4-containing vesicles to the cell membrane and incorporation of GLUT4 in the cell membranes.

In DKA, due to decreased intravascular volume and decreased cutaneous blood supply, absorption of subcutaneously administered insulin is not reliable. Therefore IV is preferred to subcutaneous delivery to achieve instant action of insulin in an insulin-deprived acute emergency state of DKA.

There are short-acting, rapid-acting, intermediate-acting, and long-acting preparations of insulin available. For IV administration, only regular insulin (short-acting) is used. Longer-acting insulin preparations are needed, along with short/rapid-acting insulins when insulin is administered subcutaneously by syringe or insulin pen. All types of insulins act by the same mechanism as already explained.

A Inhibition of the activity of dipeptidyl peptidase-4 would be the mechanism of action of antidiabetic drugs of the gliptin subclass (e.g., sitagliptin).

C Insulin inhibits, not activates, the gluconeogenesis pathway.

D Insulin binds to its cell membrane receptor and activates, not inhibits, tyrosine kinase activity.

▶ *Learning objective:* Describe the physiological effects of insulin on glucose, fat, and protein metabolism.

6.   Answer: A

Insulin promotes anabolism and inhibits catabolism, and its major function is to promote storage of ingested nutrients. Insulin inhibits intracellular lipolysis of stored triglycerides in adipocytes by inhibiting intracellular lipase (hormone-sensitive lipase). In DKA, insulin deficiency causes activation of hormone-sensitive lipase, resulting in increased fatty acid flux to liver and ketogenesis. Administration of insulin will promote glucose utilization by the cells and decrease ketogenesis in the liver by decreasing fatty acid flux from the adipose tissue.

B Glucose entry into the brain is independent of insulin action.

C Increased renal excretion of glucose occurs when glucose in the renal tubules surpasses tubular reabsorption capacity. By decreasing plasma glucose levels, insulin would decrease renal tubular glucose concentration, thus reducing, not increasing, renal excretion of glucose.

D Glucose is freely filtered by the renal glomerulus. Insulin does not regulate this process. The net amount of renal excretion of glucose is regulated by tubular reabsorption, which, under normal physiology, is nil, because all the filtered glucose is reabsorbed from the renal tubules.

E Increased catabolism of skeletal muscles occurs in the absence of insulin.

▶ *Learning objective:* Describe the effects of ketoacidosis on serum and intracellular potassium levels.

7. Answer: B

In DKA, total body potassium depletion occurs due to polyuria and vomiting. However, hyperkalemia occurs primarily because of a lack of insulin that causes the following:

▶ A decrease of the activity of the Na^+/K^+ pump
▶ A decrease of glucose entry inside the cells with the concomitant potassium entry
▶ Metabolic acidosis, due to ketogenesis, that shifts cellular potassium to the extracellular space

Replenishing body fluids and replacement of insulin in DKA increase glucose utilization, suppress ketogenesis, and correct acidosis. Therefore, it is important to monitor plasma potassium levels while treating DKA and replace potassium accordingly to prevent hypokalemia.

A An increased activity of the Na^+/K^+ pump would decrease, not increase, plasma potassium concentration.

C Decreased excretion of potassium in the urine would occur in advanced chronic renal failure.

D, E Increased potassium reabsorption from renal tubules and increased absorption from the intestinal tract are not the causes of hyperkalemia seen in ketoacidosis.

▶ *Learning objective:* Describe why only rapid-acting insulin is sufficient to control hyperglycemia in a type 1 diabetic patient by using an insulin pump.

8. Answer: A

An insulin pump is an electronic device that allows administration of insulin subcutaneously as a continuous subcutaneous infusion to provide basal insulin levels in between meals as well as insulin boluses to control postprandial hyperglycemia. Because the device can administer insulin continuously to provide basal levels of insulin, there is no need for an intermediate-acting (isophane) or a long-acting insulin (glargine, detemir). Therefore, the insulin pump needs only a rapid-acting insulin (lispro, aspart, or glulisine) or the short-acting insulin (regular insulin).

B, C, D See above explanation.

E Regular insulin could be correct, too, as far as the type of insulin needed in an insulin pump is concerned, but current insulin pumps use rapid-acting insulins, such as lispro and aspart insulin.

▶ *Learning objective:* Describe different types of insulin preparations and their therapeutic application in the management of DM1.

9. Answer: E

Insulin preparations are subdivided according to their duration as follows:

▶ Rapid-acting: lispro, aspart, glulisine
▶ Short-acting: regular insulin
▶ Intermediate-acting: isophane insulin
▶ Long-acting: glargine, detemir

Regular insulin is a human recombinant insulin that has the same number and sequence of amino acids as found in endogenous human insulin. *Insulin analogues* are insulin preparations that are also recombinant insulins, but the sequence of amino acids is slightly different from that in human endogenous insulin. Modification in the sequence of amino acids in insulin has provided pharmacokinetic benefits. For example, when injected subcutaneously, rapid-acting insulin analogues have faster onset of action compared to regular insulin. Of course, the onset of action is immediate when any of the insulin preparations is injected IV.

Older intermediate-acting and longer-acting insulin preparations were formulated by complexing certain molecules with the regular insulin. For example, isophane insulin, an intermediate-acting insulin, is prepared by complexing insulin with protamine. Upon subcutaneous injection, insulin is released slowly from the complexes to enter into the circulation in order to provide basal levels of insulin. These insulin preparations have delayed onset of action (1–3 hours) and a longer duration of action (10–12 hours to > 24 hours) that make intermediate or long-acting insulins appropriate for providing basal levels of insulins. These are not appropriate for controlling postprandial hyperglycemia, as rapid rise of insulin levels, to match postprandial glucose surge in plasma, is not achieved. Newer long-acting insulins (glargine, detemir) are insulin analogues that have a duration of action longer than a day. They do not need to be combined with other molecules to allow their prolonged release from the injected site.

In contrast to insulin administration via insulin pump, when insulin is administered subcutaneously by using a syringe or pen, a patient would need different types of insulins to control both postprandial (after meals) and basal levels (between meals) of plasma glucose. There is a surge in plasma glucose levels after eating. A parallel and rapid rise in plasma insulin levels is required to control this surge. Rapid-acting insulins take about 10 to 15 minutes for onset of their action after subcutaneous injection, so they can be administered as a bolus injection 10 to 15 minutes before eating a meal. The short-acting insulin (regular insulin) would need to be administered about 30 minutes before a meal. Most patients are prescribed rapid-acting insulins for controlling postprandial hyperglycemia. For "tight glycemic control," a rapid-acting insulin is injected before each meal. Between meals, a continuous supply of lower amounts of insulin is required to maintain normal homeostasis. This is achieved by either intermediate-acting or long-acting insulins. An example of an insulin regimen for a patient who is taking insulin by using syringe would be to take insulin lispro before each meal (before breakfast, lunch, and dinner) to control postprandial hyperglycemia, and insulin glargine at bedtime to provide basal insulin for 24 hours.

A, B, C, D None of these insulin regimes ensures an appropriate control of both postprandial and basal levels of plasma glucose.

▶ *Learning objective:* Describe the appropriate precautions to be taken while on insulin therapy to prevent its adverse effects.

10. Answer: A

Hypoglycemia is a major adverse effect of insulin therapy. It is more common in patients who are on *intensive insulin therapy* to achieve *tight glycemic control.* Hypoglycemia occurs due to a mismatch between carbohydrate intake and insulin dose. When a patient takes the usual dose of insulin at the usual time but eats less than the usual portion of food, extra insulin would keep acting, even after glucose levels drop to near normal. This continued action of insulin drops plasma glucose even further, leading to hypoglycemia. In case of delaying a meal after taking insulin at the usual time, excessive insulin action would result in hypoglycemia. It is critical to avoid development of hypoglycemia, particularly in children, because frequent hypoglycemia episodes impact normal development of the brain.

B Regular exercise is good, but excessive exercise would require either increased calorie intake or insulin dose adjustment to prevent development of hypoglycemia. So excessive exercise is not going to have any therapeutic advantages.

C If a type 1 diabetic patient indulges in overeating, the insulin dose would need to be raised accordingly to deal with the extra glucose. Insulin, due to its anabolic effects, causes weight gain. Thus overeating and the resulting increased insulin requirements would both make the patient overweight, which would adversely affect diabetes.

D The insulin pump needs to be switched on all the time to deliver basal (in between the meals) insulin and insulin boluses before meals.

E Oral antidiabetic drugs do not work in a patient with absolute deficiency of insulin. Treatment of DM1 requires replacement therapy with insulin.

▶ *Learning objective:* Describe the causes of early morning hyperglycemia in a type 1 diabetic patient on insulin therapy.

11. Answer: B

One of the causes of early morning (pre-breakfast) hyperglycemia in a type 1 diabetic patient who is on insulin therapy can be due to administration of less than the required dose of basal insulin at bedtime. In the dawn phenomenon, prebreakfast hyperglycemia develops due to waning of overnight basal insulin levels and is not accompanied by nocturnal hypoglycemia. In patients who administer insulin by using a syringe or an insulin pen, early morning hyperglycemia due to the dawn phenomenon can be treated by increasing the dose of bedtime basal insulin. Usually patients who develop the dawn phenomenon while being on isophane insulin do better when switched to glargine. This is likely due to glargine's longer duration of action. In D.A., who is using an insulin pump, early morning hyperglycemia can be treated by stepping up the basal insulin infusion rate at around 4 to 5 a.m.; the exact time for stepping up the infusion rate can be determined by monitoring the blood glucose level in the middle of the night.

A Somogyi's effect refers to prebreakfast hyperglycemia accompanied with 3 to 4 a.m. hypoglycemia (nocturnal hypoglycemia) that is caused by administration of more than the required dose of basal insulin at bedtime. This nocturnal hypoglycemia evokes a surge of counterregulatory hormones to produce high blood glucose levels by 7 a.m. Early morning hyperglycemia due to Somogyi's effect can be treated by reducing the dose of basal insulin

(intermediate- or long-acting insulin) at bedtime.

C Raynaud's phenomenon is characterized by recurrent ischemia of the fingers and toes, usually in response to cold.

D Lazarus's syndrome is the spontaneous return of circulation after failed cardiopulmonary resuscitation.

E Sheehan's syndrome, also called postpartum hypopituitarism, is hypopituitarism due to ischemic necrosis of the anterior pituitary caused by blood loss during childbirth or postpartum hemorrhage.

▶ *Learning objective:* Describe the adverse effects of insulin therapy.

12. Answer: D

Hypoglycemia is a major adverse effect of insulin therapy. It occurs due to a mismatch between carbohydrate intake and the insulin dose. When a patient takes the usual dose of insulin at the usual time but eats less than the usual portion of food, extra insulin will keep acting even after glucose levels drop to near normal. This continued action of insulin drops plasma glucose even further, leading to hypoglycemia. Similarly, hypoglycemia can develop from unusual physical exertion without supplemental calories or without a decrease in insulin dose. Symptoms of hypoglycemia include profuse perspiration, chills and shakes, palpitation, and blurred vision. A patient is usually able to identify these symptoms and eat something promptly to receive instant glucose in order to prevent untoward outcomes. In D.A.'s case, he was on intensive insulin therapy via insulin pump. He might have skipped his meal, and most likely he continued taking his usual dose of insulin while playing, the factors that contributed toward development of hypoglycemia. He was a new patient who freshly started insulin therapy, and, because he was engrossed in playing, he failed to identify the symptoms of hypoglycemia and passed out.

A, B Hyperosmolar hyperglycemic state (HHS) and DKA are two of the most serious and life-threatening acute complications of diabetes. They each represent an extreme in the hyperglycemic spectrum. Both can cause coma, and both are characterized by very high glucose levels. D.A.'s history and the fact that he responded well and quickly to dextrose infusion confirm that HHS and DKA had nothing to do with his faint.

C Hyperkalemia can occur in an acute insulin deficiency state of DKA. D.A. was on intensive insulin therapy, so hyperkalemia was unlikely.

E Diabetic nephropathy is a chronic, long-standing complication of diabetes. It cannot cause fainting.

Case 49

Type 2 Diabetes Mellitus

D.M., A 42-year-old woman, presented to her family physician with fatigue lasting most of the day, and curdy vaginal secretions. She said that she needed to wake up multiple times at night for urination and also that she was not feeling fresh in the morning. She was also feeling thirsty all the time. She said she had been noticing these changes for the past month or so.

The patient revealed that she had suffered from similar vaginal symptoms twice, earlier that year. Both times, she was given a vaginal pessary for the treatment. Her father, who was 69 years old, and her first cousin, 40 years old, were on treatment for type 2 diabetes mellitus. Her mother had died 2 years ago at the age of 61 after suffering a massive stroke.

Physical examination showed a Caucasian woman who appeared obese. Her body mass index (BMI) was 32. Her vital signs were blood pressure 138/88 mm Hg, pulse 88 bpm, respirations 18/min.

A blood exam was ordered with the following pertinent results:

- Hemoglobin (Hb): 12 g/dL (normal 12–16)
- White blood cell count (WBC): 9,000 /μL (normal 4,500–11,000)
- Hemoglobin A_{1c} (HbA_{1c}): 9.2% (normal < 6%)
- Fasting blood sugar: 160 mg/dL (normal 70–110)
- 2-h postprandial blood sugar: 260 mg/dL (normal < 140)
- Sodium (Na^+): 138 mEq/L (normal 136–145)
- Potassium (K^+): 4.0 mEq/L (normal 3.5–5.0)
- Calcium (Ca^{2+}): 9.8 mg/dL (normal 9.5–11.0)
- Creatinine: 1.1 mg/dL (normal 0.6–1.2)
- Blood urea nitrogen (BUN): 8 mg/dL (normal 7–20)
- Total bilirubin: 1.0 mg/dL (normal 0.3–1.0)
- Aspartame aminotransferase (AST): 15 U/L (normal 10–35)
- Alanine aminotransferase (ALT): 18 U/L (normal 8–20)
- Total cholesterol: 230 mg/dL (normal < 200)
- Low-density lipoprotein (LDL) cholesterol: 120 mg/dL (normal < 100)
- High-density lipoprotein (HDL) cholesterol: 38 mg/dL normal 40–50)
- Triglycerides: 350 mg/dL (normal < 150)

Based on the history, physical examination, and lab results, she was diagnosed with type 2 diabetes mellitus and vaginal candidiasis.

She was given dietary and lifestyle modification advice and was started on metformin 500 mg to be taken once a day with breakfast. She was also prescribed fluconazole 150 mg to be taken only for 1 day to treat her vaginal candidiasis.

After a week, her dose of metformin was increased to 500 mg twice a day with meals. Initially she responded reasonably well to this monotherapy with metformin, as reflected by her fasting blood glucose levels of 120 mg/dL and HbA$_{1c}$ of 7%, but within 3 years her blood glucose levels required the metformin dose to be increased to 1,000 mg twice a day.

Despite the increase in metformin doses, her HbA$_{1C}$ was remaining around 8.6%. Her physician added glimepiride to her therapy. Her daily self-monitored blood glucose readings showed improvements in her blood glucose levels as compared to previous blood glucose values. Four months later, her HbA$_{1c}$ was 7.8%. However, this improvement did not last much longer. Moreover, she was not adhering strictly to the lifestyle modification measures. At the end of 1 year with this two-drug combination therapy, her fasting blood glucose was remaining at 140 to 160 mg/dL and the HbA$_{1c}$ had raised to 8.2%. Her physician also ordered a liver function test, which was normal. D.M. did not want an injectable drug, so her physician added pioglitazone to her medications, but that was discontinued after 6 months when D.M. reported difficulty breathing while lying in bed and swelling in both her feet. Her new symptoms were appropriately managed, and her physician added sitagliptin to her continuing therapy with metformin and glimepiride. Subsequent follow-up revealed her HbA$_{1c}$ to be 7.8%.

One year later, she experienced severe pain in the right lower quadrant of her abdomen. She was diagnosed with acute appendicitis and was admitted for surgery to remove her appendix. During her surgery and the duration of hospitalization, an appropriate drug was used to control her blood glucose levels. She was discharged from the hospital after 4 days with the same oral antidiabetic drugs she was taking before surgery.

During her follow-up visit 6 months later, she complained of an increased urge to drink fluids and increased frequency of urination. Her HbA$_{1c}$ was 8.4%, and fasting blood glucose was 136 mg/dL. At this point, her physician added insulin to her therapy.

Questions

1. D.M. was diagnosed with type 2 diabetes mellitus (DM2), and her fasting blood glucose (FBG) levels at the time of diagnosis were 160 mg/dL. Which of the following metabolic processes most likely plays a predominant role in elevating FBG levels in DM2?

A. Ketogenesis

B. Gluconeogenesis

C. Glycogenesis

D. Lipogenesis

2. DM2 is characterized by insulin-resistance in the peripheral tissues. Which of the following processes most likely mediates this resistance?

A. Increased insulin secretion

B. Decreased glucagon levels

C. Increased FFAs

D. Increased amino acid delivery to liver

E. Decreased Insulin secretion

3. Certain lab tests were ordered for D.M. Her blood glucose levels and HbA$_{1c}$ assisted in making a diagnosis of DM 2. In addition to these test results, which of the following lab results was required for the prescription of an appropriate antidiabetic therapy for this patient?

A. White blood cells

B. Serum creatinine

C. Hemoglobin

D. LDL cholesterol

E. Calcium

4. D.M. was prescribed metformin along with advice for lifestyle changes. Which of the following actions most likely mediated the antidiabetic effect of the drug in the patient's disease?

A. Decreased breakdown of glycogen

B. Decreased intestinal glucose absorption

C. Increased insulin secretion from pancreas

D. Increased glucose excretion in urine

E. Decreased glucose output from the liver

5. D.M. was instructed to take metformin with food. Which of the following was the primary reason for this instruction?

A. To prevent abdominal discomfort

B. To improve oral bioavailability of metformin

C. To slow down renal excretion of metformin

D. To avoid degradation of metformin by gastric acid

E. To decrease fat absorption from the gastrointestinal tract

6. D.M. was prescribed fluconazole for treating her vaginal candidiasis. Which of the following molecular actions on fungal cells most likely mediated the therapeutic effect of the drug in the patient's disease?

A. Inhibition of the activity of squalene epoxidase

B. Formation of pores in the fungal cell wall

C. Inhibition of ergosterol synthesis

D. Inhibition of thymidylate synthase

E. Inhibition of DNA synthesis

7. D.M.'s physician decided to add glimepiride to her therapy. Which of the following actions most likely mediated the therapeutic effect of the drug in the patient's disease?

A. Blockade of adenosine triphosphate (ATP)-sensitive potassium channels

B. Transcription of genes related to glucose utilization

C. Inhibition of α-glucosidase

D. Blockade of glucagon receptors

E. Activation of insulin receptors

8. D.M.'s physician added pioglitazone to her therapy after evaluating her glycemic control. Which of the following effects most likely occurred in response to pioglitazone?

A. Decreased pancreatic beta cell mass

B. Increased circulating FFAs

C. Decreased expression of GLUT-4

D. Increased adiponectin levels

E. Increased insulin secretion

437

9. D.M.'s physician stopped her therapy with pioglitazone. An increased risk of which of the following complications most likely suggested the decision to stop this drug?

A. Glomerulonephritis

B. Hepatotoxicity

C. Heart failure

D. Anaphylactic reaction

E. Hypoglycemia

10. Sitagliptin was added to D.M.'s combination therapy with metformin and glimepiride, after pioglitazone was discontinued. Which of the following molecular actions most likely mediated the therapeutic effect of this drug?

A. Inhibition of dipeptidyl peptidase-4

B. Inhibition of α-glycosidase

C. Activation of AMP-activated protein kinase

D. Activation of glucagon-like peptide (GLP)-1 receptors

E. Blockade of ATP-sensitive K$^+$ channels

F. Phosphorylation of tyrosine kinase receptor

11. D.M. had undergone surgery for appendicitis. Which of the following drugs was most likely used during surgery and her hospitalization to control her blood glucose levels?

A. Glimepiride

B. Metformin

C. Acarbose

D. Insulin

E. Sitagliptin

12. A gliptin drug that acts by decreasing the degradation of endogenous incretins was added to D.M.'s combination therapy. Which of the following drugs acts directly by activating the incretin receptors and could be an alternative to sitagliptin for D.M.?

A. Pramlintide

B. Exenatide

C. Glargine

D. Miglitol

E. Glyburide

13. D.M.'s physician tried different combinations of antidiabetic drugs in order to achieve optimal glycemic control. Which of the following is a microvascular complication, the risk of which is reduced dramatically with tight glycemic control in a DM2 patient?

A. Nephropathy

B. Coronary artery disease

C. Stroke

D. Peripheral vascular disease

E. Intestinal ischemia

Answers and Explanations

▶ *Learning objective:* Describe the pathophysiology of DM2.

1. Answer: B

Under normal physiological conditions, during a fasting state, appropriate blood glucose levels (normal FBG 70–110 mg/dL) are maintained by gluconeogenesis in the liver and the kidneys. About 85% of glucose is derived from the liver, and the rest comes from the kidneys. Appropriate levels of glucose are essential to provide a constant supply of energy to the brain. During a fasting state, 75% of the glucose disposal takes place in the brain and splanchnic tissues and the remaining in the skeletal muscles.

During a fasting state, as the plasma glucose levels decline, glucagon is secreted by the alpha cells of the pancreas. Glucagon opposes insulin action and activates the gluconeogenesis pathway to maintain a normal range of blood glucose levels. In the fed state, carbohydrate ingestion increases blood glucose levels, which stimulates insulin release. Insulin, in addition to facilitating glucose uptake by the peripheral tissues, suppresses glucagon secretion, and so gluconeogenesis stops.

DM2 is characterized by the following:

▶ Defective insulin secretion
▶ Insulin resistance, particularly in three major organs (liver, muscle, and fat).

Due to relative insulin deficiency, glucagon secretion and its action on the liver remain unchecked, resulting in continuously increased gluconeogenesis, thus leading to increased levels of FBG (> 126 mg/dL). In addition, this also contributes to elevated postprandial blood glucose levels. Increased blood glucose levels in response to a meal plus the increased glucose output from the liver (due to continuously increased gluconeogenesis) would cause sustained postprandial hyperglycemia (> 200 mg/dL).

A Ketogenesis is the synthesis of ketone bodies. Due to deficiency of insulin, their levels increase alarmingly in the circulation in order to provide alternate sources of energy. This causes diabetic ketoacidosis, which is more common in DM1 than in DM2.

C Glycogen synthesis is impaired in the absence of insulin. Moreover, glycogen synthesis uses glucose, and so glucose output into the circulation would not increase.

D Insulin is a potent inhibitor of lipolysis. After ingestion of food, insulin levels increase, which inhibits lipolysis of triglycerides to free fatty acids (FFAs) in the adipose tissue. FFAs serve as an important energy source during fasting. In DM2, due to relative deficiency of insulin, lipolysis, not lipogenesis, is increased, resulting in increased FFAs in the circulation.

▶ *Learning objective:* Identify a biochemical process that can cause insulin resistance.

2. Answer: C

Insulin is a potent inhibitor of lipolysis. After ingestion of food, insulin levels increase, which inhibits lipolysis of triglycerides to FFAs in the adipose tissue. FFAs serve as an important energy source during fasting. In DM2, due to relative deficiency of insulin, lipolysis is increased resulting in increased FFAs in the circulation. Chronically elevated FFAs cause insulin resistance in the peripheral organs and impairment of insulin secretion.

A In DM2, initially there can be increased insulin secretion and hyperinsulinemia to compensate for the peripheral

resistance to insulin, but this is not the cause of insulin resistance.

B Glucagon levels increase in the presence of relative deficiency of insulin in DM2.

D Increased amino acid delivery to liver is a consequence of insulin resistance, it does not cause insulin resistance. These amino acids are utilized in the gluconeogenesis pathway.

E DM2 is characterized by defective insulin secretion, and insulin resistance; particularly in three major organs (liver, muscle, and fat). DM2 is a progressive disorder in which there can be a relative deficiency of insulin (hyperinsulinemia in the presence of insulin resistance), and eventually insulin secretion is decreased. However, decrease in insulin is not the cause of insulin resistance.

▶ *Learning objective:* Describe the importance of knowing results of the kidney function test before prescribing an appropriate drug therapy for DM2.

3. Answer: B

D.M.'s HbA_{1c} levels indicate that her blood sugars were elevated for at least the past 3 months. Many patients with long-standing hyperglycemia due to previously undiagnosed DM2 have already developed chronic complications of hyperglycemia, including microvascular and macrovascular complications. The development and progression of microvascular complications (nephropathy, retinopathy, and neuropathy) is directly linked to duration and level of hyperglycemia. This is why it is important to check kidney function (serum creatinine, BUN) in diabetic patients. Another important reason for assessing renal function is that many antidiabetic drugs undergo clearance via the renal route. An impaired renal function can be a contraindication for their use. Drug therapy of most DM2 patients is initiated with metformin, unless there is any contraindication. One of the contraindications of metformin is impaired renal function.

A, C, D, E These lab results are not needed for an appropriate antidiabetic treatment of this patient.

▶ *Learning objective:* Describe the mechanism of action of metformin.

4.   Answer: E

Metformin is recommended as the first-line therapy for DM2 unless the patient has a contraindication for its use. Metformin activates adenosine monophosphate (AMP)-activated protein kinase and reduces gluconeogenesis to decrease glucose output from the liver. This action causes a decrease in FBG levels. Metformin also decreases peripheral resistance to insulin, but the exact mechanisms of this effect are not clear.

Metformin reduces HbA_{1c} by 1.5 to 2% and FBG levels by 60 to 80 mg/dL. It also exerts favorable effects on the lipid profile by decreasing plasma triglycerides and LDL cholesterol by about 8 to 15%. The drug also decreases body weight by 2 to 3 kg, which is good for obese DM2 patients, as most of them are.

A Decrease in glycogen breakdown is not a metformin direct effect. This may occur when tissues regain insulin sensitivity, so in the fed state insulin will act to enhance glucose uptake and convert it to storage forms (glycogen). Otherwise it has been shown that metformin does not affect glycogenolysis directly, but rather it can reduce both glycogenesis and gluconeogenesis.

B Metformin does not affect intestinal glucose absorption. Some other antidiabetic drugs can achieve this effect either by decreasing gastric motility or by inhibiting gastrointestinal enzymes required to break down complex carbohydrates.

C Metformin does not act on the pancreas to increase insulin secretion. That's why hypoglycemia with monotherapy with metformin is rare.

D Metformin decreases plasma glucose levels, so the amount of glucose filtered by the glomerulus and excreted in urine will decrease, not increase.

▶ *Learning objective:* Describe the adverse effects of metformin.

5.   Answer: A

About 20 to 30% of patients on metformin experience its gastrointestinal adverse effects, such as abdominal discomfort, anorexia, nausea, vomiting, and diarrhea. These adverse effects are dose-related and transient, lessening in severity over several weeks. Chances of these adverse effects can be minimized by taking the drug with or right after meals. Starting metformin with the lowest doses is also helpful in minimizing the risk of gastrointestinal adverse effects. That's why initially D.M. was prescribed metformin at the lowest dose of 500 mg once a day. Over a period of time his daily dose was increased to a maximum effective dose of 2,000 mg. However, D.M. did not experience the appropriate therapeutic effect of metformin, even at the maximum dose, so her physician added another drug to her therapy.

Metformin can rarely cause lactic acidosis. The conditions that predispose a DM2 patient to this adverse effect are those conditions that either increase lactic acid synthesis or impair disposal of lactic acid. Lactic acid production increases in hypoperfusion states and hypoxia-inducing conditions, such as congestive heart failure, pulmonary diseases, shock, and septicemia. Severe liver disease and alcohol consumption also compromise removal of lactic acid from the body.

B Metformin's oral bioavailability is approximately 50 to 60%. This is not affected by food.

C Metformin is not metabolized in the body and is excreted unchanged in the urine. Taking it with food has no effect on its renal excretion.

D Metformin is not gastric acid labile.

E Metformin does not decrease fat absorption from the gastrointestinal tract. Its positive effects on the lipid profile are due to its actions in the liver and insulin sensitizing effects in the periphery.

▶ *Learning objective:* Describe the mechanism of action of fluconazole.

6.   Answer: C

Fluconazole is an azole antifungal agent. Azoles inhibit fungal ergosterol synthesis by inhibiting cytochrome P-450 (CYP-450) C 14α-demethylase. Because ergosterol is an important component of the fungal cell membrane, the ultimate effect is a disruption of this membrane. An important indication of fluconazole is *Candida* infection.

A Terbinafine inhibits squalene epoxidase in susceptible fungi.

B Amphotericin B binds to ergosterol in the cell membrane of susceptible fungi to create pores in the fungal cell membrane.

D, E Flucytosine is an antifungal agent that is converted into 5-fluorouracil inside the fungal cell. Fluorouracil inhibits fungal DNA and RNA synthesis by inhibiting thymidylate synthase.

▸ *Learning objective:* Describe the mechanism of action of sulfonylureas.

7. Answer: A

Glimepiride is a sulfonylurea agent. Sulfonylureas bind to sulfonylurea receptors (which are a component of ATP-sensitive potassium channels) and blocks ATP-sensitive K^+ channels in the cell membrane of pancreatic beta cells. Inhibition of these channels changes resting potential of these cells, leading to opening of voltage-gated calcium channels, which results in calcium influx and release of preformed insulin. Because these agents stimulate insulin secretion, they are also called insulin secretagogues.

Sulfonylureas also reduce serum glucagon concentrations. This effect appears to involve indirect inhibition of glucagon secretion due to enhanced release of both insulin and somatostatin, which inhibit secretions from the pancreatic alpha cells.

These drugs are also called hypoglycemic agents because they cause a decrease in glycemic levels by increasing insulin secretion from the pancreas. If food is delayed while the patient is on these drugs, hypoglycemia occurs as an adverse effect.

For appropriate control of glycemia in diabetic patients, an HbA_{1c} goal of < 7% is considered optimal to reduce the risk of chronic complications of diabetes mellitus. DM2 is a progressive disorder in which pancreatic beta cell function declines with increased duration of the disorder. It is not unusual for a DM2 patient who fails to respond to monotherapy after initially attaining a favorable glycemic control

with it. When this occurs, a DM2 patient requires a combination drug therapy.

According to the *stepped-care approach* for treating DM2, when monotherapy fails to achieve optimal glycemic control, it is recommended to add another antidiabetic drug (step 2 of the stepped-care approach), rather than substituting for the first drug (which is metformin for most patients). Similarly, step 3 of the approach recommends adding a third drug (noninsulin drug or insulin, depending on the patient's glucose control, blood glucose levels, and HbA_{1c}). Eventually, most patients would require insulin therapy as the disease advances and beta cell failure progresses. Insulin therapy, initially as add-on therapy, can be considered when HbA_{1c} levels stay above 8%. Usually an intermediate- or long-acting insulin, such as insulin glargine, detemir, or isophane, is added at bedtime.

B Transcription of genes related to glucose utilization would be the mechanism of antidiabetic action of thiazolidinediones (TZDs).

C Inhibition of α-glucosidase would be the mechanism of antidiabetic action of acarbose and miglitol.

D Glimepiride can indirectly reduce glucagon secretion but has no effect on glucagon receptors.

E Insulin receptors are activated only by binding insulin.

▸ *Learning objective:* Describe the mechanism of action of TZDs.

8. Answer: D

Pioglitazone and rosiglitazone are thiazolidinedione TZD derivatives. The major site of action of these drugs is the adipose tissue, where they bind to the nuclear peroxisome proliferator activated receptor-γ (PPAR-γ). PPAR-γ regulates the transcription of several insulin-responsive genes. Activation of PPAR-γ results in the following:

▸ Decreased lipolysis of triglycerides to FFAs, thus reducing flux of fatty acids to skeletal muscles. This results in a decrease of insulin resistance.
▸ Activation of adiponectin, one of the adipokines in the adipose tissue. Adiponectin is associated

441

with increased insulin sensitivity by elevating AMP kinase.

The overall effect is a reduction in insulin resistance and an enhanced tissue sensitivity to insulin. TZDs are also called insulin sensitizers and are euglycemics because they do not cause hypoglycemia. They are metabolized by the CYP-450 system in the liver. Their maximal clinical effect becomes apparent only after 6 to 12 weeks.

A TZDs do not decrease pancreatic beta cell mass. This cell mass is already decreasing progressively in DM2. It is not proved yet, but it appears that TZDs may actually prolong beta cell survival.

B TZDs decrease, not increase, the levels of circulating FFAs, thereby decreasing insulin resistance in the insulin-sensitive tissues.

C Stimulation of PPAR-γ is associated with increase, not decrease, in GLUT-4 expression, which in turn would stimulate glucose uptake by the cells, especially skeletal muscle cells.

E TZD's major site of action is adipose tissue. It does not act as an insulin secretagogue to increase insulin release.

▶ *Learning objective:* Describe the adverse effects and contraindications of pioglitazone.

9. Answer: C

Increased risk of developing or exacerbating heart failure has been noted with the use of pioglitazone. Increase in plasma volume has been reported in response to TZDs, which might contribute to heart failure. D.M. developed pedal edema and coughing on lying down. These are the symptoms of heart failure. TZDs are contraindicated in patients who have symptoms of heart failure.

A Glomerulonephritis is not associated with TZDs.

B D.M.'s symptoms were not consistent with hepatotoxicity. An earlier TZD agent, troglitazone, was withdrawn because it was associated with significant incidents of hepatotoxicity. With rosiglitazone or pioglitazone, hepatotoxicity has been reported very rarely. Nevertheless, a baseline liver function is recommended before starting therapy with TZDs. D.M.'s liver function was normal when pioglitazone was started.

D Hypersensitivity reactions to TZDs, including an anaphylactic reaction, have been reported rarely, but the patient's symptoms did not indicate a hypersensitivity reaction.

E TZDs are insulin sensitizers. They do not cause hypoglycemia as monotherapy, but hypoglycemia can occur, when given in combination with insulin secretagogues. Hypoglycemia usually presents with a feeling of intense hunger, palpitations, and profuse sweating. D.M. did not develop these symptoms in response to pioglitazone combination therapy.

▶ *Learning objective:* Describe the mechanism of action of gliptin antidiabetic drugs.

10. Answer: A

Sitagliptin is a gliptin drug. These agents act by inhibiting the activity of dipeptidyl peptidase-4 (DPP-4), the enzyme that catalyzes the degradation of endogenous incretins.

Incretins are gut hormones, and their release is stimulated in response to mixed meals. Two important incretins are GLP-1 and glucose-dependent insulinotropic peptide (GIP).

GLP-1 is secreted by L cells in the distal intestinal mucosa. It is shown to exert the following effects:

▶ Stimulate insulin secretion. The insulin secretion effect, called the insulinotropic effect, is glucose dependent. Glucose levels must be higher than 90 mg/dL for GLP-1 to enhance insulin secretion.
▶ Suppresses glucagon secretion
▶ Slows gastric emptying
▶ Reduces food intake by increasing satiety

These effects together limit postprandial glucose excursions.

GIP is secreted by K cells in the jejunum. Like GLP-1, GIP increases insulin secretion, but it has no effect on glucagon secretion, gastric emptying, and satiety.

Both gut hormones have a short half-life (< 10 minutes). They are rapidly inactivated by the action of DPP-4.

In DM2 the levels of GLP-1 are found to be lower than normal. DPP-4 inhibitors, such as sitagliptin, raise the levels of endogenous incretins by inhibiting the enzyme that catalyzes their degradation.

B Inhibition of α-glycosidase would be the mechanism of action of acarbose and miglitol.

C Activation of AMP-activated protein kinase would be the mechanism of action of metformin.

D Activation of GLP-1 receptors would be the mechanism of action of exenatide.

E Blockade of ATP-sensitive K⁺ channels would be the mechanism of action of sulfonylureas and meglitinide analogues.

F Phosphorylation of tyrosine kinase receptor would be the mechanism of action of insulin.

▶ *Learning objective:* Describe the indications of insulin therapy in a patient with DM2.

11. Answer: D

During stressful situations (surgery, trauma, acute severe infections), levels of counter-regulatory hormones, such as cortisol, increase multifold to deal with stress. In a nondiabetic patient, these mechanisms would act to meet the body's extra demand for glucose. However, in a DM2 patient these mechanisms would further elevate the levels of hyperglycemia to such unpredictable extents that it would become difficult to achieve glycemic control with antidiabetic drugs other than insulin. Therefore, in such stressful situations, even a DM2 patient with previously well controlled glycemic levels is switched to insulin therapy. With insulin it is much easier to control glycemic levels.

Insulin is used for treating a DM2 patient in the following situations as well:

▶ When combination therapy with other antidiabetic drugs fails to achieve optimal glycemic control
▶ When a patient with long-lasting DM2 may have lost most pancreatic beta cells. This patient would need replacement therapy with insulin similar to that needed in DM1.
▶ During pregnancy, insulin is preferred in a DM2 patient over oral antidiabetic drugs. Insulin is a peptide and does

not cross the placenta; thus it does not affect fetal glucose metabolism.

A, B, C, E All these antidiabetic drugs are not appropriate for optimal control of glycemic levels during surgery or other stressful situations.

▶ *Learning objective:* Describe the pharmacology of incretin-mimetic agents.

12. Answer: B

In DM2, the levels of GLP-1 are found to be lower than normal. There are two types of drugs available to help restore the incretin effect:

▶ GLP-1 agonists, also called incretin mimetics, such as exenatide, which acts by binding to GLP-1 receptors
▶ DPP-4 inhibitors, such as sitagliptin, which raise the levels of endogenous incretins by inhibiting their degradation

Exenatide is an incretin mimetic approved by the U.S. Food and Drug Administration in 2005 to be administered subcutaneously as an adjunctive therapy in DM2 patients who have not achieved adequate glycemic control by a sulfonylurea drug, metformin, or a combination of the two. In 2009, it was also approved for use as a monotherapy. Exenatide exerts the following effects:

▶ Increases insulin secretion when glucose levels are elevated (glucose-dependent insulin secretion, eliminating the risk of hypoglycemia)
▶ Suppresses glucagon secretion
▶ Slows gastric emptying (slows the rate of glucose entry into the circulation)
▶ Decreases appetite

Common adverse effects of the drug include nausea (~ 44%), vomiting, and diarrhea.

A Pramlintide is an amylin analogue approved for subcutaneous administration to DM1 patients, and DM2 patients who use insulin. Amylin is a small peptide hormone that is released by the pancreatic beta cells along with insulin in response to a meal. It slows gastric emptying and suppresses glucagon secretion.

C Glargine is a long-acting insulin that is used to provide basal levels of insulin in patients with DM1 and in patients with DM2 who need insulin therapy.

D Miglitol is an inhibitor of α-glucosidase, an enzyme located on the brush border of intestinal cells that is involved in the breakdown of starches and disaccharides into simple sugars.

E Glyburide is an insulin secretagogue from the sulfonylurea class of drugs.

▶ *Learning objective:* Describe the effect of tight glycemic control on the chronic complications of diabetes mellitus.

13.   Answer: A

Studies have concluded that tight glycemic control with the goal of keeping HbA$_{1c}$ < 7% dramatically decreases the risk of microvascular complications (retinopathy, nephropathy, neuropathy) of DM, but the effect of tight glycemic control on reduction of macrovascular complication is not very clear. Macrovascular complications seem to be multifactorial. Insulin resistance and resulting hyperinsulinemia in DM2 are thought to contribute to the development of hypertension, dyslipidemia, and platelet dysfunction, all of which are risk factors for atherosclerosis and contribute toward pathogenesis of macrovascular complications (coronary artery disease, stroke, peripheral vascular disease).

B, C, D, E These are all macrovascular disorders, not microvascular.

Urinary Tract Infection

W.A., a 57-year-old woman, complained to her physician of burning on urination over the past 2 days. Past medical history of the patient indicated that she had been suffering from gastro-esophageal reflux disease for 10 years, for which she had been taking over-the-counter antacids. The patient had been diagnosed with three urinary tract infections over the past 9 months, each successfully treated with trimethoprim–sulfamethoxazole. W.A. had no other medical problems. She did not smoke and denied use of illicit drugs but admitted to drinking two or three glasses of wine every day. W.A. was retired from work as a school teacher and lived at home with her husband.

The patient reported that she had some suprapubic pain and an urgent need to urinate, and she was voiding a small volume of urine. She had to urinate seven or eight times at night, and she also noted that her preceding urinary tract infections as well as her present symptoms seemed to have started soon after sexual intercourse.

Physical examination showed a woman in no acute distress, with the following vital signs: blood pressure 134/78 mm Hg, heart rate 72 bpm, respirations 12/min, temperature 97.3°F (36.3°C). No costovertebral angle percussion tenderness was found. Pelvic examination showed mild suprapubic tenderness and no vaginal discharge or lesions.

Some lab exams were ordered with the following results:

Urinalysis

- Osmolality: 700 mOsm/kg
- pH: 5.5
- Protein: negative
- Blood: positive
- Glucose: negative
- Ketones: negative
- Bilirubin: negative
- Nitrite: positive
- White blood cell count (WBC): 2/high-power field (HPF) (normal < 5)
- Red blood cell count (RBC): 10/HPF (normal < 3)
- Bacteria: 40/HPF (normal < 20)
- Sediment: gram-positive and gram-negative bacteria

Blood hematology

- Red blood cell count (RBC): $4.2 \times 10^6/\mu L$ (normal 4.0–6.0)
- Hemoglobin (Hb): 11 g/dL (normal, women 12–16)
- Hematocrit (Hct): 40% (normal 36–48)
- White blood cell count (WBC): $11 \times 10^3/\mu L$ (normal 4–10)
- Platelets: $250 \times 10^3/\mu L$ (normal 130–400)

- Creatinine: 1.1 mg/dL (normal 0.6–1.2)
- Blood urea nitrogen (BUN): 30 mg/dL (normal 8–25)
- Sodium (Na⁺): 140 mEq/L (normal 135–146)
- Potassium (K⁺): 4.5 mEq/L (normal 3.6–5.3)
- Glucose: 92 mg/dL (normal 60–110)

A diagnosis of urinary tract infection (UTI) was made, and the physician prescribed a 7-day course of trimethoprim–sulfamethoxazole.

Over the next 4 days, W.A.'s UTI did not improve substantially, and the physician suspected that resistance to trimethoprim-sulfamethoxazole had developed. The therapy was changed, and a 7-day course of ciprofloxacin was prescribed. The physician instructed the patient to avoid the use of antacids during the ciprofloxacin treatment. The therapy was able to treat her symptoms completely.

Four months later W.A. was admitted to the emergency department with fever, chills, sweats, nausea, and frequent vomiting. Physical examination showed a woman in obvious distress with the following vital signs: blood pressure 96/60 mm Hg, heart rate 110 bpm, respirations 22/min, temperature 102.6°F (39.2°C). A strong costovertebral angle percussion tenderness was found on her left side.

A diagnosis of acute pyelonephritis was made, and urinalysis identified gram-positive cocci, gram-negative diplococci, and gram-positive and -negative rods. An emergency therapy was started that included intravenous (IV) administration of meropenem.

Questions

1. W.A. was diagnosed with UTI. Which of the following pairs of exam results of this patient are most indicative of a UTI?

A. Positive urine nitrite–hematuria

B. WBC count–bacteriuria

C. Positive urine nitrite–bacteriuria

D. Hematuria–WBC count

E. WBC count–positive urine nitrite

F. Hematuria–bacteriuria

2. From the patient's symptoms and signs, which of the following types of UTI did W.A. most likely have?

A. Acute uncomplicated cystitis

B. Chronic pyelonephritis

C. Acute pyelonephritis

D. Acute complicated urethritis

E. Chronic urethritis

3. Which of the following pairs of bacteria are the most frequent cause of UTI?

A. *Legionella pneumophila–Escherichia coli*

B. *Staphylococcus saprophyticus–Legionella pneumophila*

C. *Clostridium difficile–Staphylococcus saprophyticus*

D. *Clostridium difficile–Escherichia coli*

E. *Escherichia coli–Staphylococcus saprophyticus*

F. *Legionella pneumophila–Clostridium difficile*

4. W.A. was treated with trimethoprim–sulfamethoxazole. The inhibition of which of the following pairs of enzymes most likely mediates the therapeutic effect of the drug in the patient's disorder?

A. Dihydropteroate synthase–DNA gyrase

B. Transglycosylase–DNA gyrase

C. Dihydropteroate synthase–dihydrofolate reductase

D. DNA gyrase–dihydrofolate reductase

E. Transglycosylase–dihydropteroate synthase

F. Dihydrofolate reductase–transglycosylase

5. The trimethoprim–sulfamethoxazole therapy was not effective, and the physician suspected that resistance to sulfamethoxazole had occurred. This resistance was most likely due to which of the following mechanisms?

A. Increased permeability of bacterial cell membrane

B. Decreased sulfonamide binding to bacterial ribosomes

C. Increased production of para-aminobenzoic acid

D. Decreased sulfonamides binding to dihydrofolate reductase

E. Decreased activity if the multidrug efflux pump

6. W.A. started a therapy with ciprofloxacin. Which of the following molecular actions most likely mediated the therapeutic effect of the drug in the patient's disease?

A. Inhibition of bacterial cell wall synthesis

B. Inhibition of relaxation of supercoiled bacterial DNA

C. Stimulation of synthesis of abnormal bacterial proteins

D. Inhibition of ergosterol synthesis in bacterial cell membrane

E. Stimulation of bacterial DNA helicase

F. Stimulation of bacterial DNA–dependent RNA polymerase

7. The physician advised W.A. to avoid the use of antacids during ciprofloxacin therapy. Which of the following statements best explains why antacids should not be given to patients taking ciprofloxacin?

A. They increase the production of ciprofloxacin toxic metabolites.

B. They increase ciprofloxacin renal elimination.

C. They decrease ciprofloxacin penetration into bacterial cells.

D. They decrease ciprofloxacin crossing the intestinal wall.

447

8. Because of ciprofloxacin therapy W.A. was at increased risk of which of the following life-threatening adverse effects?

A. Acute kidney failure

B. Pseudomembranous colitis

C. Ventricular arrhythmia

D. Pulmonary thromboembolism

E. Stroke

9. W.A. started a therapy that included meropenem. Which of the following molecular actions most likely mediated the therapeutic effect of the drug in the patient's disease?

A. Misreading of the messenger RNA template code

B. Inhibition of tetrahydrofolate synthesis

C. Inhibition of RNA polymerization

D. Blockade of peptidyl-transfer RNA translocation

E. Inhibition of peptidoglycan synthesis

10. W.A. started a treatment that included meropenem, a carbapenem antibiotic with a very broad activity spectrum. Which of the following sets of activity spectrum is correct for carbapenems?

Set	Klebsiella pneumoniae	Mycoplasma pneumoniae	Legionella pneumophila	Enterococcus faecalis	Streptococcus pneumoniae
A.	Resistant	Sensitive	Sensitive	Resistant	Sensitive
B.	Sensitive	Resistant	Resistant	Resistant	Sensitive
C.	Sensitive	Sensitive	Sensitive	Sensitive	Resistant
D.	Sensitive	Resistant	Resistant	Sensitive	Sensitive

Answers and Explanations

▶ *Learning objective:* Identify the two urinary tests that are most indicative for a UTI.

1. Answer: C

Both bacteriuria and positive urinary nitrite are indicative of UTI. Bacteriuria with > 20 bacteria per HPF is indicative for UTI. Nitrites are found in urine because gram-negative bacteria contain enzymes that reduce urine nitrate to nitrite. The specificity of the urinary nitrite test is quite high, and a positive result is highly predictive of UTI.

B, D, E Usually the presence of WBC in the urine indicates a UTI, but the patient has negligible urinary WBC.

A, D, E Hematuria can occur in about half of UTIs, but the patient has negligible urinary RBC.

▶ *Learning objective:* Differentiate between acute uncomplicated cystitis and other types of UTI.

2. Answer: A

The patient was most likely suffering from acute uncomplicated cystitis. A UTI is considered

▶ **complicated** when there are underlying factors that predispose to ascending bacterial infection

▶ **uncomplicated** when it occurs without underlying abnormality or impairment of urine flow

The present patient has no factors that can predispose to ascending bacterial infection, such as a urinary catheter, anatomic abnormalities, obstruction of urine flow by calculi, or bladder neurogenic dysfunction. Therefore her UTI should be uncomplicated. In women sexual intercourse usually precedes uncomplicated cystitis, because bacteria from the gastrointestinal tract can be introduced into the urethral opening during intercourse. The postmenopausal age and the previous history of UTIs are also factors that can lead to acute uncomplicated cystitis. Both were factors in the present case.

B, C Symptoms and signs of pyelonephritis usually include chills, fever, and flank or colicky abdominal pain. Costovertebral angle percussion tenderness is generally present on the infected side. These symptoms and signs are absent in this patient.

D Urethritis in women can have symptoms and signs very close to those of cystitis, but acute complicated urethritis must have factors that predispose to ascending bacterial infection.

E A chronic disease, as defined by the U.S. National Center for Health Statistics, is a disease lasting 3 months or longer.

▶ *Learning objective:* Identify the two bacteria that are the most frequent cause of UTI.

3. Answer: E

Escherichia coli is by far the most frequent cause of UTI, accounting for 75 to 95% of cases. The second most common is *Staphylococcus saprophyticus*, which can account for 5 to 30% of cases. Other bacteria that can cause UTIs include *Proteus mirabilis*, *Klebsiella pneumoniae, Pseudomonas aeruginosa*, and *Enterococcus faecalis*. UTIs can also be caused by yeasts (*Candida albicans*), viruses (adenoviruses), and helminths (*Schistosoma haematobium*). Sexually transmitted UTIs are caused primarily by *Neisseria gonorrhoeae* and *Mycoplasma genitalium*.

A, B, C, D, F *Legionella pneumophila* and *Clostridium difficile* do not cause UTIs.

▶ *Learning objective:* Identify the two enzymes specifically inhibited by the trimethoprim–sulfamethoxazole combination.

4. Answer: C

By inhibiting dihydropteroate synthase, sulfonamides inhibit the formation of folate. By inhibiting dihydrofolate reductase, trimethoprim inhibits the formation of dihydrofolate and tetrahydrofolate.

Inhibition of these consecutive steps in the formation of tetrahydrofolate constitutes a sequential blockade and results in antibacterial synergy and decreased resistance.

A, B, D Inhibition of DNA gyrase would be the mechanism of action of fluoroquinolones.

B, E, F Inhibition of transglycosylase would be the mechanism of action of vancomycin.

▶ *Learning objective:* Explain the mechanism of resistance to sulfonamides.

5. Answer: C

Many bacteria originally sensitive to sulfonamides are resistant today. Resistance to trimethoprim–sulfamethoxazole is less frequent than resistance to either of the agents alone, but it can still occur in several cases. When resistance develops, it is usually persistent and irreversible. Mechanisms of resistance to sulfonamides include the following:

▶ Decreased affinity for sulfonamides by dihydropteroate synthetase
▶ Decreased bacterial permeability to the drug
▶ Increased production of para-aminobenzoic acid (PABA). For example, some resistant staphylococci may synthesize 70 times as much PABA as do the susceptible parental strains.

A, E These mechanisms would increase, not decrease, the bacterial sensitivity to sulfonamides.

B Sulfonamides do not act by binding to bacterial ribosomes.

D Sulfonamides do not act by binding to dihydrofolate reductase.

▶ *Learning objective:* Explain the mechanism of action of fluoroquinolones.

6. Answer: B

Ciprofloxacin is a fluoroquinolone antibiotic. Fluoroquinolones inhibit bacterial DNA synthesis by blocking the following enzymes:

▶ Topoisomerase II (also called DNA gyrase). The blockade prevents the relaxation of supercoiled DNA, which

is required for normal transcription (prevalent mechanism in gram-negative bacteria).
▶ Topoisomerase IV. The blockade interferes with separation of replicated chromosomal DNA during cell division (prevalent mechanism in gram-positive bacteria).

A Inhibition of bacterial cell wall synthesis would be the mechanism of action of β-lactam antibiotics.
C Stimulation of synthesis of abnormal bacterial proteins would be the mechanism of action of aminoglycosides.
D Inhibition of ergosterol synthesis in bacterial cell membranes would be the mechanism of action of antifungal azoles.
E Helicases are bacterial enzymes involved in DNA replication. Fluoroquinolones have no activity on these enzymes.
F This would be the mechanism of action of rifampin.

▶ *Learning objective:* Explain the interaction between antacids and fluoroquinolones.

7. Answer: D

Antacids can significantly decrease fluoroquinolone intestinal absorption (up to 70%) because certain cations (e.g., Ca^{2+}, Mg^{2+}, and Al^{3+}) can form insoluble complexes with them. The interaction can be avoided by taking the antacids 2 hours before or 4 hours after a fluoroquinolone dose, but this practice is complicated for the patient. Patients should simply avoid these products while taking fluoroquinolones.
A, B, C Antacids do not have these effects.

▶ *Learning objective:* Identify a serious adverse effect of fluoroquinolones.

8. Answer: B

Pseudomembranous colitis can occur with all antibiotics, but fluoroquinolones, clindamycin, and broad-spectrum penicillins and cephalosporins are the antibiotic classes most frequently associated with the disease. Pseudomembranous colitis can subside in 2 to 4 weeks, if properly treated, but it can have a fulminant course with a high mortality rate.

A, C, D, E Fluoroquinolones do not increase the risk of these disorders.

▶ *Learning objective:* Identify the mechanism of action of meropenem.

9. Answer: E

Meropenem is a β-lactam antibiotic from the carbapenem subclass. The patient's urinalysis indicates that her pyelonephritis was polymicrobial. Since she had had repeated UTIs, her bacteria were most likely resistant to several antibiotics; therefore a broad-spectrum antibiotic is needed. Carbapenems have the widest activity spectrum among β-lactam drugs. All β-lactam antibiotics act by inhibiting peptidoglycan synthesis.
A Misreading of the messenger RNA template code would be the mechanism of action of aminoglycosides. These drugs are not active against most gram-positive bacteria.
B Inhibition of tetrahydrofolate synthesis would be the mechanism of action of sulfonamides and trimethoprim.
C Inhibition of RNA polymerization would be the mechanism of action of rifamycins.
D Blockade of peptidyl-transfer RNA translocation would be the mechanism of action of macrolides.

▶ *Learning objective:* Identify the correct activity spectrum of carbapenems.

10. Answer: D

Carbapenems are effective against:
▶ Many gram-positive bacteria (including *Enterococcus faecalis* and *Streptococcus pneumoniae*)
▶ Many gram-negative bacteria (including *Klebsiella pneumoniae*)
Carbapenems are not effective against *Mycoplasma* sp (*Mycoplasma pneumoniae*) and *Legionella* sp (*Legionella pneumophila*)
A This would be a correct antibacterial spectrum for macrolides.
B This would be a correct antibacterial spectrum for third-/fourth-generation cephalosporins.
C This would be a correct antibacterial spectrum for fluoroquinolones.

Index

A

Abnormal heart valve, 215
Abstinence syndrome, 94
ABVD anticancer regimen,
    186
  alopecia, 186
  myelosuppression, 186
Accelerated phase, leukemia,
    179
ACE. See Angiotensin-
    converting enzyme
    (ACE)
ACE inhibitor contraindica-
    tions, 112
ACE inhibitor–induced angio-
    edema, 112
ACE inhibitors. See Angio-
    tensin-converting
    enzyme (ACE)
    inhibitors
Acetaminophen-codeine,
    256–257
Acetone increase, 428
Acetylcholine decrease, 263
Acetylcholine secretion
    (ACh), 294
ACh. See Acetylcholine secre-
    tion (ACh)
Acid. See LSD
Acidophils, 3
Acid phosphatase level, 350
Aciterin, 360
Acne treatment, 195
Acquired immunodeficiency
    syndrome (AIDS),
    206
Acromegaly, 1–7
  anterior pituitary gland
    cells, 3
    acidophils, 3
    basophils, 3
    corticotrophs, 3
    gonadotrophs, 3
    lactotrophs, 3
    somatrophs, 3
    thyrotrophs, 3
  bone overgrowth, 7
  chemoreceptor trigger
    zone (CTZ), 6
  cyclic adenosine mono-
    phosphate (cAMP)
    levels, 5
  dopamine agonists, 5

adverse effects, 6
    bromocriptine, 5
    cabergoline, 5
  GH-secreting adenoma, 3
  growth hormone (GH), 3
  hypothalamic hormones, 4
    GH-releasing hormone
      (GHRH), 4
    somatostatin (SST), 4
  macroadenoma, 4
  nonfunctional pituitary
    adenoma, 4
  octreotide, 4
    adverse effects, 6
  pegvisomant, 6
  pituitary tumor mass, 4
  prognathism, 7
  prolactinoma, 5
  prolactin release, 5
  somatostatin analogues, 4
    lanreotide, 4
    octreotide, 4
  SST receptors (SSTRs), 5
  transsphenoidal surgery, 5
Activated partial thrombo-
    plastin time (aPTT),
    32, 369
Acute angle-closure glau-
    coma, 131
Acute emesis, 186–187
Acute lymphoblastic leuke-
    mia, 9–15
  asparaginase, 14
    adverse reaction, 14
  CNS preventative therapy,
    14
    intracranial irradiation,
      14
    intrathecal administra-
      tion of anticancer
      drugs, 14
    methotrexate, 14
  cure rate, 12
  diagnosis, 12
  rasburicase mechanism of
    action, 15
  sevelamer mechanism of
    action, 15
  symptoms, 7
  treatment phases, 13
    CNS prophylaxis, 13
    consolidation, 13
    induction, 13
    maintenance, 13

    tumor lysis syndrome, 14
      catabolism, 14
      hyperphosphatemia, 14
      phosphate concentra-
        tion, 14
    vinca alkaloids, 13
      dose-limiting myelosup-
        pression, 13
      toxicities, 13
      vinblastine, 13
      vincristine, 13
      vincristine neuropathy, 13
Acute-phase reaction, 21
Acute uncomplicated cystitis,
    448
Adalimumab, 67
Addiction, 90
Addison's disease. See
    Primary adrenal
    deficiency (Addi-
    son's disease)
Adenine, 137
Adenocarcinomas, 349
Adenosine deaminase, 136
ADPKD. See Autosomal domi-
    nant gene (ADPKD)
Affinity for target channels,
    34
Afterdepolarizations, 423
Age-related acceleration in
    oocyte degenera-
    tion, 302
AIDS. See Acquired immuno-
    deficiency syn-
    drome (AIDS)
AIDS vs. HIV, 206
Albuterol
  asthma, 21
  chronic kidney disease, 75
Albuterol-induced tremor, 83
Alcohol and substance abuse,
    bipolar disorder, 40
Alcoholic liver disease, 234
Aldosterone, 172
Aldosterone receptor antago-
    nist, 333
Alkylating drug, 417
Allergic rhinitis, 20
Allopurinol treatment,
    138–139
Alloxanthine, 139
Alopecia, 186
αβ-adrenoceptor blocker,
    171

Index

α-₂ adrenoceptor agonist, 131
Alteplase
　myocardial infarction, 276
　　adverse effect, 276
　　mechanism of action, 276
　stroke, 406
Alveolar ventilation, 367
Amantadine, 288
Amenorrhea, 302
Aminoglycoside antibiotic, 263
Aminosalicylates, 65
Amiodarone
　atrial fibrillation, 35
　torsade de pointes, 423
Amlodipine, 111
Ammonia detoxification impairment, 236
Ammonia secretion, 74
Anabolic GH effects, 157
Anastrozole, 49
　adverse effects, 50
　aromatase inhibition, 49–50
Anatomical site of Crohn's disease, 63
Androgen-binding protein (ABP), 159
Androgen receptors, 158
Anemia, 77. See also Folic acid anemia; Iron deficiency anemia; Megaloblastic anemia
Anemia-induced loss of pain sensation, 249
Anesthesia, general, 115–124
　antimuscarinic drug, 122
　benzodiazepines, 118–119
　dantrolene, 123
　depolarizing neuromuscular blocking drug, 120
　glycopyrrolate, 122
　inhalational MAC, 120
　IV use, 119
　ketorolac, 123
　malignant hyperthermia, 123
　　mechanism, 123
　　pathogenesis, 123
　midazolam, 118–119
　minimum alveolar concentration (MAC), 120
　neostigmine, 122
　nitrous oxide MAC, 120
　nondepolarizing skeletal muscle relaxant, 121
　nonsteroidal anti-inflammatory drug (NSAID), 123

propofol, 119, 123
　adverse effect, 119
　ion channel action, 119
　reversible cholinesterase inhibitors, 122
　sevoflurane with nitrous oxide, 120–121
　rapid recovery from, 121
　stages, 118
　excitatory symptoms, 118
　succinylcholine, 120
　vecuronium, 121
　sequence of muscle paralysis, 121
Angiotensin-converting enzyme (ACE), 77
Angiotensin-converting enzyme (ACE) inhibitors
　heart failure, 171, 172
　stroke, 407
Angiotensin II, 172
Angiotensin II receptor antagonists, 112
Anisocytosis, 249
Angle-closure glaucoma, 128
Anovulatory cycles, 331
Anovulatory infertility, 334
ANP. See Atrial natriuretic peptide (ANP)
ANP-induced increase in cGMP, 30
Antacid drugs, 294
Anterior pituitary gland cells, 3
　acidophils, 3
　basophils, 3
　corticotrophs, 3
　gonadotrophs, 3
　lactotrophs, 3
　somatrophs, 3
　thyrotrophs, 3
Antibiotic prophylaxis, 368
Antifungal azole subclass, 205
Antimetabolite anticancer drug, 241
Antimuscarinic drug
　anesthesia, 122
　glaucoma, 130
　Parkinson's disease, 286
Antiplatelet drug
　heart failure, 278
　stroke, 406–407
Antiprotease activity, 83
Antiresorptive drugs, 305
Antithrombin III (ATIII), 368
Antiviral agent, 288
Apomorphine, 288
　adverse effect, 288–289
Apraclonidine, 131

Aprepitant, 187
aPTT. See Activated partial thromboplastin time (aPTT)
Aqueous humor, 129
　decreased production of, 129
　latanoprost mediation, 130
　primary path for outflow of, 129
　secondary pathway for outflow of, 129
Arachidonic acid, 22
Aripiprazole, 390, 391
Arthritis, 415. See also Rheumatoid arthritis
Asparaginase, 14
　adverse reaction, 14
Aspirin administration, 274
Aspirin vs. warfarin, 31
Asthma, 17–24
　albuteral, 21
　allergic rhinitis, 20
　arachidonic acid, 22
　atopy, 20
　azole subclass, 23
　β2-adrenoceptors, 21
　bronchial hyperreactivity, 20
　candidiasis, 23
　chronic obstructive pulmonary disease (COPD), 20
　clotrimazole, 23–24
　cyclic adenosine monophosphate (cAMP) levels, 21
　cytochrome P450 enzymes, 23
　expiratory reserve volume (ERV), 20
　fluticasone, 22
　forced vital capacity (FVC), 20
　glucocorticoids, 22–23
　　drug-induced oral candidiasis, 23
　hyperreactivity, 20
　IgE antibodies, 20
　inspiratory reserve volume (IRV), 20
　leukotriene receptor antagonists, 23
　　montelukast, 23
　　zafrilukast, 23
　leukotrienes, 21
　opportunistic fungal infection, 23
　pathogenesis, 21
　　acute-phase reaction, 21
　　eosinophils, 21

late-phase reaction, 21
mast cells, 21
Th2 helper cells, 21
phospholipase A2, 22
residual volume (RV), 20
spirometry, 20
tidal volume (TV), 20
Asymptomatic heart failure,
168
Atonic seizures, 99
Atopy, 20
Atrial fibrillation, 25–35
amiodarone, 35
atrial rate, 29
cardiac electrical impulses,
29–30
chronic obstructive pulmonary disorder (COPD),
31, 34
coagulation cascade, 32
coumarin anticoagulant, 32
diltiazem, 33, 34
affinity for target chan-
nels, 34
site of action, 34
electrical cardioversion
(EC), 33
flecainide, 35
heart rate, 29
hemostasis, 32
activated partial throm-
boplastin time
(aPTT), 32
international normalized
ratio (INR), 32
hyperthyroidism, 31
ibutilide, 35
left ventricular filling, 30
lightheadedness, 30
procainamide, 35
prothrombin, 32
quaternary anticholinergic
drugs, 34
rate control, 33, 34
rhythm control, 33
sotalol, 35
stroke, 31
systemic emboli, 31, 33
urinary urgency, 30
ANP-induced increase in
cGMP, 30
atrial natriuretic peptide
(ANP), 30
cyclic guanosine mono-
phosphate (cGMP),
30
vitamin K administration,
33
vitamin K synthesis inhibition, 31, 32

warfarin therapy, 31
vs. aspirin, 31
Atrial natriuretic peptide
(ANP), 30
Atrial rate, 29
ATIII. See Antithrombin III
(ATIII)
Aura phase of migraine, 254
Autoimmune attack, 262
Autoimmune disorder
psoriasis, 358
systemic lupus erythemato-
sus, 415
Autonomic control of eye, 130
ciliary muscle, 130
radial muscle, 130
sphincter muscle, 130
Autosomal dominant gene
(ADPKD), 76
Azathioprine
Crohn's disease, 67–68
myasthenia gravis, 266
Azithromycin, 324
Azole antifungal agent,
440–441
Azole subclass, 23

B

Bacteremia, 215
Bacteriuria, 448
Baroreceptor reflex, 110
Basal ganglia, 284
Basophils, 3
Benign prostatic hyperplasia,
350
Benzodiazepines, 118–119
Benztropine, 286
β_1-adrenoceptor agonist,
56–57
β_2-adrenoceptors, 21
β-lactam antibiotic
infective endocarditis, 216
liver cirrhosis, 235
UTI, 450
Betamethasone, 359
β-receptors, 149
Bile acids, 68
Bile salts, 68
Biologic DMARD advantages,
380
adverse effects, 381
Bipolar disorder, 37–41
age of onset, 39
alcohol and substance
abuse, 40
carbamazepine, 41
lithium, 40
adverse effects, 40
mechanism, 40
overdose toxicity, 40

loop diuretics, 41
olanzapine, 41
prevalence, 39
psychotic features, 39
thiazide diuretics, 41
Bismuth salt, 297
Bisphosphonate drug, 352
Bisphosphonates, 305
adverse effects, 306–307
Blast phase, leukemia, 179
Bleomycin, 188–189
lethal effect, 188–189
mechanism, 188
Blood pressure definition, 110
Blood pressure drop, 314–315
Blood pressure–lowering
goals, 109
Blood supply, large tumors,
240–241
Blood urea nitrogen (BUN), 73
Blood vessel resistance,
Poiseuille's equation
for, 111
Bone overgrowth, 7
Bone scan, 350
Botulinum toxin, 407
Bradykinin, 112
Breast cancer, 42–50
anastrozole, 49
adverse effects, 50
aromatase inhibition,
49–50
ERBB2 receptor protein, 47
family history, 46
human epidural growth
factor receptor
(EGFR), 47, 49
laminins, and metastasization, 47
lymph node correlation, 47
raloxifene, 48
raloxifene-induced venous
thromboembolism, 48
selective estrogen receptor
modulator (SERM), 48
stages, 47
tamoxifen, 48
trastuzumab
adverse effects, 49
mechanism, 49
Brimonidine, 131
Broca's aphasia, 404
Bromocriptine, 5
Bronchial hyperreactivity, 20
BUN. See Blood urea nitrogen
(BUN)
Busulfan, 179

C

Cabergoline, 5

Index

Calcipotriene, 359
Calcium channel blocker, 314
Calcium salts, 75
cAMP levels. *See* Cyclic adenos-
   ine monophosphate
   (cAMP) levels
Candidiasis, 23
Cannabinoid receptors, 90
Captopril, 407
Catabolic GH effects, 157
Ca^{2+} channel blocker, 85
Carbamazepine
   adverse effect, 101
   antiseizure action, 100
   bipolar disorder, 41
   induction of own metabo-
      lism, 103
Carbapenems, 450
Carbidopa, 286
Carbonic anhydrase inhibitor,
   131
Cardiac electrical impulses,
   29–30
Cardiac oxygen consumption
   change, 56
Cardiogenic shock, 51–57
   cardiac oxygen consump-
      tion change, 56
   cardiovascular parameter
      changes, 54
      pulmonary capillary
         wedge pressure
         (PCWP), 54
      total peripheral resistance
         (TPR), 54
   dobutamine
      β1-adrenoceptor agonist,
         56–57
      molecular mechanism, 56
   dopamine by IV infusion
      rationale, 55
   double product, 56
   stroke volume increase
      after dopamine
      administration, 56
   therapeutic window of a
      drug, 55
Cardiovascular parameter
   changes, 54
   pulmonary capillary wedge
      pressure (PCWP), 54
   total peripheral resistance
      (TPR), 54
Carvedilol, 171
   action mediating therapeu-
      tic effect, 171
   molecular mechanism, 171
Catabolism, 14
Catastrophic hemodynamic
   collapse, 366

Catecholamine-induced
   tachycardia, 314
Catecholamines, 313
CD. *See* Crohn's disease (CD)
CD4 receptors, 205
Ceftriaxone, 324
Cell apoptosis, 188
Cell wall synthesis inhibitor,
   216
Central nervous system (CNS)
   prophylaxis, 14
   intracranial irradiation, 14
   intrathecal administration
      of anticancer drugs,
      14
   methotrexate, 14
Central nervous system (CNS)
   prophylaxis, 13
Cephalosporin
   pneumonia, 324
   solid organ transplant, 397
Cerebral artery blockage, 404
cGMP. *See* Cyclic guanosine
   monophosphate
   (cGMP)
CHCs. *See* Combination
   hormonal contracep-
   tives (CHCs), 194
Chemoreceptor trigger zone
   (CTZ), 6
Chemotherapy-induced
   emesis, 186
Chlorthalidone, 138
Cholinergic crisis, 266
Cholinesterase enzymes, 265
Chromaffin cells tumor, 313
Chronic bronchitis, 82
Chronic kidney disease,
   69–78
   albuterol, 75
   ammonia secretion, 74
   anemia, 77
   angiotensin-converting
      enzyme (ACE), 77
   autosomal dominant gene
      (ADPKD), 76
   blood urea nitrogen (BUN),
      73
   calcium salts, 75
   erythropoietin production,
      77
   glomerular filtration rate
      (GFR) calculation, 73
   hematuria, 76
   hyperkalemia, 74–75
   hypermagnesemia, 74–75
   hyperphosphatemia, 75–76,
      77
   hypertension, 77
   hypocalcemia, 76

insulin-dextrose IV, 75
metabolic acidosis, 74
polyuria, 73
prostacyclin, 78
prostaglandin E2, 78
renal toxicity, 78
serum creatine (SCr), 73
sevelamer, 77–78
stages, 73
Chronic myelogenous leukemia, 177
Chronic obstructive pulmonary disease (COPD),
   20, 31, 34, 79–85
   albuterol-induced tremor,
      83
   antiprotease activity, 83
   Ca2+ channel blocker, 85
   chronic bronchitis, 82
   diltiazem, 85
   emphysema, 82
   first second of expiration
      (FEV1), 82
   ipratropium, 84
      adverse effects, 84
      with salmeterol, 84
   losartan, 83
   lung volumes and capaci-
      ties, 82
   methylxanthine, 84
      adverse effects, 85
   pH decrease, 84
   protease activity, 83
   quaternary ammonium
      antimuscarinic drugs,
      84
   salmeterol, 84
   spirometry reduction, 83
   theophylline, 84
   wheezing, 82
Chronic stable phase, leukemia, 179
Chronic viral hepatitis B, 232
Ciliary body, 129
Ciliary epithelium, 129
Ciprofloxacin, 449–450
Cisplatin, 241
   adverse effect, 242
CK-MB ratio. *See* Creatin-
   kinase-MB (CK-MB)
   ratio
Class III antiarrhythmic drugs,
   423
Clindamycin, 217
Clomiphene, 334
Clonidine, 112, 315–316
   adverse effects, 112
Clopidogrel
   myocardial infarction, 278
   stroke, 407

Clotrimazole, 23–24
Clozapine, 391
  adverse effect, 391
CNS preventative therapy.
        See Central ner-
        vous system (CNS)
        prophylaxis
CNS prophylaxis. *See* Central
        nervous system
        (CNS) prophylaxis,
        13
Coagulation cascade
  atrial fibrillation, 32
  pulmonary embolism, 366
Cobalamin deficiency. *See*
        Vitamin B$_{12}$ (cobala-
        min) deficiency
Cocaine, 90
  addiction, 90
  overdose, 90
Colchicine, 138
Combination hormonal con-
        traceptives (CHCs),
        194, 332
  adverse effects, 195
  formulations, 196
  missed dose, 197
  over 35, 199–200
  quick-start method, 197
  smokers, 199–200
Community-acquired pneu-
        monia, 323
Compensatory hyperinsu-
        linemia, 333
Complex partial seizures, 99
Concomitant treatment with
        two antibiotics, 297
Contraceptives. *See* Hormonal
        contraceptives
COPD. *See* Chronic obstructive
        pulmonary disease
        (COPD)
Corticosteroids, 181
Coumarin anticoagulant, 32
Cortical bone size, 159
Cortical spreading depression
        (CSD), 254–255
Corticotrophs, 3
Counterregulatory hormones,
        443
COX-1. *See* Cyclooxygenase
        type 1 (COX-1)
C-peptide, 430
Creatine kinase, 408
Creatine-kinase-MB (CK-MB)
        ratio, 274
Crohn's disease (CD), 59–68
  adalimumab, 67
  aminosalicylates, 65
  anatomical site of, 63

azathioprine, 67–68
bile acids, 68
bile salts, 68
diagnostic biopsy, 64
dihydrofolate reductase, 66
glucocorticoids, 65
hemocrit, low, 64
infliximab, 67
  lethal adverse effect, 67
  substitutes, 67
iron deficiency anemia, 64
loperamide action, 64
mesalamine (5-ASA), 65
methotrexate, 65, 66
metronidazole, 66
natalizumab, 68
steatorrhea, 68
T-helper cells, 66
transmural inflammation, 63
tumor necrosis factor
        (TNF)-α, 67
weight loss, 64
Crystal-induced arthritis, 137
CSD. *See* Cortical spreading
        depression (CSD)
CTZ. *See* Chemoreceptor trig-
        ger zone (CTZ)
Cyclic adenosine monophos-
        phate (cAMP) levels,
        5, 21
Cyclic guanosine monophos-
        phate (cGMP), 30,
        275
Cyclooxygenase, 378
Cyclooxygenase type 1 (COX-
        1), 274
Cyclophosphamide, 417
  adverse effect, 417
Cyclosporine
  hematopoietic cell trans-
        plantation, 180
    action, 180
    adverse effect, 180
  psoriasis, 361
    adverse effect, 361
Cytochrome P450 enzymes,
        23
Cytokines involved in RA, 376

D

Dabigatran, 369
Dacarbazine, 189
Dantrolene, 123
Darifenacin, 130
Decreasing androgen synthe-
        sis, 332–333
Delayed emesis, 187
Dental surgery, 215
Depolarizing neuromuscular
        blocking drug, 120

Diabetes. *See* Type 1 diabetes
        mellitus; Type 2
        diabetes mellitus
Diabetic ketoacidosis (DKA),
        428
Diagnostic biopsy, Crohn's
        disease, 64
Diazepam, 103
Digoxin, 172
  antidote for poisoning,
        172–173
  atropine-resistant brady-
        cardia, 172
  hyperkalemia, 172
  nausea and vomiting, 172
Dihydrofolate formation, 449
Dihydrofolate reductase, 66
Dihydropyridine drugs, 111
Dilation of large arterial and
        venous meningeal
        vessels, 254
Diltiazem, 33, 34
  affinity for target channels,
        34
  COPD, 85
  site of action, 34
Diplopia, 262
Direct thrombin inhibitors,
        369
Disease-modifying anti-
        rheumatic drugs
        (DMARDs), 378
Diuresis, 398
Diuretic-induced hypokale-
        mia, 169
DKA. *See* Diabetic ketoacido-
        sis (DKA)
DM1. *See* Type 1 diabetes
        mellitus (DM1)
DM2. *See* Type 2 diabetes
        mellitus
DNA-dependent RNA-poly-
        merase, 208
Dobutamine
  β1-adrenoceptor agonist,
        56–57
  molecular mechanism, 56
Dopamine, 286
Dopamine agonists, 5
  adverse effects, 6
  bromocriptine, 5
  cabergoline, 5
Dopamine by IV infusion
        rationale, 55
Dopamine hypothesis, schizo-
        phrenia, 387–388
Dopamine increase, 90
Dopamine receptor agonist,
        285
Dorzolamide, 131

Dose-limiting myelosuppression, 13
Double product, 56
Double-stranded DNA antibody test, 415
Doxorubicin, 187–188
  lethal effect, 188
Drospirenone, 197
Drug abuse, 87–94
  cocaine, 90
    addiction, 90
    overdose, 90
  dopamine increase, 90
  heroin-induced miosis, 93
    Edinger-Westphal's nucleus, 93
  hypothalamic preoptic area, 90
  LSD, 92
  marijuana smoking, 90
    cannabinoid receptors, 90
    somatic indications of, 91
    therapeutic index of, 90
  median forebrain, 90
  methylenedioxymethamphetamine, 92
  naloxone, 94
    abstinence syndrome, 94
  opioid-induced respiratory depression, 93
    tolerance, 93
  phencyclidine, 92
    intoxication, 92
  reward system of the brain, 90
Drug-induced oral candidiasis, 23

E
Early morning hyperglycemia, 433
EC. See Electrical cardioversion (EC)
Edinger-Westphal's nucleus, 93
Efflux pumps, 324
EGFR. See Human epidural growth factor receptor (EGFR)
Electrical cardioversion (EC), 33
Emergency contraception, 194
Emphysema, 82
Emtricitabine, 207
Endogenous GH, 157
Endophonium, 265
Enoxaparin, 277
Entacapone, 287
Eosinophils, 21

Epilepsy, 95–103
  atonic seizures, 99
  carbamazepine, 100, 103
    adverse effect, 101
    antiseizure action, 100
    induction of own metabolism, 103
  complex partial seizures, 99
  diazepam, 103
  gabapentin, 103
  glutamatergic neurons increase in excitatory activity, 98
  inhibitory GABA neurons decrease in activity, 98
  lamotrigine, 102
    adverse effect, 102
  levetiracetam, 102
  lorazepam, 103
  myoclonic seizures, 99
  nystagmus, 100
  petit mal seizures, 99
  phenytoin, 99
    adverse effect, 100
    anticonvulsant effect, 99
    dose-dependent elimination, 100
  posttetanic potentiation inhibition, 100
  vs. seizures
  status epilepticus, 103
  tonic-clonic seizures, 99
    autonomic signs, 99
  topiramate, 102
  valporic acid, 101
    adverse effect, 101
    mechanism, 101
ERBB2 receptor protein, 47
Erectile dysfunction, 160
Ergotamine, 256
  -induced vasospasm, 256
Erlotinib, 242–243
  adverse effect, 243
ERV. See Expiratory reserve volume (ERV)
Erythrocyte sedimentation rate (ESR), 137
Erythrodermic, 358
Erythromycin, 296
Erythropoiesis deficiency, 248
Erythropoietin production, 77
ESR. see Erythrocyte sedimentation rate (ESR)
Essential hypertension. See Hypertension, essential
Estrogen, 194
Estrogen level decline, 303

Etanercept, 381
Ethambutol, 208
Euthyroid state, 148–149
Excess androgen production, 330
Exenatide, 443
Exophthalmos, 150
Expiratory reserve volume (ERV), 20
Extended-cycle contraceptives, 198
Extrinsic coagulation pathway, 367
Eye autonomous receptors, 129

F
Family history
  breast cancer, 46
  pheochronomocytoma, 314
  psoriasis, 359
Febuxostat, 139
Fenoldopam, 113
Ferratin, 223
FEV_1. See First second of expiration (FEV_1)
Fibrinolytic drug, 406
Filgrastim, 150
Final common pathway, 367
First second of expiration (FEV_1), 82
5-ASA. See Mesalamine (5-ASA)
$5-HT_{2A}$ receptors, 391
Flaccid skeletal muscle paralysis and acetylcholine, 267
Flecainide, 35
Fluconazole, 205
Fludarabine
  DM2, 441–442
  hematopoietic cell transplantation, 179
Fluoroquinolones
  pneumonia, 323
  UTIs, 449–450
    adverse effects, 450
    antacid interactions, 450
Flutamide, 352
  adverse effect, 352
Fluticasone, 22
Focal brain infarction, 404
Folate formation, 449
Folic acid anemia, 249
Follicle-stimulating hormone (FSH), 159, 160
Forced vital capacity (FVC), 20
FSH. See Follicle-stimulating hormone (FSH)

Furosemide, 169, 235
  adverse effects, 170
  decrease of kidney concen-
    trating ability, 169
  site of action, 169
  underlying therapeutic
    effect, 169
FVC. See Forced vital capacity
    (FVC)

G

Gabapentin, 103
Ganciclovir, 209
Gastric mucosal defense
    decrease, 295
Gemcitabine, 241
General anesthesia. See Anes-
    thesia, general
Gentamicin, 263
GFR calculation. See Glomer-
    ular filtration rate
    (GFR) calculation
GH. See Growth hormone
    (GH)
GH-releasing hormone
    (GHRH), 4
GHRH. See GH-releasing hor-
    mone (GHRH)
GH-secreting adenoma, 3
Glargine, 433
Glaucoma, 125–132
  acute angle-closure glau-
    coma, 131
  α-2 adrenoceptor agonist,
    131
  angle-closure glaucoma, 128
  antimuscarinic drug, 130
  apraclonidine, 131
  aqueous humor, 129
    decreased production of,
      129
    latanoprost mediation,
      130
    primary path for outflow
      of, 129
    secondary pathway for
      outflow of, 129
  autonomic control, 130
    ciliary muscle, 130
    radial muscle, 130
    sphincter muscle, 130
  brimonidine, 131
  carbonic anhydrase inhibi-
    tor, 131
  ciliary body, 129
  ciliary epithelium, 129
  darifenacin, 130
  dorzolamide, 131
  eye autonomous receptors,
    129

  hyperosmotic agent,
    131–132
  intraocular pressure (IOP),
    130
  latanoprost, 130
  mannitol, 131–132
  muscarinic agonist, 131
  open-angle glaucoma, 128
  optic neuropathy, 128
  pilocarpine, 131
  prostaglandin F2α ana-
    logue, 130
Gleason grading system, 350
Glimepiride, 441
Gliptin drugs, 442
Glomerular filtration rate
    (GFR) calculation, 73
Glomerulonephritis, 415
Glucocorticoids
  asthma, 22–23
  Crohn's disease, 65
  Hodgkin's lymphoma, 187
  myasthenia gravis, 266
  psoriasis, 359
Gluconeogenesis, 438
Glutamatergic neurons
    increase in excit-
      atory activity, 98
Glutamate hypothesis,
    schizophrenia, 388
Glutamate-mediated excito-
    toxicity, 405
Glycopyrrolate, 122
Gonadotrophs, 3
Gonadotropins, 335
Gout, 133–141
  adenine, 137
  adenosine deaminase, 136
  allopurinol treatment,
    138–139
  alloxanthine, 139
  chlorthalidone, 138
  colchicine, 138
  crystal-induced arthritis,
    137
  erythrocyte sedimentation
    rate (ESR), 137
  febuxostat, 139
  granulocyte migration, 138
  guanine, 137
  hyperuricemia, 137
  inosine, 136
  monosodium urate crystals,
    137
  NSAIDs use, 140
  opioid use, 140
  pegloticase, 140–141
  probenecid, 139
  purine drug, 139
  purines, 137

  recombinant mammalian
    uricase, 140–141
  renal colic, 140
  Stevens-Johnson's syn-
    drome, 140
  synovial fluid, 137
  thiazide-like diuretic, 138
  uric acid production, 136
  uric acid stones, 140
  uricosuric agent, 139–140
  white blood count (WBC),
    137
Graft-versus-host disease,
    180
Gram-negative bacteria, 450
Gram-positive bacteria, 450
Gram-positive bacterial infec-
    tion, 214
Granulocyte migration, 138
Graves' disease, 143–152
  β-receptors, 149
  euthyroid state, 148–149
  exophthalmos, 150
  filgrastim, 150
  hepatitis, 149
  hypothalamus-pituitary-
    thyroid axis, 147
  levothyroxine, 151
  methimazole, 148
  myxedema coma, 151–152
  prednisone, 150
  propylthiouracil, 148
  radioactive iodine (131I),
    150
  radioiodine uptake (RAIU)
    test, 148
  recombinant granulocyte-
    colony stimulating
    factor (G-CSG), 150
  thioamide agents, 149
    adverse reactions, 149
  thioamide drugs, 148
  thyroid growth-stimulating
    immunoglobulin
    (TGI), 147
  thyroid-stimulating hor-
    mone (TSH) receptors,
    146
  thyroid-stimulating immu-
    noglobulin (TSI),
    146–147
  thyroid storm, 149
  thyrotoxicosis, 149
  TSH-binding inhibitor
    immunoglobulin
    (TBII), 147
Growth hormone (GH), 3
Growth retardation and
    hypogonadism,
    153–161

Index

anabolic GH effects, 157
androgen-binding protein (ABP), 159
androgen receptors, 158
catabolic GH effects, 157
cortical bone size, 159
endogenous GH, 157
erectile dysfunction, 160
follicle-stimulating hormone (FSH), 159, 160
human chorionic gonadotropin (HCG), 160
Kallmann's syndrome, 159
Klinefelter's syndrome, 159
luteinizing hormone, 159, 160
phosphodiesterase 5 (PDE5) inhibitors, 160, 161
Prader-Willis syndrome, 159
primary hypogonadism, 157
recombinant human growth hormone (rhGH), 156
secondary hypogonadism, 157
Sheehan's syndrome, 159
sildenafil, 160
somatomedins, 157
somatropin, 156, 157
spermatogenesis, 160
tadalafil, 160
tertiary hypogonadism, 157
testosterone replacement therapy, 158
Turner's syndrome, 160
Guanine, 137
Guttate, 358
Gynecomastia
    heart failure, 170–171
    prostate cancer, 352
    schizophrenia, 390

H

HAART. See Highly active antiretroviral therapy (HAART)
Haloperidol, 389
    adverse effect, 389
HbA₁c, 439, 444
HCG. See Human chorionic gonadotropin (HCG)
HCl. See Hydrochloric acid (HCl)
Heart action phases, 422
Heart action repolarization, 422
Heart failure, 163–174
    aldosterone, 172

αβ-adrenoceptor blocker, 171
angiotensin-converting enzyme (ACE) inhibitors, 171, 172
angiotensin II, 172
asymptomatic heart failure, 168
carvedilol, 171
    action mediating therapeutic effect, 171
    molecular mechanism, 171
digoxin, 172
    antidote for poisoning, 172–173
    atropine-resistant bradycardia, 172
    hyperkalemia, 172
    nausea and vomiting, 172
diuretic-induced hypokalemia, 169
furosemide, 169
    adverse effects, 170
    decrease of kidney concentrating ability, 169
    site of action, 169
    underlying therapeutic effect, 169
gynecomastia, 170–171
high risk heart failure, 168
loop diuretics, 169
    low GFR, 170
    vs. thiazide diuretics, 170
low-output systolic heart failure, 167
mean blood pressure decrease in systolic heart failure, 167
nocturia, 168
orthopnea, 168
refractory heart failure, 168
spironolactone, 170–171
spironolactone use, 172
stages, 168
symptomatic heart failure, 168
Heart rate, 29
Heart transplant. See Solid organ transplant
Hematopoietic cell transplantation, 175–181
accelerated phase, 179
blast phase, 179
busulfan, 179
chronic myelogenous leukemia, 177
chronic stable phase, 179
corticosteroids, 181

cyclosporine, 180
    action, 180
    adverse effect, 180
fludarabine, 179
graft-versus-host disease, 180
host-versus-graft disease, 180
imatinib, 178
    adverse effect, 178
    failure of, 178
    mechanism of action, 178
myeloablative preparative regimen, 179
nephrotoxicity, 180
nilotinib, 178
oncogene of Philadelphia chromosome, 177
purine analogue, 179
Hematuria, 76
Heme, 222–223
Heme moieties, 222
Hemocrit, low, 64
Hemoglobin, 222
Hemostasis, 32
    activated partial thromboplastin time (aPTT), 32
    international normalized ratio (INR), 32
Heparin-induced inhibition, 368
Hepatic artery, 231
Hepatic encephalopathy, 232
Hepatitis, 149
HER inhibitors. See Human epidermal growth factor receptor (HER) inhibitors
Heroin
    Edinger-Westphal's nucleus, 93
    and HIV, 205
    induced miosis, 93
HHM. See Humora-hypocalcemia of malignancy (HHM)
Highly active antiretroviral therapy (HAART), 206
High risk heart failure, 168
HIV infection. See Human immunodeficiency virus (HIV) infection
HIV vs. AIDS, 206
Hodgkin's lymphoma, 183–189
    ABVD anticancer regimen, 186
    alopecia, 186
    myelosuppression, 186

acute emesis, 186–187
aprepitant, 187
bleomycin, 188–189
    lethal effect, 188–189
    mechanism, 188
cell apoptosis, 188
chemotherapy-induced emesis, 186
dacarbazine, 189
delayed emesis, 187
doxorubicin, 187–188
    lethal effect, 188
glucocorticoids, 187
ondansetron, 187
stages, 185–186
Stenberg's cells, 185
vinblastine, 189
Hormonal contraceptives, 191–200
acne treatment, 195
combination hormonal contraceptives (CHCs), 194
    adverse effects, 195
    formulations, 196
    missed dose, 197
    over 35, 199–200
    quick-start method, 197
    smokers, 199–200
drospirenone, 197
emergency contraception, 194
estrogen, 194
extended-cycle contraceptives, 198
levonorgestrel, 194
ovarian cancer, 199
Plan B-One Step, 194
progestin, 194
    pharmacology, 199
synthetic progestins, 196
    clinical applications, 196
venous thromboembolism (VTE), 198
Hormone replacement therapy (HRT), 304
adverse effects, 306
Host-versus-graft disease, 180
Hot flash, 302, 303, 304
HRT. See Hormone replacement therapy (HRT)
Human chorionic gonadotropin (HCG), 160
Human epidermal growth factor receptor (HER) inhibitors, 242–243
Human epidural growth factor receptor (EGFR), 47, 49

Human immunodeficiency virus (HIV) infection, 201–209
antifungal azole subclass, 205
CD4 receptors, 205
DNA-dependent RNA-polymerase, 208
emtricitabine, 207
ethambutol, 208
fluconazole, 205
ganciclovir, 209
heroin addiction, 205
highly active antiretroviral therapy (HAART), 206
HIV vs. AIDS, 206
integrase strand transfer, 208
isoniazid, 208
isoniazid-induced adverse effects, 208–209
lopinavir, 207
miconazole, 205
mycolic acid, 208
nonnucleoside reverse transcriptase inhibitors (NNRTIs), 206
nucleoside analogue, 209
nucleoside or nucleotide reverse transcriptase inhibitors (NRTIs), 206
nucleotide reverse transcriptase inhibitor, 207
oral candidiasis, 205
protease inhibitors, 207
pyridoxine, 208
raltegravir, 208
reverse transcriptase inhibitors, 206
rifampin, 208
ritonavir, 207
tenofovir, 207
tuberculosis, 208
Humora-hypocalcemia of malignancy (HHM), 240
Hydrochloric acid (HCl), 294, 296
Hydroxychloroquine, 378, 418
adverse effect, 379
Hydrochlorothiazide, 112
Hyperandrogenism, 330
Hyperglycemia, 315, 316
Hyperinsulinemia, 331
Hyperkalemia, 74–75
Hypermagnesemia, 74–75
Hyperosmotic agent, 131–132

Hyperphosphatemia, 14, 75–76, 77
Hyperprolactinemia, 390
Hyperreactivity, 20
Hypertension, 31, 77
Hypertension, essential, 105–113
ACE inhibitor contraindications, 112
ACE inhibitor–induced angioedema, 112
amlodipine, 111
angiotensin II receptor antagonists, 112
baroreceptor reflex, 110
blood pressure definition, 110
blood pressure–lowering goals, 109
bradykinin, 112
clonidine, 112
    adverse effects, 112
dihydropyridine drugs, 111
fenoldopam, 113
frequency, US population, 109
hydrochlorothiazide, 112
hypertensive crisis, 113
mean blood flow, 110
mean blood pressure, 109
Na+/Cl– symporter, 111
nitroprusside, 113
pathogenesis of, 110
Poiseuille's equation for blood vessel resistance, 111
renal retention of excess sodium, 110
system vascular resistance (SVR), 110
thiazides, 111
vasodilation mechanism, 111
Hypertensive crisis, 113
Hyperthyroidism, 31
Hyperuricemia, 137
Hypocalcemia, 76
Hypoglycemia, 432
Hypoglycemic agents, 441
Hypogonadism. See Growth retardation and hypogonadism
Hypokalemia, 233
Hypothalamic hormones, 4
GH-releasing hormone (GHRH), 4
somatostatin (SST), 4
Hypothalamic preoptic area, 90

Index

Hypothalamus-pituitary-thyroid axis, 147

I

Ibulitide, 35
ICP. *See* Intrinsic coagulation pathway (ICP)
Idaruciumab, 369–370
IgE antibodies, 20
IgG. *See* Immunoglobulin G (IgG)
Imatinib, 178
  adverse effect, 178
  failure of, 178
  mechanism of action, 178
Immune system dysregulation, 358
Immunoglobulin G (IgG), 264
Immunopathological phenomena, 215
Immunosuppressant drug, 361
Immunosuppressive therapy, 416
Inappropriate gonadotropin secretion, 330
Increased V/Q ratio, 367
Increasing synthesis of SHBG, 332
Incretin-mimetic agents, 443
Infective endocarditis, 211–217
  abnormal heart valve, 215
  bacteremia, 215
  β-lactam antibiotic, 216
  cell wall synthesis inhibitor, 216
  clindamycin, 217
  dental surgery, 215
  gram-positive bacterial infection, 214
  immunopathological phenomena, 215
  lincosamide antibiotic, 217
  minor oral trauma, 215
  penicillin G, 216
  septic embolization, 215
  sustained bacteremia, 215
  valvular destruction, 215
  vancomycin, 216
    activity spectrum, 217
    adverse effects, 216
    mechanism of action, 216
    site of action, 216
Infliximab
  Crohn's disease, 67
    lethal adverse effect, 67
    substitutes, 67
  psoriasis, 361
Inhalational MAC, 120

Inhibitory GABA neurons decrease in activity, 98
Inosine, 136
INR. *See* International normalized ratio (INR)
INR prothrombin time test. *See* International normalized ratio (INR) prothrombin time test
Inspiratory reserve volume (IRV), 20
Insulin, 430
  adverse effects, 432, 433
  intensive therapy, 432
  mechanism of action, 430
  physiological effects, 430–431
  rapid acting, 431
Insulin-dextrose IV, 75
Insulin pump, 431–432
Insulin resistance, 333
Insulin therapy, 443
Integrase strand transfer, 208
Intensive care immune-suppressed patients, 323
International normalized ratio (INR), 32
International normalized ratio (INR) prothrombin time test, 234
Intestinal absorption of iron, 224
  heme iron, 224
  inorganic iron, 224
Intracranial irradiation, 14
Intraoccular pressure (IOP), 130
Intrathecal administration of anticancer drugs, 14
Intrinsic coagulation pathway (ICP), 367
Inverse lesions, 358
IOP. *See* Intraoccular pressure (IOP)
Ipratropium, 84
  adverse effects, 84
  with salmeterol, 84
Iron deficiency anemia, 64, 219–226
  ferratin, 223
  heme, 222–223
  heme moieties, 222
  hemoglobin, 222
  intestinal absorption, 224
    heme iron, 224
    inorganic iron, 224
  IV iron administration, 225

NSAID-induced gastric damage, 223
  local action, 223
  systemic action, 224
oral iron therapy, 225
  gastrointestinal adverse effects, 226
physiological compensation for anemia, 224
quaternary structure of hemoglobin, 223
relaxed (R) configuration, 223
serum transferrin, 225
target organs, 225
tense (T) configuration, 223
tissue factors that increase hemoglobin, 223
IRV. *See* Inspiratory reserve volume (IRV)
Ischemia, 314
Ischemic pain, 272
Ischemic stroke, 404
Isoniazid, 208
Isoniazid-induced adverse effects, 208–209
Isoproterenol
  solid organ transplantation, 398
  torsade de pointes, 422

J

Jaundice, 233
Juvenile idiopathic arthritis, 375

K

Kallmann's syndrome, 159
Ketoacidosis, 431
Ketorolac, 123
Klinefelter's syndrome, 159

L

Labetalol
  pheochromocytoma, 317
  stroke, 405
Lactotrophs, 3
Lamotrigine, 102
  adverse effect, 102
Laminins, and metastasization, 47
Lanreotide, 4
Latanoprost, 130
Late-phase reaction, 21
Leflunomide, 380
Left ventricular filling, 30
Letrozole, 335
  adverse effects, 335
Leukotriene receptor antagonists, 23

montelukast, 23
zafrilukast, 23
Leukotrienes, 21
Leuprolide, 351
   adverse effect, 352
Levetiracetam, 102
Levodopa, 285, 286
   adverse effect, 287
   wearing-off and on-off
      reactions, 287
Levofloxacin, 323
Levonorgestrel, 194
Levothyroxine, 151
LH/FSH ratio, 331
Lightheadedness, 30
Lincosamide antibiotic, 217
Lipolysis, 439
Lisinopril, 278
   adverse effect, 279
   molecular mechanism, 278
Lithium, 40
   adverse effects, 40
   mechanism, 40
   overdose toxicity, 40
Liver cell failure, 232
Liver cirrhosis, 227–236
   alcoholic liver disease, 234
   ammonia detoxification
      impairment, 236
   β-lactam antibiotic, 235
   chronic viral hepatitis B,
      232
   furosemide, 235
   hepatic artery, 231
   hepatic encephalopathy,
      232
   hypokalemia, 233
   international normalized
      ratio (INR) prothrom-
      bin time test, 234
   jaundice, 233
   liver cell failure, 232
   meropenem, 235
   morphological changes
      characterizing, 331
   neutrophil count, 234
   portal hypertension, 232
   portal vein, 231
   propranolol, 235–236
   secondary hyperaldosteron-
      ism, 233
   spider angiomas, 233
   spironolactone, 234
LMWH. See Low-molecular-
      weight heparin
      (LMWH)
Loop diuretics, 169
   bipolar disorder, 41
   low GFR, 170
   vs. thiazide diuretics, 170

Loperamide action, 64
Lopinavir, 207
Lorazepam, 103
Losartan, 83
Lovastatin
   solid organ transplantation,
      399
   stroke, 408
      adverse effect, 408
Low-molecular-weight hepa-
      rin (LMWH), 277
Low-output systolic heart
      failure, 167
LSD, 92
Lung cancer, 237–243
   antimetabolite anticancer
      drug, 241
   blood supply, large tumors,
      240–241
   cisplatin, 241
      adverse effect, 242
   erlotinib, 242–243
      adverse effect, 243
   gemcitabine, 241
   human epidermal growth
      factor receptor (HER)
      inhibitors, 242–243
   humora-hypocalcemia of
      malignancy (HHM),
      240
   monoclonal antibodies, 243
   paclitaxel, 242
      adverse effect, 242
   platinum analogues, 241
   smoking and, 240
   squamous cell cancer, 240
   taxane derivatives, 242
   tyrosine kinase inhibitors,
      243
Lung infiltrate, 323
Lung volumes and capaci-
      ties, 82
Luteinizing hormone, 159,
      160
Lymph node correlation,
      breast cancer, 47

M

MAC. See Minimum alveolar
      concentration (MAC)
Macroadenoma, 4
Macrolide antibiotic, 296
Macrovascular complications
      of DM2, 444
Magnesium sulfate, 424
Main pulmonary artery
      occlusion, 366
Malignant hyperthermia, 123
   mechanism, 123
   pathogenesis, 123

Mannitol, 131–132
Marijuana smoking, 90
   cannabinoid receptors, 90
   somatic indications of, 91
   therapeutic index of, 90
Mast cells, 21
Mean blood flow, 110
Mean blood pressure, 109
   decrease in systolic heart
      failure, 167
Median forebrain, 90
Megaloblastic anemia,
      245–250
   anemia-induced loss of pain
      sensation, 249
   anisocytosis, 249
   erythropoiesis deficiency,
      248
   folic acid anemia, 249
   poikilocytosis, 249
   tetrahydrofolate synthesis
      impairment, 249–250
   vitamin B12 (cobalamin)
      deficiency, 248
      antianemic action of, 250
      available supply, 249
      length of therapy, 250
      oral dosage efficacy, 250
Meropenem
   liver cirrhosis, 235
   UTIs, 450
Mesalamine (5-ASA), 65
Mesocortical neuronal path-
      way, 388–389
Mesolimbic neuronal path-
      way, 388–389
Metabolic acidosis, 74
Metformin
   DMS2, 440
      adverse effects, 440
   polycystic ovarian syn-
      drome, 333, 334
Methimazole, 148
Methotrexate
   acute lymphoblastic leuke-
      mia, 14
   Crohn's disease, 65, 66
   psoriasis, 360
   rheumatoid arthritis, 379
      adverse effects, 379
Methylenedioxymetham-
      phetamine, 92
Methylprednisolone-induced
      gastric damage, 397
Methylxanthine
   COPD, 84
      adverse effects, 85
Methoxsalen, 360
Metoclopramide, 256
Metronidazole, 66

peptic ulcer disease, 296
Metoprolol, 277–278
Metyrosine, 316
Miconazole, 205
Microvascular complications of DM2, 444
Midazolam, 118–119
Migraine, 251–258
  acetaminophen-codeine, 256–257
  aura phase, 254
  cortical spreading depression (CSD), 254–255
  dilation of large arterial and venous meningeal vessels, 254
  ergotamine, 256
    -induced vasospasm, 256
  metoclopramide, 256
  neurovascular theory, 254
  NSAIDs and, 255
    gastric disorder, 255
  oral contraceptive risk, 255
  predisposition, 254
  prevalence in women, 253–254
  prodrome, 254
  prophylactic treatment, 257
    antiepileptic drugs, 257
    β-blockers, 257
  scintillating scotomas preceding, 254
  sumatriptan, 257
  valporic acid, 258
    prenatal risks, 258
  vasodilation, 255
Milrinone, 396–397
Miniature excitatory postsynaptic potentials (EPSPs), 264
Minimum alveolar concentration (MAC), 120
Minor oral trauma, 215
Monoclonal antibodies, 243
Monomorphic ventricular tachycardia, 421
Monosodium urate crystals, 137
Montelukast, 23
Muscarinic agonist, 131
Myasthenia gravis, 259–267
  acetylcholine decrease, 263
  aminoglycoside antibiotic, 263
  autoimmune attack, 262
  azathioprine, 266
    adverse effect, 266
  cholinergic crisis, 266
  cholinesterase enzymes, 265

diplopia, 262
endophonium, 265
flaccid skeletal muscle paralysis and acetylcholine, 267
gentamicin, 263
glucocorticoids, 266
immunoglobulin G (IgG), 264
miniature excitatory postsynaptic potentials (EPSPs), 264
nicotinic muscular postsynaptic receptors, 262
presynaptic acetylcholine stores, 263
ptosis, 262–263
pyridostigmine, 265
  atropine counteraction of side effect, 265
  side effects, 265, 266
skeletal muscle fiber, 263
thymus hyperplasia, 264
thymus involvement, 264
Mycolic acid, 208
Mycophenolate mofetil
  solid organ transplantation, 399
  systemic lupus erythematosus, 417, 418
Myeloablative preparative regimen, 179
Myelosuppression, 186
Myocardial infarction, 269–279
  alteplase, 276
    adverse effect, 276
    mechanism of action, 276
  antiplatelet drug, 278
  aspirin administration, 274
  clopidogrel, 278
  creatine-kinase-MB (CK-MB) ratio, 274
  cyclic guanosine monophosphate (cGMP), 275
  cyclooxygenase type 1 (COX-1), 274
  enoxaparin, 277
  ischemic pain, 272
  lisinopril, 278
    adverse effect, 279
    molecular mechanism, 278
  low-molecular-weight heparin (LMWH), 277
  metoprolol, 277–278
  nitrates, 275
  nitroglycerin, 275
  opioids, 275–276

platelet ADP receptor inhibitor, 278
S3 gallop, 273–274
sympathetic nervous system activation, 273
troponin 1, 274
Myoclonic seizures, 99
Myopathy, 408
Myxedema coma, 151–152

N

Na⁺/Cl⁻ symporter, 111
Naloxone, 94
  abstinence syndrome, 94
Natalizumab, 68
Necrosis of cerebral infarct, 405
Neostigmine, 122
Nephritis, 416
Nephrotoxicity, 180
Neurovascular theory of migraines, 254
Neutrophil count, 234
Nicotinic muscular postsynaptic receptors, 262
Nifedipine, 314
Nigrostriatal neuronal pathway, 388–389
Nigrostriatal pathway, 389
Nilotinib, 178
Nitrates, 275
Nitroglycerin
  myocardial infarction, 275
  solid organ transplant, 398
Nitroprusside, 113
Nitrous oxide MAC, 120
NNRTIs. See Nonnucleoside reverse transcriptase inhibitors (NNRTIs)
Nocturia, 168
Nonbiologic DMARD, 380
  adverse effect, 380
Nondepolarizing skeletal muscle relaxant, 121
Nonfunctional pituitary adenoma, 4
Nonnucleoside reverse transcriptase inhibitors (NNRTIs), 206
Nonselective β-adrenoceptor agonist, 398
Nonsteroidal anti-inflammatory drug (NSAID)
  anesthesia, 123
  gout, 140
  migraine, 255
  rheumatoid arthritis, 378
Nonsustained ventricular tachycardia, 421

NRTIs. *See* Nucleoside or nucleotide reverse transcriptase inhibitors (NRTIs)
NSAID. *See* Nonsteroidal anti-inflammatory drug (NSAID)
NSAID-induced gastric damage, 223, 255
  local action, 223
  systemic action, 224
Nucleoside analogue, 209
Nucleoside or nucleotide reverse transcriptase inhibitors (NRTIs), 206
Nucleotide reverse transcriptase inhibitor, 207
Nystagmus, 100

O

Octreotide, 4
  adverse effects, 6
Olanzapine, 41
Omeprazole
  peptic ulcer disease, 295, 296
  solid organ transplant, 397
Oncogene of Philadelphia chromosome, 177
Ondansetron, 187
Open-angle glaucoma, 128
Opioid-induced respiratory depression, 93
  tolerance, 93
Opioid use for pain, 140, 275–276
Opportunistic fungal infection, 23
Optic neuropathy, 128
Oral candidiasis, 205
Oral contraceptive risk and migraine, 255
Oral iron therapy, 225
  gastrointestinal adverse effects, 226
Orthopnea, 168
Osmotic diuresis, 429
Osteoporosis, 304
Ovarian cancer, 199
Ovarian dysfunction, 330
Ovarian follicle degeneration, 304
Overdose
  cocaine, 91
  lithium, 40
  opioid, 94
  phencyclidine, 92
  warfarin, 33

P

Paclitaxel, 242
  adverse effect, 242
Pamidronate, 352, 353
  adverse effect, 353
Parkinson's disease, 281–289
  amantadine, 288
  antimuscarine drug, 286
  antiviral agent, 288
  apomorphine, 288
    adverse effect, 288–289
  basal ganglia, 284
  benztropine, 286
  carbidopa, 286
  dopamine, 286
  dopamine receptor agonist, 285
  entacapone, 287
  levodopa, 285, 286
    adverse effect, 287
  pramipexole, 285
    adverse effect, 285–286
  presynaptic neuronal and glial cell protein, 284
  rasagiline, 285
  selective irreversible inhibitors of monoamine oxidase, 285
  striatum, 284
  synuclein, 284
  synucleinopathy, 284
  wearing–off and on-off reactions, 287
Paroxetine, 307
Pathological lesions, 358
PCOS. *See* polycystic ovarian syndrome
PCWP. *See* Pulmonary capillary wedge pressure (PCWP)
PDE5 inhibitors. *See* Phosphodiesterase 5 (PDE5) inhibitors
Pegloticase, 140–141
Pegvisomant, 6
Penicillin G, 216
Peptic ulcer disease, 291–297
  acetylcholine secretion (Ach), 294
  antacid drugs, 294
  bismuth salt, 297
  concomitant treatment with two antibiotics, 297
  erythromycin, 296
  gastric mucosal defense decrease, 295
  hydrochloric acid (HCl), 294, 296

macrolide antibiotic, 296
metronidazole, 296
omeprazole, 295, 296
proton pump inhibitors, 295, 296
somatostatin, 295
triple therapy, 297
Perimenopause and osteoporosis, 299–307
  age-related acceleration in oocyte degeneration, 302
  amenorrhea, 302
  antiresorptic drugs, 305
  bisphosphonates, 305
    adverse effects, 306–307
  estrogen level decline, 303
  hormone replacement therapy (HRT), 304
    adverse effects, 306
  hot flash, 302, 303, 304
  menopause, 302
    genitourinary atrophy, 303
    vasomotor symptoms, 303
  osteoporosis, 304
  ovarian follicle degeneration, 304
  paroxetine, 307
  progestin, 304
  selective serotonin reuptake inhibitors (SSRIs), 307
  serotonin and norepinephrine reuptake inhibitors (SNRIs), 307
  urinary tract infections, 306
  vaginal atrophy, 306
  venlafaxine, 307
Petit mal seizures, 99
pH decrease with COPD, 84
Phencyclidine, 92
  intoxication, 92
Phenoxybenzamine, 316
Phenytoin, 99
  adverse effect, 100
  anticonvulsant effect, 99
  dose-dependent elimination, 100
Pheochromocytoma, 309–317
  blood pressure drop, 314–315
  calcium channel blocker, 314
  catecholamine-induced tachycardia, 314
  catecholamines, 313
  chromaffin cells tumor, 313
  clonidine, 314–316
  family history, 314

Index

hyperglycemia, 315, 316
ischemia, 314
labetalol, 317
metyrosine, 316
nifedipine, 314
phenoxybenzamine, 316
propranolol, 317
pseudoephedrine paroxysmal symptoms, 313
symptoms, 313
Phosphate concentration, 14
Phosphodiesterase 5 (PDE5) inhibitors, 160, 161
Phosphodiesterase inhibitor, 396
Phospholipase A_2, 22
Physiological compensation for anemia, 224
Pilocarpine, 131
Pioglitazone, 441–442
adverse effects, 442
Pituitary tumor mass, 4
Plan B-One Step, 194
Plaque, 358
Platelet ADP receptor inhibitor, 278
Platinum analogues, 241
Pleuritic chest pain, 367
Pneumonia, 319–324
azithromycin, 324
ceftriaxone, 324
cephalosporins, 324
community-acquired pneumonia, 323
efflux pumps, 324
fluoroquinolones, 323
intensive care immune-suppressed patients, 323
levofloxacin, 323
lung infiltrate, 323
transport proteins, 324
Poikilocytosis, 249
Poiseuille's equation for blood vessel resistance, 111
Polycystic ovarian syndrome, 327–335
aldosterone receptor antagonist, 333
anovulatory cycles, 331
anovulatory infertility, 334
clomiphene, 334
combined hormonal contraceptives (CHC), 332
compensatory hyperinsulinemia, 333
decreasing androgen synthesis, 332–333
excess androgen production, 330

gonadotropins, 335
hyperandrogenism, 330
hyperinsulinemia, 331
inappropriate gonadotropin secretion, 330
increasing synthesis of SHBG, 332
insulin resistance, 333
letrozole, 335
adverse effects, 335
LH/FSH ratio, 331
metformin, 333, 334
ovarian dysfunction, 330
spironolactone, 333
Polymorphic ventricular tachycardia, 421
Polyuria, 73
Portal hypertension, 232
Portal vein, 231
Positive urinary nitrate, 448
Posttetanic potentiation inhibition, 100
Prader-Willis syndrome, 159
Pramipexole, 285
adverse effect, 285–286
Prednisone, 150
Preproinsulin, 428–429
Presynaptic acetylcholine stores, 263
Presynaptic neuronal and glial cell protein, 284
Primary adrenal deficiency (Addison's disease), 337–346
acute adrenal crisis, 345
aldosterone, 343–344
aldosterone deficiency, 341, 342
autoimmune adrenalitis, 341, 342
autoimmunity, 341
corticotrophin-releasing hormone (CRH), 341–342
cortisol, 344
cortisol deficiency, 341
fludrocortisone, 343, 345
glucocorticoids, 345–346
Graves' disease, 342
Hashimoto's thyroiditis, 342
hemorrhage, 341
homeostasis, 344
hydrocortisone, 353
adverse effects, 345
infection, 341
mineralocorticoid replacement, 343
Primary hypogonadism, 157
Probenecid, 139

Procainamide, 35
Prodrome, 254
Progestin, 194
perimenopause, 304
pharmacology, 199
synthetic, 196
Prognathism, 7
Progressive dyspnea, 366
Prolactinoma, 5
Prolactin release, 5
Prophylactic treatment for migraine, 257
antiepileptic drugs, 257
β-blockers, 257
Propofol, 119
adverse effect, 119
antiemetic properties, 123
ion channel action, 119
Propranolol, 235–236
liver cirrhosis, 235–236
pheochromcytoma, 317
Propylthiouracil, 148
Prostacyclin, 78
Prostaglandin E_2, 78
Prostaglandin $F_{2\alpha}$ analogue, 130
Prostaglandins, 378
Prostate cancer, 347–353
acid phosphatase level, 350
adenocarcinomas, 349
benign prostatic hyperplasia, 350
bisphosphonate drug, 352
bone scan, 350
flutamide, 352
adverse effect, 352
Gleason grading system, 350
Gn-RH agonist, 351
gynecomastia, 352
leuprolide, 351
adverse effect, 352
pamidronate, 352, 353
adverse effect, 353
peripheral zone, 350
prostate-specific antigen (PSA), 350
urinary problems, 350
Prostate-specific antigen (PSA), 350
Protamine sulfate, 368
Protease activity, 83
Protease inhibitors
HIV, 207
pulmonary embolism, 368
Prothrombin, 32
Proton pump inhibitors, 295, 296
PSA. See Prostate-specific antigen (PSA)

Pseudoephedrine paroxysmal symptoms, 313
Psoralens, 360
Psoriasis, 355–361
  aciterin, 360
  autoimmune disorder, 358
  betamethasone, 359
  calcipotriene, 359
  cyclosporine, 361
    adverse effect, 361
  erythrodermic, 358
  family history, 358
  glucocorticoids, 359
  guttate, 358
  immune system dysregulation, 358
  immunosuppressant drug, 361
  infliximab, 361
  inverse, 358
  methotrexate, 360
  methoxsalen, 360
  pathological lesions, 358
  plaque, 358
  psoralens, 360
  pustular, 358
  retinoid, 360
  salicylic acid, 359
  tumor necrosis factor-α (TNF-α) inhibitor, 361
  types, 358
Psychotic features, bipolar disorder, 39
Ptosis, 262–263
Pulmonary capillary wedge pressure (PCWP), 54
Pulmonary embolism 363–370
  activated partial thromboplastin time, 369
  alveolar ventilation, 367
  antibiotic prophylaxis, 368
  antithrombin III (ATIII), 368
  catastrophic hemodynamic collapse, 366
  coagulation cascade, 366
  dabigatran, 369
  direct thrombin inhibitors, 369
  extrinsic coagulation pathway, 367
  final common pathway, 367
  heparin-induced inhibition, 368
  idarucizumab, 369–370
  increased V/Q ratio, 367
  intrinsic coagulation pathway (ICP), 367
  main pulmonary artery occlusion, 366

  pleuritic chest pain, 367
  progressive dyspnea, 366
  protamine sulfate, 368
  protease inhibitor, 368
  tachycardia, 368
  thromboembolism, 366
  unfractionated heparin, 369
  vascular endothelial growth factor (VEGF), 367
Purine analogue, 179
Purine drug, 139
Purines, 137
Pustular lesions, 358
Pyridostigmine, 265
  atropine counteraction of side effect, 265
  side effects, 265, 266
Pyridoxine, 208

Q

Quaternary ammonium antimuscarinic drugs, 84
Quaternary anticholinergic drugs, 34
Quaternary structure of hemoglobin, 223
QT interval increase, 423
QT interval prolongation, 423

R

RA. See Rheumatoid arthritis (RA)
Radioactive iodine (¹³¹I), 150
Raloxifene, 48
Raloxifene-induced venous thromboembolism, 48
Raltegravir, 208
Rapid-acting insulin, 431
Rasagiline, 285
Rasburicase mechanism of action, 15
Rate control, 33, 34
R configuration. See Relaxed (R) configuration
Recombinant granulocyte-colony stimulating factor (G-CSG), 150
Recombinant human growth hormone (rhGH), 156
Recombinant mammalian uricase, 140–141
Refractory heart failure, 168
Relaxed (R) configuration, 223
Renal colic, 140
Renal retention of excess sodium, 110
Renal toxicity, 78
Residual volume (RV), 20

Retinoid, 360
Reverse transcriptase inhibitors, 206
Reversible cholinesterase inhibitors, 122
Reward system of the brain, 90
Rheumatoid arthritis (RA), 371–381
  biologic DMARD advantages, 380
    adverse effects, 381
  clinical and laboratory data criteria, 376
  cyclooxygenase, 378
  cytokines involved, 376
  disease-modifying antirheumatic drugs (DMARDs), 378
  etanercept, 381
  hydroxychloroquine, 378
    adverse effect, 379
  joints involved in, 376
  juvenile idiopathic arthritis, 375
  leflunomide, 380
  methotrexate, 379
    adverse effect, 379
  nonbiologic DMARD, 380
    adverse effect, 380
  NSAIDs and, 378
  onset age, 375
  percentage of population affected, 375
  prostaglandins, 378
  radiographic hallmarks, 376
  Sjögren's syndrome, 377
  subcutaneous necrotizing granulomas, 377
  synovial lining, 376
  TNF-α inhibitor, 381
rhGH. See Recombinant human growth hormone (rhGH)
Rhythm control, 33
Rifampin, 208
Ritonavir, 207
Rosiglitazone, 441–442
RV. See Residual volume (RV)

S

Salicylic acid, 359
Salmeterol, 84
Schizophrenia, 383–391
  aripiprazole, 390, 391
  clozapine, 391
    adverse effect, 391
  dopamine hypothesis, 387–388
  5-HT2A receptors, 391

Index

glutamate hypothesis, 388
gynecomastia, 390
haloperidol, 389
    adverse effect, 389
hyperprolactinemia, 390
mesocortical neuronal
    pathway, 388–389
mesolimbic neuronal path-
    way, 388–389
negative symptoms, 387
nigrostriatal neuronal path-
    way, 388–389
partial agonists, 390
positive symptoms, 387
serotonin hypothesis, 388
tardive dyskinesia, 389–390
target symptoms, 386
tuberoinfundibular neuro-
    nal pathway, 388–389
Scintillating scotomas pre-
    ceding migraine, 254
SCr. See Serum creatine (SCr)
Secondary hyperaldosteron-
    ism, 233
Secondary hypogonadism,
    157
Seizures vs. epilepsy, 98
Selective estrogen receptor
    modulator (SERM),
    48
Selective irreversible inhibi-
    tors of monoamine
    oxidase, 285
Selective serotonin reuptake
    inhibitors (SSRIs),
    307
Septic embolization, 215
SERM. See Selective estrogen
    receptor modulator
    (SERM)
Serotonin and norepineph-
    rine reuptake inhibi-
    tors (SNRIs), 307
Serotonin hypothesis, schizo-
    phrenia, 388
Serum creatine (SCr), 73
Serum transferrin, 225
Sevelamer, 77–78
Sevelamer mechanism of
    action, 15
Sevoflurane with nitrous
    oxide, 120–121
    rapid recovery from, 121
Sheehan's syndrome, 159
Sildenafil, 160
Sirolimus, 400
Sitagliptin, 442
Sjögren's syndrome, 377
SLE. See Systemic lupus ery-
    thematosus (SLE)

Smoking and lung cancer, 240
SNRIs. See Serotonin and
    norepinephrine
    reuptake inhibitors
    (SNRIs)
Solid organ transplant,
    393–400
    cephalosporin, 397
    diuresis, 398
    isoproterenol, 398
    lovastatin, 399
    methylprednisolone-
        induced gastric dam-
        age, 397
    milrinone, 396–397
    mycophenolate mofetil, 399
    nitroglycerin, 398
    nonselective
        β-adrenoceptor ago-
        nist, 398
    omeprazole, 397
    phosphodiesterase inhibi-
        tor, 396
    sirolimus, 400
    statins, 399
    tacrolimus, 399
        adverse effects, 400
    trimethoprim-sulfamethox-
        azole, 397
    vancomycin, 397
Somatomedins, 157
Somatostatin (SST)
    acromegaly, 4
    peptic ulcer disease, 295
Somatostatin analogues, 4
    lanreotide, 4
    octreotide, 4
Somatrophs, 3
Somatropin, 156, 157
Sotalol, 35, 424
Spermatogenesis, 160
Spider angiomas, 233
Spirometry, 20
Spirometry reduction, 83
Spironolactone
    heart failure, 170–171
    liver cirrhosis, 234
    polycystic ovarian syn-
        drome, 333
Spironolactone use, 172
Squamous cell cancer, 240
SSRIs. See Selective serotonin
    reuptake inhibitors
    (SSRIs)
SST. See Somatostatin (SST)
SST receptors (SSTRs), 5
SSTRs. See SST receptors
    (SSTRs)
Stages
    anesthesia, 118

breast cancer, 47
chronic kidney disease, 73
heart failure, 168
Hodgkin's lymphoma,
    185–186
leukemia, 179
Statins
    solid organ transplantation,
        399
    stroke, 408
Status epilepticus, 103
Steatorrhea, 68
Stenberg's cells, 185
Stevens-Johnson's syndrome,
    140
S3 gallop, 273–274
Striatum, 284
Stroke, 31, 401–409
    ACE inhibitors, 407
    alteplase, 406
    antiplatelet therapy,
        406–407
    botulinum toxin, 407
    Broca's aphasia, 404
    captopril, 407
    cerebral artery blockage,
        404
    clopidogrel, 406
    creatine kinase, 408
    fibrinolytic drug, 406
    focal brain infarction, 404
    glutamate-mediated excito-
        toxicity, 405
    ischemic stroke, 404
    labetalol, 405
    lovastatin, 408
        adverse effect, 408
    myopathy, 408
    necrosis of cerebral infarct,
        405
    regular, 404
    statins, 408
    transient ischemic attack,
        404
Stroke volume increase after
    dopamine adminis-
    tration, 56
Subcutaneous necrotizing
    granulomas, 377
Succinylcholine, 120
Sulfonamides, 449
Sulfonylureas, 441
Sumatriptan, 257
Sustained bacteremia, 215
Sustained ventricular tachy-
    cardia, 421
SVR. See System vascular
    resistance (SVR)
Sympathetic nervous system
    activation, 273

Symptomatic heart failure, 168
Synovial fluid, 137
Synovial lining, 376
Synthetic progestins, 196
 clinical applications, 196
Synuclein, 284
Synucleinopathy, 284
Systemic emboli, 31, 33
Systemic glucocorticoids, 416
Systemic lupus erythematosus (SLE), 411–418
 alkylating drug, 417
 arthritis, 415
 associated disorders, 418
 autoimmune disorder, 415
 cyclophosphamide, 417
  adverse effect, 417
 double-stranded DNA antibody test, 415
 glomerulonephritis, 415
 hydroxychloroquine, 418
 immunosuppressive therapy, 416
 mycophenolate mofetil, 417, 418
 nephritis, 416
 risk factors, 414
 symptoms, signs, lab results, 416
 systemic glucocorticoids, 416
 T-helper cells, 415
 vasculitis, 415
System vascular resistance (SVR), 110

T

Tachycardia, 368
Tacrolimus, 399
 adverse effects, 400
Tadalafil, 160
Tamoxifen, 48
Tardive dyskinesia, 389–390
Target organs for iron, 225
Taxane derivatives, 242
TBII. See TSH-binding inhibitor immunoglobulin (TBII)
T configuration. See Tense (T) configuration
TDS. See Torsade de pointes (TDS)
Tenofovir, 207
Tense (T) configuration, 223
Tertiary hypogonadism, 157
Testosterone replacement therapy, 158
Tetrahydrofolate formation, 449

Tetrahydrofolate synthesis impairment, 249–250
TGI. See Thyroid growth-stimulating immunoglobulin (TGI), 147
Therapeutic window of a drug, 55
Thiazide diuretics, 41
Thiazide-like diuretic, 138
Thiazides, 111
T-helper cells
 Crohn's disease, 66
 systemic lupus erythematosus, 415
Theophylline, 84
Thiazolidinediones (TZDs), 441, 442
Thioamide agents, 149
 adverse reactions, 149
Thioamide drugs, 148
Thromboembolism, 366
T_h2 helper cells, 21
Thymus hyperplasia, 264
Thymus involvement, 264
Thyroid growth-stimulating immunoglobulin (TGI), 147
Thyroid-stimulating hormone (TSH) receptors, 146
Thyroid-stimulating immunoglobulin (TSI), 146–147
Thyroid storm, 149
Thyrotoxicosis, 149
Thyrotrophs, 3
Tidal volume (TV), 20
Tight glycemic control
 DM1, 432
 DM2, 444
Tissue factors that increase hemoglobin, 223
TNF-α. See Tumor necrosis factor (TNF)-α
TNF-α inhibitor. See Tumor necrosis factor-α (TNF-α) inhibitor
Tonic-clonic seizures, 99
 autonomic signs, 99
Topiramate, 102
Torsade de pointes (TDS), 419–424
 afterdepolarizations, 423
 amiodarone, 423
  adverse effects, 423
 class III antiarrhythmic drugs, 423
 heart action phases, 422
 heart action repolarization, 422

isoproterenol, 424
magnesium sulfate, 424
monomorphic ventricular tachycardia, 421
nonsustained ventricular tachycardia, 421
polymorphic ventricular tachycardia, 421
QT interval increase, 423
QT interval prolongation, 423
sotalol, 424
sustained ventricular tachycardia, 421
ventricular fibrillation, 424
Total peripheral resistance (TPR), 54
TPR. See Total peripheral resistance (TPR), 54
Transient ischemic attack, 404
Transmural inflammation, 63
Transport proteins, 324
Transsphenoidal surgery, 5
Trimethoprim-sulfamethoxazole
 solid organ transplantation, 397
 UTIs, 449
Triple therapy, 297
Troponin 1, 274
TSH-binding inhibitor immunoglobulin (TBII), 147
TSH receptors. See Thyroid-stimulating hormone (TSH) receptors
TSI. See Thyroid-stimulating immunoglobulin (TSI)
Tuberculosis, 208
Tuberoinfundibular neuronal pathway, 388–389
Tumor lysis syndrome, 14
 catabolism, 14
 hyperphosphatemia, 14
 phosphate concentration, 14
Tumor necrosis factor (TNF)-α, 67
Tumor necrosis factor-α (TNF-α) inhibitor
 psoriasis, 361
 rheumatoid arthritis, 381
Turner's syndrome, 160
Type 1 diabetes mellitus (DM1), 425–434
 acetone increase, 428
 C-peptide, 430
 diabetic ketoacidosis (DKA), 428

early morning hyperglyce-
mia, 433
glargine, 433
hypoglycemia, 432
insulin, 430
adverse effects, 432, 433
mechanism of action, 430
physiological effects,
430–431
insulin pump, 431–432
intensive insulin therapy,
432
ketoacidosis, 431
osmotic diuresis, 429
preproinsulin, 428–429
rapid-acting insulin, 431
tight glycemic control, 432
Type 2 diabetes mellitus,
435–444
azole antifungal agent,
440–441
counterregulatory hor-
mones, 443
exenatide, 443
fluconazole, 441–442
glimepiride, 441
gliptin drugs, 442
gluconeogenesis, 438
HbA1C, 439, 444
hypoglycemic agents, 441
incretin-mimetic agents,
443
insulin therapy, 443
lipolysis, 439
macrovascular complica-
tions of DM2, 444
metformin, 440
adverse effects, 440
microvascular complica-
tions of DM2, 444
pathophysiology, 438
pioglitazone, 441–442
adverse effects, 442
rosiglitazone, 441–442
sitagliptin, 442
sulfonylureas, 441
thiazolidinediones (TZDs),
441, 442
tight glycemic control, 444
Tyrosine kinase inhibitors,
243

TZDs. *See* Thiazolidinediones
(TZDs)

U

Unfractionated heparin, 369
Uric acid production, 136
Uric acid stones, 140
Uricosuric agent, 139–140
Urinary problems, 350
Urinary tract infections, 306,
445–450
acute uncomplicated cystitis, 448
bacterial causes, 449
bacteriuria, 448
β-lactam antibiotic, 450
carbapenems, 450
ciprofloxacin, 449–450
dihydrofolate formation,
449
fluoroquinolones, 449–450
adverse effects, 450
antacid interactions, 450
folate formation, 449
gram-negative bacteria, 450
gram-positive bacteria, 450
meropenem, 450
positive urinary nitrate, 448
sulfonamides, 449
tetrahydrofolate, formation,
449
trimethoprim-sulfamethox-
azole combination,
449
Urinary urgency, 30
UTI. *See* Urinary tract infection (UTI)

V

Vaginal atrophy, 306
Valporic acid, epilepsy, 101
adverse effect, 101
mechanism, 101
Valporic acid, migraine, 258
prenatal risks, 258
Valvular destruction, 215
Vancomycin
infective endocarditis, 216
activity spectrum, 217
adverse effects, 216
mechanism of action, 216

site of action, 216
solid organ transplant, 397
Vascular endothelial growth
factor (VEGF), 367
Vasculitis, 415
Vasodilation, 255
Vasodilation mechanism, 111
Vecuronium, 121
sequence of muscle paraly-
sis, 121
VEGF. *See* Vascular endothe-
lial growth factor
(VEGF)
Venlafaxine, 307
Venous thromboembolism
(VTE), 198
Ventricular fibrillation, 424
Vinblastine, 13, 189
Vinca alkaloids, 13
dose-limiting myelosup-
pression, 13
toxicities, 13
vinblastine, 13
vincristine, 13
Vincristine, 13
Vincristine neuropathy, 13
Vitamin B_{12} (cobalamin)
deficiency, 248
antianemic action of, 250
available supply, 249
length of therapy, 250
oral dosage efficacy, 250
Vitamin K administration, 33
Vitamin K synthesis inhibition, 31, 32
VTE. *See* Venous thromboem-
bolism (VTE)

W

Warfarin therapy, 31
WBC. *See* White blood count
(WBC)
Weight loss, Crohn's disease,
64
Wheezing, 82
White blood count (WBC),
137

Z

Zafrilukast, 23